Fourth Edition

Plastic Surgery

Breast

Volume Five

Content Strategist: Belinda Kuhn
Content Development Specialists: Louise Cook, Sam Crowe, Alexandra Mortimer
e-products, Content Development Specialist: Kim Benson
Project Managers: Anne Collett, Andrew Riley, Julie Taylor
Designer: Miles Hitchen
Illustration Managers: Karen Giacomucci, Amy Faith Heyden
Marketing Manager: Melissa Fogarty
Video Liaison: Will Schmitt

Fourth Edition

Plastic Surgery

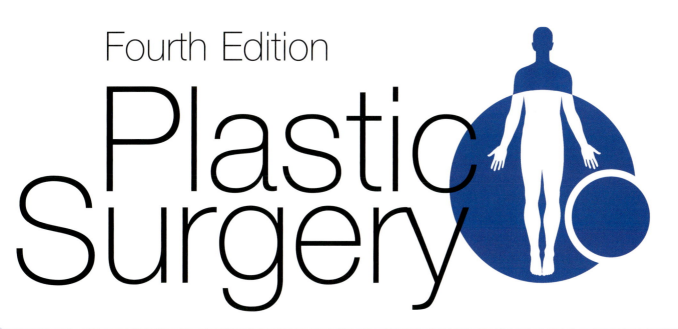

Breast

Volume Five

Volume Editor

Maurice Y. Nahabedian
MD, FACS
Professor and Chief
Section of Plastic Surgery
MedStar Washington Hospital Center
Washington DC, USA;
Vice Chairman
Department of Plastic Surgery
MedStar Georgetown University Hospital
Washington DC, USA

Editor-in-Chief

Peter C. Neligan
MB, FRCS(I), FRCSC, FACS
Professor of Surgery
Department of Surgery, Division of Plastic Surgery
University of Washington
Seattle, WA, USA

Multimedia Editor

Daniel Z. Liu
MD
Plastic and Reconstructive Surgeon
Cancer Treatment Centers of America at
Midwestern Regional Medical Center
Zion, IL, USA

For additional online figures, videos and video lectures visit Expertconsult.com

ELSEVIER   London, New York, Oxford, Philadelphia, St Louis, Sydney 2018

ELSEVIER

First edition 1990
Second edition 2006
Third edition 2013
Fourth edition 2018

Notices

Knowledge and best practice in this field are constantly changing. As new research and experience broaden our understanding, changes in research methods, professional practices, or medical treatment may become necessary.

Practitioners and researchers must always rely on their own experience and knowledge in evaluating and using any information, methods, compounds, or experiments described herein. In using such information or methods they should be mindful of their own safety and the safety of others, including parties for whom they have a professional responsibility.

With respect to any drug or pharmaceutical products identified, readers are advised to check the most current information provided (i) on procedures featured or (ii) by the manufacturer of each product to be administered, to verify the recommended dose or formula, the method and duration of administration, and contraindications. It is the responsibility of practitioners, relying on their own experience and knowledge of their patients, to make diagnoses, to determine dosages and the best treatment for each individual patient, and to take all appropriate safety precautions.

To the fullest extent of the law, neither the Publisher nor the authors, contributors, or editors, assume any liability for any injury and/or damage to persons or property as a matter of products liability, negligence or otherwise, or from any use or operation of any methods, products, instructions, or ideas contained in the material herein.

Volume 5 ISBN: 978-0-323-35709-8
Volume 5 Ebook ISBN: 978-0-323-35710-4
6 volume set ISBN: 978-0-323-35630-5

your source for books,
journals and multimedia
in the health sciences

www.elsevierhealth.com

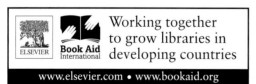

Working together
to grow libraries in
developing countries

www.elsevier.com • www.bookaid.org

The
publisher's
policy is to use
**paper manufactured
from sustainable forests**

Printed in Canada
Last digit is the print number: 9 8 7 6 5 4 3 2 1

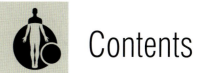

Contents

Volume One: Principles
edited by Geoffrey C. Gurtner

Volume Three: Craniofacial, Head and Neck Surgery, and Pediatric Plastic Surgery

Part 1: Head, neck, and craniofacial surgery: edited by Eduardo D. Rodriguez

Part 2: Pediatrics: edited by Joseph E. Losee

Section I: Clefts

Volume Five: Breast

edited by Maurice Y. Nahabedian

Section I: Aesthetic Breast Surgery

Section II: Reconstructive Breast Surgery

Volume Six: Hand and Upper Extremity

edited by James Chang

Video Contents

Lecture Video Contents

Preface to the Fourth Edition

When I wrote the preface to the 3rd edition of this book, I remarked how honored and unexpectedly surprised I was to be the Editor of this great series. This time 'round, I'm equally grateful to carry this series forward. When Elsevier called me and suggested it was time to prepare the 4th edition, my initial reaction was that this was way too soon. What could possibly have changed in Plastic Surgery since the 3rd edition was launched in 2012? As it transpires, there have been many developments and I hope we have captured them in this edition.

We have an extraordinary specialty. A recent article by Chadra, Agarwal and Agarwal entitled "Redefining Plastic Surgery" appeared in *Plastic and Reconstructive Surgery—Global Open*. In it they gave the following definition: "Plastic surgery is a specialized branch of surgery, which deals with deformities, defects and abnormalities of the organs of perception, organs of action and the organs guarding the external passages, besides innovation, implantation, replantation and transplantation of tissues, and aims at restoring and improving their form, function and the esthetic appearances." This is an all-encompassing but very apt definition and captures the enormous scope of the specialty.[1]

In the 3rd edition, I introduced volume editors for each of the areas of the specialty because the truth is that one person can no longer be an expert in all areas of this diverse specialty, and I'm certainly not. I think this worked well because the volume editors not only had the expertise to present their area of subspecialty in the best light, but they were tuned in to what was new and who was doing it. We have continued this model in this new edition. Four of the seven volume editors from the previous edition have again helped to bring the latest and the best to this edition: Drs Gurtner, Song, Rodriguez, Losee, and Chang have revised and updated their respective volumes with some chapters remaining, some extensively revised, some added, and some deleted. Dr. Peter Rubin has replaced Dr. Rick Warren to compile the Aesthetic volume (Vol. 2). Dr. Warren did a wonderful job in corralling this somewhat disparate, yet vitally important, part of our specialty into the Aesthetic volume in the 3rd edition but felt that the task of doing it again, though a labor of love, was more than he wanted to take on. Similarly, Dr. Jim Grotting who did a masterful job in the last edition on the Breast volume, decided that doing a major revision should be undertaken by someone with a fresh perspective and Dr. Maurice Nahabedian stepped into that breach. I hope you will like the changes you see in both of these volumes.

Dr. Allen Van Beek was the video editor for the last edition and he compiled an impressive array of movies to complement the text. This time around, we wanted to go a step further and though we've considerably expanded the list of videos accompanying the text (there are over 170), we also added the idea of lectures accompanying selected chapters. What we've done here is to take selected key chapters and include the images from that chapter, photos and artwork, and create a narrated presentation that is available online; there are annotations in the text to alert the reader that this is available. Dr. Daniel Liu, who has taken over from Dr. Van Beek as multimedia editor (rather than video editor) has done an amazing job in making all of this happen. There are over 70 presentations of various key chapters online, making it as easy as possible for you, the reader, to get as much knowledge as you can, in the easiest way possible from this edition. Many of these presentations have been done by the authors of the chapters; the rest have been compiled by Dr. Liu and myself from the content of the individual chapters. I hope you find them useful.

The reader may wonder how this all works. To plan this edition, the Elsevier team, headed by Belinda Kuhn, and I, convened a face-to-face meeting in San Francisco. The volume editors, as well as the London based editorial team, were present. We went through the 3rd edition, volume by volume, chapter by chapter, over an entire weekend. We decided what needed to stay, what needed to be added, what needed to be revised, and what needed to be changed. We also decided who should write the various chapters, keeping many existing authors, replacing others, and adding some new ones; we did this so as to really reflect the changes occurring within the specialty. We also decided on practical changes that needed to be made. As an example, you will notice that we have omitted the complete index for the 6 Volume set from Volumes 2-6 and highlighted only the table of contents for that particular volume. The complete index is of course available in Volume 1 and fully searchable online. This allowed us to save several hundred pages per volume, reducing production costs and diverting those dollars to the production of the enhanced online content.

In my travels around the world since the 3rd edition was published, I've been struck by what an impact this publication has had on the specialty and, more particularly, on training. Everywhere I go, I'm told how the text is an important part of didactic teaching and a font of knowledge. It is gratifying to see that the 3rd edition has been translated into Portuguese, Spanish, and Chinese. This is enormously encouraging. I hope this 4th edition continues to contribute to the specialty, remains a resource for practicing surgeons, and continues to prepare our trainees for their future careers in Plastic Surgery.

Peter C. Neligan
Seattle, WA
September, 2017

---

[1] Chandra R, Agarwal R, Agarwal D. Redefining Plastic Surgery. *Plast Reconstr Surg Glob Open*. 2016;4(5):e706.

List of Editors

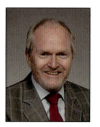

Editor-in-Chief
Peter C. Neligan, MB, FRCS(I), FRCSC, FACS
Professor of Surgery
Department of Surgery, Division of Plastic Surgery
University of Washington
Seattle, WA, USA

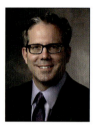

Volume 1: Principles
Geoffrey C. Gurtner, MD, FACS
Johnson and Johnson Distinguished Professor of
Surgery and Vice Chairman,
Department of Surgery (Plastic Surgery)
Stanford University
Stanford, CA, USA

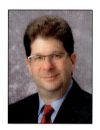

Volume 2: Aesthetic
J. Peter Rubin, MD, FACS
UPMC Professor of Plastic Surgery
Chair, Department of Plastic Surgery
Professor of Bioengineering
University of Pittsburgh
Pittsburgh, PA, USA

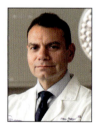

Volume 3: Craniofacial, Head and Neck Surgery
Eduardo D. Rodriguez, MD, DDS
Helen L. Kimmel Professor of Reconstructive
Plastic Surgery
Chair, Hansjörg Wyss Department of Plastic
Surgery
NYU School of Medicine
NYU Langone Medical Center
New York, NY, USA

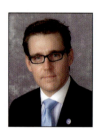

Volume 3: Pediatric Plastic Surgery
Joseph E. Losee, MD
Ross H. Musgrave Professor of Pediatric Plastic
Surgery
Department of Plastic Surgery
University of Pittsburgh Medical Center;
Chief Division of Pediatric Plastic Surgery
Children's Hospital of Pittsburgh
Pittsburgh, PA, USA

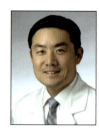

Volume 4: Lower Extremity, Trunk, and Burns
David H. Song, MD, MBA, FACS
Regional Chief, MedStar Health
Plastic and Reconstructive Surgery
Professor and Chairman
Department of Plastic Surgery
Georgetown University School of Medicine
Washington, DC, USA

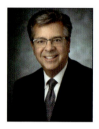

Volume 5: Breast
Maurice Y. Nahabedian, MD, FACS
Professor and Chief
Section of Plastic Surgery
MedStar Washington Hospital Center
Washington, DC, USA;
Vice Chairman
Department of Plastic Surgery
MedStar Georgetown University Hospital
Washington, DC, USA

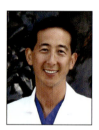

Volume 6: Hand and Upper Extremity
James Chang, MD
Johnson & Johnson Distinguished
Professor and Chief
Division of Plastic and Reconstructive Surgery
Stanford University Medical Center
Stanford, CA, USA

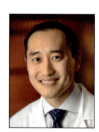

Multimedia editor
Daniel Z. Liu, MD
Plastic and Reconstructive Surgeon
Cancer Treatment Centers of America at Midwestern Regional Medical Center
Zion, IL, USA

List of Contributors

The editors would like to acknowledge and offer grateful thanks for the input of all previous editions' contributors, without whom this new edition would not have been possible.

VOLUME ONE

Hatem Abou-Sayed, MD, MBA
Vice President
Physician Engagement
Interpreta, Inc.
San Diego, CA, USA

Paul N. Afrooz, MD
Resident
Plastic and Reconstructive Surgery
University of Pittsburgh Medical Center
Pittsburgh, PA, USA

Claudia R. Albornoz, MD, MSc
Research Fellow
Plastic and Reconstructive Surgery
Memorial Sloan Kettering Cancer Center
New York, NY, USA

Nidal F. Al Deek, MD
Doctor of Plastic and Reconstructive Surgery
Chang Gung Memorial Hospital
Taipei, Taiwan

Amy K. Alderman, MD, MPH
Private Practice
Atlanta, GA, USA

Louis C. Argenta, MD
Professor of Plastic and Reconstructive Surgery
Department of Plastic Surgery
Wake Forest Medical Center
Winston Salem, NC, USA

Stephan Ariyan, MD, MBA
Emeritus Frank F. Kanthak Professor of Surgery,
Plastic Surgery, Surgical Oncology,
Otolaryngology
Yale University School of Medicine;
Associate Chief
Department of Surgery;
Founding Director, Melanoma Program
Smilow Cancer Hospital, Yale Cancer Center
New Haven, CT, USA

Tomer Avraham, MD
Attending Plastic Surgeon
Mount Sinai Health System
Tufts University School of Medicine
New York, NY, USA

Aaron Berger, MD, PhD
Clinical Assistant Professor
Division of Plastic Surgery
Florida International University School of Medicine
Miami, FL, USA

Kirsty Usher Boyd, MD, FRCSC
Assistant Professor Surgery (Plastics)
Division of Plastic and Reconstructive Surgery
University of Ottawa
Ottawa, Ontario, Canada

Charles E. Butler, MD, FACS
Professor and Chairman
Department of Plastic Surgery
Charles B. Barker Endowed Chair in Surgery
The University of Texas MD Anderson Cancer Center
Houston, TX, USA

Peter E. M. Butler, MD, FRCSI, FRCS, FRCS(Plast)
Professor
Plastic and Reconstructive Surgery
University College and Royal Free London
London, UK

Yilin Cao, MD, PhD
Professor
Shanghai Ninth People's Hospital
Shanghai Jiao Tong University School of Medicine
Shanghai, China

Franklyn P. Cladis, MD, FAAP
Associate Professor of Anesthesiology
Department of Anesthesiology
The Children's Hospital of Pittsburgh of UPMC
Pittsburgh, PA, USA

Mark B. Constantian, MD
Private Practice
Surgery (Plastic Surgery)
St. Joseph Hospital
Nashua, NH, USA

Daniel A. Cuzzone, MD
Plastic Surgery Fellow
Hanjörg Wyss Department of Plastic Surgery
New York University Medical Center
New York, NY, USA

Gurleen Dhami, MD
Chief Resident
Department of Radiation Oncology
University of Washington
Seattle, WA, USA

Gayle Gordillo, MD
Associate Professor
Plastic Surgery
The Ohio State University
Columbus, OH, USA

Geoffrey C. Gurtner, MD, FACS
Johnson and Johnson Distinguished Professor
of Surgery and Vice Chairman,
Department of Surgery (Plastic Surgery)
Stanford University
Stanford, CA, USA

Phillip C. Haeck, MD
Surgeon
Plastic Surgery
The Polyclinic
Seattle, WA, USA

The late Bruce Halperin[†], MD
Formerly Adjunct Associate Professor of Anesthesia
Department of Anesthesia
Stanford University
Stanford, CA, USA

Daniel E. Heath
Lecturer
School of Chemical and Biomedical Engineering
University of Melbourne
Parkville, Victoria, Australia

Joon Pio Hong, MD, PhD, MMM
Professor
Plastic Surgery
Asan Medical Center, University of Ulsan
Seoul, South Korea

Michael S. Hu, MD, MPH, MS
Postdoctoral Fellow
Division of Plastic Surgery
Department of Surgery
Stanford University School of Medicine
Stanford, CA, USA

C. Scott Hultman, MD, MBA
Professor and Chief
Division of Plastic and Reconstructive Surgery
University of North Carolina
Chapel Hill, NC, USA

Amir E. Ibrahim
Division of Plastic Surgery
Department of Surgery
American University of Beirut Medical Center
Beirut, Lebanon

Leila Jazayeri, MD
Microsurgery Fellow
Plastic and Reconstructive Surgery
Memorial Sloan Kettering Cancer Center
New York, NY, USA

Brian Jeffers
Student
Bioengineering
University of California Berkeley
Berkeley, CA USA

Lynn Jeffers, MD, FACS
Private Practice
Oxnard, CA, USA

Mohammed M. Al Kahtani, MD, FRCSC
Clinical Fellow
Division of Plastic Surgery
Department of Surgery
University of Alberta
Edmonton, Alberta, Canada

Gabrielle M. Kane, MB, BCh, EdD, FRCPC
Associate Professor
Radiation Oncology
University of Washington
Seattle, WA, USA

Raghu P. Kataru, PhD
Senior Research Scientist
Memorial Sloan-Kettering Cancer Center
New York, NY, USA

Carolyn L. Kerrigan, MD, MSc, MHCDS
Professor of Surgery
Surgery
Dartmouth–Hitchcock Medical Center
Lebanon, NH, USA

Timothy W. King, MD, PhD, FAAP, FACS
Associate Professor with Tenure
Departments of Surgery and Biomedical
Engineering;
Director of Research, Division of Plastic Surgery
University of Alabama at Birmingham (UAB)
Craniofacial and Pediatric Plastic Surgery
Children's of Alabama – Plastic Surgery;
Chief, Plastic Surgery Section
Birmingham VA Hospital
Birmingham, AL, USA

Brian M. Kinney, MD, FACS, MSME
Clinical Assistant Professor of Plastic Surgery
University of Southern California
School of Medicine
Los Angeles, CA, USA

W. P. Andrew Lee, MD
The Milton T. Edgerton MD, Professor and
Chairman
Department of Plastic and Reconstructive
Surgery
Johns Hopkins University School of Medicine
Baltimore, MD, USA

Sherilyn Keng Lin Tay, MBChB, MSc, FRCS(Plast)
Consultant Plastic Surgeon
Canniesburn Plastic Surgery Unit
Glasgow Royal Infirmary
Glasgow, UK

Daniel Z. Liu, MD
Plastic and Reconstructive Surgeon
Cancer Treatment Centers of America at
Midwestern Regional Medical Center
Zion, IL, USA

Wei Liu, MD, PhD
Professor
Plastic and Reconstructive Surgery
Shanghai Ninth People's Hospital
Shanghai Jiao Tong University School of
Medicine
Shanghai, China

Michael T. Longaker, MD, MBA, FACS
Deane P. and Louise Mitchell Professor and Vice
Chair
Department of Surgery
Stanford University
Stanford, CA, USA

H. Peter Lorenz, MD
Service Chief and Professor, Plastic Surgery
Lucile Packard Children's Hospital
Stanford University School of Medicine
Stanford, CA, USA

Susan E. Mackinnon, MD
Sydney M. Shoenberg Jr. and Robert H.
Shoenberg Professor
Department of Surgery, Division of Plastic and
Reconstructive Surgery
Washington University School of Medicine
St. Louis, MO, USA

Malcolm W. Marks, MD
Professor and Chairman
Department of Plastic Surgery
Wake Forest University School of Medicine
Winston-Salem, NC, USA

Diego Marre, MD
Fellow
O'Brien Institute
Department of Plastic and Reconstructive
Surgery
St. Vincent's Hospital
Melbourne, Australia

David W. Mathes, MD
Professor and Chief of the Division of Plastic
and Reconstructive Surgery
University of Colorado
Aurora, CO, USA

Evan Matros MD, MMSc
Plastic Surgeon
Memorial Sloan-Kettering Cancer Center
New York, NY, USA

Isabella C. Mazzola, MD
Attending Plastic Surgeon
Klinik für Plastische und Ästhetische Chirurgie
Klinikum Landkreis Erding
Erding, Germany

Riccardo F. Mazzola, MD
Plastic Surgeon
Department of Specialistic Surgical Sciences
Fondazione Ospedale Maggiore Policlinico, Ca'
Granda IRCCS
Milano, Italy

Lindsay D. McHutchion, MS, BSc
Anaplastologist
Institute for Reconstructive Sciences in Medicine
Edmonton, Alberta, Canada

Babak J. Mehrara, MD, FACS
Associate Member, Associate Professor of
Surgery (Plastic)
Memorial Sloan Kettering Cancer Center
Weil Cornell University Medical Center
New York, NY, USA

Steven F. Morris, MD, MSc, FRCSC
Professor of Surgery
Department of Surgery
Dalhousie University
Halifax, Nova Scotia, Canada

Wayne A. Morrison, MBBS, MD, FRACS
Professorial Fellow
O'Brien Institute
Department of Surgery, University of Melbourne
Department of Plastic and Reconstructive
Surgery, St. Vincent's Hospital
Melbourne, Australia

Peter C. Neligan, MB, FRCS(I), FRCSC, FACS
Professor of Surgery
Department of Surgery, Division of Plastic
Surgery
University of Washington
Seattle, WA, USA

Andrea J. O'Connor, BE(Hons), PhD
Associate Professor
Department of Chemical and Biomolecular
Engineering
University of Melbourne
Parkville, Victoria, Australia

Rei Ogawa, MD, PhD, FACS
Professor and Chief
Department of Plastic
Reconstructive and Aesthetic Surgery
Nippon Medical School
Tokyo, Japan

Dennis P. Orgill, MD, PhD
Professor of Surgery
Harvard Medical School
Medical Director, Wound Care Center;
Vice Chairman for Quality Improvement
Department of Surgery
Brigham and Women's Hospital
Boston, MA, USA

Cho Y. Pang, PhD
Senior Scientist
Research Institute
The Hospital for Sick Children;
Professor
Departments of Surgery/Physiology
University of Toronto
Toronto, Ontario, Canada

Ivo Alexander Pestana, MD, FACS
Associate Professor
Plastic and Reconstructive Surgery
Wake Forest University
Winston Salem, NC, USA

Giorgio Pietramaggior, MD, PhD
Swiss Nerve Institute
Clinique de La Source
Lausanne, Switzerland

Andrea L. Pusic, MD, MHS, FACS
Associate Professor
Plastic and Reconstructive Surgery
Memorial Sloan Kettering Cancer Center
New York, NY, USA

Russell R. Reid, MD, PhD
Associate Professor
Surgery/Section of Plastic and Reconstructive
Surgery
University of Chicago Medicine
Chicago, IL, USA

Neal R. Reisman, MD, JD
Chief
Plastic Surgery
Baylor St. Luke's Medical Center
Houston, TX, USA

Joseph M. Rosen, MD
Professor of Surgery
Plastic Surgery
Dartmouth–Hitchcock Medical Center
Lebanon, NH, USA

Sashwati Roy, MS, PhD
Associate Professor
Surgery, Center for Regenerative Medicine and
Cell based Therapies
The Ohio State University
Columbus, OH, USA

J. Peter Rubin, MD, FACS
UPMC Professor of Plastic Surgery
Chair, Department of Plastic Surgery
Professor of Bioengineering
University of Pittsburgh
Pittsburgh, PA, USA

Karim A. Sarhane, MD
Department of Surgery
University of Toledo Medical Center
Toledo, OH, USA

David B. Sarwer, PhD
Associate Professor of Psychology
Departments of Psychiatry and Surgery
University of Pennsylvania School of Medicine
Philadelphia, PA, USA

Saja S. Scherer-Pietramaggiori, MD
Plastic and Reconstructive Surgeon
Plastic Surgery
University Hospital Lausanne
Lausanne, Vaud, Switzerland

Iris A. Seitz, MD, PhD
Director of Research and International
Collaboration
University Plastic Surgery
Rosalind Franklin University;
Clinical Instructor of Surgery
Chicago Medical School
Chicago, IL, USA

Jesse C. Selber, MD, MPH, FACS
Associate Professor, Director of Clinical
Research
Department of Plastic Surgery
MD Anderson Cancer Center
Houston, TX, USA

Chandan K. Sen, PhD
Professor and Director
Center for Regenerative Medicine and Cell-
Based Therapies
The Ohio State University Wexner Medical
Center
Columbus, OH, USA

Wesley N. Sivak, MD, PhD
Resident in Plastic Surgery
Department of Plastic Surgery
University of Pittsburgh
Pittsburgh, PA, USA

M. Lucy Sudekum
Research Assistant
Thayer School of Engineering at Dartmouth
College
Hanover, NH, USA

**G. Ian Taylor, AO, MBBS, MD, MD(Hon
Bordeaux), FRACS, FRCS(Eng), FRCS(Hon
Edinburgh), FRCSI(Hon), FRSC(Hon
Canada), FACS(Hon)**
Professor
Department of Plastic Surgery
Royal Melbourne Hospital;
Professor
Department of Anatomy
University of Melbourne
Melbourne, Victoria, Australia

Chad M. Teven, MD
Resident
Section of Plastic and Reconstructive Surgery
University of Chicago
Chicago, IL, USA

Ruth Tevlin, MB BAO BCh, MRCSI, MD
Resident in Surgery
Department of Plastic and Reconstructive
Surgery
Stanford University School of Medicine
Stanford, CA, USA

E. Dale Collins Vidal, MD, MS
Chief
Section of Plastic Surgery
Dartmouth–Hitchcock Medical Center
Lebanon, NH, USA

Derrick C. Wan, MD
Associate Professor
Division of Plastic Surgery
Department of Surgery
Director of Maxillofacial Surgery
Lucile Packard Children's Hospital
Stanford University School of Medicine
Stanford, CA, USA

Renata V. Weber, MD
Assistant Professor Surgery (Plastics)
Division of Plastic and Reconstructive Surgery
Albert Einstein College of Medicine
Bronx, NY, USA

Fu-Chan Wei, MD
Professor
Department of Plastic Surgery
Chang Gung Memorial Hospital
Taoyuan, Taiwan

Gordon H. Wilkes, BScMed, MD
Clinical Professor of Surgery
Department of Surgery University of Alberta
Institute for Reconstructive Sciences in Medicine
Misericordia Hospital
Edmonton, Alberta, Canada

**Johan F. Wolfaardt, BDS,
MDent(Prosthodontics), PhD**
Professor
Division of Otolaryngology – Head and Neck
Surgery
Department of Surgery
Faculty of Medicine and Dentistry;
Director of Clinics and International Relations
Institute for Reconstructive Sciences in Medicine
University of Alberta
Covenant Health Group
Alberta Health Services
Alberta, Canada

Kiryu K. Yap, MBBS, BMedSc
Junior Surgical Trainee & PhD Candidate
O'Brien Institute
Department of Surgery, University of Melbourne
Department of Plastic and Reconstructive
Surgery, St. Vincent's Hospital
Melbourne, Australia

Andrew Yee
Research Assistant
Division of Plastic and Reconstructive Surgery
Washington University School of Medicine
St. Louis, MO, USA

Elizabeth R. Zielins, MD
Postdoctoral Research Fellow
Surgery
Stanford University School of Medicine
Stanford, CA, USA

VOLUME TWO

Paul N. Afrooz, MD
Resident
Plastic and Reconstructive Surgery
University of Pittsburgh Medical Center
Pittsburgh, PA, USA

Jamil Ahmad, MD, FRCSC
Director of Research and Education
The Plastic Surgery Clinic
Mississauga;
Assistant Professor
Surgery
University of Toronto
Toronto, Ontario, Canada

Lisa E. Airan, MD
Aesthetic Dermatologist NYC
Private Practice;
Associate Clinical Professor Department of
Dermatology
Mount Sinai School of Medicine
New York, NY, USA

Gary J. Alter, MD
Assistant Clinical Professor
Division of Plastic Surgery
University of California
Los Angeles, CA, USA

Al S. Aly, MD
Professor of Plastic Surgery
Aesthetic and Plastic Surgery Institute University
of California Irvine
Orange, CA, USA

Khalid Al-Zahrani, MD, SSC-PLAST
Assistant Professor
Consultant Plastic Surgeon
King Khalid University Hospital
King Saud University
Riyadh, Saudi Arabia

Bryan Armijo, MD
Plastic Surgery Chief Resident
Department of Plastic and Reconstructive
Surgery
Case Western Reserve/University Hospitals
Cleveland, OH, USA

Daniel C. Baker, MD
Professor of Surgery
Institute of Reconstructive Plastic Surgery
New York University Medical Center
Department of Plastic Surgery
New York, NY, USA

Fritz E. Barton Jr., MD
Clinical Professor
Department of Plastic Surgery
UT Southwestern Medical Center
Dallas, TX, USA

Leslie Baumann, MD
CEO
Baumann Cosmetic and Research Institute
Miami, FL, USA

Miles G. Berry, MS, FRCS(Plast)
Consultant Plastic and Aesthetic Surgeon
Institute of Cosmetic and Reconstructive
Surgery
London, UK

Trevor M. Born, MD
Division of Plastic Surgery
Lenox Hill/Manhattan Eye Ear and Throat
Hospital North Shore-LIJ Hospital
New York, NY, USA;
Clinical Lecturer
Division of Plastic Surgery
University of Toronto Western Division
Toronto, Ontario, Canada

Terrence W. Bruner, MD, MBA
Private Practice
Greenville, SC, USA

Andrés F. Cánchica, MD
Chief Resident of Plastic Surgery
Plastic Surgery Service Dr. Osvaldo Saldanha
São Paulo, Brazil

Joseph F. Capella, MD
Chief Post-bariatric Body Contouring
Division of Plastic Surgery
Hackensack University Medical Center
Hackensack, NJ, USA

Robert F. Centeno, MD, MBA
Medical Director
St. Croix Plastic Surgery and MediSpa;
Chief Medical Quality Officer
Governor Juan F. Luis Hospital and Medical
Center
Christiansted, Saint Croix, United States Virgin
Islands

Ernest S. Chiu, MD, FACS
Associate Professor of Plastic Surgery
Department of Plastic Surgery
New York University
New York, NY, USA

Jong Woo Choi, MD, PhD, MMM
Associate Professor
Department of Plastic and Reconstructive
Surgery
Seoul Asan Medical Center
Seoul, South Korea

Steven R. Cohen, MD
Senior Clinical Research Fellow, Clinical
Professor
Plastic Surgery
University of California
San Diego, CA;
Director
Craniofacial Surgery
Rady Children's Hospital, Private Practice,
FACES+ Plastic Surgery, Skin and Laser Center
La Jolla, CA, USA

Sydney R. Coleman, MD
Assistant Clinical Professor
Plastic Surgery
New York University Medical Center
New York;
Assistant Clinical Professor
Plastic Surgery
University of Pittsburgh Medical Center
Pittsburgh, PA, USA

Mark B. Constantian, MD
Private Practice
Surgery (Plastic Surgery)
St. Joseph Hospital
Nashua, NH, USA;
Adjunct Clinical Professor
Surgery (Plastic Surgery)
University of Wisconsin School of Medicine
Madison, WI, USA;
Visiting Professor
Plastic Surgery
University of Virginia Health System
Charlottesville, VA, USA

Rafael A. Couto, MD
Plastic Surgery Resident
Department of Plastic Surgery
Cleveland Clinic
Cleveland, OH, USA

Albert Cram, MD
Professor Emeritus
University of Iowa
Iowa City Plastic Surgery
Coralville, IO, USA

Phillip Dauwe, MD
Department of Plastic Surgery
University of Texas Southwestern Medical
School
Dallas, TX, USA

Dai M. Davies, FRCS
Consultant and Institute Director
Institute of Cosmetic and Reconstructive
Surgery
London, UK

Jose Abel De la Peña Salcedo, MD, FACS
Plastic Surgeon
Director
Instituto de Cirugia Plastica S.C.
Huixquilucan
Estado de Mexico, Mexico

Barry DiBernardo, MD, FACS
Clinical Associate Professor, Plastic Surgery
Rutgers, New Jersey Medical School
Director New Jersey Plastic Surgery
Montclair, NJ, USA

Felmont F. Eaves III, MD, FACS
Professor of Surgery, Emory University
Medical Director, Emory Aesthetic Center
Medical Director, EAC Ambulatory Surgery
Center
Atlanta, GA, USA

Marco Ellis, MD
Director of Craniofacial Surgery
Northwestern Specialists in Plastic Surgery;
Adjunct Assistant Professor
University of Illinois Chicago Medical Center
Chicago, IL, USA

Dino Elyassnia, MD
Associate Plastic Surgeon
Marten Clinic of Plastic Surgery
San Francisco, CA, USA

Julius Few Jr., MD
Director
The Few Institute for Aesthetic Plastic Surgery;
Clinical Professor
Plastic Surgery
University of Chicago Pritzker School of
Medicine
Chicago, IL, USA

Osvaldo Ribeiro Saldanha Filho, MD
Professor of Plastic Surgery
Plastic Surgery Service Dr. Osvaldo Saldanha
São Paulo, Brazil

Jack Fisher, MD
Associate Clinical Professor
Plastic Surgery
Vanderbilt University
Nashville, TN, USA

Nicholas A. Flugstad, MD
Flugstad Plastic Surgery
Bellevue, WA, USA

James D. Frame, MBBS, FRCS, FRCSEd, FRCS(Plast)
Professor of Aesthetic Plastic Surgery
Anglia Ruskin University
Chelmsford, UK

Jazmina M. Gonzalez, MD
Bitar Cosmetic Surgery Institute
Fairfax, VA, USA

Richard J. Greco, MD
CEO
The Georgia Institute For Plastic Surgery
Savannah, GA, USA

Ronald P. Gruber, MD
Adjunct Associate Clinical Professor
Division of Plastic and Reconstructive Surgery
Stanford University
Stanford, CA
Clinical Association Professor
Division of Plastic and Reconstructive Surgery
University of California San Francisco
San Francisco, CA, USA

Bahman Guyuron, MD, FCVS
Editor in Chief, Aesthetic Plastic Surgery Journal
Emeritus Professor of Plastic Surgery
Case School of Medicine
Cleveland, OH, USA

Joseph P. Hunstad, MD, FACS
Associate Consulting Professor
Division of Plastic Surgery
The University of North Carolina at Chapel Hill;
Private Practice
Huntersville/Charlotte, NC, USA

Clyde H. Ishii, MD, FACS
Assistant Clinical Professor of Surgery
John A. Burns School of Medicine;
Chief, Department of Plastic Surgery
Shriners Hospital
Honolulu Unit
Honolulu, HI, USA

Nicole J. Jarrett, MD
Department of Plastic Surgery
University of Pittsburgh
Pittsburgh, PA, USA

Elizabeth B. Jelks, MD
Private Practice
Jelks Medical
New York, NY, USA

Glenn W. Jelks, MD
Associate Professor
Department of Ophthalmology
Department of Plastic Surgery
New York University School of Medicine
New York, NY, USA

Mark Laurence Jewell, MD
Assistant Clinical Professor Plastic Surgery
Oregon Health Science University
Portland, OR, USA

David M. Kahn, MD
Clinical Associate Professor of Plastic Surgery
Department of Surgery
Stanford University School of Medicine
Stanford, CA, USA

Michael A. C. Kane, BS, MD
Attending Surgeon
Plastic Surgery
Manhattan Eye, Ear, and Throat Hospital
New York, NY, USA

David L. Kaufman, MD, FACS
Private Practice Plastic Surgery
Aesthetic Artistry Surgical and Medical Center
Folsom, CA, USA

Jeffrey Kenkel, MD
Professor and Chairman
Department of Plastic Surgery
UT Southwestern Medical Center
Dallas, TX, USA

Kyung S. Koh, MD, PhD
Professor of Plastic Surgery
Asan Medical Center, University of Ulsan School
of Medicine
Seoul, South Korea

Tracy Leong, MD
Dermatology
Rady Children's Hospital - San Diego;
Sharp Memorial Hospital;
University California San Diego Medical Center
San Diego;
Private Practice, FACES+ Plastic Surgery, Skin
and Laser Center
La Jolla, CA, USA

Steven M. Levine, MD
Assistant Professor of Surgery (Plastic)
Hofstra Medical School, Northwell Health,
New York, NY, USA

Michelle B. Locke, MBChB, MD
Senior Lecturer in Surgery
Department of Surgery
University of Auckland Faculty of Medicine and
Health Sciences;
South Auckland Clinical Campus
Middlemore Hospital
Auckland, New Zealand

Alyssa Lolofie
University of Utah
Salt Lake City, UT, USA

Timothy J. Marten, MD, FACS
Founder and Director
Marten Clinic of Plastic Surgery
San Francisco, CA, USA

Bryan Mendelson, FRCSE, FRACS, FACS
The Centre for Facial Plastic Surgery
Toorak, Victoria, Australia

Constantino G. Mendieta, MD, FACS
Private Practice
Miami, FL, USA

Drew B. Metcalfe, MD
Division of Plastic and Reconstructive Surgery
Emory University
Atlanta, GA, USA

Gabriele C. Miotto, MD
Emory School of Medicine
Atlanta, GA, USA

Foad Nahai, MD
Professor of Surgery
Division of Plastic and Reconstructive Surgery
Department of Surgery
Emory University School of Medicine
Emory Aesthetic Center at Paces
Atlanta, Georgia, USA

Suzan Obagi, MD
Associate Professor of Dermatology
Dermatology
University of Pittsburgh;
Associate Professor of Plastic Surgery
Plastic Surgery
University of Pittsburgh
Pittsburgh, PA, USA

Sabina Aparecida Alvarez de Paiva, MD
Resident of Plastic Surgery
Plastic Surgery Service Dr. Ewaldo Bolivar de
Souza Pinto
São Paulo, Brazil

Galen Perdikis, MD
Assistant Professor of Surgery
Division of Plastic Surgery
Emory University School of Medicine
Atlanta, GA, USA

Jason Posner, MD, FACS
Private Practice
Boca Raton, FL, USA

Dirk F. Richter, MD, PhD
Clinical Professor of Plastic Surgery
University of Bonn
Director and Chief
Dreifaltigkeits-Hospital
Wesseling, Germany

Thomas L. Roberts III, FACS
Plastic Surgery Center of the Carolinas
Spartanburg, SC, USA

Jocelyn Celeste Ledezma Rodriguez, MD
Private Practice
Guadalajara, Jalisco, Mexico

Rod J. Rohrich, MD
Clinical Professor and Founding Chair
Department of Plastic Surgery
Distinguished Teaching Professor
University of Texas Southwestern Medical Center
Founding Partner
Dallas Plastic Surgery Institute
Dallas, TX, USA

E. Victor Ross, MD
Director of Laser and Cosmetic Dermatology
Scripps Clinic
San Diego, CA, USA

J. Peter Rubin, MD, FACS
Chief
Plastic and Reconstructive Surgery
University of Pittsburgh Medical Center;
Associate Professor
Department of Surgery
University of Pittsburgh
Pittsburgh, PA, USA

Ahmad N. Saad, MD
Private Practice
FACES+ Plastic Surgery
Skin and Laser Center
La Jolla, CA, USA

Alesia P. Saboeiro, MD
Attending Physician
Private Practice
New York, NY, USA

Cristianna Bonnetto Saldanha, MD
Plastic Surgery Service Dr. Osvaldo Saldanha
São Paulo, Brazil

Osvaldo Saldanha, MD, PhD
Director of Plastic Surgery Service Dr. Osvaldo
Saldanha;
Professor of Plastic Surgery Department
Universidade Metropolitana de Santos
- UNIMES
São Paulo, Brazil

Renato Saltz, MD, FACS
Saltz Plastic Surgery
President
International Society of Aesthetic Plastic Surgery
Adjunct Professor of Surgery
University of Utah
Past-President, American Society for Aesthetic
Plastic Surgery
Salt Lake City and Park City, UT, USA

Paulo Rodamilans Sanjuan MD
Chief Resident of Plastic Surgery
Plastic Surgery Service Dr. Ewaldo Boliar de
Souza Pinto
São Paulo, Brazil

Nina Schwaiger, MD
Senior Specialist in Plastic and Aesthetic
Surgery
Department of Plastic Surgery
Dreifaltigkeits-Hospital Wesseling
Wesseling, Germany

Douglas S. Steinbrech, MD, FACS
Gotham Plastic Surgery
New York, NY, USA

Phillip J. Stephan, MD
Clinical Faculty
Plastic Surgery
UT Southwestern Medical School;
Plastic Surgeon
Texoma Plastic Surgery
Wichita Falls, TX, USA

David Gonzalez Sosa, MD
Plastic and Reconstructive Surgery
Hospital Quirónsalud Torrevieja
Alicante, Spain

James M. Stuzin, MD
Associate Professor of Surgery
(Plastic) Voluntary
University of Miami Leonard M. Miller School of
Medicine
Miami, FL, USA

Daniel Suissa, MD, MSc
Clinical Instructor
Section of Plastic and Reconstructive Surgery
Yale University
New Haven, CT, USA

Charles H. Thorne, MD
Associate Professor of Plastic Surgery
Department of Plastic Surgery
NYU School of Medicine
New York, NY, USA

Ali Totonchi, MD
Assistant Professor
Plastic Surgery
Case Western Reserve University;
Medical Director Craniofacial Deformity Clinic
Plastic Surgery
MetroHealth Medical center
Cleveland, OH, USA

Jonathan W. Toy, MD, FRCSC
Program Director, Plastic Surgery Residency
Program Assistant Clinical Professor
University of Alberta
Edmonton, Alberta, Canada

Matthew J. Trovato, MD
Dallas Plastic Surgery Institute
Dallas, TX, USA

Simeon H. Wall Jr., MD, FACS
Director
The Wall Center for Plastic Surgery;
Assistant Clinical Professor
Plastic Surgery
LSU Health Sciences Center at Shreveport
Shreveport, LA, USA

Joshua T. Waltzman, MD, MBA
Private Practice
Waltzman Plastic and Reconstructive Surgery
Long Beach, CA, USA

Richard J. Warren, MD, FRCSC
Clinical Professor
Division of Plastic Surgery
University of British Columbia
Vancouver, British Columbia, Canada

Edmund Weisberg, MS, MBE
University of Pennsylvania
Philadelphia, PA, USA

Scott Woehrle, MS BS
Physician Assistant
Department of Plastic Surgery
Jospeh Capella Plastic Surgery
Ramsey, NJ, USA

**Chin-Ho Wong, MBBS, MRCS, MMed(Surg),
FAMS(Plast Surg)**
W Aesthetic Plastic Surgery
Mt Elizabeth Novena Specialist Center
Singapore

Alan Yan, MD
Former Fellow
Adult Reconstructive and Aesthetic
Craniomaxillofacial Surgery
Division of Plastic and Reconstructive Surgery
Massachusetts General Hospital
Boston, MA, USA

Michael J. Yaremchuk, MD
Chief of Craniofacial Surgery
Massachusetts General Hospital;
Clinical Professor of Surgery
Harvard Medical School;
Program Director
Harvard Plastic Surgery Residency Program
Boston, MA, USA

James E. Zins, MD
Chairman
Department of Plastic Surgery
Dermatology and Plastic Surgery Institute
Cleveland Clinic
Cleveland, OH, USA

VOLUME THREE

Neta Adler, MD
Senior Surgeon
Department of Plastic and Reconstructive
Surgery
Hadassah University Hospital
Jerusalem, Israel

Ahmed M. Afifi, MD
Assistant Professor of Plastic Surgery
Department of Surgery
University of Wisconsin
Madison, WI, USA;
Associate Professor
Department of Plastic Surgery
Cairo University
Cairo, Egypt

Marta Alvarado, DDS, MS
Department of Orthodontics
Facultad de Odontología
Universidad de San Carlos de Guatemala
Guatemala

Eric Arnaud, MD
Pediatric Neurosurgeon and Co-Director
Unité de Chirurgie Craniofaciale
Hôpital Necker Enfants Malades
Paris, France

Stephen B. Baker, MD, DDS
Associate Professor and Program Director
Co-Director Inova Hospital for Children
Craniofacial Clinic
Department of Plastic Surgery
Georgetown University Hospital
Georgetown, WA, USA

Scott P. Bartlett, MD
Professor of Surgery
Surgery
University of Pennsylvania;
Chief Division of Plastic Surgery
Surgery
Children's Hospital of Philadelphia
Philadelphia, PA, USA

Bruce S. Bauer, MD
Chief
Division of Plastic Surgery
NorthShore University HealthSystem
Highland Park;
Clinical Professor of Surgery
Department of Surgery
University of Chicago Pritzker School of
Medicine
Chicago, IL, USA

Adriane L. Baylis, PhD
Speech Scientist
Section of Plastic and Reconstructive Surgery
Nationwide Children's Hospital
Columbus, OH, USA

Mike Bentz, MD, FAAP, FACS
Interim Chairman
Department of Surgery
University of Wisconsin;
Chairman Division of Plastic Surgery
Department of Surgery
University of Wisconsin
Madison, WI, USA

Craig Birgfeld, MD, FACS
Associate Professor, Pediatric Plastic and
Craniofacial Surgery
Seattle Children's Hospital
Seattle, WA, USA

William R. Boysen, MD
Resident Physician, Urology
University of Chicago Medicine
Chicago, IL, USA

James P. Bradley, MD
Professor and Chief
Section of Plastic and Reconstructive Surgery
Temple University
Philadelphia, PA, USA

Edward P. Buchanan, MD
Division of Plastic Surgery
Baylor College of Medicine
Houston, TX, USA

Michael R. Bykowski, MD, MS
Plastic Surgery Resident
Plastic Surgery
University of Pittsburgh Medical Center
Pittsburgh, PA, USA

Edward J. Caterson, MD, PhD
Director of Craniofacial Surgery
Division of Plastic Surgery
Brigham and Women's Hospital
Boston, MA, USA

Rodney K. Chan, MD
Chief Plastic and Reconstructive Surgery
Clinical Division and Burn Center
United States Army Institute of Surgical
Research
Joint Base San Antonio, TX, USA

Edward I. Chang, MD
Assistant Professor
Department of Plastic Surgery
The University of Texas M. D. Anderson Cancer
Center
Houston, TX, USA

Constance M. Chen, MD, MPH
Director of Microsurgery
Plastic and Reconstructive Surgery
New York Eye and Ear Infirmary of Mt Sinai;
Clinical Assistant Professor
Plastic and Reconstructive Surgery
Weil Medical College of Cornell University;
Clinical Assistant Professor
Plastic and Reconstructive Surgery
Tulane University School of Medicine
New York, NY, USA

Yu-Ray Chen, MD
Professor of Surgery
Plastic and Reconstructive Surgery
Chang Gung Memorial Hospital
Taoyuan City, Taiwan

Philip Kuo-Ting Chen, MD
Professor
Craniofacial Center
Chang Gung Memorial Hospital
Taoyuan City, Taiwan

Ming-Huei Cheng, MD, MBA
Professor
Division of Reconstructive Microsurgery
Department of Plastic and Reconstructive
Surgery
Chang Gung Memorial Hospital
Taoyuan City, Taiwan

Gerson R. Chinchilla, DDS MS
Director
Department of Orthodontics
Facultad de Odontología
Universidad de San Carlos de Guatemala
Guatemala

Peter G. Cordeiro, MD
Chief
Plastic and Reconstructive Surgery
Memorial Sloan Kettering Cancer Center;
Professor of Surgery
Surgery
Weil Medical College of Cornell University
New York, NY, USA

Alberto Córdova-Aguilar, MD, MPH
Attending Plastic Surgeon
Surgery
Faculty of Medicine Ricardo Palma University
Lima, Peru

Edward H. Davidson, MA(Cantab), MBBS
Resident Plastic Surgeon
Department of Plastic Surgery
University of Pittsburgh
Pittsburgh, PA, USA

Sara R. Dickie, MD
Clinician Educator
Surgery
University of Chicago Hospital Pritzker School of Medicine;
Attending Surgeon
Section of Plastic and Reconstructive Surgery
NorthShore University HealthSystem
Northbrook, IL, USA

Risal S. Djohan, MD
Microsurgery Fellowship Program Director
Plastic Surgery
Cleveland Clinic;
Surgery ASC Quality Improvement Officer
Plastic Surgery
Cleveland Clinic
Cleveland, OH, USA

Amir H. Dorafshar, MBChB, FACS, FAAP
Associate Professor
Plastic and Reconstructive Surgery
Johns Hopkins Medical Institute;
Assistant Professor
Plastic Surgery
R Adams Cowley Shock Trauma Center
Baltimore, MD, USA

Jeffrey A. Fearon, MD
Director
The Craniofacial Center
Dallas, TX, USA

Alexander L. Figueroa, DMD
Craniofacial Orthodontist
Rush Craniofacial Center
Rush University Medical Center
Chicago, IL, USA

Alvaro A. Figueroa, DDS, MS
Co-Director
Rush Craniofacial Center
Rush University Medical Center
Chicago, IL, USA

David M. Fisher, MB, BCh, FRCSC, FACS
Medical Director Cleft Lip and Palate Program
Plastic Surgery
Hospital for Sick Children;
Associate Professor
Surgery
University of Toronto
Toronto, Ontario, Canada

Roberto L. Flores, MD
Associate Professor of Plastic Surgery
Director of Cleft Lip and Palate
Hansjörg Wyss Department of Plastic Surgery
NYU Langone Medical Center
New York, NY, USA

Andrew Foreman, B. Physio, BMBS(Hons), PhD, FRACS
Consultant Surgeon, Department of
Otolaryngology - Head and Neck Surgery
University of Adelaide,
Royal Adelaide Hospital,
Adelaide, SA, Australia

Patrick A. Gerety, MD
Assistant Professor of Surgery
Division of Plastic and Reconstructive Surgery
Indiana University and Riley Hospital for Children
Philadelphia, PA, USA

Jesse A. Goldstein, MD
Chief Resident
Department of Plastic Surgery
Georgetown University Hospital
Washington, DC, USA

Arun K. Gosain, MD
Chief
Division of Plastic Surgery
Ann and Robert H. Lurie Children's Hospital of Chicago
Chicago, IL, USA

Lawrence J. Gottlieb, MD
Professor of Surgery
Department of Surgery
Section of Plastic and Reconstructive Surgery
University of Chicago
Chicago, IL, USA

Arin K. Greene, MD, MMSc
Department of Plastic and Oral Surgery
Boston Children's Hospital;
Associate Professor of Surgery
Harvard Medical School
Boston, MA, USA

Patrick J. Gullane, MD, FRCS
Wharton Chair in Head and Neck Surgery
Professor of Surgery, Department of
Otolaryngology - Head and Neck Surgery
University of Toronto
Toronto, Ontario, Canada

Mohan S. Gundeti, MB, MCh, FEBU, FRCS(Urol), FEAPU
Associate Professor of Urology in Surgery and Pediatrics, Director Pediatric Urology, Director Centre for Pediatric Robotics and Minimal Invasive Surgery
University of Chicago and Pritzker Medical School Comer Children's Hospital
Chicago, IL, USA

Eyal Gur, MD
Professor of Surgery, Chief
Department of Plastic and Reconstructive Surgery
The Tel Aviv Sourasky Medical Center
Tel Aviv, Israel

Bahman Guyuron, MD, FCVS
Editor in Chief, Aesthetic Plastic Surgery Journal;
Emeritus Professor of Plastic Surgery
Case School of Medicine
Cleveland, OH, USA

Matthew M. Hanasono, MD
Associate Professor
Department of Plastic Surgery
The University of Texas MD Anderson Cancer Center
Houston, TX, USA

Toshinobu Harada, PhD
Professor in Engineering
Department of Systems Engineering
Faculty of Systems Engineering
Wakayama University
Wakayama, Japan

Jill A. Helms, DDS, PhD
Professor
Surgery
Stanford University
Stanford, CA, USA

David L. Hirsch, MD, DDS
Director of Oral Oncology and Reconstruction
Lenox Hill Hospital/Northwell Health
New York, NY, USA

Jung-Ju Huang, MD
Associate Professor
Division of Microsurgery
Plastic and Reconstructive Surgery
Chang Gung Memorial Hospital
Taoyuan, Taiwan

William Y. Hoffman, MD
Professor and Chief
Division of Plastic and Reconstructive Surgery
UCSF
San Francisco, CA, USA

Larry H. Hollier Jr., MD
Division of Plastic Surgery
Baylor College of Medicine
Houston, TX, USA

Richard A. Hopper, MD, MS
Chief
Division of Craniofacial Plastic Surgery
Seattle Children's Hospital;
Surgical Director
Craniofacial Center
Seattle Children's Hospital;
Associate Professor
Department of Surgery
University of Washington
Seattle, WA, USA

Gazi Hussain, MBBS, FRACS
Clinical Senior Lecturer
Macquarie University
Sydney, Australia

Oksana Jackson, MD
Assistant Professor
Plastic Surgery
Perelman School of Medicine at the University of Pennsylvania;
Assistant Professor
Plastic Surgery
The Children's Hospital of Philadelphia
Philadelphia, PA, USA

Syril James, MD
Clinic Marcel Sembat
Boulogne-Billancourt
Paris, France

Leila Jazayeri, MD
Microsurgery Fellow
Plastic and Reconstructive Surgery
Memorial Sloan Kettering Cancer Center
New York, NY, USA

Sahil Kapur, MD
Assistant Professor
Department of Plastic Surgery
University of Texas - MD Anderson Cancer
Center
Houston, TX, USA

Henry K. Kawamoto Jr., MD, DDS
Clinical Professor
Surgery Division of Plastic Surgery
UCLA
Los Angeles, CA, USA

David Y. Khechoyan, MD
Division of Plastic Surgery
Baylor College of Medicine
Houston, TX, USA

Richard E. Kirschner, MD
Section Chief
Plastic and Reconstructive Surgery
Nationwide Children's Hospital;
Senior Vice Chair
Plastic Surgery
The Ohio State University Medical College
Columbus, OH, USA

John C. Koshy, MD
Division of Plastic Surgery
Baylor College of Medicine
Houston, TX, USA

Michael C. Large, MD
Urologic Oncologist
Urology of Indiana
Greenwood, IN, USA

Edward I. Lee, MD
Division of Plastic Surgery
Baylor College of Medicine
Houston, TX, USA

Jamie P. Levine, MD
Chief of Microsurgery
Associate Professor
Plastic Surgery
NYU Langone Medical Center
New York, NY, USA

Jingtao Li, DDS, PhD
Consultant Surgeon
Oral and Maxillofacial Surgery
West China Hospital of Stomatology
Chengdu, Sichuan, People's Republic of China

Lawrence Lin, MD
Division of Plastic Surgery
Baylor College of Medicine
Houston, TX, USA

Joseph E. Losee, MD
Ross H. Musgrave Professor of Pediatric Plastic
Surgery
Department of Plastic Surgery
University of Pittsburgh Medical Center;
Chief, Division of Pediatric Plastic Surgery
Children's Hospital of Pittsburgh
Pittsburgh, PA, USA

David W. Low, MD
Professor of Surgery
Division of Plastic Surgery
Perelman School of Medicine at the University
of Pennsylvania;
Clinical Associate
Department of Surgery
Children's Hospital of Philadelphia
Philadelphia, PA, USA

Ralph T. Manktelow, MD, FRCSC
Professor of Surgery,
The University of Toronto,
Toronto, Ontario, Canada

Paul N. Manson, MD
Distinguished Service Professor
Plastic Surgery
Johns Hopkins University
Baltimore, MD, USA

David W. Mathes, MD
Professor and Chief of the Division of Plastic
and Reconstructive Surgery
Surgery Division of Plastic and Reconstructive
Surgery
University of Colorado
Aurora, CO, USA

Frederick J. Menick, MD
Private Practitioner
Tucson, AZ, USA

Fernando Molina, MD
Director
Craniofacial Anomalies Foundation A.C.
Mexico City;
Professor of Plastic Reconstructive and
Aesthetic Surgery
Medical School
Universidad La Salle
Mexico City, Distrito Federal, Mexico

Laura A. Monson, MD
Division of Plastic Surgery
Baylor College of Medicine
Houston, TX, USA

Reid V. Mueller, MD
Associate Professor
Plastic Surgery
Oregon Health and Science University
Portland, OR, USA

John B. Mulliken, MD
Professor
Department of Plastic and Oral Surgery
Boston Children's Hospital
Harvard Medical School
Boston, MA, USA

Gerhard S. Mundinger, MD
Assistant Professor
Craniofacial, Plastic, and Reconstructive Surgery
Louisiana State University Health Sciences
Center
Children's Hospital of New Orleans
New Orleans, LA, USA

Blake D. Murphy, BSc, PhD, MD
Craniofacial Fellow
Plastic Surgery
Nicklaus Children's Hospital
Miami, FL, USA

**Peter C. Neligan, MB, FRCS(I), FRCSC,
FACS**
Professor of Surgery
Department of Surgery, Division of Plastic
Surgery
University of Washington
Seattle, WA, USA

M. Samuel Noordhoff, MD, FACS
Emeritus Professor in Surgery
Chang Gung University
Taoyuan City, Taiwan

Giovanna Paternoster, MD
Unité de chirurgie crânio-faciale du departement
de neurochirurgie
Hôpital Necker Enfants Malades
Paris, France

Jason Pomerantz, MD
Assistant Professor
Surgery
University of California San Francisco;
Surgical Director
Craniofacial Center
University of California San Francisco
San Francisco, CA, USA

Julian J. Pribaz, MD
Professor of Surgery
University of South Florida, Morsani College of
Medicine
Tampa General Hospital
Tampa, FL, USA

Chad A. Purnell, MD
Division of Plastic Surgery
Lurie Children's Hospital of Northwestern
Feinberg School of Medicine
Chicago, IL, USA

Russell R. Reid, MD, PhD
Associate Professor
Surgery/Section of Plastic and Reconstructive
Surgery
University of Chicago Medicine
Chicago, IL, USA

Eduardo D. Rodriguez, MD, DDS
Helen L. Kimmel Professor of Reconstructive
Plastic Surgery
Chair, Hansjörg Wyss Department of Plastic
Surgery
NYU School of Medicine
NYU Langone Medical Center
New York, NY, USA

Craig Rowin, MD
Craniofacial Fellow
Plastic Surgery
Nicklaus Children's Hospital
Miami, FL, USA

Ruston J. Sanchez, MD
Plastic and Reconstructive Surgery Resident
University of Wisconsin
Madison, WI, USA

Lindsay A. Schuster, DMD, MS
Director Cleft-Craniofacial Orthodontics
Pediatric Plastic Surgery
Children's Hospital of Pittsburgh of UMPC;
Clinical Assistant Professor of Plastic Surgery
Department of Plastic Surgery
University of Pittsburgh School of Medicine
Pittsburgh, PA, USA

Jeremiah Un Chang See, MD
Plastic Surgeon
Department of Plastic and Reconstructive
Surgery
Penang General Hospital
Georgetown, Penang, Malaysia

Pradip R. Shetye, DDS, BDS, MDS
Assistant Professor (Orthodontics)
Hansjörg Wyss Department of Plastic Surgery
NYU Langone Medical Center
New York, NY, USA

Roman Skoracki, MD
Plastic Surgery
The Ohio State University
Columbus, OH, USA

Mark B. Slidell, MD, MPH
Assistant Professor of Surgery
Department of Surgery
Section of Pediatric Surgery
University of Chicago Medicine Biological
Sciences
Chicago, IL, USA

Michael Sosin, MD
Research Fellow
Department of Plastic Surgery Institute of
Reconstructive Plastic Surgery
NYU Langone Medical Center
New York, NY, USA;
Research Fellow
Division of Plastic Reconstructive and
Maxillofacial Surgery
R Adams Cowley Shock Trauma Center
University of Maryland Medical Center
Baltimore, MD, USA;
Resident
Department of Surgery
Medstar Georgetown University Hospital
Washington, DC, USA

**Youssef Tahiri, MD, MSc, FRCSC, FAAP,
FACS**
Associate Professor
Pediatric Plastic & Craniofacial Surgery
Cedars Sinai Medical Center
Los Angeles, CA, USA

Peter J. Taub, MD
Professor
Surgery Pediatrics Dentistry and Medical
Education
Surgery Division of Plastic and Reconstructive
Surgery
Icahn School of Medicine at Mount Sinai
New York, NY, USA

Jesse A. Taylor, MD
Mary Downs Endowed Chair of Pediatric
Craniofacial Treatment and Research;
Director, Penn Craniofacial Fellowship;
Co-Director, CHOP Cleft Team
Plastic, Reconstructive, and Craniofacial Surgery
The University of Pennsylvania and
Children's Hospital of Philadelphia
Philadelphia, PA, USA

Kathryn S. Torok, MD
Assistant Professor
Pediatric Rheumatology
University of Pittsburgh
Pittsburgh, PA, USA

Ali Totonchi, MD
Assistant Professor
Plastic Surgery
Case Western Reserve University;
Medical Director Craniofacial Deformity Clinic
Plastic Surgery
MetroHealth Medical Center
Cleveland, OH, USA

Kris Wilson, MD
Division of Plastic Surgery
Baylor College of Medicine
Houston, TX, USA

S. Anthony Wolfe, MD
Plastic Surgery
Miami Children's Hospital
Miami, FL, USA

Akira Yamada, MD, PhD
Professor of Plastic Surgery
World Craniofacial Foundation
Dallas, TX, USA;
Clinical Assistant Professor
Plastic Surgery
Case Western Reserve University
Cleveland, OH, USA

Peirong Yu, MD
Professor
Plastic Surgery
M. D. Anderson Cancer Center;
Adjunct Professor
Plastic Surgery
Baylor College of Medicine
Houston, TX, USA

**Ronald M. Zuker, MD, FRCSC, FACS,
FRCSEd(Hon)**
Professor of Surgery
Department of Surgery
University of Toronto;
Staff Plastic and Reconstructive Surgeon
Department of Surgery
SickKids Hospital
Toronto, Ontario, Canada

VOLUME FOUR

Christopher E. Attinger, MD
Professor, Interim Chairman
Department of Plastic Surgery
Center for Wound Healing
Medstar Georgetown University Hospital
Washington, DC, USA

Lorenzo Borghese, MD
Plastic Surgeon
Chief of International Missions
Ospedale Pediatrico Bambino Gesù
Rome, Italy

Charles E. Butler, MD, FACS
Professor and Chairman
Department of Plastic Surgery
Charles B. Barker Endowed Chair in Surgery
The University of Texas M. D. Anderson Cancer
Center
Houston, TX, USA

David W. Chang, MD
Professor of Surgery
University of Chicago
Chicago, IL, USA

Karel Claes, MD
Department of Plastic and Reconstructive
Surgery
Ghent University Hospital
Ghent, Belgium

Mark W. Clemens II, MD, FACS
Associate Professor
Plastic Surgery
MD Anderson Cancer Center,
Houston, TX, USA

Shannon M. Colohan, MD, MSc
Assistant Professor of Surgery
University of Washington
Seattle, WA, USA

Peter G. Cordeiro, MD
Chief
Plastic and Reconstructive Surgery
Memorial Sloan Kettering Cancer Center
New York, NY, USA

Salvatore D'Arpa, MD, PhD
Department of Plastic and Reconstructive
Surgery
Ghent University Hospital
Ghent, Belgium

Michael V. DeFazio, MD
Department Plastic Surgery
MedStar Georgetown University Hospital
Washington, DC, USA

A. Lee Dellon, MD, PhD
Professor of Plastic Surgery
Professor of Neurosurgery
Johns Hopkins University
Baltimore, MD, USA

Sara R. Dickie, MD
Clinical Associate of Surgery
University of Chicago Hospitals
Pritzker School of Medicine
Chicago, IL, USA

Ivica Ducic, MD, PhD
Clinical Professor of Surgery
GWU Washington Nerve Institute
McLean, VA, USA

Gregory A. Dumanian, MD
Stuteville Professor of Surgery
Division of Plastic Surgery
Northwestern Feinberg School of Medicine
Chicago, IL, USA

John M. Felder III, MD
Fellow in Hand Surgery
Plastic Surgery
Washington University in Saint Louis
St. Louis, MO, USA

Goetz A. Giessler, MD, PhD
Professor Director
Plastic-Reconstructive, Aesthetic and Hand
Surgery
Gesundheit Nordhessen
Kassel, Germany

Kevin D. Han, MD
Department of Plastic Surgery
MedStar Georgetown University Hospital
Washington, DC, USA

Piet Hoebeke
Department of Urology
Ghent University Hospital
Ghent, Belgium

Joon Pio Hong, MD, PhD, MMM
Professor of Plastic Surgery
Asan Medical Center, University of Ulsan
Seoul, South Korea

Michael A. Howard, MD
Clinical Assistant Professor of Surgery
Plastic Surgery
NorthShore University HealthSystem/University
of Chicago
Chicago, IL, USA

Jeffrey E. Janis, MD, FACS
Professor of Plastic Surgery, Neurosurgery,
Neurology, and Surgery;
Executive Vice Chairman, Department of Plastic
Surgery;
Chief of Plastic Surgery, University Hospitals
Ohio State University Wexner Medical Center
Columbus, OH, USA

Leila Jazayeri, MD
Microsurgery Fellow
Plastic and Reconstructive Surgery
Memorial Sloan Kettering Cancer Center
New York, NY, USA

Grant M. Kleiber, MD
Assistant Professor of Surgery
Division of Plastic and Reconstructive Surgery
Washington University School of Medicine
St. Louis, MO, USA

Stephen J. Kovach III, MD
Assistant Professor
Division of Plastic Surgery
University of Pennsylvania
Philadelphia, PA, USA

Robert Kwon, MD
Southwest Hand and Microsurgery
3108 Midway Road, Suite 103
Plano, TX, USA

**Raphael C. Lee, MS, MD, ScD, FACS,
FAIMBE**
Paul and Allene Russell Professor
Plastic Surgery, Dermatology, Anatomy and
Organismal Biology, Molecular Medicine
University of Chicago
Chicago, IL, USA

L. Scott Levin, MD, FACS
Chairman of Orthopedic Surgery
Department of Orthopaedic Surgery
University of Pennsylvania School of Medicine
Philadelphia, PA, USA

Otway Louie, MD
Associate Professor
Surgery
University of Washington Medical Center
Seattle, WA, USA

Nicolas Lumen, MD, PhD
Head of Clinic
Urology
Ghent University Hospital
Ghent, Belgium

Alessandro Masellis, MD
Plastic Surgeon
Euro-Mediterranean Council for Burns and Fire
Disasters
Palermo, Italy

Michele Masellis, MD
Former Chief of Department of Plastic and
Reconstructive Surgery and Burn Therapy
Department of Plastic and Reconstructive
Surgery and Burn Therapy - ARNAS Ospedale
Civico e Benfratelli
Palermo, Italy

Stephen M. Milner, MB BS, BDS
Professor of Plastic Surgery
Surgery
Johns Hopkins School of Medicine
Baltimore, MD, USA

Arash Momeni, MD
Fellow, Reconstructive Microsurgery
Division of Plastic Surgery
University of Pennsylvania Health System
Philadelphia, PA, USA

Stan Monstrey, MD, PhD
Department of Plastic and Reconstructive
Surgery
Ghent University Hospital
Ghent, Belgium

**Venkateshwaran N, MBBS, MS, DNB, MCh,
MRCS(Intercollegiate)**
Consultant Plastic Surgeon
Jupiter Hospital
Thane, India

Rajiv P. Parikh, MD, MPHS
Resident Physician
Department of Surgery, Division of Plastic and
Reconstructive Surgery
Washington University School of Medicine
St. Louis, MO, USA

Mônica Sarto Piccolo, MD, MSc, PhD
Director
Pronto Socorro para Queimaduras
Goiânia, Goiás, Brazil

Nelson Sarto Piccolo, MD
Chief
Division of Plastic Surgery
Pronto Socorro para Queimaduras
Goiânia, Goiás, Brazil

Maria Thereza Sarto Piccolo, MD, PhD
Scientific Director
Pronto Socorro para Queimaduras
Goiânia, Goiás, Brazil

Vinita Puri, MS, MCh
Professor and Head
Department of Plastic, Reconstructive Surgery
and Burns
Seth G S Medical College and KEM Hospital
Mumbai, Maharashtra, India

Andrea L. Pusic, MD, MHS, FACS
Associate Professor
Plastic and Reconstructive Surgery
Memorial Sloan Kettering Cancer Center
New York, NY, USA

Vinay Rawlani, MD
Division of Plastic Surgery
Northwestern Feinberg School of Medicine
Chicago, IL, USA

Juan L. Rendon, MD, PhD
Clinical Instructor Housestaff
Department of Plastic Surgery
The Ohio State University Wexner Medical
Center
Columbus, OH, USA

Michelle C. Roughton, MD
Assistant Professor
Division of Plastic and Reconstructive Surgery
University of North Carolina at Chapel Hill
Chapel Hill, NC, USA

Hakim K. Said, MD, FACS
Associate Professor
Division of Plastic surgery
University of Washington
Seattle, WA, USA

Michel Saint-Cyr, MD, FRSC(C)
Professor
Plastic Surgery
Mayo Clinic
Rochester, MN, USA

Michael Sauerbier, MD, PhD
Professor, Chair
Department for Plastic, Hand, and
Reconstructive Surgery
Academic Hospital Goethe University Frankfurt
am Main
Frankfurt am Main, Germany

Loren S. Schechter, MD
Associate Professor and Chief
Division of Plastic Surgery
Chicago Medical School
Morton Grove, IL, USA

David H. Song, MD, MBA, FACS
Regional Chief, MedStar Health
Plastic and Reconstructive Surgery
Professor and Chairman
Department of Plastic Surgery
Georgetown University School of Medicine
Washington, DC, USA

Yoo Joon Sur, MD, PhD
Associate Professor
Department of Orthopedic Surgery
The Catholic University of Korea, College of
Medicine
Seoul, Korea

Chad M. Teven, MD
Resident
Section of Plastic and Reconstructive Surgery
University of Chicago
Chicago, IL, USA

VOLUME FIVE

Jamil Ahmad, MD, FRCSC
Director of Research and Education
The Plastic Surgery Clinic
Mississauga, Ontario, Canada;
Assistant Professor of Surgery
University of Toronto
Toronto, Ontario, Canada

Robert J. Allen Sr., MD
Clinical Professor of Plastic Surgery
Department of Plastic Surgery
New York University Medical Center
Charleston, NC, USA

Ryan E. Austin, MD, FRCSC
Plastic Surgeon
The Plastic Surgery Clinic
Mississauga, ON, Canada

Brett Beber, BA, MD, FRCSC
Plastic and Reconstructive Surgeon
Lecturer, Department of Surgery
University of Toronto
Toronto, Ontario, Canada

Philip N. Blondeel, MD
Professor of Plastic Surgery
Department of Plastic Surgery
University Hospital Ghent
Ghent, Belgium

Benjamin J. Brown, MD
Gulf Coast Plastic Surgery
Pensacola, FL, USA

Mitchell H. Brown, MD, MEd, FRCSC
Plastic and Reconstructive Surgeon
Associate Professor, Department of Surgery
University of Toronto
Toronto, Ontario, Canada

M. Bradley Calobrace, MD, FACS
Plastic Surgeon
Calobrace and Mizuguchi Plastic Surgery Center
Departments of Surgery, Divisions of Plastic
Surgery
Clinical Faculty, University of Louisville and
University of Kentucky
Louisville, KY, USA

Grant W. Carlson, MD
Wadley R. Glenn Professor of Surgery
Emory University
Atlanta, GA, USA

Bernard W. Chang, MD
Chief of Plastic and Reconstructive Surgery
Mercy Medical Center
Baltimore, MD, USA

Mark W. Clemens II, MD, FACS
Assistant Professor Plastic Surgery
M. D. Anderson Cancer Center
Houston, TX, USA

Robert Cohen MD, FACS
Medical Director
Plastic Surgery
Scottsdale Center for Plastic Surgery
Paradise Valley, AZ and;
Santa Monica, CA, USA

Amy S. Colwell, MD
Associate Professor
Harvard Medical School
Massachusetts General Hospital
Boston, MA, USA

Edward H. Davidson, MA(Cantab), MB, BS
Resident Plastic Surgeon
Department of Plastic Surgery
University of Pittsburgh Medical Center
Pittsburgh, PA, USA

Emmanuel Delay, MD, PhD
Unité de Chirurgie Plastique et Reconstructrice
Centre Léon Bérard
Lyon, France

Francesco M. Egro, MB ChB, MSc, MRCS
Department of Plastic Surgery
University of Pittsburgh Medical Center
Pittsburgh, PA, USA

Neil A. Fine, MD
President
Northwestern Specialists in Plastic Surgery;
Associate Professor (Clinical) Surgery/Plastics
Northwestern University Fienberg School of
Medicine
Chicago, IL, USA

Jaime Flores, MD
Plastic and Reconstructive Microvascular
Surgeon
Miami, FL, USA

Joshua Fosnot, MD
Assistant Professor of Surgery
Division of Plastic Surgery
The Perelman School of Medicine
University of Pennsylvania Health System
Philadelphia, PA, USA

Allen Gabriel, MD
Clinical Associate Professor
Department of Plastic Surgery
Loma Linda University Medical Center
Loma Linda, CA, USA

Michael S. Gart, MD
Resident Physician
Division of Plastic Surgery
Northwestern University Feinberg School of
Medicine
Chicago, IL, USA

Matthew D. Goodwin, MD
Plastic Surgeon
Plastic Reconstructive and Cosmetic Surgery
Boca Raton Regional Hospital
Boca Raton, FL, USA

Samia Guerid, MD
Cabinet
50 rue de la République
Lyon, France

Moustapha Hamdi, MD, PhD
Professor of Plastic and Reconstructive Surgery
Brussels University Hospital
Vrij Universitaire Brussels
Brussels, Belgium

Alexandra M. Hart, MD
Emory Division of Plastic and Reconstructive
Surgery
Emory University School of Medicine
Atlanta, GA, USA

Emily C. Hartmann, MD, MS
Aesthetic Surgery Fellow
Plastic and Reconstructive Surgery
University of Southern California
Los Angeles, CA, USA

Nima Khavanin, MD
Resident Physician
Department of Plastic and Reconstructive
Surgery
Johns Hopkins Hospital
Baltimore, MD, USA

John Y. S. Kim, MD
Professor and Clinical Director
Department of Surgery
Division of Plastic Surgery
Northwestern University Feinberg School of
Medicine
Chicago, IL, USA

Steven Kronowitz, MD
Owner, Kronowitz Plastics
PLLC;
University of Texas, M. D. Anderson Medical
Center
Houston, TX, USA

John V. Larson, MD
Resident Physician
Division of Plastic and Reconstructive Surgery
Keck School of Medicine of USC
University of Southern California
Los Angeles, CA, USA

Z-Hye Lee, MD
Resident
Department of Plastic Surgery
New York University Medical Center
New York, NY, USA

Frank Lista, MD, FRCSC
Medical Director
The Plastic Surgery Clinic
Mississauga, Ontario, Canada;
Assistant Professor Surgery
University of Toronto
Toronto, Ontario, Canada

Albert Losken, MD, FACS
Professor of plastic surgery and Program
Director
Emory Division of Plastic and Reconstructive
Surgery
Emory University School of Medicine
Atlanta, GA, USA

**Charles M. Malata, BSc(HB), MB ChB,
LRCP, MRCS, FRCS(Glasg), FRCS(Plast)**
Professor of Academic Plastic Surgery
Postgraduate Medical Institute
Faculty of Health Sciences
Anglia Ruskin University
Cambridge and Chelmsford, UK;
Consultant Plastic and Reconstructive Surgeon
Department of Plastic and Reconstructive
Surgery
Cambridge Breast Unit at Addenbrooke's
Hospital
Cambridge University Hospitals NHS
Foundation Trust
Cambridge, UK

Jaume Masià, MD, PhD
Chief and Professor of Plastic Surgery
Sant Pau University Hospital
Barcelona, Spain

G. Patrick Maxwell, MD, FACS
Clinical Professor of Surgery
Department of Plastic Surgery
Loma Linda University Medical Center
Loma Linda, CA, USA

James L. Mayo, MD
Microsurgery Fellow
Plastic Surgery
New York University
New York, NY, USA

Roberto N. Miranda, MD
Professor
Department of Hematopathology
Division of Pathology and Laboratory Medicine
MD Anderson Cancer Center
Houston, TX, USA

**Colin M. Morrison, MSc (Hons) FRCSI
(Plast)**
Consultant Plastic Surgeon
St. Vincent's University Hospital
Dublin, Ireland

Maurice Y. Nahabedian, MD, FACS
Professor and Chief
Section of Plastic Surgery
MedStar Washington Hospital Center
Washington DC, USA;
Vice Chairman
Department of Plastic Surgery
MedStar Georgetown University Hospital
Washington DC, USA

James D. Namnoum, MD
Clinical Professor of Plastic Surgery
Atlanta Plastic Surgery
Emory University School of Medicine
Atlanta, GA, USA

Maria E. Nelson, MD
Assistant Professor of Clinical Surgery
Department of Surgery, Division of Upper GI/
General Surgery, Section of Surgical Oncology
Keck School of Medicine
University of Southern California
Los Angeles, CA, USA

Julie Park, MD
Associate Professor of Surgery
Section of Plastic Surgery
University of Chicago
Chicago, IL, USA

Ketan M. Patel, MD
Assistant Professor of Surgery
Division of Plastic and Reconstructive Surgery
Keck Medical Center of USC
University of Southern California
Los Angeles, CA, USA

**Nakul Gamanlal Patel, BSc(Hons),
MBBS(Lond), FRCS(Plast)**
Senior Microsurgery Fellow
St. Andrew's Centre for Plastic Surgery
Broomfield Hospital
Chelmsford, UK

Gemma Pons, MD, PhD
Head
Microsurgery Unit
Plastic Surgery
Hospital de Sant Pau
Barcelona, Spain

Julian J. Pribaz, MD
Professor of Surgery
Brigham and Women's Hospital
Harvard Medical School
Boston, MA, USA

**Venkat V. Ramakrishnan, MS, FRCS,
FRACS(Plast Surg)**
Consultant Plastic Surgeon
St. Andrew's Centre for Plastic Surgery
Broomfield Hospital
Chelmsford, UK

Elena Rodríguez-Bauzà, MD
Plastic Surgery Department
Hospital Santa Creu i Sant Pau
Barcelona, Spain

Michael R. Schwartz, MD
Board Certified Plastic Surgeon
Private Practice
Westlake Village, CA, USA

Stephen F. Sener, MD
Professor of Surgery, Clinical Scholar
Chief of Breast, Endocrine, and Soft Tissue
Surgery
Department of Surgery, Keck School of
Medicine of USC
Chief of Surgery and Associate Medical Director
Perioperative Services
LAC+USC (LA County) Hospital
Los Angeles, CA, USA

Joseph M. Serletti, MD, FACS
The Henry Royster–William Maul Measey
Professor of Surgery and Chief
Division of Plastic Surgery
University of Pennsylvania Health System
Philadelphia, PA, USA

Deana S. Shenaq, MD
Chief Resident
Department of Surgery - Plastic Surgery
The University of Chicago Hospitals
Chicago, IL, USA

Kenneth C. Shestak, MD
Professor, Department of Plastic Surgery
University of Pittsburgh Medical Center
Pittsburgh, PA, USA

Ron B. Somogyi, MD MSc FRCSC
Plastic and Reconstructive Surgeon
Assistant Professor, Department of Surgery
University of Toronto
Toronto, ON, Canada

David H. Song, MD, MBA, FACS
Regional Chief, MedStar Health
Plastic and Reconstructive Surgery
Professor and Chairman
Department of Plastic Surgery
Georgetown University School of Medicine
Washington, DC, USA

The late Scott L. Spear†, MD
Formerly Professor of Plastic Surgery
Division of Plastic Surgery
Georgetown University
Washington, MD, USA

Michelle A. Spring, MD, FACS
Program Director
Glacier View Plastic Surgery
Kalispell Regional Medical Center
Kalispell, MT, USA

W. Grant Stevens, MD, FACS
Clinical Professor of Surgery
Marina Plastic Surgery Associates;
Keck School of Medicine of USC
Los Angeles, CA, USA

Elizabeth Stirling Craig, MD
Plastic Surgeon and Assistant Professor
Department of Plastic Surgery
University of Texas
MD Anderson Cancer Center
Houston, TX, USA

Simon G. Talbot, MD
Assistant Professor of Surgery
Brigham and Women's Hospital
Harvard Medical School
Boston, MA, USA

Jana Van Thielen, MD
Plastic Surgery Department
Brussels University Hospital
Vrij Universitaire Brussel (VUB)
Brussels, Belgium

Henry Wilson, MD, FACS
Attending Plastic Surgeon
Private Practice
Plastic Surgery Associates
Lynchburg, VA, USA

Kai Yuen Wong, MA, MB BChir, MRCS, FHEA, FRSPH
Specialist Registrar in Plastic Surgery
Department of Plastic and Reconstructive
Surgery
Cambridge University Hospitals NHS
Foundation Trust
Cambridge, UK

VOLUME SIX

Hee Chang Ahn, MD, PhD
Professor
Department of Plastic and Reconstructive
Surgery
Hanyang University Hospital School of Medicine
Seoul, South Korea

Nidal F. Al Deek, MD
Surgeon
Plastic and Reconstructive Surgery
Chang Gung Memorial Hospital
Taipei, Taiwan

Kodi K. Azari, MD, FACS
Reconstructive Transplantation Section Chief
Professor
Department of Orthopedic Surgery
UCLA Medical Center
Santa Monica, CA, USA

Carla Baldrighi, MD
Staff Surgeon
Pediatric Surgery Meyer Children's Hospital
Pediatric Hand and Reconstructive Microsurgery
Unit
Azienda Ospedaliera Universitaria Careggi
Florence, Italy

Gregory H. Borschel, MD, FAAP, FACS
Assistant Professor
University of Toronto Division of Plastic and
Reconstructive Surgery;
Assistant Professor
Institute of Biomaterials and Biomedical
Engineering;
Associate Scientist
The SickKids Research Institute
The Hospital for Sick Children
Toronto, Ontario, Canada

Kirsty Usher Boyd, MD, FRCSC
Assistant Professor
Division of Plastic Surgery, University of Ottawa
Ottawa, Ontario, Canada

Gerald Brandacher, MD
Scientific Director
Department of Plastic and Reconstructive
Surgery
Johns Hopkins University School of Medicine
Baltimore, MD, USA

Lesley Butler, MPH
Clinical Research Coordinator
Charles E. Seay, Jr. Hand Center
Texas Scottish Rite Hospital for Children
Dallas, TX, USA

Ryan P. Calfee, MD
Associate Professor
Department of Orthopedic Surgery
Washington University School of Medicine
St. Louis, MO, USA

Brian T. Carlsen, MD
Associate Professor
Departments of Plastic Surgery and Orthopedic
Surgery
Mayo Clinic
Rochester, MN, USA

David W. Chang, MD
Professor
Division of Plastic and Reconstructive Surgery
The University of Chicago Medicine
Chicago, IL, USA

James Chang, MD
Johnson & Johnson Distinguished Professor
and Chief
Division of Plastic and Reconstructive Surgery
Stanford University Medical Center
Stanford, CA, USA

Robert A. Chase, MD
Holman Professor of Surgery – Emeritus
Stanford University Medical Center
Stanford, CA, USA

Alphonsus K. S. Chong, MBBS, MRCS, MMed(Orth), FAMS (Hand Surg)
Senior Consultant
Department of Hand and Reconstructive
Microsurgery
National University Health System
Singapore;
Assistant Professor
Department of Orthopedic Surgery
Yong Loo Lin School of Medicine
National University of Singapore
Singapore

David Chwei-Chin Chuang, MD
Senior Consultant, Ex-President, Professor
Department of Plastic Surgery
Chang Gung University Hospital
Tao-Yuan, Taiwan

Kevin C. Chung, MD, MS
Chief of Hand Surgery
Michigan Medicine
Charles B G De Nancrede Professor, Assistant
Dean for Faculty Affairs
University of Michigan Medical School
Ann Arbor, Michigan, USA

Christopher Cox, MD
Attending Surgeon
Kaiser Permanente
Walnut Creek, CA, USA

Catherine Curtin, MD
Associate Professor
Department of Surgery Division of Plastic
Surgery
Stanford University
Stanford, CA, USA

Lars B. Dahlin, MD, PhD
Professor and Consultant
Department of Clinical Sciences, Malmö – Hand
Surgery
University of Lund
Malmö, Sweden

Kenneth W. Donohue, MD
Hand Surgery Fellow
Division of Plastic Surgery
Department of Orthopedic Surgery
Baylor College of Medicine
Houston, TX, USA

Gregory A. Dumanian, MD, FACS
Stuteville Professor of Surgery
Division of Plastic Surgery
Northwestern Feinberg School of Medicine
Chicago, IL, USA

William W. Dzwierzynski, MD
Professor and Program Director
Department of Plastic Surgery
Medical College of Wisconsin
Milwaukee, WI, USA

Simon Farnebo, MD, PhD
Associate Professor and Consultant Hand
Surgeon
Department of Plastic Surgery, Hand Surgery
and Burns
Institution of Clinical and Experimental
Medicine, University of Linköping
Linköping, Sweden

Ida K. Fox, MD
Assistant Professor of Plastic Surgery
Department of Surgery
Division of Plastic and Reconstructive Surgery
Washington University School of Medicine
St. Louis, MO, USA

Paige M. Fox, MD, PhD
Assistant Professor
Department of Surgery, Division of Plastic and
Reconstructive Surgery
Stanford University Medical Center
Stanford, CA, USA

Jeffrey B. Friedrich, MD
Professor of Surgery and Orthopedics
Department of Surgery, Division of Plastic
Surgery
University of Washington
Seattle, WA, USA

Steven C. Haase, MD, FACS
Associate Professor
Department of Surgery, Section of Plastic
Surgery
University of Michigan Health
Ann Arbor, MI, USA

Elisabet Hagert, MD, PhD
Associate Professor
Department of Clinical Science and Education
Karolinska Institute;
Chief Hand Surgeon
Hand Foot Surgery Center
Stockholm, Sweden

Warren C. Hammert, MD
Professor of Orthopedic and Plastic Surgery
Chief, Division of Hand Surgery
Department of Orthopedics and Rehabilitation
University of Rochester
Rochester, NY, USA

Isaac Harvey, MD
Clinical Fellow
Department of Pediatric Plastic and
Reconstructive Surgery
Hospital for SickKids
Toronto, Ontario, Canada

Vincent R. Hentz, MD
Emeritus Professor of Surgery and Orthopedic
Surgery (by courtesy)
Stanford University
Stanford, CA, USA

Jonay Hill, MD
Clinical Assistant Professor
Anesthesiology, Perioperative and Pain Medicine
Stanford University School of Medicine
Stanford, CA, USA

Steven E. R. Hovius, MD, PhD
Former Head, Department of Plastic,
Reconstructive and Hand Surgery
Erasmus MC
University Medical Center
Rotterdam, the Netherlands;
Xpert Clinic, Hand and Wrist Center
The Netherlands

Jerry I. Huang, MD
Associate Professor
Department of Orthopedics and Sports
Medicine
University of Washington;
Program Director
University of Washington Hand Fellowship
University of Washington
Seattle, WA, USA

Marco Innocenti, MD
Associate Professor of Plastic Surgery,
University of Florence;
Director, Reconstructive Microsurgery
Department of Oncology
Careggi University Hospital
Florence, Italy

Neil F. Jones, MD, FRCS
Professor and Chief of Hand Surgery
University of California Medical Center;
Professor of Orthopedic Surgery;
Professor of Plastic and Reconstructive Surgery
University of California Irvine
Irvine, CA, USA

Ryosuke Kakinoki, MD, PhD
Professor of Hand Surgery and Microsurgery,
Reconstructive, and Orthopedic Surgery
Department of Orthopedic Surgery
Faculty of Medicine
Kindai University
Osakasayama, Osaka, Japan

Jason R. Kang, MD
Chief Resident
Department of Orthopedic Surgery
Stanford Hospital & Clinics
Redwood City, CA, USA

Joseph S. Khouri, MD
Resident
Division of Plastic Surgery, Department of
Surgery
University of Rochester
Rochester, NY, USA

Todd Kuiken, MD, PhD
Professor
Departments of PM&R, BME, and Surgery
Northwestern University;
Director, Neural Engineering Center for Artificial
Limbs
Rehabilitation Institute of Chicago
Chicago, IL, USA

Donald Lalonde, BSC, MD, MSc, FRCSC
Professor of Surgery
Division of Plastic and Reconstructive Surgery
Saint John Campus of Dalhousie University
Saint John, New Brunswick, Canada

W. P. Andrew Lee, MD
The Milton T. Edgerton MD, Professor and
Chairman
Department of Plastic and Reconstructive
Surgery
Johns Hopkins University School of Medicine
Baltimore, MD, USA

Anais Legrand, MD
Postdoctoral Research Fellow
Plastic and Reconstructive Surgery
Stanford University Medical Center
Stanford, CA, USA

Terry Light, MD
Professor
Department of Orthopedic Surgery
Loyola University Medical Center
Maywood, IL, USA

Jin Xi Lim, MBBS, MRCS
Senior Resident
Department of Hand and Reconstructive
Microsurgery
National University Health System
Singapore

Joseph Lopez, MD, MBA
Resident, Plastic and Reconstructive Surgery
Department of Plastic and Reconstructive
Surgery
Johns Hopkins University School of Medicine
Baltimore, MD, USA

Susan E. Mackinnon, MD
Sydney M. Shoenberg, Jr. and Robert H.
Shoenberg Professor
Department of Surgery, Division of Plastic and
Reconstructive Surgery
Washington University School of Medicine
St. Louis, MO, USA

Brian Mailey, MD
Assistant Professor of Surgery
Institute for Plastic Surgery
Southern Illinois University
Springfield, IL, USA

Steven J. McCabe, MD, MSc, FRCS(C)
Director of Hand and Upper Extremity Program
University of Toronto
Toronto Western Hospital
Toronto, Ontario, Canada

Kai Megerle, MD, PhD
Assistant Professor
Clinic for Plastic Surgery and Hand Surgery
Technical University of Munich
Munich, Germany

Amy M. Moore, MD
Assistant Professor of Surgery
Division of Plastic and Reconstructive Surgery
Department of Surgery
Washington University School of Medicine
St. Louis, MO, USA

Steven L. Moran, MD
Professor and Chair of Plastic Surgery
Division of Plastic Surgery, Division of Hand and
Microsurgery;
Professor of Orthopedics
Rochester, MN, USA

Rebecca L. Neiduski, PhD, OTR/L, CHT
Dean of the School of Health Sciences
Professor of Health Sciences
Elon University
Elon, NC, USA

David T. Netscher, MD
Program Director, Hand Surgery Fellowship;
Clinical Professor, Division of Plastic Surgery
and Department of Orthopedic Surgery
Baylor College of Medicine;
Adjunct Professor of Clinical Surgery (Plastic
Surgery)
Weill Medical College
Cornell University
Houston, TX, USA

Michael W. Neumeister, MD
Professor and Chairman
Division of Plastic Surgery
Springfield Illinois University School of Medicine
Springfield, IL, USA

Shelley Noland, MD
Assistant Professor
Division of Plastic Surgery
Mayo Clinic Arizona
Phoenix, AZ, USA

Christine B. Novak, PT, PhD
Associate Professor
Department of Surgery, Division of Plastic and
Reconstructive Surgery
University of Toronto
Toronto, Ontario, Canada

Scott Oates, MD
Deputy Department Chair;
Professor
Department of Plastic Surgery, Division of
Surgery
The University of Texas MD Anderson Cancer
Center
Houston, TX, USA

Kerby Oberg, MD, PhD
Associate Professor
Department of Pathology and Human Anatomy
Loma Linda University School of Medicine
Loma Linda, CA, USA

Scott Oishi, MD
Director, Charles E. Seay, Jr. Hand Center
Texas Scottish Rite Hospital for Children;
Professor, Department of Plastic Surgery and
Department of Orthopedic Surgery
University of Texas Southwestern Medical Center
Dallas, TX, USA

William C. Pederson, MD, FACS
President and Fellowship Director
The Hand Center of San Antonio;
Adjunct Professor of Surgery
The University of Texas Health Science Center at
San Antonio
San Antonio, TX, USA

Dang T. Pham, MD
General Surgery Resident
Department of Surgery
Houston Methodist Hospital
Houston, TX, USA

Karl-Josef Prommersberger, MD, PhD
Chair, Professor of Orthopedic Surgery
Clinic for Hand Surgery
Bad Neustadt/Saale, Germany

Carina Reinholdt, MD, PhD
Senior Consultant in Hand Surgery
Center for Advanced Reconstruction of
Extremities
Sahlgrenska University Hospital/ Mölndal
Mölndal, Sweden;
Assistant Professor
Department of Orthopedics
Institute for Clinical Sciences
Sahlgrenska Academy
Goteborg, Sweden

Justin M. Sacks, MD, MBA, FACS
Director, Oncological Reconstruction;
Assistant Professor
Department of Plastic and Reconstructive
Surgery
Johns Hopkins School of Medicine
Baltimore, MD, USA

Douglas M. Sammer, MD
Associate Professor of Plastic and Orthopedic
Surgery
Chief of Plastic Surgery at Parkland Memorial
Hospital
Program Director Hand Surgery Fellowship
University of Texas Southwestern Medical Center
Dallas, TX, USA

Subhro K. Sen, MD
Clinical Associate Professor
Plastic and Reconstructive Surgery
Robert A. Chase Hand and Upper Limb Center
Stanford University School of Medicine
Stanford, CA, USA

**Pundrique R. Sharma, MBBS, PhD and
FRCS (Plast)**
Consultant Plastic Surgeon
Department for Plastic and Reconstructive
Surgery
Alder Hey Children's Hospital
Liverpool, UK

Randolph Sherman, MD, FACS
Vice Chair
Department of Surgery
Cedars-Sinai Medical Center
Los Angeles, CA, USA

Jaimie T. Shores, MD
Clinical Director, Hand/Arm Transplant Program
Department of Plastic and Reconstructive
Surgery
Johns Hopkins University School of Medicine
Baltimore, MD, USA

Vanila M. Singh, MD, MACM
Clinical Associate Professor
Anesthesiology, Perioperative and Pain Medicine
Stanford University School of Medicine
Stanford, CA, USA

Jason M. Souza, MD, LCDR, MC, USN
Staff Plastic Surgeon, United States Navy
Walter Reed National Military Medical Center
Bethesda, MD, USA

Amir Taghinia, MD, MPH
Attending Surgeon
Department of Plastic and Oral Surgery
Boston Children's Hospital;
Assistant Professor of Surgery
Harvard Medical School
Boston, MA, USA

David M. K. Tan, MBBS
Senior Consultant
Department of Hand and Reconstructive
Microsurgery
National University Health System
Singapore;
Assistant Professor
Department of Orthopedic Surgery
Yong Loo Lin School of Medicine
National University Singapore
Singapore

Jin Bo Tang, MD
Professor and Chair
Department of Hand Surgery;
Chair, The Hand Surgery Research Center
Affiliated Hospital of Nantong University
Nantong, The People's Republic of China

Johan Thorfinn, MD, PhD
Senior Consultant of Plastic Surgery, Burn Unit;
Co-Director
Department of Plastic Surgery, Hand Surgery
and Burns
Linköping University Hospital
Linköping, Sweden

Michael Tonkin, MBBS, MD, FRACS(Orth), FRCS(Ed Orth)
Professor of Hand Surgery
Department of Hand Surgery and Peripheral
Nerve Surgery
Royal North Shore Hospital
The Children's Hospital at Westmead
University of Sydney Medical School
Sydney, New South Wales, Australia

Joseph Upton III, MD
Staff Surgeon
Department of Plastic and Oral Surgery
Boston Children's Hospital;
Professor of Surgery
Harvard Medical School
Boston, MA, USA

Francisco Valero-Cuevas, PhD
Director
Brain-Body Dynamics Laboratory;
Professor of Biomedical Engineering;
Professor of Biokinesiology and Physical
Therapy;
(By courtesy) Professor of Computer Science
and Aerospace and Mechanical Engineering
The University of Southern California
Los Angeles, CA, USA

Christianne A. van Nieuwenhoven, MD, PhD
Plastic Surgeon/Hand Surgeon
Plastic and Reconstructive Surgery
Erasmus Medical Centre
Rotterdam, the Netherlands

Nicholas B. Vedder, MD
Professor of Surgery and Orthopedics
Chief of Plastic Surgery Vice Chair
Department of Surgery
University of Washington
Seattle, WA, USA

Andrew J. Watt, MD
Attending Hand and Microvascular Surgeon;
Associate Program Director, Buncke Clinic Hand
and Microsurgery Fellowship;
Adjunct Clinical Faculty, Stanford University
Division of Plastic and Reconstructive Surgery
The Buncke Clinic
San Francisco, CA, USA

Fu-Chan Wei, MD
Professor
Department of Plastic Surgery
Chang Gung Memorial Hospital
Taoyuan, Taiwan

Julie Colantoni Woodside, MD
Orthopedic Surgeon
OrthoCarolina
Gastonia, NC, USA

Jeffrey Yao, MD
Associate Professor
Department of Orthopedic Surgery
Stanford Hospital & Clinics
Redwood City, CA, USA

Acknowledgments

My wife, Gabrielle Kane, has always been my rock. She not only encourages me in my work but gives constructive criticism bolstered by her medical expertise as well as by her knowledge and training in education. I can never repay her. The editorial team at Elsevier have made this series possible. Belinda Kuhn leads the group of Alexandra Mortimer, Louise Cook, and the newest addition to the team, Sam Crowe. The Elsevier production team has also been vital in moving this project along. The volume editors, Geoff Gurtner, Peter Rubin, Ed Rodriguez, Joe Losee, David Song, Mo Nahabedian, Jim Chang, and Dan Liu have shaped and refined this edition, making vital changes to keep the series relevant and up-to-date. My colleagues in the University of Washington, headed by Nick Vedder, have provided continued encouragement and support. Finally, and most importantly, the residents and fellows who pass through our program keep us on our toes and ensure that we give them the best possible solutions to their questions.

Peter C. Neligan, MB, FRCS(I), FRCSC, FACS

The current edition of the Breast volume represents a complete, thorough and up-to-date body of knowledge as it relates to all aspects of aesthetic and reconstructive surgery of the breast. I have invited academic and private practice thought leaders and experts in breast surgery from around the globe to share their knowledge and expertise that will undoubtedly serve as a valuable resource for all surgeons. I would like to thank every one of them for their hard work, time, and diligence in preparing these chapters.

There are several individuals that I would like to personally acknowledge. Dr. Scott Spear has been my greatest mentor and friend, whose inspiration and teaching has guided me for the past 12 years at Georgetown University. His untimely and unexpected passing on March 16, 2017 is a loss to our specialty and all that knew him. I would also like to thank the 66 chief residents and all the students that I have had the privilege to mentor and train over the past 22 years. They have challenged and inspired me with their ideas, innovations, and brilliance. Finally, none of this would have been possible without the love and support of my wife and two daughters: Anissa, Danielle, and Sophia Nahabedian who have enabled me to realize the importance of family and to prioritize wisely.

Maurice Nahabedian, MD

Dedicated to future plastic surgeons. Take up the torch and lead us forward!

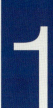

Breast anatomy for plastic surgeons

John V. Larson, Maria E. Nelson, Stephen F. Sener and Ketan M. Patel

SYNOPSIS

- Size, shape, symmetry, proportionality, and location of the breast on the chest wall all impact the attractiveness of the breast.
- Breast shape is dependent on numerous factors, including fat and glandular content, skin and connective tissue compliment, and muscular and skeletal shape.
- Knowledge of the anatomy of the breast and its associated structures, as well as careful surgical technique, is extremely important in minimizing operative complications and achieving successful patient outcomes.

Introduction

Comprehensive knowledge of breast anatomy enables safe and effective performance of the many aesthetic and reconstructive breast procedures. Augmentation mammoplasty, reduction mammoplasty, mastopexy, as well as post-mastectomy reconstruction all require a thorough understanding of normal as well as pathologic anatomy. Vascular and soft-tissue anatomy may allow for the execution of procedures with greater reliability and predictability in outcomes, and minimize the occurrence of complications.

Embryology and breast development

Understanding the development of the chest wall and breast allows for a better understanding of disease processes, natural changes to the breast, and the superficial manifestations of chest wall abnormalities. Starting in the fourth week of gestation, ectoderm and underlying mesoderm begin the process of proliferating and differentiating into skin. It is during this time that the glandular component of the breast also begins to differentiate. Paired ectodermal thickenings, termed mammary ridges, develop on the ventral surface of the embryo, extend from the axilla to the groin, and later disappear except at the level of the fourth intercostal space on the anterolateral chest wall (Fig. 1.1). The mammary ridge begins proliferating into a primary mammary bud, which then propagates downward into the underlying dermis and begins to branch, resulting in secondary buds which eventually develop into the mammary lobules. As these buds continue lengthening and branching, small lumina develop within the buds forming the lactiferous ducts. At term, approximately 20 lobes of glandular tissue have formed, each containing a lactiferous duct. While the inward proliferation of ectoderm results in mammary glands, the mesoderm surrounding this area also proliferates, creating the circular and longitudinally oriented smooth muscle fibers of the nipple. Finally, the surrounding areola is formed by ectoderm.

The female breast undergoes several age-related anatomic and physiologic changes (Fig. 1.2). As previously stated, the glandular tissue of the breast is organized into approximately 20 major lobes, each made up of lobules that contain milk-producing acini. Following a brief period of activity shortly after birth in response to maternal prolactin production, breast development is quiescent until puberty, with ducts and stromal structures enlarging in proportion to body size but no lobular development occurring. During puberty, rapid growth of the breast is primarily due to deposition of fat and connective tissue, although some growth of the ductal

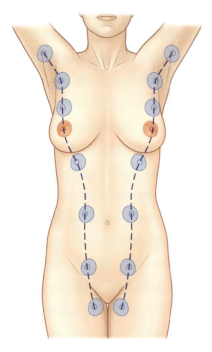

Fig. 1.1 The milk lines. *(Reproduced with permission from Standring S (ed). Gray's Anatomy, 40th edn. London: Churchill Livingston; 2008.)*

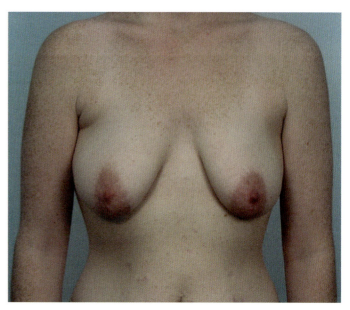

Fig. 1.3 Clinical example of a patient with moderate ptosis. The nipple areolar complex is below the level of the inframammary fold at the lower aspect of the breast.

Breast dimensions and architecture

system also occurs. Generally, parenchymal growth has extended to its mature borders by age fourteen and is complete by age twenty. During pregnancy, the glandular component completes differentiation and reaches functional maturity with the formation of secretory alveoli. During lactation, this alveolar epithelium is stimulated by maternal hormones to produce milk. As the woman ages, however, glandular tissue begins to atrophy. The breast lobules involute, with a reduction in the number and size of acini per lobule.[1,2] Over time, the glandular elements of the breast are progressively replaced with fat and connective tissue. This increased fatty tissue accumulation coupled with the attenuation of fascial support results in a softer consistency to the breast and progressive ptosis with age (Fig. 1.3).

The appearance of the breast is a crucial aspect defining the female form. While size, shape, symmetry, proportionality, and location of the breast on the chest wall all impact the attractiveness of the breast, it is important to understand that the appearance of the ideal breast is fairly subjective. Each patient will have their own views pertaining to the appearance of their breasts, which should be given consideration when planning any operative intervention.

Breast shape is dependent on numerous factors, including fat and glandular content, skin and connective tissue compliment, and muscular and skeletal shape (Fig. 1.4). The borders of the breast include the clavicle superiorly, the inframammary fold inferiorly, the sternum medially, and the anterior border of the latissimus dorsi laterally. The breast tissue that extends

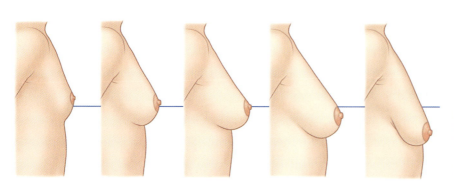

Fig. 1.2 Stages in breast development. Pre- and post-pubertal development and structure of the female breast demonstrating changes in the shape and contour of the breast. *(Reproduced with permission from Standring S (ed). Gray's Anatomy, 40th edn. London: Churchill Livingston; 2008.)*

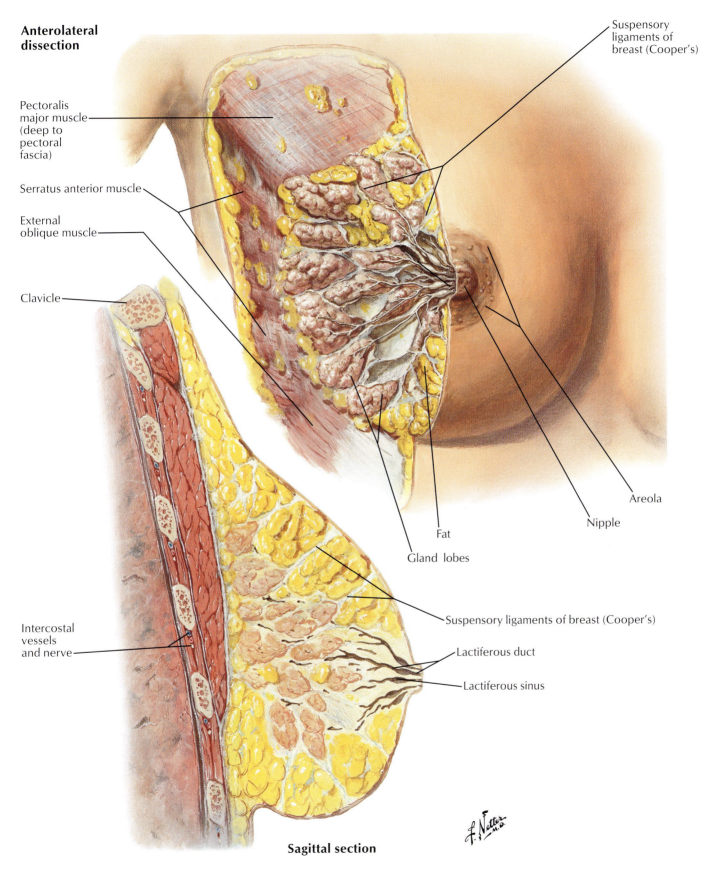

Anterolateral dissection

Pectoralis major muscle (deep to pectoral fascia)

Serratus anterior muscle

External oblique muscle

Clavicle

Intercostal vessels and nerve

Suspensory ligaments of breast (Cooper's)

Areola

Nipple

Fat

Gland lobes

Suspensory ligaments of breast (Cooper's)

Lactiferous duct

Lactiferous sinus

Sagittal section

Fig. 1.4 Structure of the breast. *(© Elsevier Inc. All Rights Reserved.)*

laterally through the axillary fascia into the axillary fat pad is referred to as the "tail of Spence". Important landmarks of the breast include the upper pole of the breast, location of the nipple areolar complex, inframammary fold, and lateral breast fold. In the nonptotic breast, the breast mound is situated over the pectoralis major muscle between the second and sixth ribs.[3] The upper pole of the breast extends from just below the clavicle to the level of the nipple. The contour should be neither concave nor convex, but a plane that extends out to the point of maximum projection of the breast at the level of the nipple. In the ideal breast form, the nipple areolar complex should be located above the level of the inframammary fold. The inframammary fold is a defining feature in the shape of the female breast, and an extremely important landmark in breast surgery. However, the anatomy and tissue components of the inframammary fold remain controversial. Some authors have suggested that the inframammary fold is produced by a supporting ligament running between the dermis in the fold region to a variety of locations on the ribcage or pectoral fascia.[4-6] Others have reported that there is no evidence of any ligamentous structure, but instead describe the fold as an intrinsic dermal structure consisting of arrangements of collagen.[7] Alternatively, other authors describe the fold as different configurations of deep fascia being fused with superficial fascia, or the superficial fascial layer inserting into the dermis.[8]

Statistical standards for breast dimensions have been reported by various authors[9-15] (Fig. 1.5). The distance from the sternal notch to the nipple is 19–21 cm. The distance from the midclavicular line to the nipple is also 19–21 cm. The distance from nipple to the inframammary fold is 5–7 cm. The distance from the nipple to the midline is 9–11 cm. Although these measurements are useful as guidelines for modifying the breast, they must be individualized for each patient based on size, shape, proportionality, differences in chest wall anatomy, and patient preference.

Blood supply

The breast has a rich and redundant vascular supply from multiple arterial sources (Fig. 1.6). Blood supply to the skin is robust, supplied by the subdermal plexus which communicates through perforators with the deeper vessels supplying the breast parenchyma. This collateralization provides redundant vascular supply to the overlying skin. The breast parenchyma is supplied by the internal mammary artery perforators, lateral thoracic artery, anterolateral and anteromedial intercostal perforators, and the thoracoacromial artery (Figs. 1.7–1.9).[16,17] The redundancy in arterial supply allows for the safe division of breast tissue as long as one or more of the vascular axes are preserved, allowing for breast parenchymal flaps to be based on any of the various vascular pedicles.

The internal mammary artery, or internal thoracic artery, is a paired artery which after arising from the subclavian artery courses along each side of the sternum. The internal mammary perforators branch from the internal mammary artery and enter the superior medial portion of the breast via the second through sixth intercostal spaces, and provide approximately 60% of the vascular supply for the breast. The second and third perforators are the largest caliber of these perforating vessels and are the preferred recipient vessels for free tissue reconstruction using the internal mammary perforators.[18,19] The lateral thoracic artery, or external mammary artery, supplies the superolateral aspect of the breast. This vessel is a primary branch of the axillary artery and enters the breast after following the lower border of the pectoralis minor muscle and passing around the lateral border of the pectoralis major muscle. The lateral aspect of the breast is supplied by perforators from the anterolateral intercostal arteries. These vessels perforate the serratus anterior just lateral to the pectoral border and enter the breast at the anterior margin of the latissimus dorsi muscle. The inferior central aspect of the breast is supplied by anteromedial intercostal perforators. After the anterior intercostal arteries branch from the internal thoracic artery, anteromedial intercostal perforators pass from deep to superficial to supply the breast parenchyma and nipple areolar complex. Finally, the thoracoacromial artery

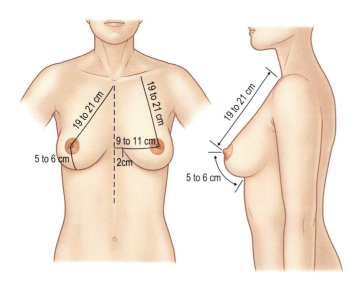

Fig. 1.5 Statistical standards for the dimensions of the breast.

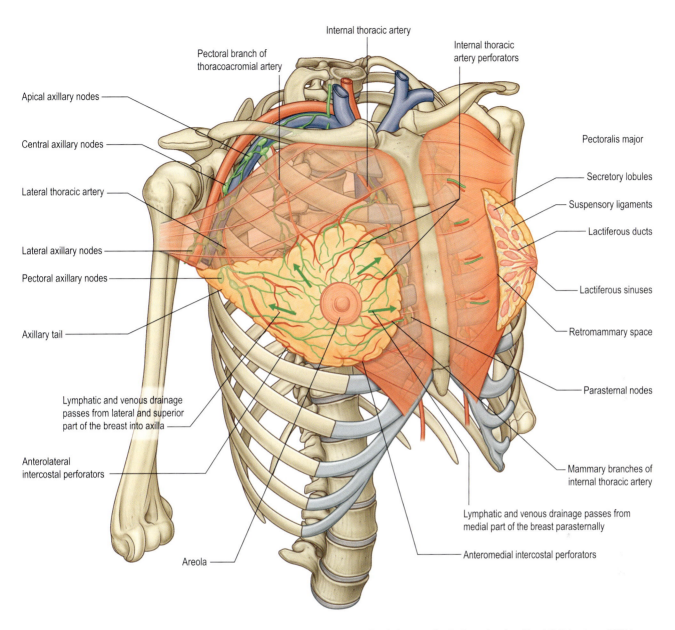

Fig. 1.6 The relations of the breast. *(Reproduced with permission from Drake R, et al. Gray's Anatomy for Students. London: Churchill Livingstone; 2005.)*

arises from the axillary artery and divides into a pectoral branch, which descends between the pectoralis minor and major muscles. This artery supplies the superior aspect of the breast and anastomoses with the anterior intercostal branches of the internal thoracic artery and with the lateral thoracic artery.

Venous drainage of the breast is via two systems. The subdermal venous plexus above the superficial fascia represents the superficial system and anastomoses with the deep system. The deep system parallels the arterial supply, with the veins paired to their respective arteries. Venous perforators following the internal mammary perforators drain via the internal mammary vein to the brachiocephalic vein, or innominate vein. The lateral thoracic veins drain via the axillary vein into the superior vena cava.

Innervation

Sensory innervation to the breast includes the anterolateral and anteromedial branches of thoracic intercostal nerves, as well as the cervical plexus. Branches of the cervical plexus course superficially in the subcutaneous tissue and provide sensory innervation to the superior medial aspect of the breast. Anterolateral and anteromedial branches of the thoracic intercostal nerves are responsible for the majority of breast sensation, which occurs in a dermatomal pattern (Fig. 1.10). The third through sixth anterolateral intercostal nerves pass through the interdigitations of the serratus muscles to enter the lateral aspect of the breast, providing sensation to the lateral portion of the breast extending to and

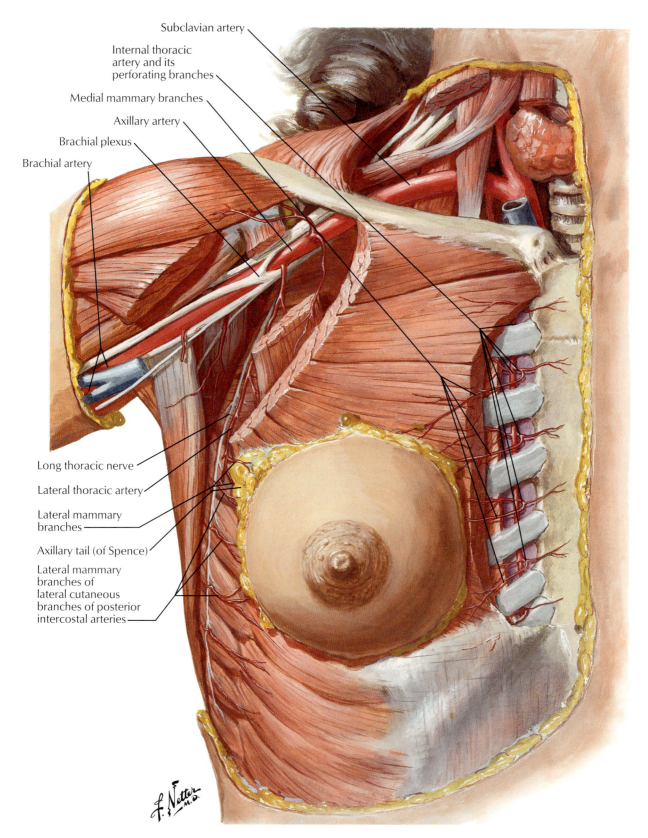

Subclavian artery

Internal thoracic artery and its perforating branches

Medial mammary branches

Axillary artery

Brachial plexus

Brachial artery

Long thoracic nerve

Lateral thoracic artery

Lateral mammary branches

Axillary tail (of Spence)

Lateral mammary branches of lateral cutaneous branches of posterior intercostal arteries

Fig. 1.7 Blood supply to the breast. *(© Elsevier Inc. All Rights Reserved.)*

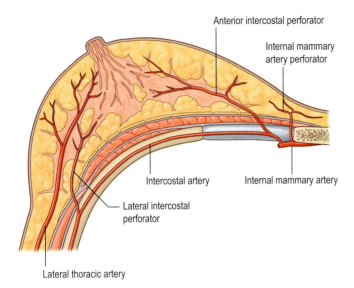

Fig. 1.8 Blood supply to the breast: cross-sectional view.

including the nipple areolar complex. Likewise, the second through sixth anteromedial intercostal nerves enter the medial aspect of the breast parenchyma alongside the internal mammary perforating vessels, providing innervation to the medial breast and nipple areolar complex.[20,21]

Nipple areolar complex

The nipple areolar complex is the focal point of the breast, normally located at the prominence of the breast mound. The nipple itself is covered by keratinizing

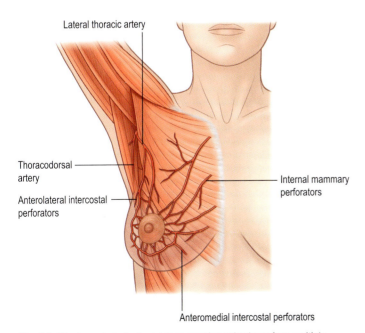

Fig. 1.9 Blood supply to the breast demonstrating redundancy from multiple arterial sources.

stratified squamous epithelium continuous with that overlying the skin of the breast, and may project as much as 1 cm or more, with a diameter of approximately 4–7 mm (Fig. 1.11). The nipple contains many lactiferous sinus openings, each of which drains a lactiferous duct which extends from the lactiferous sinus opening on the surface of the nipple down to the parenchyma. The lining of the ducts transitions from stratified squamous epithelium on the surface of the nipple, to stratified cuboidal epithelium within the lactiferous sinuses, to simple cuboidal epithelium within the lactiferous ducts. The areola comprises the pigmented skin surrounding the nipple and is approximately 4–5 cm in diameter, although diameters outside this range commonly occur. It consists of keratinized, stratified squamous epithelium and contains lactiferous sinus openings, sebaceous glands, and Montgomery glands. Deep to the nipple and areola are smooth muscle fibers arranged in a circumferential and radial distribution, which attach to the thick connective tissue of the areola and produce nipple erection.

Achieving proper location and maintaining nipple function are crucial when performing breast surgery. Pedicles employed during reduction mammoplasty or mastopexy, for example, are based on preservation of the blood supply to the nipple. Fortunately, the vascular supply to the nipple is robust and redundant, supplied by both the subdermal plexus as well as the previously mentioned parenchymal vessels.[22] Thus, preservation of a vascular pedicle from underlying parenchyma will maintain the viability of the nipple. Nipple sensation also must be considered. Innervation of the nipple is primarily from the lateral cutaneous branch of the fourth intercostal nerve via two branches, one which passes superficial to the gland and the other which passes through the retromammary space.[23] Contributions from the third and fifth intercostal nerves also provide some nipple sensation.

Connective tissue

Intricate fascial layers derived from the superficial fascial system support the breast tissue (Fig. 1.12). Breast parenchyma is fixed in placed by the superficial fascial system. This superficial fascial system extends cephalad from the abdomen and separates into a superficial and deep layer which envelopes the breast tissue and maintains its attachment to the breast wall.[24,25] The superficial layer of superficial fascia envelopes the glandular tissue deep to the dermal layer and can be difficult to distinguish from the dermis. However, subcutaneous adipose tissue between the dermis and the superficial layer distinguish the two layers. The deep layer of superficial

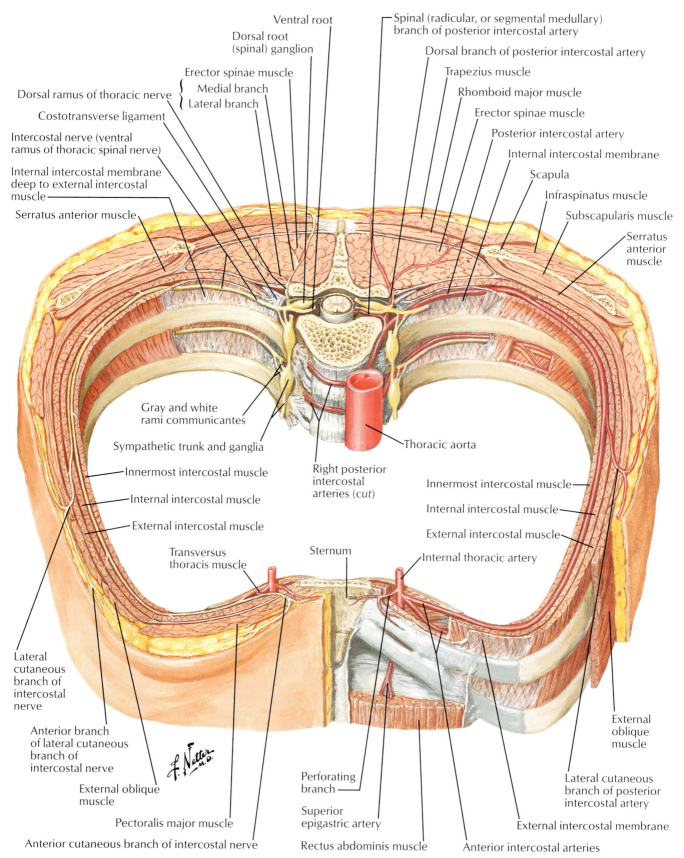

Fig. 1.10 Cross-sectional image demonstrating vasculature and sensory innervation to the breast: anterolateral and anteromedial branches of thoracic intercostal nerves.
(© Elsevier Inc. All Rights Reserved.)

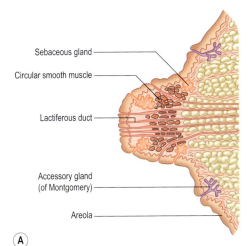

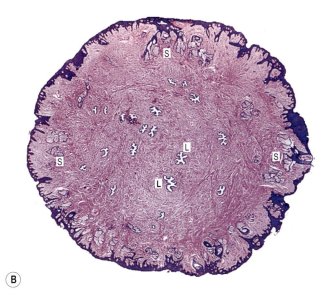

Fig. 1.11 (A) Cross-section of the nipple. **(B)** There is a layer of stratified squamous epithelium over the nipple surface; approximately 20 lactiferous ducts (L) open onto the surface; sebaceous glands (S) are deep to the epidermis. (A, reproduced with permission from Standring S (ed). Gray's Anatomy, *40th edn.* London: Churchill Livingstone; 2008; B, from Kerr JB. Atlas of Functional Histology. London: Mosby; 1999, with permission from Dr. J.B. Kerr, Monash University.)

Parenchyma

The glandular tissue of the breast functions to produce milk in the postpartum period. It consists of alveoli, the secretory units of the gland, clustered together into approximately 20 lobes separated by connective tissue and fat. These alveoli are connected by interlobular ducts which join to form approximately 20 primary lactiferous ducts. Beneath the nipple, the dilated lactiferous ducts form lactiferous sinuses which open onto the nipple areolar complex. As previously stated, the ducts are lined with cuboidal cells which transition to stratified squamous epithelium in the lactiferous sinuses. This glandular parenchyma is distributed within a significant amount of adipose tissue.[26] Although widely variable, adipose tissue generally comprises a considerable amount of the total breast volume at approximately 50–70%.[27] In most breasts, between the dermis and the breast parenchyma exists a consistent and distinct layer

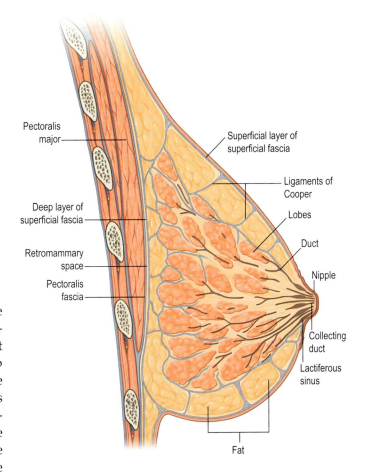

Fig. 1.12 Cross-section of the breast demonstrating the superficial fascial system, which separates into a superficial and deep layer and envelopes the breast tissue. (Reproduced with permission from Standring S (ed). Gray's Anatomy, *40th edn.* London: Churchill Livingstone; 2008.)

fascia diverges at the level of the sixth rib, where the inframammary fold is the inferior border of the parenchyma, and sits on the deep surface of the breast just superficial to the pectoralis fascia. Between the deep layer of superficial fascia and the pectoralis fascia is the retromammary space filled with loose tissue that allows the breast to move over the chest wall. Cooper's ligaments provide numerous interconnections between the deep and superficial layers. These ligaments penetrate the deep layer of superficial fascia and invest into the breast parenchyma to the superficial layer of superficial fascia. With age, the suspensory structure becomes more attenuated, resulting in progressive breast ptosis.

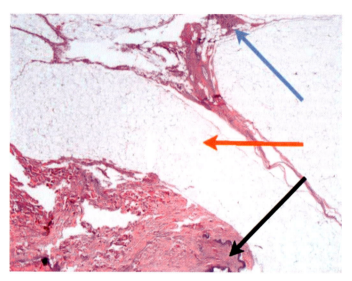

Fig. 1.13 Photomicrograph demonstrating the relationship among the epidermis (black arrow), subcutaneous tissue (red arrow), and most superficial breast lobule (blue arrow). Hematoxylin and eosin staining, 2× magnification. *(Reproduced with permission from Larson D, Basir Z, Bruce T. Is oncologic safety compatible with a predictably viable mastectomy skin flap? Plast Reconstr Surg. 2011;127:27–33.)*

By providing muscle coverage for breast implants, the pectoralis major serves an extremely important role in both aesthetic and reconstructive breast surgery. In the setting of breast reconstruction, coverage of the implant decreases the risk of implant exposure, where post-mastectomy skin and underlying subcutaneous tissues are often thin. Additionally, the muscle decreases implant palpability by providing added tissue between the implant and skin. However, subpectoral placement of the implant can cause the implant to ripple and be detected during contraction of the muscle. Releasing the pectoralis muscle from its inferior and medial attachments can serve to decrease this problem. Furthermore, inferior release of the pectoralis muscle allows lower positioning of the implant to be achieved, resulting in a more aesthetic appearance.

The pectoralis minor is a flat and fan-shaped muscle which lies between the pectoralis major and the chest wall and extends from its origin on the anterolateral surface of the third through fifth ribs to its insertion on the coracoid process of the scapula. Blood supply to the muscle is either directly from the axillary artery or as a branch from the thoracoacromial artery or lateral thoracic artery. Innervation is derived from both the medial and lateral pectoral nerves. Although not commonly utilized in breast surgery, the pectoralis minor muscle

of subcutaneous tissue with a thickness of approximately 1 cm (Fig. 1.13).[28] By identifying and preserving this layer during skin-sparing mastectomy, the oncologic surgeon can perform an oncologically safe resection while also achieving predictably viable skin flaps which contain little to no breast parenchyma. Leaving this layer of subcutaneous tissue not only maintains the viability of the skins flaps but also enhances the final reconstructive outcome by providing a uniform layer of tissue beneath the skin flaps.

Musculature

The muscles associated with the anterior chest wall include the pectoralis major, pectoralis minor, serratus anterior, rectus abdominis, and the external oblique (Fig. 1.14). While primarily attached to the pectoralis major, the breast tissue also has attachments with the serratus anterior, external oblique, and the superior portion of the rectus abdominis.

The pectoralis major muscle is a broad muscle that extends from its origin on the medial clavicle, lateral sternum, and second through sixth ribs to its insertion on the upper humerus on the lateral side of the intertubercular sulcus. The muscle acts to flex, adduct, and rotate the arm medially. It has a primary vascular supply based on the thoracoacromial artery and a secondary supply via the lateral thoracic artery, intercostal perforators, and internal mammary perforators. The muscle is innervated by the medial and lateral pectoral nerves, which enter posteriorly and laterally.

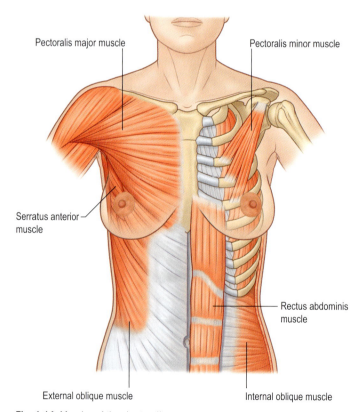

Fig. 1.14 Muscles of the chest wall.

has been used as an innervated free flap in the field of facial reanimation.[29]

The serratus anterior runs along the anterolateral chest wall, extending from its origin at the anterolateral aspect of the first through eighth ribs to its insertion on the medial aspect of the scapula. Its vascular supply is derived equally from the lateral thoracic artery, which supplies the superior part of the muscle, and branches from the thoracodorsal artery, which supplies the inferior part. The muscle is responsible for rotation of the scapula, raising the point of the shoulder and drawing the scapula inward toward the body. Innervation of the serratus anterior is provided by the long thoracic nerve. One must be careful during axillary lymph node dissection to avoid transecting this nerve, as its loss results in "winging" as the scapula moves upward and outward away from the body. Because the serratus anterior underlies the lateral aspect of the breast, blunt elevation of the pectoralis major laterally for implant placement can elevate a small portion of the serratus muscle. During breast reconstruction, complete muscle coverage of the implant often necessitates that the serratus anterior be partially elevated.

The rectus abdominis is an elongated muscle that runs from its origin at the pubic symphysis, pubic crest, and pubic tubercle to its insertion at the xiphoid process and costal cartilages of the fifth through seventh ribs. Breast tissue attaches to the superior limit of the rectus abdominis, delineating the inferior border of the breast. The function of the muscle includes compression of the abdomen and flexion of the spine. Innervation is segmental from the seventh through twelfth intercostal nerves, while blood supply to the muscle is provided by two dominant pedicles, the superior and inferior deep epigastric arteries. The superior epigastric artery, a terminal branch of the internal mammary artery, supplies the upper portion of the muscle, whereas the inferior epigastric artery runs superiorly on the posterior surface of the rectus and penetrates the rectus at the arcuate line to supply the lower portion. Additionally, many small segmental contributions are provided by the lower six intercostal arteries.

The rectus abdominis is particularly important in breast reconstruction as it relates to the transverse rectus abdominis myocutaneous (TRAM) flap, one of the most common forms of autologous tissue reconstruction to date.[30,31] With regard to implant-based reconstruction, in attempting to achieve complete coverage with muscle, the rectus fascia can be elevated to place the implant sufficiently caudal.

The external oblique muscle is a broad muscle originating from the fifth through twelfth ribs and inserting along the anterior half of the iliac crest, the pubic tubercle, and the aponeurosis of the linea alba from the xiphoid to the pubis. This muscle borders the inferolateral aspect of the breast. It acts to compress the abdomen, flex and laterally rotate the spine, and depress the ribs. Innervation to the muscle is provided by the seventh through eleventh intercostal nerves and the subcostal nerve. It receives its blood supply in a segmental fashion from the inferior eight posterior intercostal arteries. During implant-based reconstruction, the external oblique along with the rectus abdominis may be elevated to provide inferior coverage and proper placement of the implant.

Skeletal support

Breast shape and symmetry are dependent on normal skeletal support. Deformities of the chest wall such as pectus excavatum or pectus carinatum can lead to alterations in breast projection. Likewise, spinal abnormalities such as scoliosis can affect the appearance of breast symmetry.[32] Poland syndrome can lead to unilateral underdevelopment or absence of the pectoralis muscle, as well as abnormalities to the breast and nipple. While abnormalities of the underlying chest wall may be difficult to appreciate, they are extremely important to consider when evaluating the breasts during preoperative planning. Any pre-existing spinal curvature or chest wall deformities must be recognized and demonstrated to the patient, as these may become more noticeable postoperatively and affect the patient's perception of the appearance and symmetry of their breasts.

Lymphatics

The lymphatic anatomy of the breast has been extensively investigated, particularly for its role in breast cancer dissemination. Lymphatic drainage of the breast includes a network of both superficial and deep lymphatic drainage (Fig. 1.15). Superficial lymphatic drainage originates from the periareolar lymphatic plexus, while deep lymphatic drainage originates from each lactiferous duct and lobule, and then penetrates the deep fascia of the underlying musculature. The predominance of lymph drainage of the breast originates from the lymphatic vessels within the breast lobules which then flow to the subareolar plexus. From this plexus, lymphatic drainage takes place through several routes. Lymphatic drainage from the lateral and superior aspect of the breast courses around the inferior edge of the pectoralis major muscle and communicates with the pectoral group of axillary nodes. Additional lymphatics course through the pectoral muscles to the apical lymph nodes. From the axillary lymph nodes, lymph

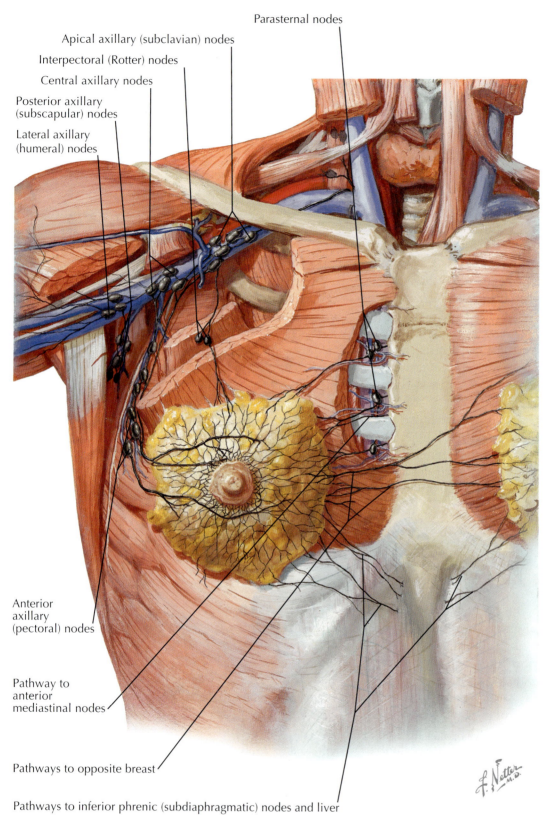

Parasternal nodes

Apical axillary (subclavian) nodes

Interpectoral (Rotter) nodes

Central axillary nodes

Posterior axillary (subscapular) nodes

Lateral axillary (humeral) nodes

Anterior axillary (pectoral) nodes

Pathway to anterior mediastinal nodes

Pathways to opposite breast

Pathways to inferior phrenic (subdiaphragmatic) nodes and liver

Fig. 1.15 Lymphatic drainage of the breast. *(© Elsevier Inc. All Rights Reserved.)*

drains into the subclavian and supraclavicular lymph nodes. Lymphatic drainage from the medial aspect of the breast drains to the parasternal nodes, which then drains into the bronchomediastinal trunks.

Considerations for the plastic surgeon

Recipient sites for free tissue transfer

The selection of suitable recipient vessels is an important requirement when free tissue transfer is used for breast reconstruction. The internal mammary arteries are very common recipient vessels. The internal mammary vessel may be preferred in delayed cases, especially in patients who have had adjuvant radiation, as dissection of axillary vessels can be very difficult. The use of the internal mammary vessels facilitates shaping the medial portion of the breast as compared to the thoracodorsal vessels. Distal to the fourth rib, the internal mammary veins become smaller (<2 mm) and bifurcate, thus making suitable outflow less predictable. Therefore, the third rib is a common level of access. The thoracodorsal vessels have been used; however, the thoracodorsal artery can be small (<2 mm) and lateralization of the flap may occur as the pedicle may be tethered toward the axilla. Use of the axillary vessels has also been reported. However, the axillary vessels may limit flap movement and shaping of the breast.

Deformities of the breast and chest wall

Pediatric chest wall and breast anomalies present as a wide spectrum of irregularities.[33] Chest wall anomalies include Poland syndrome, pectus excavatum, pectus carinatum, and various sternal anomalies. Breast abnormalities can be categorized into three groups, including hypoplastic, hyperplastic, and deformational anomalies. Hypoplastic and deformational anomalies are characterized by breast tissue paucity and include Poland syndrome, breast hypoplasia, tuberous breast, anthelia, and amastia. These anomalies often benefit from breast augmentation techniques and are frequently associated with significant reoperative rates. Hyperplastic anomalies are characterized by excess breast tissue and include gynecomastia, polymastia, polythelia, and juvenile hypertrophy. Treatment for these anomalies often requires breast reduction techniques and is less likely to require re-operation.

As previous stated, Poland syndrome is a severe form of chest wall and breast hypoplasia that includes absence of the pectoralis major and minor muscles and syndactyly of the ipsilateral hand.[33] The condition can also include absence of multiple ribs, chest wall depression, athelia, amastia, absence of the latissimus dorsi muscle, and limited subcutaneous chest wall fat. Treatment options include autologous tissue utilizing either pedicled or free latissimus dorsi or rectus abdominis musculocutaneous flaps, or implant-based reconstruction alone or in combination with autologous tissue.

Radiation changes to the breast and soft tissue

Although radiation dosimetry has improved in the past several decades, radiation injury nevertheless results in damage to the breast and soft tissue, which may lead to significant wound-healing problems during breast reconstruction.[34] Theorized mechanisms of radiation-induced injury include direct cellular damage with chromosomal alteration, and the microvascular occlusion theory. Irradiation may lead to permanent damage to fibroblasts and fibroblast stem cells, including ultrastructural damage to mitochondria, rough endoplasmic reticulum, and nuclei. It may also inhibit wound healing by preventing stem cells from replicating and providing new blood vessels in the zone of injury. The progression of radiation injury has been described as biphasic. Acute effects of irradiation occur in the first days to weeks of therapy and involve cellular death in rapidly proliferating cells. The resultant effects on breast skin include edema from leaking capillaries, inflammation, and desquamation. Delayed effects on the soft tissue of the breast may occur after several months to years, resulting in atrophy and fibrosis with replacement of the adipose tissue with collagen. During preoperative planning for breast reconstruction, communication with the radiation oncologist regarding the timing and technique of radiation are extremely important in order to minimize complications and optimize aesthetic outcomes for these patients.

Partial breast reconstruction

Due to the rising popularity of breast conservation therapy for the management of breast cancer, plastic surgeons are increasingly performing reconstruction on partial mastectomy defects. Many reconstructive techniques exist, and the decision concerning which to use depends on breast size, tumor location and size, extent and location of the resection, timing of the reconstruction in relation to radiation therapy, and patient desires.[35,36] Generally, women with defects in smaller, nonptotic breasts benefit from volume replacement techniques using local or distant flaps. Conversely, women with moderate or large-sized breasts are often amenable to reshaping procedures using local tissue rearrangement techniques, usually mastopexy or reduction techniques. As this often removes enough breast tissue and skin to change breast size and nipple position, these volume reduction procedures often require a procedure to the contralateral breast to achieve symmetry.

Role of lymphatics in mapping and biopsy of sentinel lymph nodes

The management of staging the axilla was transformed in clinically node negative early breast cancer patients with the use of sentinel lymph node biopsy (SLNB).[37] The concept of the sentinel lymph node evolved from the observation that a primary tumor is drained by an afferent lymphatic channel that courses to the first, "sentinel", lymph node in the specific regional lymphatic basin.[38] This was originally described by Morton and colleagues in the study of melanoma.[39,40] Subsequent studies by Giuliano and colleagues showed that mapping lymphatic channels with isosulfan blue dye identified the sentinel node with 100% accuracy, predicting the status of the axilla in breast cancer patients.[41,42] In addition to the isosulfan blue dye technique, there are other technical approaches for sentinel node identification, including preoperative injection of technetium sulfur colloid (Tc-99) with lymphoscintigraphy, and the combination of isosulfan blue dye and radio-isotope techniques.[43–45] Sentinel lymph node dissection is performed with injection of 3–5 mL of dye (classically isosulfan blue) and/or radiolabeled colloid into the subareolar plexus, intradermally or peritumor region. There is ongoing debate about the best site of injection.[42,46] Preoperative lymphoscintigraphy, although not mandatory, can be used to identify the sentinel lymph node and document patterns of lymphatic drainage. When injecting technetium sulfur colloid into the parenchyma surrounding the tumor, the mapping can go either to the axillary or internal mammary nodes, whereas injections performed into the periareolar dermis almost uniformly map to the axillary nodes.

Conclusion

Although breast size and shape vary among patients, knowing the anatomy of the breast facilitates safe surgical planning. When the breasts are carefully examined, significant asymmetries are revealed in most patients, which must be recognized and demonstrated to the patient, as these may be difficult to correct and can become noticeable in the postoperative period. Knowledge of the anatomy of the breast and its associated structures, as well as careful surgical technique, is extremely important in minimizing operative complications and achieving successful patient outcomes.

🌐 Access the complete reference list online at **http://www.expertconsult.com**

11. Tepper OM, Unger JG, Small KH, et al. Mammometrics: the standardization of aesthetic and reconstructive breast surgery. *Plast Reconstr Surg.* 2010;125:393–400. *This article summarizes three-dimensional breast photography and its potential for establishing a standardized method for breast analysis, in an effort to guide operative planning and better analyze surgical results.*

22. Nakajima H, Imanishi N, Aiso S. Arterial anatomy of the nipple-areola complex. *Plast Reconstr Surg.* 1995;96:843–845. *The publication examines the blood supply to the nipple-areola complex, demonstrating that branches of the external mammary artery (lateral thoracic artery) and internal mammary artery provide the dominant blood supply to the nipple-areola complex via small vessels that traverse the subcutaneous tissue.*

25. Lockwood TE. Reduction mammaplasty and mastopexy with superficial fascial system suspension. *Plast Reconstr Surg.* 1999;103:1411–1420. *This paper describes the anatomy of the superficial fascial system of the breast, and describes a technique for implementing superficial fascial system suspension during reduction mammoplasty and mastopexy.*

27. Lejour M. Evaluation of fat in breast tissue removed by vertical mammaplasty. *Plast Reconstr Surg.* 1997;99:386–393. *This publication evaluated the relative fat content versus glandular tissue of the breast by examining breast parenchyma specimens removed during reduction mammaplasty. The study found that breast fat is highly variable between patients, and increases with age, body mass, and total volume of the breast.*

28. Larson D, Basir Z, Bruce T. Is oncologic safety compatible with a predictably viable mastectomy skin flap? *Plast Reconstr Surg.* 2011;127:27–33. *This paper describes the subcutaneous tissue layer between the dermis and the parenchyma of the breast. The authors propose that by preserving the subcutaneous tissue layer during mastectomy, an oncologically safe resection can be performed while also achieving predictably viable skin flaps.*

Preoperative evaluation and consultation for breast augmentation

Michael R. Schwartz

SYNOPSIS

- Ensure thorough valuation of each patient's individual goals and expectations.
- Ensure a thorough medical history is completed with focus on the breast.
- Examination should include physical exam, 3D imaging, and implant sizing.
- Individualized systematic preoperative planning based on each patient's unique choices and examination including incision choice, pocket selection, and implant selection.

Introduction

Breast augmentation has remained one of the most popular surgical procedures performed in women in the United States. Over 285 000 procedures were performed in 2014, second only to liposuction.[1] Patients may present with either primary or secondary hypoplasia. Primary hypoplasia includes those patients with developmentally small breasts and those with some form of chest wall deformity including Poland syndrome and others. Secondary or involutional hypoplasia often occurs in the postpartum patient and may also be attributed to atrophic changes seen in extreme weight loss patients.

Discussion of the patient's goals in augmentation is an imperative part of the preoperative evaluation. There is ample evidence that inadequate breast appearance can adversely affect self-esteem and body image, and this can be improved with augmentation mammoplasty.[2] It is imperative that the patient–surgeon interaction establishes a realistic expectation within the consultative framework.

Historical perspective

The evolution of breast augmentation has been one of subjective to objective course. The simple choice of implant size has been replaced with the objective measurement and planning of a detailed and patient-specific operation. The goals of improved safety, longevity, and natural look and feel have supplanted the old standard of size enhancement alone.

In the past, the options for breast implant selection were limited to a spectrum varied only by a paralleled increase in volume and base diameter. This produced a very wide unflattering look in patients with larger implants, or devices that were essentially folded into smaller pockets with the potential for shell failure over time.

Eventually, manufacturers developed additional profiles of implants that included different base diameters for each selected volume. In other words low, moderate, high, and even ultra high projection devices (Fig. 2.1). This allowed a more individualized fit of the implant onto each patient's chest wall and led to the introduction of the concept of base diameter and dimensional planning into the vocabulary of breast surgery. Unfortunately, these advances in device design have also led to the use of overly large implants with subsequent tissue damage and atrophy, higher complication rates, and re-operation.[3]

As a parallel to the US Food and Drug Administration (FDA) demand for data in the silicone implant "crisis",

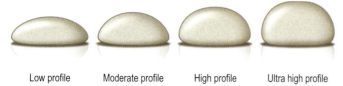

Fig. 2.1 Round implants showing different profile shapes (low profile to ultra high profile).

Low profile   Moderate profile   High profile   Ultra high profile

many critical surgeons began developing more systematic approaches to the breast augmentation process,[4–6] the goals of which include the critical analysis of objective measurements to better predict the outcome of each patient's surgical experience, and to minimize operative risk of this elective procedure. Surgeons today need to understand these varied approaches and consider how they apply to their personal technical and aesthetic principles. As always, there can be no one correct technique, but each analysis system contributes significant critical detail to the breast surgeon's ability to provide reproducibly beautiful, safe results. Important aspects of several of these will be discussed.

Finally, FDA approval of shaped and highly cohesive breast implants in the United States in 2012 and 2013 ushered in an era of additional options in both reconstructive and aesthetic breast surgery.[7] Today the breast augmentation patient has more options, increased safety, and better potential outcomes as a result of this significant advance in implant technology[8–10] (Fig. 2.2).

Consultation process

Today's electronic medical record (EMR) affords the physician the opportunity to have a very complete medical history before the patient enters the office (Fig. 2.3). The electronic documents can be customized to gather a complete breast and family history. Preoperative mammography should be obtained for patients over age 35 as per standard guidelines or at any age in patients with significant risk factors. While beyond the scope of most consultations, plastic surgeons should have a basic understanding of modern genetic testing for the breast cancer genes as this is a common question raised during the consultation.

Patients have most often spent a great deal of time on Internet research, and this is rarely accurate or productive. It is the author's strong recommendation to focus on your own information process and steer away from a long discussion on "what ifs" from less reliable sources. A key component of the initial consultation is to ascertain that the patient has realistic expectations for the procedure.

The next portion of the discussion should focus on the patient's goals. This should include not only her desired size but also the shape of her desired breast. Should it be natural or augmented in its appearance? There is certainly no consensus, but a recent paper clearly shows a majority preference toward a slightly fuller lower pole of the breast, a straight upper pole with

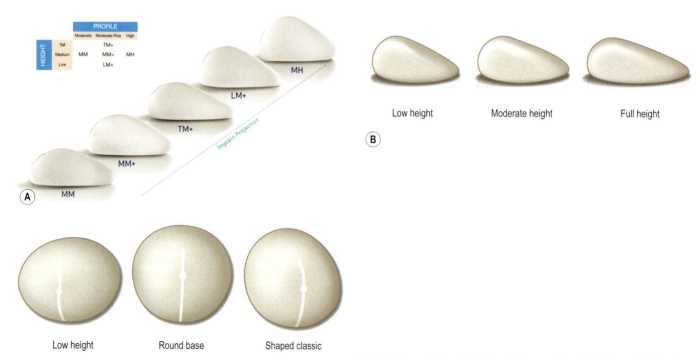

Fig. 2.2 Shaped implants. **(A)** Mentor Memory Shape. **(B)** Allergan 410 (low to full height). **(C)** Sientra HSC 2 Shaped (low height, round base, shaped classic).

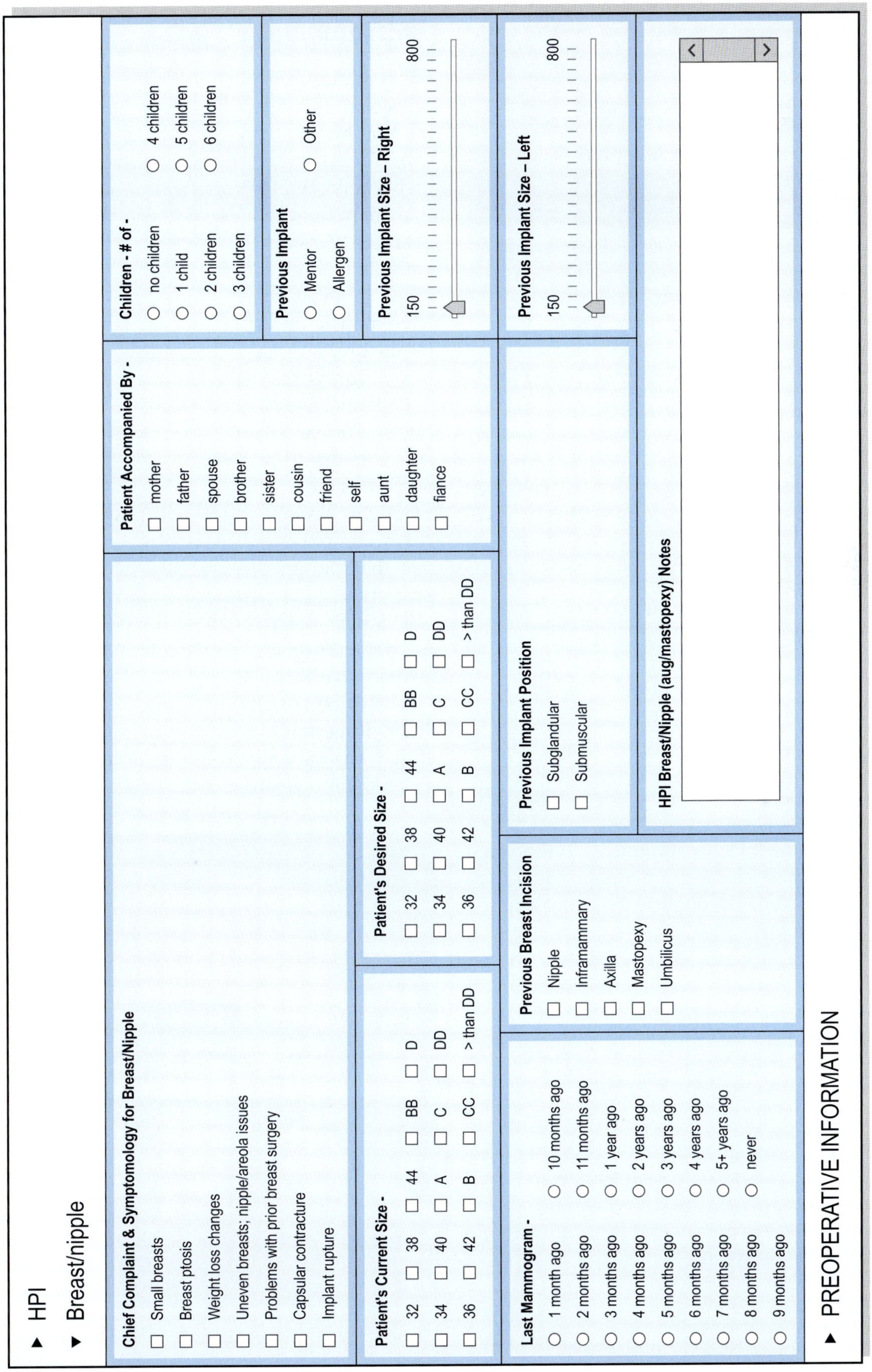

▲ HPI

▼ Breast/nipple

Chief Complaint & Symptomology for Breast/Nipple

- ☐ Small breasts
- ☐ Breast ptosis
- ☐ Weight loss changes
- ☐ Uneven breasts; nipple/areola issues
- ☐ Problems with prior breast surgery
- ☐ Capsular contracture
- ☐ Implant rupture

Patient's Current Size -

☐ 32	☐ 38	☐ 44	☐ BB	☐ D
☐ 34	☐ 40	☐ A	☐ C	☐ DD
☐ 36	☐ 42	☐ B	☐ CC	☐ > than DD

Last Mammogram -

- ○ 1 month ago   ○ 10 months ago
- ○ 2 months ago   ○ 11 months ago
- ○ 3 months ago   ○ 1 year ago
- ○ 4 months ago   ○ 2 years ago
- ○ 5 months ago   ○ 3 years ago
- ○ 6 months ago   ○ 4 years ago
- ○ 7 months ago   ○ 5+ years ago
- ○ 8 months ago   ○ never
- ○ 9 months ago

Patient Accompanied By -

- ☐ mother
- ☐ father
- ☐ spouse
- ☐ brother
- ☐ sister
- ☐ cousin
- ☐ friend
- ☐ self
- ☐ aunt
- ☐ daughter
- ☐ fiance

Patient's Desired Size -

☐ 32	☐ 38	☐ 44	☐ BB	☐ D
☐ 34	☐ 40	☐ A	☐ C	☐ DD
☐ 36	☐ 42	☐ B	☐ CC	☐ > than DD

Previous Breast Incision

- ☐ Nipple
- ☐ Inframammary
- ☐ Axilla
- ☐ Mastopexy
- ☐ Umbilicus

Previous Implant Position

- ☐ Subglandular
- ☐ Submuscular

HPI Breast/Nipple (aug/mastopexy) Notes

Children - # of -

- ○ no children   ○ 4 children
- ○ 1 child   ○ 5 children
- ○ 2 children   ○ 6 children
- ○ 3 children

Previous Implant

- ○ Mentor   ○ Other
- ○ Allergen

Previous Implant Size – Right

150   800

Previous Implant Size – Left

150   800

▲ PREOPERATIVE INFORMATION

Fig. 2.3 Example of EMR that can be customized to practice preferences.

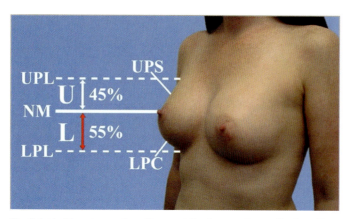

Fig. 2.4 Ideal breast proportions. Representative three-quarters profile view with standard breast parameters as used in the survey: upper pole to lower pole ratio, nipple angulation, and contour of upper and lower poles. The visible breast has an upper pole to lower pole ratio of 45:55, straight upper pole, and convex lower pole. U, upper pole; L, lower pole; UPL, upper pole line; LPL, lower pole line; NM, nipple meridian; UPS, upper pole slope; LPC, lower pole convexity. *(Reproduced with permission from Mallucci P, Branford OA. population analysis of the perfect breast: a morphometric analysis.* Plast Reconstr Surg. *2014;134:436–447.)*

a slight up-turn to the nipple at the most projecting portion[11] (Fig. 2.4).

Patient examination

Complete physical examination should include each patient's height, weight, and current bra size. Clear documentation of any chest wall and spinal deformities are essential. Documentation of asymmetry of breast size, shape, nipple position, inframammary fold (IMF) position, shoulder position, and axillary breast tissue fullness and quality are all key components. A thorough breast examination to exclude any masses or adenopathy should be completed. The quality of the breast tissue and skin should be noted (Fig. 2.5).

Multiple evaluation systems exist to guide the surgeon in the preoperative process. Key components of all include base diameter, sternal notch to nipple distance, nipple to IMF distance, intermammary distance, and upper pole skin pinch. This should be recorded accurately in the patient's chart (Fig. 2.6). Each evaluation system mentioned previously uses a differing technique to assess the elasticity and quantity of the skin envelope. This should be clearly assessed on each patient and each breast. A complete description of each evaluation system is not possible, but there are several key components that demand further discussion.

Base diameter

All the modern systems for selecting breast implants place an essential weight on respecting the patient's inherent breast base diameter; that is, the distance from the medial breast to the anterior axillary line. There is

no consensus as to what size implant in relation to the patient's starting base diameter is best. The author's preference is to select an implant that is always within 1 cm of the patient's natural base diameter. This allows for enough width to give the breast an adequate shape, but not so much that medial or lateral stretch would cause tissue damage.

For some surgeons there is truly no flexibility to exceed this measurement, and this has led to a nearly dictatorial practice of breast augmentation. They propose that violating the patient's intrinsic base diameter leads to inevitable and irreversible tissue damage with subsequent complications including implant visibility, rippling, loss of nipple sensation, and early implant malposition and ptosis. All of these lead to a significantly higher complication and re-operation rates.[3] This author agrees in principle, but as always, there are significant exceptions including the constricted breast, tubular deformity, and severe hypoplasia that require a more aggressive and individualized approach through the consultative and surgical process.

Measurement of the breast envelope

Anterior–posterior skin stretch, nipple to fold stretch, medial and lateral skin pinch, and other similar measurements are unique attempts to categorize the quality, the volume, and elasticity of each patient's breast envelope. Each surgeon needs to decide which technique

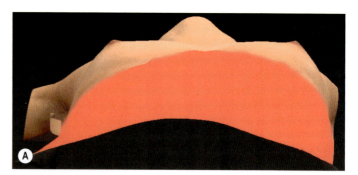

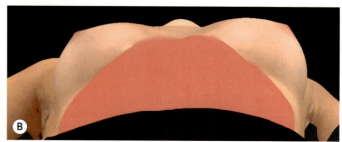

Fig. 2.5 Important differences in chest wall shape. **(A)** Flat chest wall: any implant placed in this patient is likely to remain centralized with effective volume enhancement. **(B)** Round chest wall: high profile implants will tend to fall laterally early. Textured implants may stay in position more effectively. In addition, part of the volume added effectively flattens the chest and contributes less to final volume. These patients may need additional implant size to obtain their desired result.

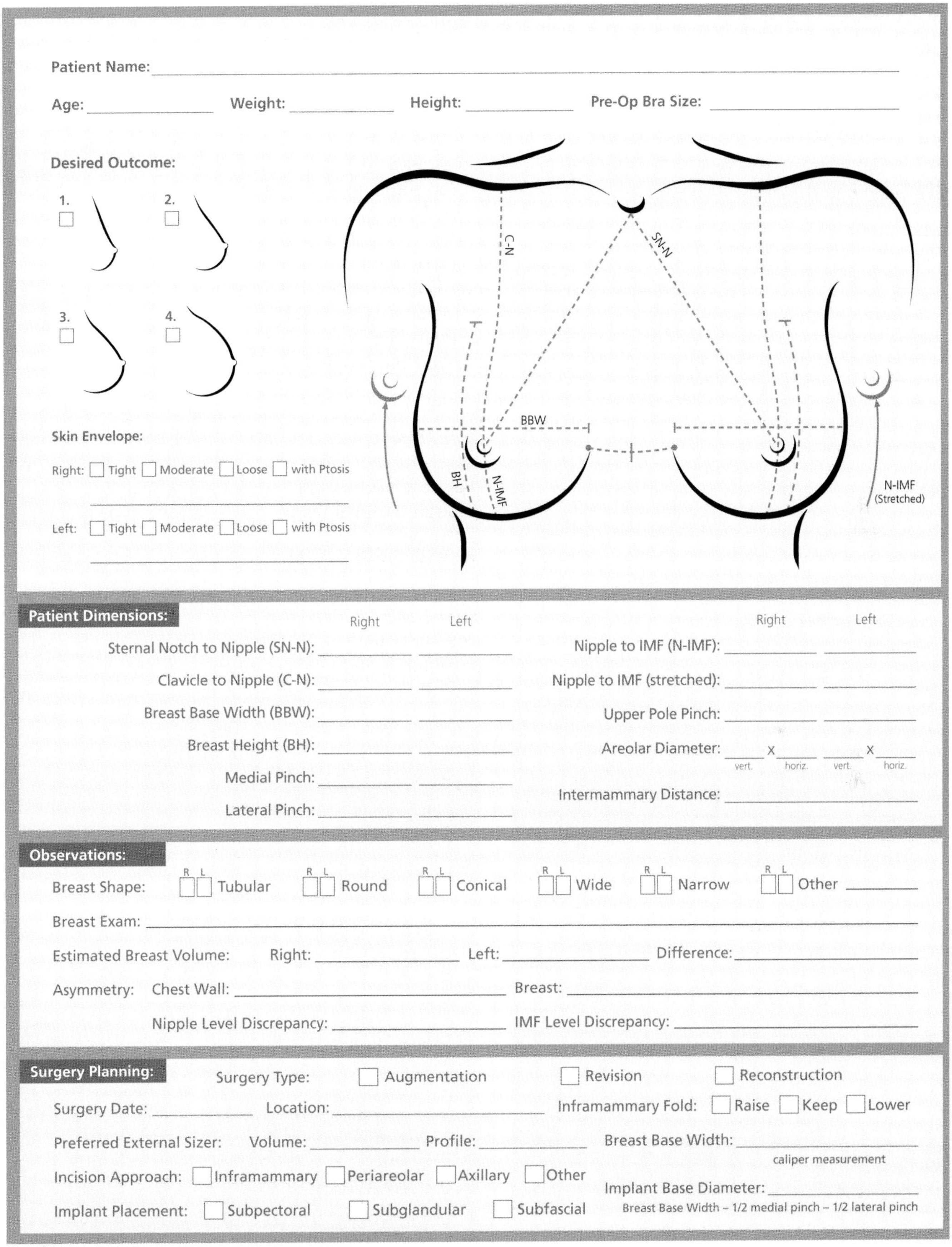

Patient Name: _____

Age: _____   Weight: _____   Height: _____   Pre-Op Bra Size: _____

Desired Outcome:

1. ☐   2. ☐

3. ☐   4. ☐

Skin Envelope:

Right: ☐ Tight ☐ Moderate ☐ Loose ☐ with Ptosis

_____

Left: ☐ Tight ☐ Moderate ☐ Loose ☐ with Ptosis

_____

(Diagram labels: C-N, SN-N, BBW, BH, N-IMF, N-IMF (Stretched))

Patient Dimensions:

	Right	Left		Right	Left
Sternal Notch to Nipple (SN-N):	_____	_____	Nipple to IMF (N-IMF):	_____	_____
Clavicle to Nipple (C-N):	_____	_____	Nipple to IMF (stretched):	_____	_____
Breast Base Width (BBW):	_____	_____	Upper Pole Pinch:	_____	_____
Breast Height (BH):	_____	_____	Areolar Diameter:	___ x ___	___ x ___
Medial Pinch:	_____	_____		vert. horiz.	vert. horiz.
Lateral Pinch:	_____	_____	Intermammary Distance:	_____	

Observations:

Breast Shape: ☐R ☐L Tubular   ☐R ☐L Round   ☐R ☐L Conical   ☐R ☐L Wide   ☐R ☐L Narrow   ☐R ☐L Other _____

Breast Exam: _____

Estimated Breast Volume: Right: _____   Left: _____   Difference: _____

Asymmetry: Chest Wall: _____   Breast: _____

Nipple Level Discrepancy: _____   IMF Level Discrepancy: _____

Surgery Planning:

Surgery Type: ☐ Augmentation   ☐ Revision   ☐ Reconstruction

Surgery Date: _____   Location: _____   Inframammary Fold: ☐ Raise ☐ Keep ☐ Lower

Preferred External Sizer: Volume: _____   Profile: _____   Breast Base Width: _____
caliper measurement

Incision Approach: ☐ Inframammary ☐ Periareolar ☐ Axillary ☐ Other

Implant Base Diameter: _____

Implant Placement: ☐ Subpectoral   ☐ Subglandular   ☐ Subfascial   Breast Base Width – 1/2 medial pinch – 1/2 lateral pinch

Fig. 2.6 One of several optional forms available for recording patient measurements and surgical planning.

they will utilize to perform this evaluation, and practice it diligently. The error of either over- or under-filling the breast will be quickly recognized, and the young breast surgeon can avoid these problems through the experience of senior breast surgeons. The systematic approaches provide a means to adjust the breast implant volumes selected to compensate for either a tighter or looser skin envelope to produce a more satisfactory result (Fig. 2.7).

Pinch thickness

The upper pole pinch thickness is an essential component in the evaluation process. This will assist in the proper selection of both implant type and pocket during the patient analysis. Thickness of other portions of the breast parenchyma can also be considered when selecting an implant size, diameter, and considering when

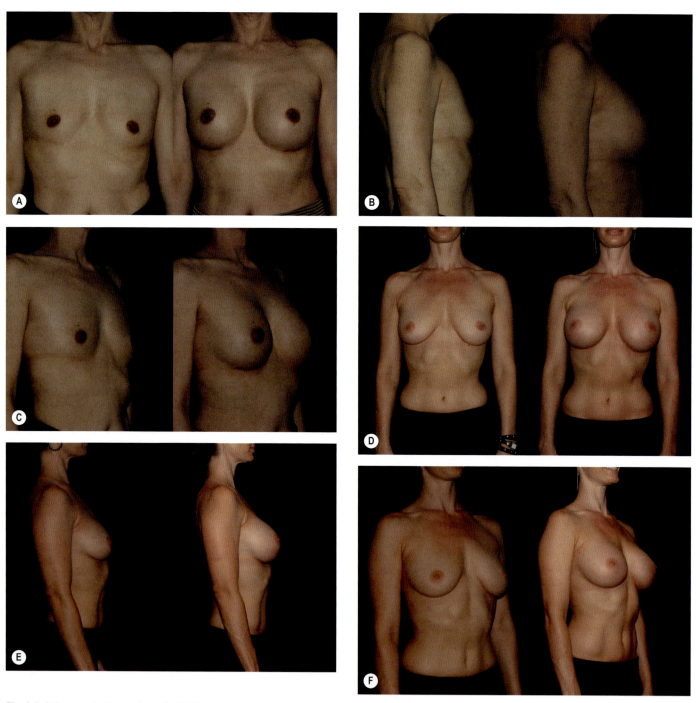

Fig. 2.7 Differences in skin envelope. **(A–C)** This patient has a tight skin envelope, minimal breast tissue, and chest wall asymmetry. Sientra shaped classic implants, submuscular position (right: 400 cc; left: 350 cc). **(D–F)** This patient has a loose skin envelope and moderate breast tissue. Mentor Moderate plus round smooth silicone implants in a subglandular position (right: 300 cc; left: 275 cc).

tissue modification such as mastopexy may be necessary. Briefly, when soft-tissue pinch is less than 2 cm in the upper pole, the implant will be less visible and palpable in the submuscular position. In addition, a shaped cohesive or saline implant fits better in the submuscular plane in this situation as well.

3D imaging

Once a thorough physical examination has been completed, the patient can undergo 3D imaging where measurements can be taken, and subsequent simulations can be performed. *An imperative in the 3D process is that size should not be selected by this technique, only confirmed.* Selecting a breast implant size via imaging violates all the principles of safe preoperative planning. The design of the imaging software is to make any size implant look good despite the patient's anatomy.

With this as a preface, it has become clear that as a measurement and predictive tool, 3D imaging is a useful clinical and marketing tool for the aesthetic breast surgeon. Multiple studies have confirmed the accuracy and patient satisfaction of 3D imaging to be as high as 90% (Fig. 2.8).[12]

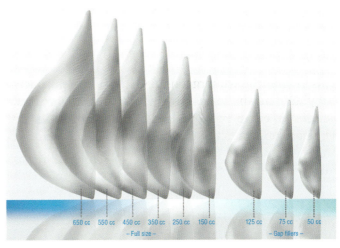

Fig. 2.9 Volumetric sizers are used for patients to try on sizes. Implants do not fill bras or T-shirts correctly and give erroneous size estimates.

Sizers

There is no best way to size breast implants. This again falls into the category of experience, systematic approach, and preference. The author's preference is patient-based within the limits of each individual's base diameter. Patients are allowed to use a commonly available volumetric sizing system (Fig. 2.9). This is placed in a tight sports bra for volume only (not shape). The patient's selected size is then imaged on the 3D imaging system based on her other measurements.

Implant selection

Simplistically, there are three choices in implant selection: saline vs. silicone, smooth vs. textured, and round vs. anatomic. Once the combinations of these are considered including the different heights and projections and brands available, the combinations are essentially too numerous to count. Each surgeon must evaluate the currently available safety data, patient characteristics, measurements, costs, and their own surgical technique to select the best implant for each situation.

The author's preference based on current data is to use a textured implant in almost all situations. The decrease in capsular contracture[13] and the author's perception of implant positional stability are the main basis for this decision. In addition, the use of shaped and highly cohesive gel implants dictate the need for texturing to prevent rotation and implant malposition.

Incision selection

Four incisions have been classically described for breast augmentation: inframammary, transaxillary, periareolar, and transumbilical. The risks and benefits of each of these incisions should be discussed with the patient, and then the best recommendation should be made based

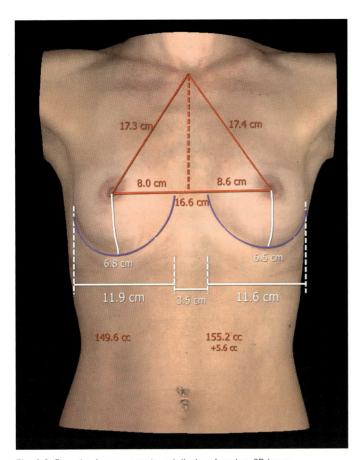

Fig. 2.8 Example of measurements and display of modern 3D image.

on implant selection, surgeon preference and ability, patient preference, and ideal surgical technique.

Inframammary incision

This incision allows complete visualization of the pocket in either the submuscular or subglandular plane. It can be used in either primary or secondary breast surgery. The incision needs to be planned in the projected fold, and recommended techniques exist to predict this accurately. The length of the incision will vary with implant type, longer with the newer cohesive gel implants.

Periareolar incision

Hidden at the junction of the areolar pigment and breast skin, this incision is best in lightly pigmented patients. Patients who have a sharp demarcation in their areolar pigment also tend to have a well-hidden scar compared with those whose pigment fades into the breast skin. This incision is helpful when adjusting the inframammary fold, or for scoring the breast tissue in patients with constricted breast deformity. Recent literature has shown a higher risk of both infection and capsular contracture with this incision especially with the use of textured devices. Additional disadvantages include more difficult visualization and inability to place silicone or cohesive implants with small areola diameters (<40 mm).

Transaxillary approach

The transaxillary incision can be used to perform either saline or silicone augmentation. In the past this has been used with blunt technique as well, but today this should all but be condemned as the risk of increased hematoma, pocket irregularity, and unnecessary tissue injury are significant. With the endoscopic technique, this approach can also be used to place newer more cohesive implants, although this can require a larger axillary incision and tunnel. This incision avoids a scar on the breast but limits the manipulation of the breast tissue and likely requires a second incision for any revisionary procedures.

Transumbilical incision

Again there is no incision on the breast mound, but this incision can only be used with saline implants. Again, blunt dissection and inability to use for revision also limit its utility.

Pocket selection

Submuscular

This location has been shown to have a decreased incidence of capsular contracture – at least with smooth implants. Studies have shown better ability to perform mammography, which is important in all patients, but especially in those with a strong family history of breast cancer. In patients with thin soft tissue, the implant will be less visible and palpable. This is especially significant with both saline and the newer more cohesive silicone implants.

Negative aspects of submuscular placement include increased risk of animation deformity in patients with significant pectoral muscle development and/or larger implants, increased postoperative pain, and the risk of long-term "piston deformity" with smooth and especially saline implants (lateral and inferior malposition).

When the submuscular plane is used, the dual plane technique[14] can be adapted to achieve outcomes similar to subglandular effects but maintain better upper pole coverage. This technique allows additional manipulation of lower pole and glandular tissue. It is helpful in the correction of the more ptotic breast, asymmetry of the breast envelope, and asymmetry of nipple position (Fig. 2.10). In using the dual plane, it is essential that the surgeon maintain medial attachment of pectoral muscle to avoid window shade deformity medially.

Subglandular

This plane remains an excellent option for breast augmentation with better correction of ptosis and likely similar risk of capsular contracture with textured implants. There is clearly a higher risk of capsular contracture with smooth implants in recent literature.

Subfascial

This dissection plane separates the breast tissue from implant with a theoretical decrease in capsular contracture. It also can eliminate the risk of animation deformity and in theory has ideal properties. This plane is more common outside the United States and requires a more difficult dissection plane.

Who decides what's best – surgeon or patient?

Author's personal algorithm[15]

In the author's practice, patients are allowed to try on size, and then all measurements are performed. Implants are selected with the following algorithm:

1. Base diameter is measured. This should not be violated by more than 1 cm either smaller or larger to create an attractive breast. Exceptions are the tuberous, constricted, or truly absent breast.

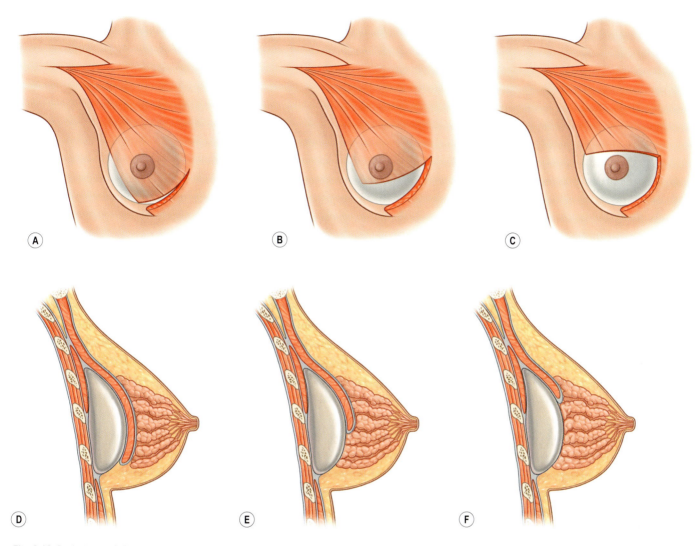

Fig. 2.10 Dual plane technique.

2. Sternal notch to nipple distance is measured to assess breast height:
   a. >21 cm – tall height implant
   b. 18–21 cm – moderate height implant or round device
   c. <18 cm – oval implant

   (This can be adjusted based on the patient's axillary fullness, goals for shape, pectoral muscle development, and chest shape.)

3. Projection is used to fill the skin envelope. This is assessed by measuring the nipple to inframammary fold distance with the breast skin on stretch. High, moderate, or low projection implants are selected based on the patient's skin envelope and size goals as much as possible.

4. Once the base diameter, implant height, and projection are selected, the volume is predetermined. Patients must be counseled when their size goal is either too large (a smaller implant must be used) or too small (a mastopexy must be performed). There is limited flexibility as patients are told that while they are the consumer, it is still my role to be the doctor. The beauty of the newest implants is their longevity and the fact they should be much less likely to require revision surgery due to device failure. Therefore, both the patient's and physician's decisions should also prevent this.

As a procedure driven by patient demand, many patients shop for a surgeon who will perform breast augmentation regardless of size and tissue limitations. This leads to short-term satisfaction, but long-term patient complications.

I believe each surgeon needs to decide his or her own philosophy on breast augmentation: patient choice or surgeon choice. If you allow the patient to dictate the

Table 2.1 How two surgeons might treat the same patient

Surgeon A		Surgeon B	
Base diameter	11.0 cm	Base diameter	12.3 cm
Height	Moderate	Volume	385
Projection	Moderate	Height	Moderate
Volume	255 cc	Projection	High
(See discussion in text below)			

volume that they can select for their augmentation, then the surgeon cannot determine at least one or more of the implant characteristics. In other words, if you measure all the characteristics of the patient's tissue, then the volume of the implant they can accommodate is predetermined. If not, then the surgeon is not in control of the procedure.

As you develop your personal technique for breast augmentation, you must honestly decide which methods suit your patient philosophy, risk aversion, and surgical technique. You must build your consultation, surgical principles, and practice around this concept. An example of how two surgeons might treat the same patient helps to illustrate the point (Table 2.1).

The first surgeon measures all characteristics of the patient's breast – diameter, height (for a shaped implant), tissue envelope (in this case selecting a round, moderate projecting device) – and therefore, from one company's catalog, can only select a 255 cc implant to fit into this breast properly.

The second surgeon allows the patient to "select" a 400 cc size implant. In trying to keep similar measurements, he must make significant compensation. The closest implant to match this size request is a high profile implant, 385 cc with a larger base diameter than the patient's actual size. As discussed above, in some patients over time this will lead to abnormal tissue stretch, thinning, wrinkling, problems with bottoming out, implant malposition, and therefore a higher re-operation rate. Even in the hands of the best surgeons, these complications are statistically significant.

While some patients will have a successful long-term result in both of these scenarios, others in the "patient size selection" model will not. As surgeons and physicians, we must live by the goal of "First do no harm".

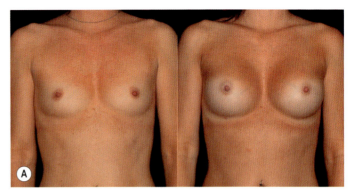

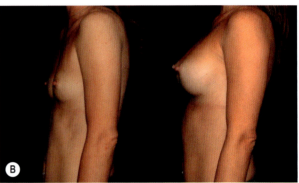

Fig. 2.11 A 24-year-old patient shown before and six months after Sientra round base silicone submuscular breast augmentation (320 cc). This patient with small breasts and a tight skin envelope still has a very natural enhancement with a result similar to the 45%/55% ratio discussed earlier.

Reasonable breast enhancement with safety and longevity is an admirable goal. High re-operation and complication rates, unnatural size, and appearance demand a critical re-evaluation of both the patient's and surgeon's goals in augmentation mammoplasty (Fig. 2.11).

Conclusion

Breast augmentation has evolved from a subjective surgery with a high incidence of complications, to an objectively determined cognitive and aesthetic procedure. New implants and better data supporting dimensionally planned, meticulously performed surgery have allowed the plastic surgeon to improve both safety and cosmetic outcome. The modern breast surgeon should strive to master these options and details in pursuit of the ideal result for each patient.

🌐 Access the complete reference list online at **http://www.expertconsult.com**

3. Tebbetts JB, Teitelbaum S. High- and extra-high-projection breast implants: potential consequences for patients. *Plast Reconstr Surg.* 2010;126:2150–2159. *Surgeons should carefully review this paper to understand the potential damage of a poorly selected or oversized implant. It is essential to understand how patient goals may not produce safe long term results.*

4. Tebbetts JB, Adams WP. Five critical decisions in breast augmentation using five measurements in 5 minutes: the high five decision support process. *Plast Reconstr Surg.* 2005;116:2005–2016. *This classic paper presents a system of analysis and planning for breast augmentation. Its principles should be clearly understood by all aesthetic breasts surgeons.*

13. Stevens WG, Nahabedian MY, Calobrace MB, et al. Risk factor analysis for capsular contracture: a 5-year Sientra study analysis using round, smooth, and textured implants for breast augmentation. *Plast Reconstr Surg.* 2013;132:1115–1123. *This review of the largest FDA manufacturer cohort shows clearly the differences in implant pocket, texturing and incision selections. It should be reviewed as part of the consultative and decision making process.*

14. Tebbetts JB. Dual plane breast augmentation: optimizing implant-soft-tissue relationships in a wide range of breast types. *Plast Reconstr Surg.* 2001;107:1255–1272. *The modern breast surgeon needs to understand the power of the dual plane technique. Its facility to shape the breast in many situations will improve any surgeons outcomes.*

15. Schwartz MR. Algorithm and techniques for using Sientra's silicone gel shaped implants in primary and revision breast augmentation. *Plast Reconstr Surg.* 2014;134:S18–S27. *This is the authors preferred technique for the evaluation, planning and procedure for breast augmentation. Text and Video provide a clear demonstration of this method.*

3

Device considerations in breast augmentation

G. Patrick Maxwell and Allen Gabriel

SYNOPSIS

- Breast augmentation is the most common aesthetic procedure performed in the United States and perhaps in the world.
- In preparing for a breast augmentation, one must understand each patient's goals and expectations and see if they can be achieved.
- Three important variables have to be addressed prior to the surgery:
    1. Incision length and placement (inframammary, periareolar, transaxillary, transumbilical)
    2. Pocket plane (subfascial, subglandular, submuscular, subpectoral with dual plane 1, 2, 3)
    3. Implant choice (saline vs. silicone, round vs. anatomic, smooth vs. textured).
- Biodimensional planning is utilized for preoperative exam.

 Access the Historical Perspective section online at
http://www.expertconsult.com

Introduction

Glandular hypomastia may occur as a developmental or involutional process and affects a significant number of women. Developmental hypomastia is often seen as primary mammary hypoplasia or as a sequela of thoracic hypoplasia (Poland syndrome) or other chest wall deformity. Involutional hypomastia may develop in the postpartum setting and may be exacerbated by breastfeeding or significant weight loss. When compared to the norm, inadequate breast volume may lead to a negative body image, feelings of inadequacy, and to low self-esteem.[1] These disturbances may adversely affect a patient's interpersonal relationships, sexual fulfillment, and quality of life.[2]

There has been a steady increase in breast augmentation surgery with the emerging importance of body image, changes in societal expectations, and the increasing acceptance of aesthetic surgery. In the United States alone, augmentation mammaplasty was performed in over 330 000 patients in 2014 and was the most frequently performed cosmetic surgical procedure in women.[3] In this chapter, we review the history of breast augmentation, operative planning and technique, and some perioperative and late complications of the procedure. The evolution of modern breast implants is described.

Basic science/disease process

Evolution of saline implants

The use of inflatable saline-filled breast implants was first reported in 1965 by Anon in France.[7] The saline-filled implant was developed in order to allow the non-inflated implant to be introduced through a relatively small incision, and then inflating the implant *in situ*.[8]

Saline-filled implants are manufactured with a range of recommended fill volumes. Mild breast asymmetry may be corrected by taking advantage of this range of recommended fill volumes during placement of the implants. Underfilling saline-filled implants may lead to increased deflation rates due to folding or friction subjected to the implant shell, and is not recommended. Underfilling saline-filled implants may also lead to a wrinkled appearance or *rippling* with the breast in certain positions. Saline-filled implants have historically performed better when slightly overfilled and when placed under thicker soft-tissue coverage. Although these implants may be slightly overfilled, aggressive overfilling may lead to a more spherical shape and *scalloping* along the implant edge with knuckle-like palpability and unnatural firmness. Another potential disadvantage of saline-filled implants is that the consistency of these implants on palpation is similar to that of water instead of the more viscous feel of natural breast tissue.

Evolution of silicone implants

The first generation silicone gel-filled implant introduced in 1962 by Cronin and Gerow was manufactured by Dow Corning Corporation.[9] The shell of the first generation implant was constructed using a thick, smooth silicone elastomer as a two-piece envelope with a seam along the periphery. The shell was filled with a moderately viscous silicone gel. The implant was anatomically shaped (teardrop) and had several Dacron fixation patches on the posterior aspect to help maintain the proper position of the implant. These early devices had a relatively high contracture rate, due to the quality of the shells and the lack of cohesivity of the gel, which then encouraged implant manufacturers to develop second-generation silicone gel-filled implants.[11]

In the 1970s, the second-generation silicone implants were developed in an effort to reduce the incidence of capsular contracture with a thinner, seamless shell and without Dacron patches incorporated into the shell. These implants were round in shape and filled with a less viscous silicone gel to provide a more natural feel. However, the second-generation breast implants were plagued by diffusion or *bleed* of microscopic silicone molecules into the periprosthetic intracapsular space due to their thin, permeable shell and low viscosity silicone gel filler. This diffused silicone produced an oily, sticky residue surrounding the implant within the periprosthetic capsule that was noticeable during explantation of older silicone-filled implants.[12]

The development of the third-generation silicone gel-filled implants in the 1980s focused on improving the strength and permeability of the shell in order to reduce silicone gel *bleed* from intact implants and to reduce implant rupture and subsequent gel migration. The manufacturers designed new implant shells that consisted of multilayered silicone elastomer. These third-generation prostheses reduced gel bleed by introducing a barrier layer and a thicker shell that significantly lowered the device shell failure rate.

After the FDA required the temporary restriction of third-generation silicone gel implants from the American market in 1992,[13–18] the *fourth- and fifth-generation* gel devices evolved. These silicone gel breast implants were designed under more stringent ASTM (American Society for Testing Methodology)[19] and FDA-influenced criteria for shell thickness and gel cohesiveness. Furthermore, they were manufactured with improved quality control[20] and with a wider variety of surface textures and implant shapes. They are currently available from all three breast implant manufacturers in the United States (Sientra, Allergan, and Mentor).[21–25]

During the same time the concept of anatomically shaped implants was introduced with the *fifth-generation* silicone gel implants.[26] In addition to having a textured surface, these anatomically shaped implants are filled with a more cohesive gel. The FDA approved fifth-generation implants from all of the US manufacturers in the following order: Sientra (2012), Allergan, and Mentor (both 2013). Each manufacturer was approved for a variety of shapes and styles with Sientra offering five styles of the HSC+ line, four 410 implant styles from Allergan, and one Contour Profile Gel (CPG) implant from Mentor.[22,27,28]

To further understand the evolution of silicone-filled implants, implant characteristics will be further reviewed, as the resultant breast form is not only dependent on the soft-tissue envelope (in augmentation and reconstruction) and the breast parenchyma (in augmentation) but also on the following implant characteristics: surface, filler, shell, and implant shape.

Surface

Surface characteristics have undergone changes and evolved with all three manufacturers working towards the common goal of utilizing texture to possibly minimize or even disrupt capsule formation.[29,30] The evolution of textured implants began with polyurethane-coated implants reporting lower capsular contracture rates.[31] These *foam*-coated implants were eventually removed voluntarily from the US market because of concerns related to difficulty associated with complete removal and the theoretical concern of malignant transformation associated with the polyurethane coating. Polyurethane foams are thought to undergo partial chemical degradation under physiologic conditions releasing compounds that could become carcinogens in experimental animals but are not known human carcinogens.[32]

In the 1980s, manufacturers shifted their focus from polyurethane-covered shells to textured silicone shells with different pore sizes. Of all the textured surfaces currently in use, none are created in the same manner and each manufacturer has a proprietary process in place. One of the critical issues during the evolution of the texture is to find a way to stabilize the implant in the breast pocket. Studies have demonstrated that the pore size is critical to allow for tissue adherence leading to the "adhesive effect" and implant stabilization.[33] It was not clear if the pore size correlated with a reduction in capsular contracture; however, it did correlate with implant stabilization.[33] Danino *et al.* compared the Biocell texture with pore diameter of 600–800 μm with a depth of 150–200 μm to Siltex pore diameter of 70–150 μm. It was noted that Siltex pores lead to *no* "adhesive effect".[33]

The manufacturing process of textured surface implants can be complex while smooth surface implants are made by dipping a mandrel into liquid silicone creating multilayers, followed by allowing the surface to cure in a laminar flow oven. Additional steps beyond creating smooth surface implants are involved in the creation of textured implants.[34] Sientra's Silimed implant (Sientra Inc., Santa Barbara, CA), named as TRUE Texture, avoids the use of sodium chloride, sugar, soak/scrub, or pressure stamping.[28,35,36] Small hollow pores are formed with minimal thin cell webbing that reduces particle formation. The Biocell (Allergan Inc., Irvine, CA) texture is created using a "loss-salt" technique,[34] which includes a layer of salt crystals with a thin overcoat of silicone followed by curing in a laminar flow oven.[34] The Siltex surface (Mentor Corp., Santa Barbara, CA), on the other hand, is created by "imprint stamping",[34] which dips the chuck into uncured silicone, pushing it into polyurethane foam and finalizing the imprint with pressure.[34]

Filler

Silicone is a mixture of semi-inorganic polymeric molecules composed of varying length chains of polydimethyl siloxane $[(CH3)2\text{-}SiO]$ monomers. The physical properties of silicones are quite variable depending on the average polymer chain length and the degree of cross-linking between the polymer chains.[37] *Liquid* silicones are polymers with a relatively short average length and very little cross-linking. They have the consistency of an oily fluid and are frequently used as lubricants in pharmaceuticals and medical devices. Silicone *gels* can be produced of varying viscosity by progressively increasing the length of the polymer chains or the degree of cross-linking.

When enough filler cross-linking is achieved to the degree that the silicone gel implant will maintain its dimensions and form (i.e., gel distribution within the shell), the cohesive gel implant is considered to be "form stable", although this terminology has recently been questioned as no gel implant on the market is truly form stable. Form stable may more appropriately refer to the ability of an implant to maintain shape. Technology

exists to measure the cohesivity of the silicone gel of commercially available devices and was utilized to measure the stiffness of both Allergan and Mentor shaped and round implants. This study showed that the 410 implant (Allergan Inc.) had the stiffest gel representing the highest cohesivity compared to the CPG implant (Mentor).[27] In a separate study it was found that the Sientra form-stable implant was the least cohesive when compared to both the CPG and 410 implants. It is important to note that cohesivity represents only a single characteristic of the implant, and one must take into account various implant features in order to evaluate the implant as a whole.[27] In this same study it was demonstrated that Allergan's round implants were the least cohesive as compared to Mentor's round implants and Sientra's implants were the most cohesive as compared to both Allergan's and Mentor's round implants.

In the past, the effect of the filler material has been shown to have an effect on capsular contracture rates.[38–41] However, these studies compared the third-generation silicone implants to saline implants, and therefore the current implants may have other outcomes since fourth-generation silicone breast implant safety and long-term outcomes have been described.[22,23,25,27,28]

Shell

Extensive chemical cross-linking of the silicone gel polymer will produce a solid form of silicone referred to as an *elastomer* with a flexible, rubber-like quality. Silicone elastomers are used for the manufacture of facial implants, tissue expanders, and the outer shell of all breast prostheses. The introduction of shell modifications, such as barrier layers and triple shell elastomer to protect the gel, have led to safer implants.[22,23,27,28,42] The elastomeric shell characteristics are also dependent on the relationship of the gel and shell. Shell characteristics also depend on the thickness and how the internal gel is bonded to the shell that leads to stability of the final shape.

Implant shape

The maintenance of gel distribution within the shell helps to preserve the form stability.[42] The more cohesive the gel, the higher the gel–shell fill ratio, and the more enhanced bonding of the gel to the shell will lead to more improved shape maintenance. The gel–shell fill ratio varies among the manufacturers and can produce visual clinical differences and may result in rippling and upper pole collapse if not used in the proper patient. It is important to note that all types of implants in the round portfolio of US manufacturers vary in the gel–shell fill ratio within the different profiles (i.e., low, moderate, high). Magnetic resonance imaging (MRI) study showed that shell rippling is still noted in a prone position in of one of the most cohesive form stable implants.[43] Changes in shape/form in different positions are generally not clinically significant but can be a patient concern.

Diagnosis and patient presentation

The initial consultation for augmentation should begin with open-ended questions about the patient's goals and expectations for the procedure. Patients today have often spent some time researching the procedure either through friends or through the internet. The surgeon should be able to form an impression of the patient as a well-informed, psychiatrically stable person with appropriately realistic expectations for the procedure. Any concerns about the patient's level of understanding, unrealistic expectations, or self-esteem issues should be fully explored prior to proceeding with surgery. A careful medical history and physical examination is essential for the assessment of risk factors and candidacy for breast augmentation. Preoperative mammography is recommended for patients over 35 years of age or patients of any age with significant risk factors for breast cancer.

The *ideal* size and shape of the female breast is inherently subjective and relates to both personal preference and to cultural norms. However, most surgeons will agree that there are certain shared characteristics that represent the aesthetic ideal of the female breast form (Fig. 3.1). These characteristics include a profile with a sloping or full upper pole and a gently curved lower pole with the nipple areolar complex at the point of maximal projection. The breast structure itself may be thought of as the breast parenchyma resting on the anterior chest wall surrounded by a soft-tissue envelope made up of skin and subcutaneous adipose tissue. Clearly, the resulting form of the breast after augmentation mammaplasty will be determined by the dynamic interaction of the breast implant, the parenchyma, and the soft-tissue envelope.[44]

A thorough physical examination begins with observation and careful documentation of any signs of chest wall deformity or spinal curvature. It is imperative to document and draw attention to any asymmetry of breast size, nipple position, or inframammary fold (IMF) position. Careful palpation of all quadrants of the breast and axilla is required to rule out any dominant masses or suspicious lymph nodes. While palpating the breast, the surgeon should carefully assess the quantity and compliance of the parenchyma and soft-tissue envelope. The soft-tissue pinch test is a useful method of assessment in which the superior pole of the breast is gathered between the examiner's thumb and index finger and measuring the thickness of the intervening tissue. In general, a pinch test result of less than 2 cm will often indicate a need for subpectoral placement of the implant. It is also important to characterize the amount, quality, and distribution of the breast parenchyma as it may be necessary to reshape or redistribute the parenchyma to achieve the desired shape of the breast mound. The elasticity of the skin should also be characterized by observing its resistance to deflection and noting any signs of skin redundancy or stretch marks. Both manufacturers have developed a preoperative planning system to facilitate patient assessment and implant selection. In addition, the authors utilize 4D technology to assess both the patient's chest wall and soft-tissue abnormalities. Chest-wall, soft-tissue asymmetries, and combinations of both are important to identify preoperatively (Figs. 3.2–3.4). This tool is also utilized to understand the patient's perception of the desired look by showing the outcomes of utilizing different size and style implants. This is also then projected in the operating room for surgical planning.[45]

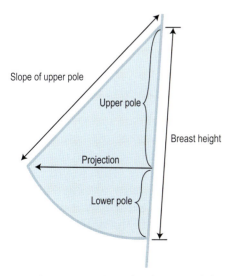

Fig. 3.1 The aesthetic breast form is composed of measurable parameters. The resultant breast form desired after surgical augmentation is determined by the dynamic interaction between the character and compliance of the soft-tissue envelope; the quality, volume, and consistency of the breast parenchyma; and the dimensions, volume, and characteristics of the breast implant. This form can be attained by the careful planning and surgical performance of a breast augmentation.

Labels in figure: Slope of upper pole; Upper pole; Breast height; Projection; Lower pole

Patient selection

Precise measurements must be taken using the IMF, the nipple areolar complex, and the suprasternal notch as key landmarks (Fig. 3.5). The surgeon should measure the breast width (BW) at its widest point, the breast height (BH), and the distance from the nipple areolar complex to the inframammary fold (N:IMF). The

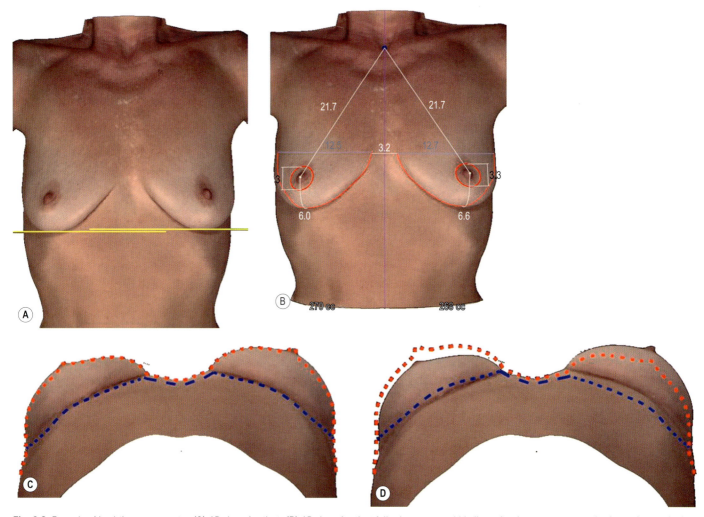

Fig. 3.2 Example of hard-tissue asymmetry. **(A)** AP view of patient. **(B)** AP view of patient following automated biodimensional measurements and volume characterization. **(C)** View of patient's chest from below. Red line delineating the soft-tissue envelope, and blue line the chest wall. **(D)** View of patient's chest from below with superimposed soft-tissue and chest wall outlines as mirror images with identification of chest wall asymmetry. Even though the volume is identical, the presenting anatomy is very different.

distance from the suprasternal notch to the nipple areolar complex (SSN:N) and the intermammary distance (IMD) should also be documented. It is often helpful to make markings on the patient in the seated position with a permanent marker just prior to surgery. It is imperative to mark the original IMF and a good idea to mark the true midline of the anterior chest.

In addition to manual measurements, 3D imaging is available to facilitate the measurement process in addition to enhancing the patient's overall experience by increasing physician–patient interaction in selecting the appropriate implant.[45] The visual display of the implant selected increases the confidence of the patient in the results that will be achieved. The 3D imaging systems can automatically measure and characterize both the soft tissue and chest wall as this is an important step in surgical planning. There are times that minor chest wall or soft-tissue asymmetries are missed by manual measurement and visualization. The system (Vectra,

Canfield Inc., Helena, MT) captures all of the asymmetries preoperatively so that appropriate preoperative planning can be performed and the patient is advised with an accurate informed consent.[45] This system is based on the biodimensional principles as previously described. As we continue to pursue increased patient safety and satisfaction while decreasing re-operation rates, this system will serve as another tool in our armamentarium to achieve these goals. This serves as an excellent consultation tool to be able to better understand what the patient expectations are with respect to choosing the size and the shape of the implant.

Informed consent

It is incumbent on the surgeon to evaluate the patient's emotional state, timing, and appropriateness of the desired outcome. It is the surgeon's responsibility to listen, educate, and evaluate; this process and the

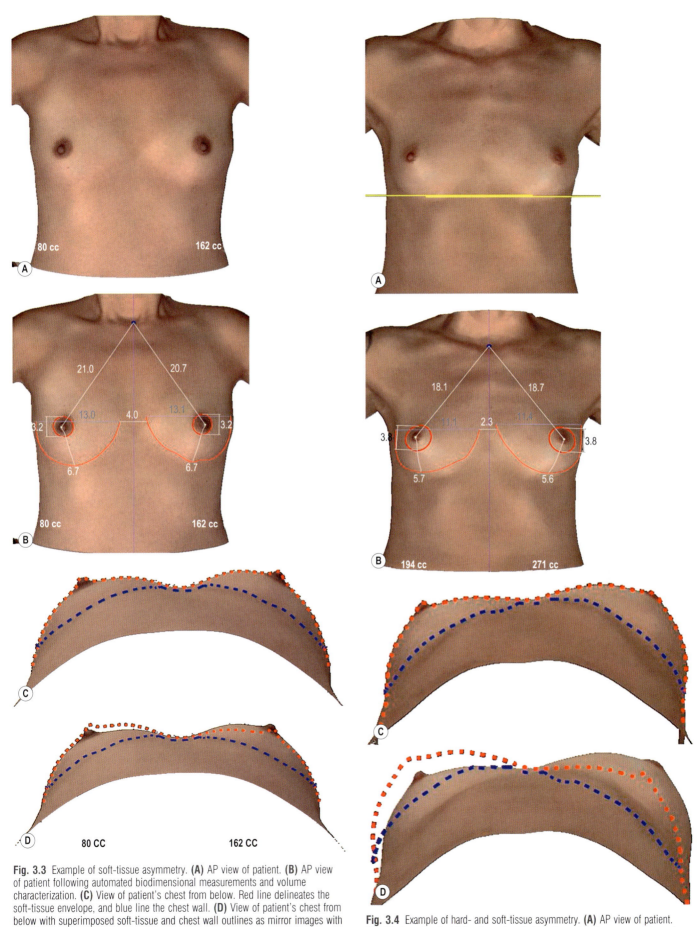

Fig. 3.3 Example of soft-tissue asymmetry. **(A)** AP view of patient. **(B)** AP view of patient following automated biodimensional measurements and volume characterization. **(C)** View of patient's chest from below. Red line delineates the soft-tissue envelope, and blue line the chest wall. **(D)** View of patient's chest from below with superimposed soft-tissue and chest wall outlines as mirror images with identification of soft-tissue asymmetry.

Fig. 3.4 Example of hard- and soft-tissue asymmetry. **(A)** AP view of patient. **(B)** AP view of patient following automated biodimensional measurements and volume characterization (C) View of patient's chest from below. Red line delineates the soft-tissue envelope, and blue line the chest wall. (D) View of patient's chest from below with superimposed soft-tissue and chest wall outlines as mirror images with identification of soft-tissue and hard tissue asymmetry..

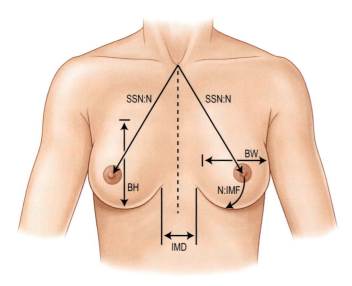

Fig. 3.5 Preoperative measures (taken before breast augmentation) include SSN to N (suprasternal notch to nipple), N to IMF (nipple to inframammary fold), BW (breast width), BH (breast height), and IMD (intermammary distance).

communication that takes place between patient and surgeon are documented in the medical record. Informed consent is not simply the signing of a paper or contract but refers to the entire process between patient and physician as well as physician extenders. To be "informed", the patient must be provided with adequate information about risks, benefits, and treatment alternatives to the proposed procedure. The authors recommend the use of official American Society of Plastic Surgeons (ASPS) informed consents. To "consent", the patient must be an adult (by age), be capable of rational communication, and be able to understand the information. The informed consent documentation must be thorough and specific to the operation and preferably the surgeon. A checklist of specifics (which must be initialed by the patient) is considered advisable. "Before and after" photographs may be shown but should be realistic. Photographs of the patient are a necessary form of documentation, requiring appropriate permission. Their confidentiality is essential unless permission is given for any use other than medical review documentation. A male surgeon should be accompanied by a female chaperone during all breast photography and examinations. Because of the multiple options in breast augmentation surgery, a second office visit is advisable. There must be a clear understanding (which is documented in the medical record) between patient and surgeon of the specific desired outcome (size, shape), the alternative ways by which this can be achieved, and the risk-to-benefit ratio of the chosen "pathway".

Operative planning

Incision length and placement

Four types of incision are commonly employed in breast augmentation: transaxillary, inframammary, periareolar, and transumbilical. After implant selection, the patient and surgeon should make the decision as to which type of incision is to be used after the options, risks, and benefits of each have been thoroughly explained. Surgeons should offer only the techniques that they are comfortable performing. The final choice should allow the surgeon optimal control and visualization to deliver the desired outcome for the specific patient and the specific implant.

The *inframammary* incision permits complete visualization of either the subpectoral or subglandular pocket and allows precise placement of virtually all implants. The technique does leave a visible scar within the inframammary fold. Smaller incisions (<3 cm) can be used for saline-filled implants, but silicone gel implants often require incisions up to 5.0–6.0 cm in length. The incision should be placed in the projected inframammary fold rather than in the existing fold to avoid visibility and widening of the subsequent scar. There are a variety of techniques described for identifying the expected IMF, and these are discussed in different chapters that discuss use of the fifth-generation gel devices.

The *periareolar* incision is placed at the areolar–cutaneous juncture and generally heals inconspicuously in lightly pigmented patients. The dissection allows easy adjustment of the inframammary fold and direct access to the lower parenchyma for scoring and release when a constricted lower pole is present. Disadvantages include limited exposure of the surgical field, transection of the parenchymal ducts (which are often colonized with *Staphylococcus epidermidis*), potentially increased risk of nipple sensitivity changes, and visible scarring on the breast mound. This technique should not routinely be used on patients with an areola diameter less than 40 mm and may not allow introduction of larger gel or enhanced cohesive gel implants. There have been some reports of possibility of increased capsular contracture rates with the use of this incision.

The *transaxillary* approach can be performed either bluntly or with the aid of an endoscope. The endoscope allows precise dissection and release of the inferior musculofascial attachments of the pectoralis major as well as direct visualization for hemostasis. This approach avoids any scarring on the breast mound and can be used with both saline and gel implants in either a subpectoral or subglandular pocket. Disadvantages include difficulty with parenchymal alterations and the probable need for a second incision on the breast mound for revisionary surgery. Precise implant placement can be more difficult with this incision, and enhanced cohesive gel and anatomic implants may be precluded.

Transumbilical breast augmentation has the obvious advantage of a single, well-hidden, remote incision. It can be used only with saline implants, however, and precise pocket dissection requires experience. The pocket is dissected bluntly, and hemostasis can be difficult from the remote access port. As with the transaxillary approach, revisions often necessitate a second incision on the breast mound.

Pocket position

The decision of subglandular/subfascial or subpectoral implant placement depends on implant selection (fill and texture) and tissue thickness (Fig. 3.6). In theory, the best position for a mammary implant is in the subglandular plane. This is the most anatomically correct position to maintain natural shape and form. The authors, however, no longer utilize the subglandular plane and instead prefer the subfascial plane. The reasons for placement of implants in the subpectoral plane are to minimize the risk of implant visibility and palpability. Risk of capsular contracture in either plane is dependent on surgical preparation and technique and not necessarily the pocket. With sound surgical techniques and appropriate postoperative management, capsular contracture can be minimized in either pocket. The authors' belief is that the subfascial pocket is more superior to subglandular, as this provides an additional durable layer between the implant and the gland.

The *subfascial* implant position has been advocated for augmentation mammaplasty in certain patients[46–50] (Fig. 3.7). Theoretically, placement of the implant in the subfascial position between the anterior fascia of the pectoralis major and the muscle itself may provide additional support to the overlying soft-tissue envelope, causing less distortion of the breast form and decreasing mobility of the implant within the pocket. The long-term outcome studies of breast augmentation employing this position are not yet available, but the procedure is gaining popularity worldwide.[47]

In patients with a pinch test result of more than 2 cm, the implant can safely be placed in the subfascial plane. Textured implants are the preferred implant for subfascial placement. If one chooses smooth gel implants for the subfascial plane, additional measures to prevent capsular contracture must be taken. These include larger pocket dissections with displacement exercises or possible dilute steroid pocket irrigation. Anatomic-shaped

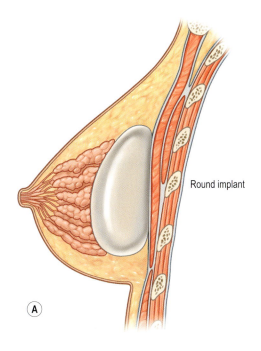

Round implant

(A)

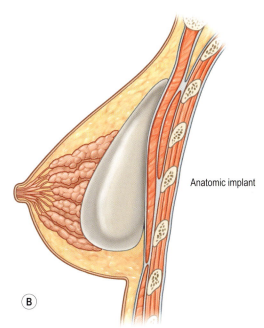

Anatomic implant

(B)

Fig. 3.6 (A,B) When ample soft tissue is present, implants may be placed in the subglandular position or subfascial position. When there is soft-tissue inadequacy, the subpectoral position is generally preferable.

textured implants are placed in the appropriate pocket as determined by soft-tissue thickness. Pockets for these implants are made only minimally larger than the footprint of the device to minimize displacement or malrotation.

When subpectoral pockets are selected, one generally divides the origin of the pectoralis major muscle just above the inframammary fold to allow better projection in the lower pole of the augmented breast and to

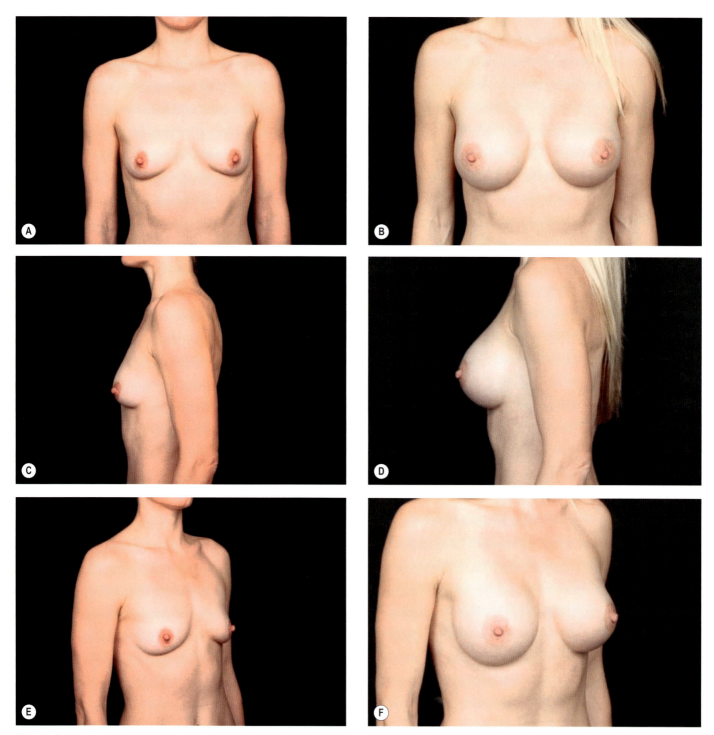

Fig. 3.7 Preoperative and postoperative views of 39-year-old female with style 410 implants at 12 months. **(A,C,E)** preoperative view, FF 425 cc. **(B,D,F)** Postoperative, FF 425 cc in a dual-plane location.

maintain a natural inframammary fold (Fig. 3.8). This places the superior portion of the implant in a subpectoral position while the inferior portion is subglandular. In constricted breasts (tuberous breasts) or ptotic breasts, for which more parenchymal surgical manipulation is necessary, or when there is a greater need for the implant to fill out the lower soft-tissue envelope, more dissection between parenchyma and muscle will allow the muscle

to cover less of the implant with a resultant greater subglandular implant coverage. Alternatively, the pectoral muscle can be divided at a higher level to give a similar result (Fig. 3.9). These pocket manipulations have been described as dual-plane maneuvers to allow varying degrees of subpectoral to subglandular implant coverage.[44] This *dual-plane* dissection allows the pectoralis muscle to retract superiorly or *window-shade*

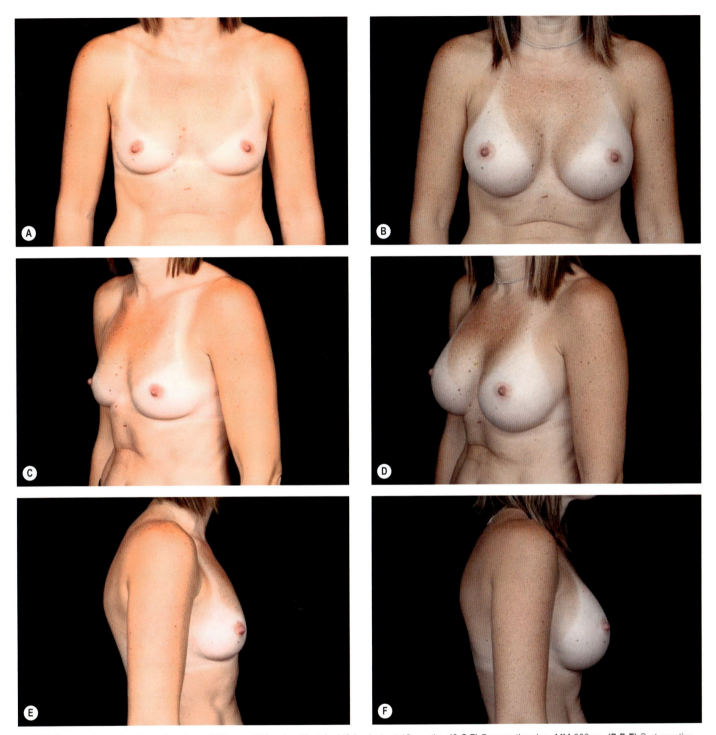

Fig. 3.8 Preoperative and postoperative views of 36-year-old female with style 410 implants at 12 months. **(A,C,E)** Preoperative view, MM 360 cc. **(B,D,F)** Postoperative, MM 360 cc in a dual-plane position.

upward while the breast parenchyma is redraped over the inferior portion of the implant avoiding deformity of the resulting augmented breast (Fig. 3.10).

Implant selection: filling material

In the US, there are two implant materials from which to choose – saline- and silicone-filled implants. The decision between a saline-filled prosthesis and a silicone gel implant is one of the patient's preferences after the surgeon's conveyance of information. Experience has shown the results of silicone gel implants in primary breast augmentation to be generally soft and to have a natural feel and appearance, assuming capsular contracture is not present. Although the authors prefer silicone gel implants, saline implants placed in the

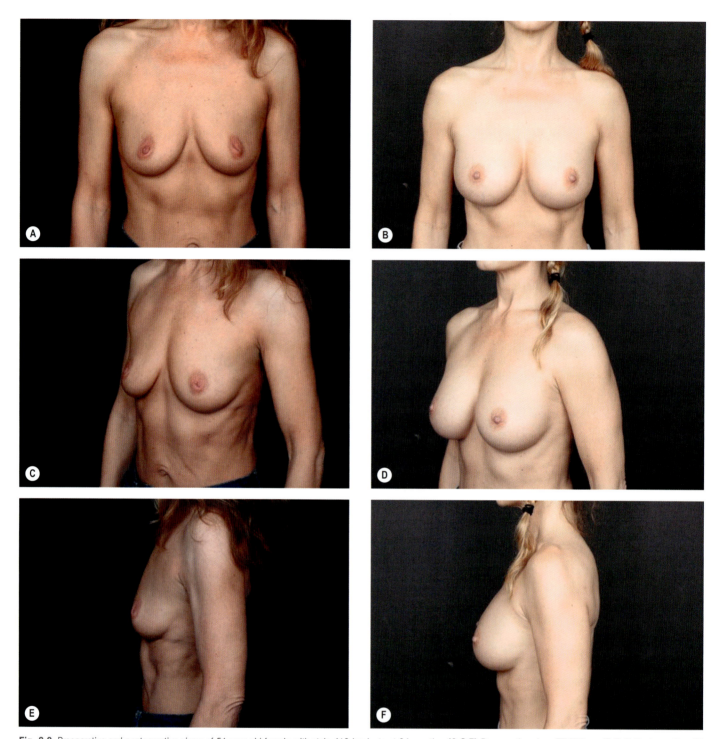

Fig. 3.9 Preoperative and postoperative views of 51-year-old female with style 410 implants at 24 months. **(A,C,E)** Preoperative view, FF 375 cc. **(B,D,F)** Postoperative, FF 375 cc in a dual-plane position.

subpectoral position can produce good results with a low incidence of capsular contracture. The thicker the soft tissue under which a saline implant is placed, the better it performs. Despite our preference for silicone gel, some patients will undoubtedly continue to have concerns about silicone-filled devices, and subpectoral saline implants have proved to be a reasonable alternative. Ultimately, the patient must feel comfortable with the implant device, so the final decision rests with the patient. The addition of shaped devices has given another option for patients to choose an implant that is more natural appearing.[51]

Implant selection: implant size

The selection of the implant size is initiated during the preoperative consultation period based on both the patient's goals and the surgeon's assessment. In general,

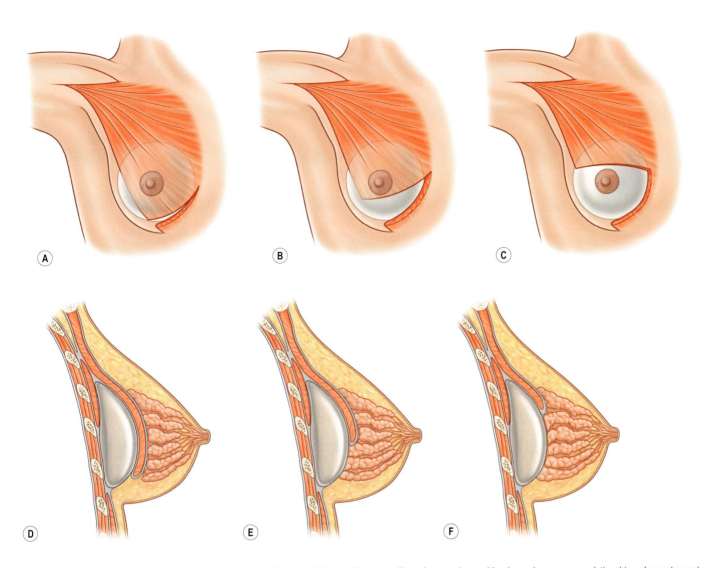

Fig. 3.10 Subpectoral implant placement generally involves release or division of the pectoralis major muscle, resulting in varying coverage relationships of muscles and parenchyma to implant. **(A,D)** For most routine breasts: *muscle division* near the inframammary fold results in muscle coverage of most of the implant. **(B,E)** Breasts with mobile parenchyma muscle interface: *muscle division* (or muscle–parenchymal detachment) to the lower areolar level results in muscle coverage of the upper half of the implant. **(C,F)** Breasts with glandular ptosis or lower pole constriction: *muscle division* (or muscle–parenchymal detachment) to the upper areolar level results in muscle coverage of the upper third of the implant.

the critical factors in selecting a specific implant size are the dimensions of the nascent breast, the compliance and characteristics of the soft-tissue envelope, and the desired volume for the resulting augmented breast. The base width of the breast is related to the width of the patient's chest and is proportional to the overall body habitus. It is imperative that this dimension is respected during augmentation in order to maintain the normal anatomical landmarks such as the lateral breast fold in the anterior axillary line and the intermammary distance (IMD). The same is true for breast height, but to a lesser degree than breast width. Violation of these landmarks may yield an unnatural and deformed appearance. Generally, the surgeon should select an implant that is slightly less wide than the existing breast. Implant manufacturers are now producing implants with varying degrees of projection for a given base width. In this way, the surgeon should be able to attain the desired amount of projection while preserving the normal aesthetic proportions of the breast (Fig. 3.11).

The patient's request for a particular breast size and shape will largely determine the dimensions of the breast implant used. In addition to a thorough discussion with the patient as to her desire for the resultant form and size, the 4D imaging system can be utilized to show the patient the outcomes based on the selection of a particular implant.

Implant selection: implant surface texture

The decision between textured and smooth-walled implants is only applicable for round implants. Anatomic implants are all textured by design to minimize malrotation (Fig. 3.12). With round implants, the choice

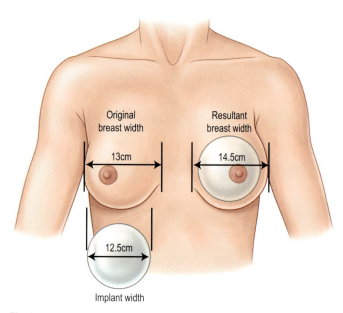

Fig. 3.11 After the width of the existing breast is measured and the desired resultant breast form is formulated, an implant is selected (generally just narrower than the original breast, shown on the patient's right) that in combination with the preoperative breast tissue will achieve the desired postoperative dimensions and form (shown on the patient's left).

between textured and smooth-walled implants is based primarily on minimizing capsular contracture. For subpectoral augmentation, either implant can probably be used with comparable results. When the device is placed in the subfascial pocket, a textured implant is preferred to minimize capsular contracture. If a smooth-walled implant is chosen, then the dissected pocket should be large enough to accommodate the implant displacement exercises (Fig. 3.13).

Implant selection: implant shape

It is important to reiterate the principle that the shape of the natural female breast is not a semicircle or a hemisphere. Dimensional analysis of the aesthetically pleasing breast form reveals a gently sloping upper pole and a curved lower pole with the nipple areolar complex at the point of maximum projection. The typical round shaped breast implant has its greatest projection centrally with the remainder of the volume distributed evenly along the base of the implant. In contrast, anatomically shaped breast implants have a flatter upper

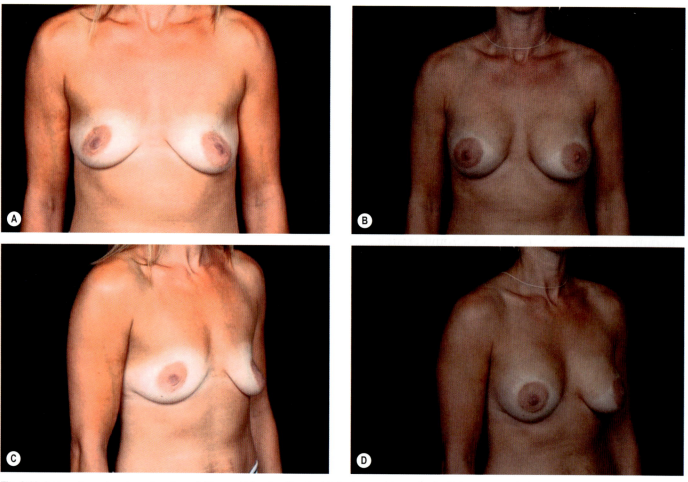

Fig. 3.12 Preoperative and postoperative views of 40-year-old female with style 410 implants at 12 months. **(A,C)** Preoperative, FM 270 cc. **(B,D)** Postoperative, FM 270 cc in a dual-plane position.

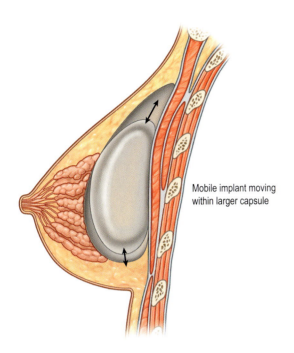

Mobile implant moving within larger capsule

Fig. 3.13 Pocket dissection.

pole with the majority of the volume and projection in the lower pole (Fig. 3.14). Thus, the anatomically shaped implant of a given base width and volume will produce less upper pole convexity than a round implant of the same base width and volume (Fig. 3.15). This characteristic of anatomically shaped implants can be extremely useful when the patient desires a significant volume augmentation but has a relatively narrow breast width.[26]

Treatment and surgical technique

Preoperative markings are made with the patient in the upright position and are useful as a reference point during the actual procedure. The surgeon should mark the chest midline in the frontal view from the suprasternal notch to the xiphoid process, the existing inframammary folds, and the likely position of the new inframammary folds as the proposed limits of the dissection. The patient is then asked to place her arms behind her head to visualize the displacement of the nipple and the true inframammary fold. The "yoga"-type stretching exercises are also reviewed with the patient at this point. Following review of the consent and the plan, the patient is taken to the operating room. The patient is then placed in the supine position, centered on the operating table with the pelvis directly over the flexion point of the bed. The arms must be well secured to the arm boards that are placed at 90-degree angles to the torso. These preparations are required so that the patient may be placed in the upright seated

position as often as needed during the procedure. The sterile preparation and draping of the anterior chest must provide visualization of the patient's shoulders as an important anatomical reference point. Triple antibiotic solution irrigation will be used for all implant cases regardless of the incision type.

Inframammary incision

The inframammary approach permits complete visualization of the implant pocket with either subglandular, subfascial, or subpectoral placement. The incision should be placed in the predicted location of the new inframammary fold that has been determined and marked preoperatively. Smaller incisions (<3 cm) may be used for inflatable saline-filled implants, but pre-filled implants (silicone gel or saline) often require incisions up to 5.0 cm in length. The incision should be designed with the majority of the incision lateral to the breast midline as this will place the resulting scar in the deepest portion of the new IMF.

The incision is made along the proposed markings, and the dissection is continued with an insulated electrocautery instrument through Scarpa's fascia. A fiberoptic headlight is worn throughout the procedure, or a variety of lighted fiberoptic retractors are available to aid illumination and direct visualization within the pocket. If the implant is to be placed in the subfascial pocket, the dissection proceeds below the pectoralis fascia but above the pectoralis major fascia. Once the fascia is identified, it will be thicker as dissection proceeds more cephalad. Several medial intercostal perforating vessels may be encountered. These should be avoided or coagulated with insulated forceps if need be. For smooth-walled implants, a larger pocket is dissected to allow mobility of the implant. For anatomic implants, the pocket is precisely dissected to snugly accommodate the implant. Care should be taken to preserve the lateral intercostal cutaneous nerves, especially the fourth

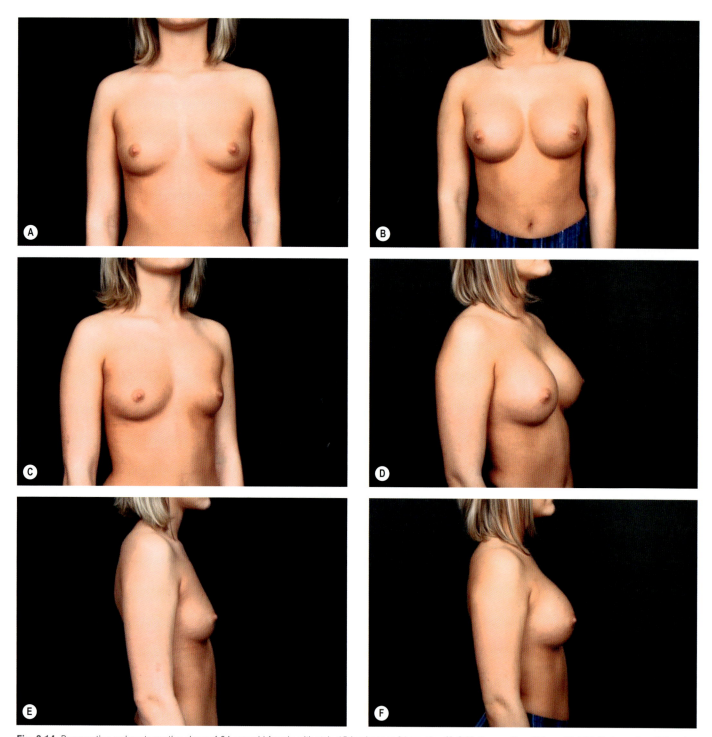

Fig. 3.14 Preoperative and postoperative views of 24-year-old female with style 15 implants at 24 months. **(A,C,E)** Preoperative, 286 cc. **(B,D,F)** Postoperative, 286 cc in a dual-plane position.

intercostal, which contains the primary sensory innervations of the nipple areolar complex.

If a subpectoral pocket is chosen, the dissection is initially carried out laterally to identify the lateral border of the pectoralis major muscle. The muscle edge can be lifted by forceps to allow easy entry into the submusculofascial plane. This plane is readily identified by the wispy areolar connective tissue and ease of dissection. An extended electrocautery instrument is used to complete the dissection. The inferior origin of the pectoralis major is released from lateral to medial at the level of the inframammary fold. Various slips of origin of the pectoralis major muscle are generally encountered and divided. Division of the pectoralis continues medially to the sternal border. Partial deep division may selectively be carried out 1–3 cm above the xiphoid, depending on which implant is to be used. Lateral dissection can be done bluntly with a finger to

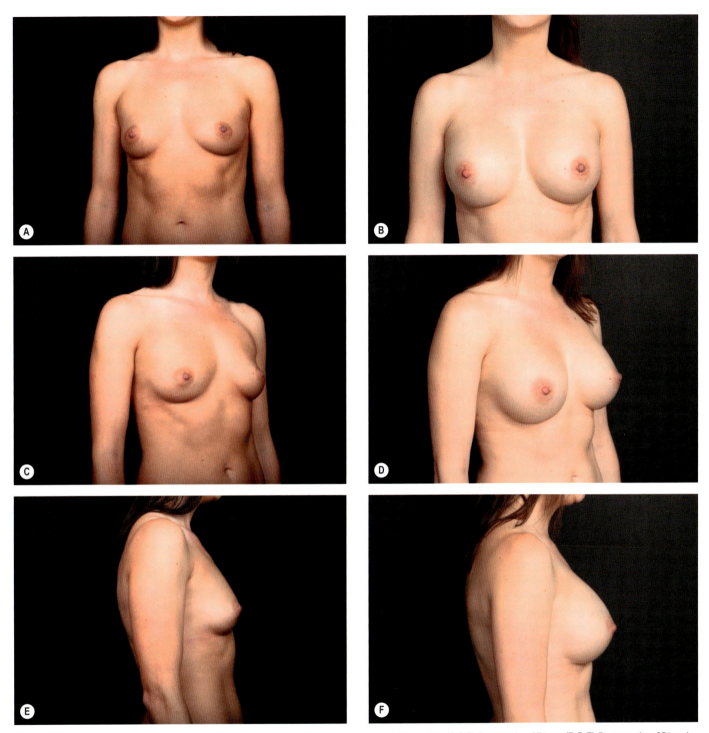

Fig. 3.15 Preoperative and postoperative views of 36-year-old female with style 15 implants at 24 months. **(A,C,E)** Preoperative, 371 cc. **(B,D,F)** Postoperative, 371 cc in a dual-plane position.

avoid injury to the lateral neurovascular bundles. The nerves can be stretched to accommodate the implant but should be preserved to minimize postoperative sensory changes. When the pectoralis major muscle is elevated, care must be taken to leave the pectoralis minor down on the chest wall. This will minimize bleeding and allow proper placement of the implant. At times, one may encounter several muscle interdigitations between the pectoralis minor and major, and these

are carefully dissected to prepare the pocket. In addition, if a dual-plane pocket is planned preoperatively, further dissection over the muscle is carried out pending the level of the desired dual plane followed by release of the pectoralis major at the inframammary fold.

Exact implant "sizers" (gel or saline) are used when available to evaluate the pockets and resultant breast form. After the sizers are in place, the patient is placed in a 90-degree upright position and evaluated from various perspectives. Any asymmetry or under-dissected areas are marked, and the patient is placed back in the supine position. Once adequate hemostasis is obtained and pocket dimensions are finalized, the pocket is irrigated with an antibiotic-containing solution,[52] and the implants are carefully placed by a minimal-touch technique.[52] The final results are assessed, again with the patient in a sitting position, and a multilayer closure is performed with absorbable suture. It is important to close off the implant pocket with a separate layer of suture before closing the skin. Once closure is complete, Steri-Strips are applied along the direction of the incisions.

Periareolar incision

The periareolar approach for augmentation mammaplasty was described by Jenny in 1972 and currently enjoys widespread use by plastic surgeons.[7] The periareolar incision is placed along the inferior portion of the areolar–cutaneous juncture. The principle advantage of this incision is that the resulting scar is usually well-camouflaged and quite inconspicuous. The periareolar approach allows easy adjustment of the IMF and direct access to the parenchyma for scoring and release when the lower pole of the breast is constricted. However, visualization and the dissection are typically inadequate with the periareolar incision in patients with areolas less than 3 cm in diameter. Other disadvantages of this approach include the potential risk of contamination if the lactiferous ducts are transected, the increased risk of changes in nipple sensitivity, and the risk of a hypopigmented scar in patients with darkly pigmented areolas.

The markings for a periareolar approach are similar to those for an inframammary augmentation. The incision is marked along the junction of the areola and the breast skin. The limits of the incision are the 3-o'clock and 9-o'clock positions.

The positioning of the patient is identical to that for an inframammary approach. It is imperative that the patient be able to fully flex at the waist for evaluation of the intraoperative appearance of the implants.

The precise incision is made. Wound edges are elevated directly up from the chest wall with an opposing pair of small sharp retractors. An insulated electrocautery unit is used to dissect straight down through the

breast parenchyma to the pectoralis major fascia. The dissection is the same as described through the inframammary incision. If the inferior pole of the breast is constricted, radial scoring of the gland in the inferior pole can allow proper redraping of the soft tissue over the implant to correct the deformity. Before final implant placement, the pocket is once again checked for hemostasis and irrigated with an antibiotic solution. The closure is particularly important with this technique. The gland must be precisely reapproximated and closed with several layers of interrupted absorbable sutures to prevent distortion of the nipple areolar complex. The skin is closed with deep everting dermal sutures and a running subcuticular absorbable monofilament. Steri-Strips are applied to the closed incision.

Transaxillary incision

The transaxillary approach was described by Hoehler in 1973 and popularized by Bostwick and others.[53] This procedure can be performed either bluntly using the Montgomery dissector, or using an endoscope for precise visualization, and dissection of the implant pocket. The transaxillary approach avoids incisional scarring directly on the breast and places the incision in the inferior and anterior area of the axilla. The transaxillary incision usually provides adequate access when placing an inflatable round breast implant and, while not precluding, is more difficult for placement of a large pre-filled implant or an anatomically shaped device. The markings for transaxillary breast augmentation are also made with the patient in the sitting or upright position. The existing and resultant inframammary folds are marked, as are the boundaries of the proposed dissection. To locate and mark the incision, the patient's arm is placed in complete adduction and the most anterior aspect of the axilla is marked. The incision should not extend beyond this line. The arm is then abducted approximately 45°, and a prominent axillary crease is identified. Any fold may be used, but preference is given to one high in the axilla, which aids in instrumentation during the procedure. For saline-filled implants, the incision should generally be 2.5–3.5 cm. Silicone implants require larger incisions. The patient is placed on the operating table in the supine position with arms abducted 90° and secured to arm boards that allow 10- to 15-degree variations in abduction and adduction from 90°. She must be able to flex 90° at the waist during the procedure. The incision is made, and small sharp retractors are used to elevate the medial aspect of the incision. Superficial subcutaneous dissection to the lateral border of the pectoralis major prevents injury to the intercostobrachial nerve. Scissor dissection is employed with use of the electrocautery and insulated forceps to control any bleeding. The fascia of the pectoralis major muscle is visualized at the lateral edge of the muscle, and the dissection is carried deep to this for a subfascial placement or deep to the muscle for subpectoral placement. One must be certain the correct plane is entered before continuing the dissection further.

For an endoscopically assisted augmentation, the endoscope is passed into the transaxillary tunnel, and the subpectoral space is seen under direct vision. This allows a more controlled release of the pectoralis major origin with a long insulated electrocautery instrument. On completion of the dissection, implant sizers are used to evaluate the pocket and identify any areas that need final adjustment. This must be done with the patient in the sitting position. The pockets are then irrigated with an antibiotic solution,[52] and the final implants are inserted. Before closure, the patient is once again placed in the sitting position for a final check of the implant position. The pectoralis muscle fascia is repaired with a single absorbable suture, and the incision is closed in one or two layers. Steri-Strips are applied to the incision.

Transumbilical

The markings for transumbilical breast augmentation are similar to those for a standard inframammary fold approach. The patient is placed on the operating table in the same manner as for an inframammary augmentation. An additional mark is made with the patient supine: a line is drawn from the umbilicus to the medial border of the areola bilaterally. An incision is made within the umbilicus, large enough to easily accommodate an index finger. An endotube with a blunt obturator is passed just above the rectus fascia along the line from the umbilicus to the areola. Care is taken to constantly palpate the progress of the obturator with the surgeon's other hand, always keeping the force up and away from the abdominal and thoracic cavities. The endotube is advanced over the costal margin. For subglandular implant placement, the force applied to the endotube is directed upward at the inframammary fold to prevent the obturator from slipping beneath the pectoralis major. The tunnel ends just cephalad to the nipple. Subpectoral positioning is possible by careful technique with use of special instruments to enter the fascial plane high laterally. The obturator is then removed, and an endoscope may be used to verify correct pocket identification. Hemostasis is also ensured. Both the endotube and endoscope are removed from the tunnel, and an expander is rolled up and placed within the incision. The expander is "milked" up the tunnel by

manual external pressure. The expander is filled with saline to 150% of the final volume of the implant. Pocket adjustments can be made manually during filling. When the expansion is complete, the expander is drained and removed from the pocket by traction on the fill tube. The implant is placed and filled in exactly the same manner as the expander. The endotube is then replaced, and an endoscope may be used to verify implant position, valve patency, and hemostasis. The incision is closed with a single layer of absorbable suture. An abdominal binder is used for compression on the abdominal tunnels.

Postoperative care

In the overwhelming majority of cases, augmentation mammaplasty is performed as an outpatient procedure. Patients are given prescriptions for oral analgesics and a 3-day course of prophylactic oral antibiotics. The patient is shown yoga-type stretching exercises of the chest to be performed on the same day following her surgery. Patients are allowed to remove operative dressings and shower as desired starting on postoperative day one. The first follow-up visit is scheduled for 1–3 days after the procedure. If smooth (non-textured) implants were used, initiation of implant mobility exercises is recommended at this time. If the patient is at risk for superior implant displacement, a circumferential elastic strap may be used to apply continuous downward pressure during the early postoperative period. Patients are usually able to return to work a few days after surgery, but are not permitted to resume rigorous exercise for 2–3 weeks. Additional follow-up visits are scheduled at 4–6 weeks, 3 months, and 1 year. The importance of postoperative photo documentation and critical analysis of the operative outcomes cannot be overemphasized. It is the author's practice to place patients on vitamin E 400 IU once a day for two years to minimize capsular contracture. Although there are no evidence-based studies in the augmentation population on the use of vitamin E, there is encouraging evidence in the treatment of radiation-induced fibrosis (RIF) in mastectomy patients with radiation-induced morbidities related to scarring.[54]

Complications

Perioperative complications

Alterations of nipple sensitivity after augmentation mammaplasty may be manifested as either anesthesia or hyperesthesia and are thought to result from traction injury, bruising, or transection of the lateral intercostal cutaneous nerves. The incidence and severity of nipple sensation changes does not vary with the surgical approach employed.[55]

Periprosthetic seroma fluid is usually resorbed by the soft tissues within the first week of surgery, and use of topical antibiotics intraoperatively has been shown to decrease the rates.[56] The authors do not use drains for primary breast augmentation.

The development of a hematoma after breast augmentation has several deleterious effects in both the early and late postoperative period including pain, blood loss, disfigurement, and capsular contracture.[57] Preoperatively, patients should receive a list of prescription and over-the-counter medications that may contribute to excessive postoperative bleeding. It is imperative that patients discontinue any medications and herbal supplements that impair clotting or platelet function at least one week prior to surgery[44,45] (Table 3.1). If a hematoma does develop in the perioperative period, immediate evacuation of the hematoma and exploration of the pocket is recommended. Unfortunately, the source of the hematoma is only rarely identified at the time of the exploration. Patients may occasionally present with a delayed hematoma 1–2 weeks or even months to years after augmentation, and frequently a history of breast trauma is elicited. Expanding hematomas require exploration and drainage regardless of the length of time from the augmentation.

Table 3.1 Herbs, herbal teas, homeopathic medicines, and dietary supplements associated with an increased risk of bleeding

Supplement type	Supplement name(s)	Treatment uses	Other side effects (in addition to intrinsic bleeding risks)	Perioperative recommendations
Herbs and herbal extracts	Garlic *Allium sativum* Ajo	Hypertension, hypercholesterolemia, fungal infections, cancer, MI prevention, PVD	Nausea, vomiting, hypoglycemia, halitosis, potentiation of warfarin, increased INR, abdominal pain, diarrhea, oral ulcers, anaphylaxis (rare)	Discontinue 7 days before surgery[7] Resume 7 days after surgery
	Ginger *Zingiber officinale*	Nausea, vomiting, GI bloating, dyspepsia, OA, RA, migraine, homeostasis restoration, weight loss	Nausea, GI bloating, worsen cholecystitis, arrhythmia (possible), hypoglycemia	Discontinue 2–3 weeks before surgery* Resume 2 weeks after surgery
	Ginseng *Panax ginseng*	Stimulant, nausea, cancer prevention, CAD, DM2, dyspepsia, colic, infections, aging, stress, homeostasis restoration	Nausea, diarrhea, headaches, hypotension, hypertension, breast tenderness, hypoglycemia, insomnia (possible), interaction with warfarin	Discontinue 7 days before surgery[7,30] Resume 2 weeks after surgery
	Ginkgo *Ginkgo biloba* Maidenhair tree	Circulatory stimulant, dementia (Alzheimer's, multi-infarct), memory enhancement, PVD, ED	Nausea, vomiting, diarrhea, GI discomfort, headaches, palpitations, potentiates warfarin	Discontinue 36 hours or more before surgery[7] Resume 7 days after surgery
	Feverfew *Tanacetum parthenium*	Fever, migraine, OA, GI upset, infertility	Oral ulcers, allergic reactions, GI discomfort and bloating	Taper and discontinue by 2–3 weeks before surgery to avoid withdrawal syndrome with abrupt cessation[52] Resume 2 weeks after surgery
	Bromelain	Inflammation, OA, autoimmune disorders, menstrual pain, digestion, gout	GI discomfort, diarrhea, tachycardia, menorrhagia (possible)	Discontinue 2–3 weeks before surgery* Resume 2 weeks after surgery
	Liquorice/licorice *Glycyrrhiza glabra*	Aphthous ulcers, peptic ulcers, cancer, OA, adrenal insufficiency	Hypokalemic paralysis, hypertension, weight loss/gain, infertility, temporary vision loss	Discontinue 2–3 weeks before surgery* Resume 2 weeks after surgery

Table 3.1 Herbs, herbal teas, homeopathic medicines, and dietary supplements associated with an increased risk of bleeding—cont'd

Supplement type	Supplement name(s)	Treatment uses	Other side effects (in addition to intrinsic bleeding risks)	Perioperative recommendations
	Red chili pepper *Capsaicin*	Analgesic, chronic neuropathy, OA, uremic pruritus, psoriasis	Burning and stinging on contact, hypoglycemia, cough	Discontinue 2–3 weeks before surgery* Resume 2 weeks after surgery
	Saw palmetto *Serenoa repens*	BPH, urinary tract infections	Nausea, vomiting, diarrhea, rhinitis, decreased libido, headache	Discontinue 2–3 weeks before surgery* Resume 2 weeks after surgery
	Oil of wintergreen Methyl salicylate	OA, joint discomfort, hypertension, inflammation, cellulite, flavoring agent	Displaces warfarin, nausea, vomiting, dizziness, increased INR	Discontinue 2–3 weeks before surgery* Resume 2 weeks after surgery
	Devil's claw *Harpagophytum procumbens*	Analgesic, fever, digestion aid, OA, appetite stimulant	Diarrhea, GI discomfort, tinnitus, headache, hypoglycemia, arrhythmia (possible)	Discontinue 2–3 weeks before surgery* Resume 2 weeks after surgery
	Chinese agrimony *Agrimonia pilosa*	Analgesic, bacterial infection, helminthic infection, diarrhea, inflammation, cough, sore throat		Discontinue 2–3 weeks before surgery* Resume 2 weeks after surgery
	Danshen *Salvia miltiorrhiza*	Atherosclerosis, stroke, angina pectoris, hypercholesterolemia, cancer, HIV, menstrual disorders, OA, insomnia, prostatitis	Hypotension, GI discomfort, reduced appetite, pruritus, seizures (possible), potentiates warfarin	Discontinue 2–3 weeks before surgery* Resume 2 weeks after surgery
	Baical skullcap root *Scutellaria baicalensis*	Anxiety, inflammation, cancer, seizures, infections, insomnia, dysentery, diarrhea, rabies, menstrual disorders	Hepatotoxicity, pneumonitis	Discontinue 2–3 weeks before surgery* Resume 2 weeks after surgery
	Geum japonicum	Diuretic, astringent, CAD, hypercholesterolemia		Discontinue 2–3 weeks before surgery* Resume 2 weeks after surgery
	Chinese peony *Paeoniae rubra*	Inflammation, GI discomfort, spasm		Discontinue 2–3 weeks before surgery* Resume 2 weeks after surgery
	Poncitrin *Poncirus trifoliata*	Constipation, diarrhea, spasm, expectorant		Discontinue 2–3 weeks before surgery* Resume 2 weeks after surgery
	Fritillaria bulbs *Fritillaria cirrhosa*	Spasm, expectorant, hypertension, cough, asthma, opium toxicity		Discontinue 2–3 weeks before surgery* Resume 2 weeks after surgery
	Japanese honeysuckle *Lonicera japonica*	Fever, headache, cough, sore throat, bacterial infection, inflammation, ulcers		Discontinue 2–3 weeks before surgery* Resume 2 weeks after surgery

Continued

Table 3.1 Herbs, herbal teas, homeopathic medicines, and dietary supplements associated with an increased risk of bleeding—cont'd

Supplement type	Supplement name(s)	Treatment uses	Other side effects (in addition to intrinsic bleeding risks)	Perioperative recommendations
Herbal formulas	Kangen-karyu	Hypertension, arteriosclerosis, memory impairment, headache		Discontinue 2–3 weeks before surgery* Resume 2 weeks after surgery
	Bak foong pill	GI disturbances, cardiovascular disturbances, gynecological dysfunction		Discontinue 2–3 weeks before surgery* Resume 2 weeks after surgery
Herbal teas	Te gastronol	GI ulcers, intestinal inflammation, colitis, gastritis, flatulence		Discontinue 2–3 weeks before surgery* Resume 2 weeks after surgery
	Seasonal tonic	Appetite suppressant		Discontinue 2–3 weeks before surgery* Resume 2 weeks after surgery
Homeopathic medicines and other dietary supplements	Guīlínggāo Tortoise jelly	Fever, acne, enhancing circulation, improving intestinal function, constipation	None documented	Discontinue 2–3 weeks before surgery* Resume 2 weeks after surgery
	Vitamin E	Peyronie's disease, bladder cancer prevention, RA, Alzheimer's disease, PMS, movement disorders	Allergic reaction, fatigue, weakness, headache, nausea, diarrhea, vision disturbance, congenital heart defects *in utero*, heart failure	Discontinue 2–3 weeks before surgery* Resume when healing is complete[3]
	Arnica montana Leopard's bane Wolf's bane	OA, sprains, joint pain, inflammation	Gastroenteritis	Discontinue 2–3 weeks before surgery* Resume 2 weeks after surgery
	Fish oil Eicosapentaenoic acid	Hypertension, hypertriglyceridemia, RA, angina pectoris, atherosclerosis	Hemorrhagic stroke, GI disturbances and bloating, diarrhea, hyperglycemia (possible)	Discontinue 2–3 weeks before surgery* Resume 2 weeks after surgery
	Chondroitin	OA	Nausea, diarrhea, constipation, GI disturbances	Discontinue 2–3 weeks before surgery* Resume 2 weeks after surgery
	Glucosamine	OA	Hypoglycemia, nausea, diarrhea, headache, insomnia, GI disturbances	Discontinue 2–3 weeks before surgery* Resume 2 weeks after surgery

CAD, coronary artery disease; DM2, diabetes mellitus Type II; ED, erectile dysfunction; GI, gastrointestinal; HIV, human immunodeficiency virus; INR, International Normalized Ratio; MI, myocardial infarction; OA, osteoarthritis; PVD, peripheral vascular disease; RA, rheumatoid arthritis. See also references 67-71.

Nonoperative management of small nonexpanding hematomas is one option, but places the patient at a higher risk of subsequent periprosthetic capsular contracture.

Postoperative wound infection may present with a spectrum of severity ranging from a mild cellulitis of the breast skin to a purulent periprosthetic space infection. The organism *Staphylococcus epidermidis* is part of the normal skin flora and is the most frequently identified pathogen in postoperative wound infections. Patients are given prophylactic antibiotics intraoperatively and postoperatively to reduce the risk of infection. Sterile technique is maintained during the procedure and the implant pocket is irrigated with an antibiotic solution containing 50 000 units of bacitracin, 1 g of cefazolin, and 80 mg of gentamicin per 500 mL of saline.[52] Further reduction of risk for bacterial contamination may be achieved by employing the *no-touch* technique in which only the surgeon handles the implant with fresh, powder-free gloves. The implant is then inserted through a sterile sleeve to minimize contact with the patient's skin and inflated using a sterile closed filling system. A significant number of postoperative wound infections will respond to oral or intravenous antibiotics if therapy is initiated very early in the course of the infection. If the infection persists or progresses, then the implant should be removed and the wound should be allowed to heal over a drain or in severe cases by secondary intention. Once the infection has totally cleared, a secondary augmentation and scar revision should be planned in 6–12 months.

Mondor's disease is a superficial thrombophlebitis of the breast that may occur in up to 1–2% of augmentation patients.[58,59] This process usually affects the veins along the inferior aspect of the breast and occurs most frequently with the inframammary approach. Fortunately, this is a self-limiting process that usually resolves with warm compresses over a period of several weeks.

Delayed complications of augmentation mammaplasty

Periprosthetic capsular contracture

One of the most common delayed complications of augmentation mammaplasty is the development of a palpable and deforming periprosthetic capsular contracture. All surgical implants undergo some degree of encapsulation due to the natural foreign body reaction by the surrounding tissues. Clinically significant periprosthetic capsular contracture is characterized by excessive scar formation that leads to firmness, distortion, and displacement of the breast implant. Histological examination of these contractures reveals circumferential linear fibrosis that is especially severe when formed in response to smooth shell implants. In 1975, Baker proposed a clinical classification system of capsular contracture after augmentation that is still commonly used to describe periprosthetic contractures[60] (Table 3.2).

While several factors have been identified which contribute to capsular contracture, the precise etiology remains unknown. The hypertrophic, circumferential linear scar probably involves stimulation of myofibroblasts that are known to be present within the periprosthetic capsule. Irritation caused by periprosthetic hematoma, seroma, or silicone gel bleed may incite the capsular contracture. Other foreign body particles such as glove powder, lint, or dust may also contribute to the

Table 3.2 Grades of capsular contracture	
Grade I	Capsular contracture of the augmented breast feels as soft as an unoperated breast.
Grade II	Capsular contracture is minimal. The breast is less soft than an unoperated breast. The implant can be palpated but is not visible.
Grade III	Capsular contracture is moderate. The breast is firmer. The implant can be palpated easily and may be distorted or visible.
Grade IV	Capsular contracture is severe. The breast is hard, tender, and painful, with significant distortion present. The capsule thickness is not directly proportional to palpable firmness, although some relationship may exist.

process.[61] Infectious etiologies have also been studied and are thought to play a role.[61] This theory describes a chronic subclinical infection located immediately adjacent to the implant shell within a microscopic biofilm that is relatively inaccessible to cellular and humoral immune function. Many strategies have been employed to prevent periprosthetic capsular contracture. One strategy has been the creation of a large implant pocket and maintenance of this oversized pocket with implant displacement exercises. The use of implants with textured surfaces has been described above and has been shown to reduce the rate of capsular contracture in breast augmentation. Other efforts have focused on minimizing operative trauma in order to reduce the risk of seroma or hematoma formation. Seromas, hematomas, and even blood staining of the periprosthetic tissues may incite capsular contracture. Any bleeding that does occur during the dissection needs to be controlled, and the staining of the tissues with blood should be diluted with copious irrigation fluid.

Leukotriene receptor antagonists that are used to treat asthma were studied in capsular contracture but are recommended to be used cautiously due to their side effects.[62,63] Specifically zafirlukast (Accolate) and montelukast (Singulair) have been shown to reverse clinical signs of capsular contracture in patients taking the medication for asthma.[62,63] Treatment of established capsular contractures usually requires operative intervention. This is discussed more completely in Chapter 4. Open capsulotomy involves scoring the capsule circumferentially, and anteriorly to adequately release and expand the soft-tissue envelope. With very thick fibrous capsules, or with calcified capsules containing silicone granulomas, it is often necessary to perform either a partial or complete capsulectomy to correct the deformity. This is often extremely effective in treating advanced grade IV capsular contractures, especially when the implant is replaced with a saline-filled or a no-bleed silicone gel-filled implant. Implant site change surgery has become popular for treating established or recurrent capsular contracture.[64–66] Revisionary surgery will be discussed in the next chapter in detail.

Implant rupture and deflation

Any defect in the silicone elastomer shell of a saline-filled breast implant will ultimately result in *deflation* of the implant. The saline filling material leaks out of the implant and is harmlessly absorbed by the surrounding tissues. Clinical recognition of deflation is usually made by the patient and virtually always requires surgical explantation and replacement of the implant. A history of recent trauma is frequently elicited with deflation, and true *spontaneous* failure of the implant shell is relatively rare.

MRI of the breast is considered the state-of-the-art technique for evaluating breast implant integrity. Modern fourth- and fifth-generation silicone gel are substantially more cohesive than the second- and third-generation gel and less likely to leak into the surrounding tissues, even when the implant shell is ruptured.

Secondary procedures

Revisionary breast surgery (secondary or tertiary), which is often performed for the late complications of breast augmentation, poses a continual challenge to plastic surgeons. These procedures are complex, challenging, and unpredictable. Over the years, we have been dealing with thinned breast tissues from large implants that have been placed either in subglandular or subpectoral space leading to some long-term complications, such as implant extrusion, gel bleed, rupture with extravasation of gel, saline implant deflation, capsular contracture, palpability, rippling, "double bubble", "snoopy breast", symmastia, and implant malposition.

Historically, our options for revision and improvement have included, replacing saline implants with gel implants, using capsular flaps to gain additional stability and coverage, or performing a site change operation. None of these procedures have resulted in complete resolution of the described complaints. The detailed management of revisionary procedures will be discussed in Chapter 17.

🌐 Access the complete reference list online at **http://www.expertconsult.com**

22. Cunningham B. The Mentor Study on Contour Profile Gel Silicone MemoryGel Breast Implants. *Plast Reconstr Surg.* 2007;120:33S–39S.

24. Cunningham B, McCue J. Safety and effectiveness of Mentor's MemoryGel implants at 6 years. *Aesthetic Plast Surg.* 2009;33:440–444. *The authors update on the post approval study for Mentor Corporation. The study shows that Mentor MemoryGel silicone breast implants represent a safe and effective choice for women seeking breast augmentation or breast reconstruction following mastectomy.*

26. Bengtson BP, Van Natta BW, Murphy DK, et al. Style 410 highly cohesive silicone breast implant core study results at 3 years. *Plast Reconstr Surg.* 2007;120:40S–48S.

41. Spear SL, Murphy DK, Slicton A, Walker PS. Inamed silicone breast implant core study results at 6 years. *Plast Reconstr Surg.* 2007;120:8S–16S, discussion 7S–8S. *The authors update on the post approval study for Allergan Corporation. The study demonstrates the safety and effectiveness of Natrelle (formerly Inamed) silicone-filled breast implants through 6 years, including a low rupture rate and high satisfaction rate.*

44. Tebbetts JB. Dual plane breast augmentation: optimizing implant-soft-tissue relationships in a wide range of breast types. *Plast Reconstr Surg.* 2001;107:1255–1272. *This article describes specific indications and techniques for a dual-plane approach to breast augmentation. Indications, operative techniques, results, and*

complications for this series of patients are presented. Dual-plane augmentation mammaplasty adjusts implant and tissue relationships to ensure adequate soft-tissue coverage while optimizing implant–soft-tissue dynamics to offer increased benefits and fewer trade-offs compared with a single pocket location in a wide range of breast types.

52. Adams WP Jr, Rios JL, Smith SJ. Enhancing patient outcomes in aesthetic and reconstructive breast surgery using triple antibiotic breast irrigation: six-year prospective clinical study. *Plast Reconstr Surg.* 2006;117:30–36. *The authors show the clinical importance of the use of triple antibiotic breast irrigation. This study shows the lower incidence of capsular contracture compared with other published reports, and its clinical efficacy supports previously published in vitro studies. Application of triple antibiotic irrigation is recommended for all aesthetic and reconstructive breast procedures and is cost effective.*

54. Magnusson M, Hoglund P, Johansson K, et al. Pentoxifylline and vitamin E treatment for prevention of radiation-induced side-effects in women with breast cancer: a phase two, double-blind, placebo-controlled randomised clinical trial (Ptx-5). *Eur J Cancer.* 2009;45:2488–2495.

60. Spear SL, Baker JL Jr. Classification of capsular contracture after prosthetic breast reconstruction. *Plast Reconstr Surg.* 1995;96:1119–1123, discussion 1124.

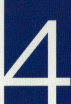

Breast augmentation

M. Bradley Calobrace

SYNOPSIS

- Breast augmentation is one of the most commonly performed aesthetic procedures in the United States and abroad.

- Preoperative assessment should determine the appropriate approach including choice of implant, breast pocket (submuscular, subfascial, subglandular, subpectoral with dual plane), incision location (inframammary, periareolar, transaxillary, transumbilical), and the need to lower the inframammary fold.

- Implant selection has expanded over the past few years to include many variables including implant fill (saline or silicone), implant shell surface (smooth or textured), implant form (round or shaped), implant dimensions (width, size, projections), and implant cohesiveness (fourth- or fifth-generation implants) with associated differences in form stability and implant softness.

- Inframammary fold positioning is critical to establishing optimal implant placement in the pocket.

- Surgical approach, implant choice, and operative technique can impact the incidence of complications, including implant malposition and capsular contracture.

Introduction

The primary indication for breast augmentation is simply inadequate volume of breast tissue, or glandular hypoplasia. This may occur from either a developmental or involutional process. Developmental hypoplasia may be either primary in nature or secondary to other developmental problems such as thoracic hypoplasia (Poland syndrome) or other chest wall deformities (pectus excavatum). Whereas developmental hypoplasia often involves deficiencies of skin, subcutaneous tissue and underlying glandular tissue, involutional changes involve hypoplasia of the glandular breast tissue with often a relative excess of skin and subcutaneous tissue.

Involutional hypoplasia usually manifests as glandular ptosis or pseudoptosis which is most associated with postpartum breast, but can likewise be affected by breastfeeding, hormonal changes and weight fluctuations. Breast augmentation is likewise performed for psychological reasons.[1] Several studies revealed that women seeking breast augmentation feel their breasts are inadequate and can create doubt as to her femininity and desirability.[2–4] Inadequate breast size as compared to the norm has been associated with low self-esteem, negative body image and feelings of inadequacy.[5] This can negatively impact interpersonal relationships, sexual fulfillment and quality of life.[6]

Access the Historical Perspective section and Table 4.1 online at

http://www.expertconsult.com

Preoperative planning

One of the most critical steps in achieving excellence in breast augmentation is the preoperative evaluation. The initial consultation should evaluate the patient's goals and expectations for the breast augmentation procedure. Patients have often done a lot of research about the procedure and the surgeon and may be seeking multiple consultations prior to making a decision. The surgeon's evaluation should be able to establish the patient as well-informed, stable and possessing reasonable expectations for the procedure. A thorough history and physical examination are essential to identify any risk factors for the procedure. Screening mammograms, although not mandatory, are usually recommended for patients aged 35 and older or even younger if a significant family history or risk factors are identified.

In the preoperative assessment, it is important to understand the goals of the patient and what type of look she finds appealing. Whereas the look of the breast is rather subjective and is undoubtedly influenced by cultural elements as well as personal preference, most would agree there are certain shared characteristics of the female breast form that create an ideal aesthetic. The characteristics including a full, sloping upper pole that leads to a fuller, gently curving lower pole. The nipple areolar complex is centralized on the breast positioned at the point of maximal projection on the breast mound above the inframammary fold. The breast mound itself is composed of parenchymal breast tissue lying on the anterior chest wall surrounded and enveloped with a soft-tissue covering made up of skin and adipose tissue (see Fig. 3.1).

A thorough evaluation of the breast form includes a complete evaluation of the breast and chest wall as well as taking precise measurements using the nipple areolar complex and inframammary fold as key landmarks. The preoperative markings create a roadmap for the planned procedure (Fig. 4.1). It is imperative to critically evaluate for asymmetries, including the chest wall, inframammary fold, volume, and nipple areolar complex position. A thorough exam for any palpable masses or lymph nodes should also be performed. A more subjective analysis includes the evaluation of the soft-tissue coverage including quality of skin and breast tissue,

amount of breast parenchyma present and the level of ptosis. This is essential in determining the optimal pocket for implant placement. The elasticity of the skin should likewise be assessed. Stretching the skin and noting redundancy as well as evaluation for looseness of the skin and stretch marks provide important information. This can greatly influence the surgical approach and implant selection.

Measurements

There are important measurements that should be a part of every evaluation for a breast augmentation (see Fig. 3.5).

Base diameter

The most important measurement is base diameter. This provides important information in implant selection, as each implant has a unique base diameter as well. It is important to realize that while each patient has a fixed breast base diameter, the *measured (actual) breast diameter*, an equally important determination is the *desired (or ideal) breast diameter* when determining implant selection. This is especially important when the breast is very narrow and the base width of the breast needs to be expanded to create an ideal breast. This measurement can be rather subjective based on the anatomy but is often the distance from the anterior axillary line to 1 cm lateral to the midline.

Sternal notch to nipple

The next measurement is the sternal notch to nipple (SN–N) distance which provides information on the length of the thorax and the position of the breast on the chest.

Breast height

It is helpful to measure the breast height to assess upper pole volume and coverage and to assess symmetry. The SN–N and breast height measurements are especially important when selecting whether to use a round implant or a shaped implant of variable heights.

Nipple to inframammary fold

A key measurement is the distance from the nipple to the inframammary fold in relaxed position and on stretch. The distance under stretch provides important information about the amount of skin available in the lower pole of the breast. Inadequate skin in the lower pole may require lowering the fold for appropriate implant positioning. On the contrary, excessive skin in the lower pole may be a determinant for pocket

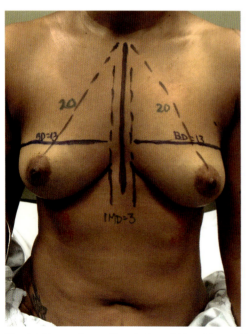

Fig. 4.1 Preoperative markings in the upright position provide critical landmarks for the planned procedure.

selection to expand the skin in the lower pole or even the need for a mastopexy.

Pinch test

The soft-tissue pinch test is useful in assessing the upper pole of the breast by pinching the tissue between the examiner's index finger and thumb. As a general rule, if the pinch is less than 2 cm, implant placement should be subpectoral to avoid upper pole wrinkling. If the tissue pinch thickness is greater than 2 cm, the subglandular/subfascial plane could also be considered.

Imaging systems

In addition to manual measurements, 3D and 4D imaging is now available and can assist in the evaluation process. Some of the systems automatically provide all the measurements. Likewise, an impressive evaluation of the soft-tissue contributions, breast shape and size and chest wall are a part of the assessment. These automated 4D systems are based on biodimensional principles and are often more accurate in visualizing small asymmetries in the chest wall and/or breast[25] (see Figs. 3.2–3.4). This evaluation has the added advantage of allowing the patient to visualize not only her breast but also the small asymmetries highlighted in the 4D evaluation. Patients can also visualize simulations of different breast implants possible for the augmentations, increasing their understanding and confidence in the final decision.

Informed consent

An appropriate informed consent requires an evaluation of the emotional state of the patient and the appropriateness of the procedure for the desired outcome. The entire consultation is part of the informed consent: listening to the patient's desires, evaluating for surgery, explaining the procedure and educating on the risk, benefits and alternatives to the planned approach. The official consent of the American Society of Plastic Surgeons can be helpful. The implant manufacturers also provide additional supplemental educational materials and patient handbooks that review all of the information included as part of a comprehensive informed consent. The informed consent must be signed and witnessed and included as part of the patient's medical record. The use of before and after photographs that fairly represent the procedure and anticipated results can be helpful. Likewise, photographing the patient is an essential part of documentation and requires appropriate permission and assurance of confidentiality. Permission to utilize the patient's photographs for

anything other than medical review is a requirement and should be documented. There are many options available in breast augmentation and many of the decisions are subjective and based on the desires of the patient for a particular outcome. It takes clear communication that is appropriately documented on the desired shape and size of the breast and the plan to achieve the result. It is often helpful to make the patient a part of that process through 4D imaging or trying on implants with sizers so the selected implant is a mutual decision between the surgeon and the patient.

Operative planning

Incision length and placement

The decision on incision placement is based on a variety of variables, including patient and surgeon preferences, anatomic considerations, implant type and size. The size of the incision depends on the location, but in general should be as small as possible and yet large enough to safely dissect the pocket and place the implant without distortion or injury to the device. In general, the length of the incision would be smaller with saline compared to silicone implants, and longer when placing more cohesive implants, larger implants and/or textured implants. Fractures of form-stable cohesive implants and rupture or distortion of silicone implants have been associated with attempting to place implants through incisions inadequate to accommodate the implant. Additionally, the quality of the scar is often better if a slightly larger scar is utilized, reducing the stretch and retraction injury placed on the scar. Incision length ranges include: 3–4.5 cm for saline implants, 4–6 cm for silicone round implants and 4.5–7 cm for shaped cohesive silicone implants.

There are four different incision options for breast augmentation: inframammary, periareolar, transaxillary and transumbilical. Each incision has distinct advantages and disadvantages that must be discussed with the patient. After implant selection, the choice of incision should be based on surgeon comfort with the technique, patient desire, and the ability to provide optimal control and visualization to achieve the desired outcome for the implant selected.

Inframammary incision

The inframammary incision is the most commonly used due to its direct access and visualization of the pocket with the least injury to surrounding structures. This incision can be used to access the subglandular, subfascial or subpectoral space and can be utilized with virtually any of the implants. The incision should be placed in the location of the planned inframammary fold position, which may be at the native fold or potentially lower if the fold is repositioned.

Periareolar incision

Although used less often in the past few years, this incision can be very useful for someone wanting to avoid a scar in the fold of the breast. It is most inconspicuous when there is a distinct border and a marked color contrast between the areolar skin and surrounding breast skin. This incision allows direct access for adjustments in the inframammary fold position and in parenchymal scoring and release often needed in constricted breast deformity. Disadvantages of this incision include transection of the ducts colonized potentially with bacteria, visible scarring in front of breast mound, possibly greater nipple sensitivity changes and limited exposure of the surgical field. Patients with smaller areolar complexes may also be inappropriate due to difficulty in implant placement, especially with larger, textured or shaped implants, as injury to the implant can occur while trying to place an implant through the longer breast tunnel associated with these incisions.

Transaxillary incision

This approach avoids any scar on the breast mound with the incision placed deep in the axillary space. The access allows pocket creation either bluntly or with the aid of an endoscope. The endoscopic approach is preferred due to the ability to maintain prospective hemostasis through direct visualization and precise release of the pectoralis muscle above the inframammary fold. Saline or silicone implants can be placed through this incision, either above or below the pectoralis muscle. The placement of shaped implants, more cohesive implants and larger implants can be more challenging and may not be possible in every situation. The use of an insertion sleeve can be very useful in providing ease of placement.

Transumbilical incision

This incision is located in the upper portion of the umbilicus and is very well hidden and remote. A clear disadvantage is only being able to place saline implants through this incision, which has made this access incision less utilized in the past few years with the increased use of silicone implants in the United States. The dissection is performed bluntly and no direct visualization is possible to provide prospective hemostasis. Revisions are generally not possible through this incision and a second incision is usually required.

Inframammary fold positioning

Predicting the final position of the inframammary fold is critical to determining the placement of all breast incisions, but especially the inframammary incision. This can be a challenging task as so many variables contribute to the final position of the fold. The inframammary fold is formed by the fusion of the anterior and posterior leaves of the superficial fascia which is intimately associated with the dermis at the lowest aspect of the inferior pole of the breast.[26] Prior to surgery, the inframammary fold (IMF) is identified and marked in the sitting position. The true IMF position is actually determined by performing an IMF expansion test. The breast is grasped and auto-rotated inferiorly to identify the inferior extent of the attachments of the inframammary fold (Fig. 4.2). This is the best predictor of where the fold will naturally sit after breast augmentation. The amount of lower pole skin required and the ultimate position of the fold is a function of many factors, including the type of implant (saline vs. silicone, round vs. shaped), size of implant, pocket location and the strength and stability of the soft tissue of the lower pole. The distance measured from the nipple to true fold under maximal stretch assesses the amount of lower pole skin available to accommodate the selected implant. An acceptable standard that has been used is an implant with a base diameter of 11 cm requires 7 cm, a base diameter of 12 cm requires 8 cm, and a base diameter of 13 cm requires 9 cm.[27] A more comprehensive evaluation has been described using tissue-based planning principles.[28] In the High Five System analysis, variables are analyzed including implant volume, patient's base

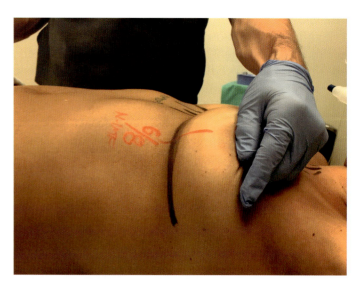

Fig. 4.2 The true fold, the best predictor of where the fold will lie postoperatively, is assessed by autorotation of the breast inferiorly to identify the inferior extent of the fascial attachments at the fold.

width, implant base width, anterior pulled skin stretch, and nipple-to-fold distance under maximal stretch. Based on the selected implant, a reference chart provides the desired nipple-to-fold distance, which if longer than the measured distance, will require IMF lowering. In determining fold position, the author has found an alternative method extremely useful. This calculation takes into consideration implant selections that may fall outside the limits of appropriate tissue-based planning. The required distance from nipple to fold is calculated as a function of implant height and implant projection, which is useful for both round and shaped implants.

Optimal N-IMF distance = ½ implant projection
+ ½ implant height

IMF Lowering = Optimal N-IMF distance
– measured N-IMF distance (maximum stretch)

If the desired nipple-to-inframammary fold (N–IMF) distance is equal or less than the measured N–IMF distance, then the fold does not require lowering. The distance can be adjusted based upon expectation for lower pole stretch postoperatively. This observation has become increasingly important as more textured round and shaped implants are being used. It is important to recognize that inframammary fold lowering is less often required when placing a smooth silicone implant, especially if higher profile or larger sized implants are used secondary to lower pole stretch over time[29,30] (Fig. 4.3). However, when placing textured implants, inframammary fold lowering may be required more often compared to smooth implants due less lower pole stretch and inferior implant descent created by the frictional component or adherence of the texture in the implant pocket.[31,32] Likewise, shaped implants are not only textured but also have a greater volume of a more cohesive gel present in the lower pole of the implant, thus requiring more lower pole skin to accommodate the implant.[33–38] Box 4.1 identifies some implant and soft-tissue characteristics that may be associated with greater need to lower the inframammary fold due to less postoperative stretching of the lower pole.[28–38]

Pocket position

There continues to be divergent thought as to the optimal pocket for breast implants. The subglandular/subfascial pocket is the most natural for the implant with avoidance of animation deformities seen with submuscular implants, enhanced correction of constricted breast or ptotic breasts, ease of dissection and less postoperative discomfort for the patient[39–42] (Fig. 4.4). The subfascial placement may have some advantages to subglandular placement. The implant is placed between the anterior fascia of the pectoralis major and the muscle itself which may provide additional support to the overlying soft-tissue envelope, less distortion of the breast form and decreasing mobility of the implant in the pocket (see Fig. 3.6). It has been widely accepted that an upper pole pinch test of 2 cm is required to place an implant in the subglandular/subfascial pocket to reduce the risk of upper pole implant visibility or wrinkling. Although data is mixed and not completely established as of yet, there is some emerging evidence that textured implants may be advantageous in the subglandular/subfascial pocket to reduce the incidence of capsular contracture.[32,43–45]

However, maximizing soft-tissue coverage whenever possible has been one of the most important guiding principles for success in breast augmentation. Inadequate coverage, often combined with heavy, oversized implants, leads to soft-tissue parenchymal atrophy, skin stretching due to the pressure and weight of the implant, and ultimately wrinkling and palpability of the implants and associated breast deformities.[29,30] The subpectoral pocket provides the greatest coverage for the implant and is performed by creating a pocket between the pectoralis major muscle and the chest wall and the advantages have included lower capsular contracture rates, enhanced coverage of the implant minimizing issues of wrinkling, creation of a more natural, sloping upper pole and enhanced support for the breast implant.[32,39,43,46,47] Undoubtedly, the issues of wrinkling and need for enhanced coverage with saline implants provided the impetus for subpectoral pockets becoming the preferred pocket by US surgeons.

The challenges with a purely subpectoral implant is greater animation distortion, the inability to expand the lower pole of a ptotic breast, and lack of exposure of the lower pole for parenchymal scoring (such as with a constricted breast deformity). Thus, the author's preferred pocket is the dual plane pocket. In all actuality, a subpectoral placement where the origin of the muscle is

---

BOX 4.1 **Characteristics associated with less stretching of the lower pole**

Textured implants

Cohesive implants

Shaped implants

Silicone compared to saline implants

Lower profile implants

Smaller implants

Tight, firm breast skin

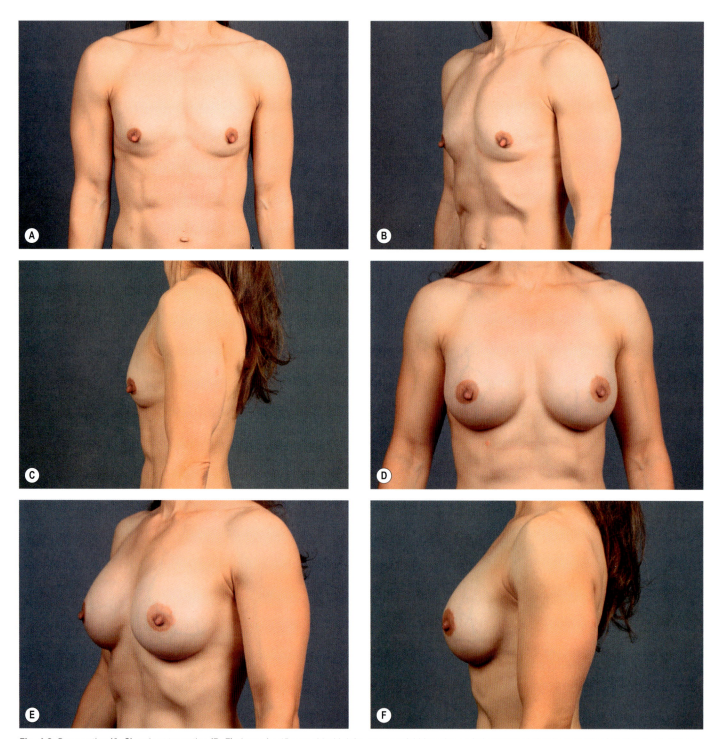

Fig. 4.3 Preoperative **(A–C)** and postoperative **(D–F)** views of a 45-year-old with inframammary fold lowering and placement of classic anatomic shaped textured 400 cc implants.

divided above the fold constitutes a level 1 dual plane, as the lower portion below the division technically places the implant in the subglandular plane (Fig. 4.5). The dual plane, initially described by Tebbetts, maximizes coverage and support of the breast implant while allowing for exposure and expansion of the lower pole when indicated.[47] In the dual plane, the pectoralis muscle covers over the superior portion of the implant and the lower portion of the implant is subglandular (Fig. 4.6). The greater the level of dual plane, the greater portion of the lower pole covering the implant is subglandular (see Fig. 3.10).

Pocket control

No matter which pocket is selected, it is helpful during the marking process to identify as accurately as

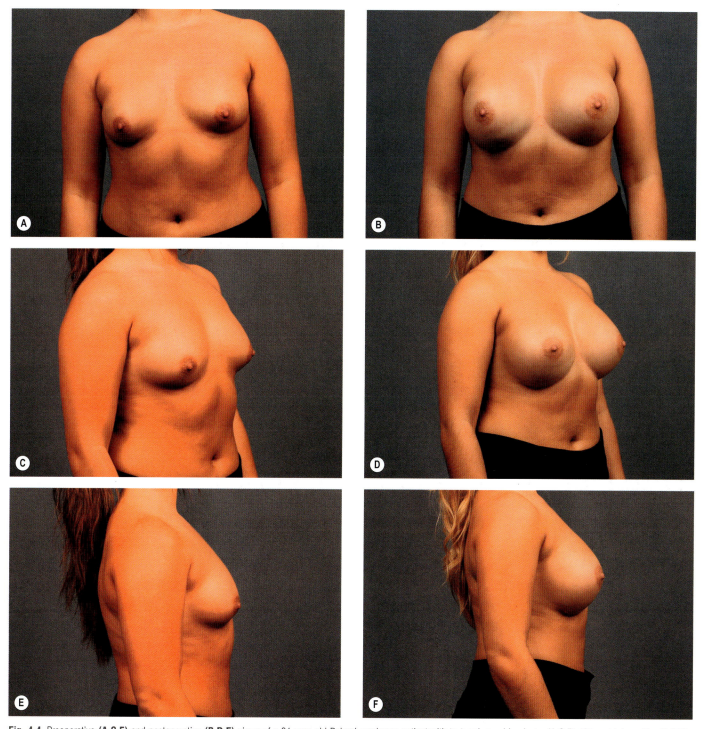

Fig. 4.4 Preoperative **(A,C,E)** and postoperative **(B,D,F)** views of a 31-year-old Poland syndrome patient with textured round implants. (A,C,E) 425 cc high profile; (B,D,F) 320 cc moderate profile in subfascial position.

possible the pocket size necessary to accommodate the selected implant. This will provide a pocket that maintains the implant in a controlled position and minimizes the risk of postoperative implant malposition. In breast augmentation with round implants, the accurate placement of the inframammary fold and control of the medial and lateral extent of the pockets provide ideal implant positioning to achieve the desired cleavage and minimize lateral migration of the implant.[31] When using a shaped implant, a controlled pocket is even more essential to minimize the risk of implant rotation postoperatively.[33,36,38] This requires not only controlling the pocket similar to a round implant, but additionally limiting the dissection of the superior pocket to snuggly accommodate the height of the shaped implant.

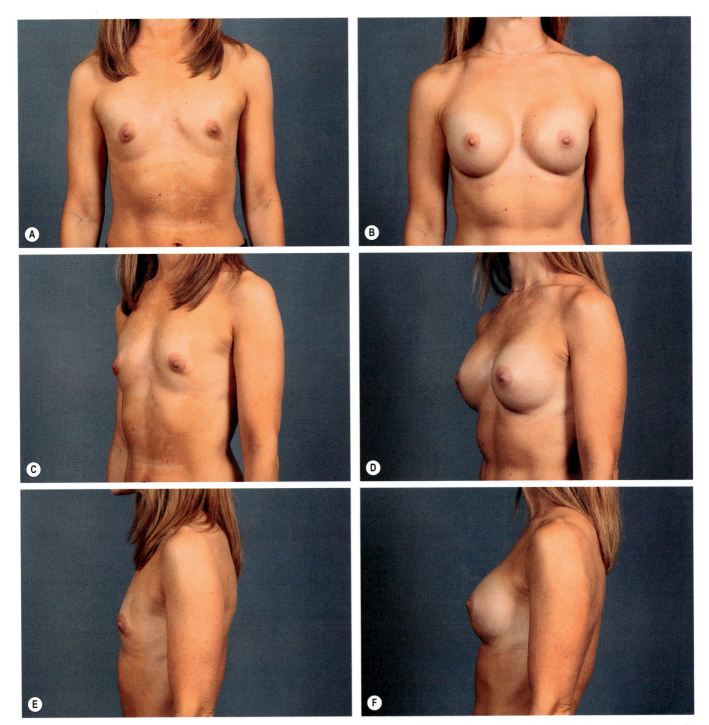

Fig. 4.5 Preoperative **(A,C,E)** and postoperative **(B,D,F)** views of a 43-year-old with smooth round 235 cc moderate profile implants in the submuscular (dual plane 1) position.

Implant selection

Filler material

In the United States there are currently two broad categories of implants based on the filler material: saline and silicone. The ultimate decision between using saline and silicone implant is ultimately the patient's after a thorough discussion of the differences, risk and benefits of each of these implants. Saline implants can be placed subpectoral with excellent aesthetic results. The incisions to place saline implants are smaller and differential fill of saline implants allows easy correction of minor breast or chest wall asymmetries. In thinner patients or when implants are placed subglandular, wrinkling becomes palpable in almost all cases and visible in some. It is generally agreed that silicone implants convey a much more natural, softer feel as compared to saline implants. Within the silicone category, there are different options

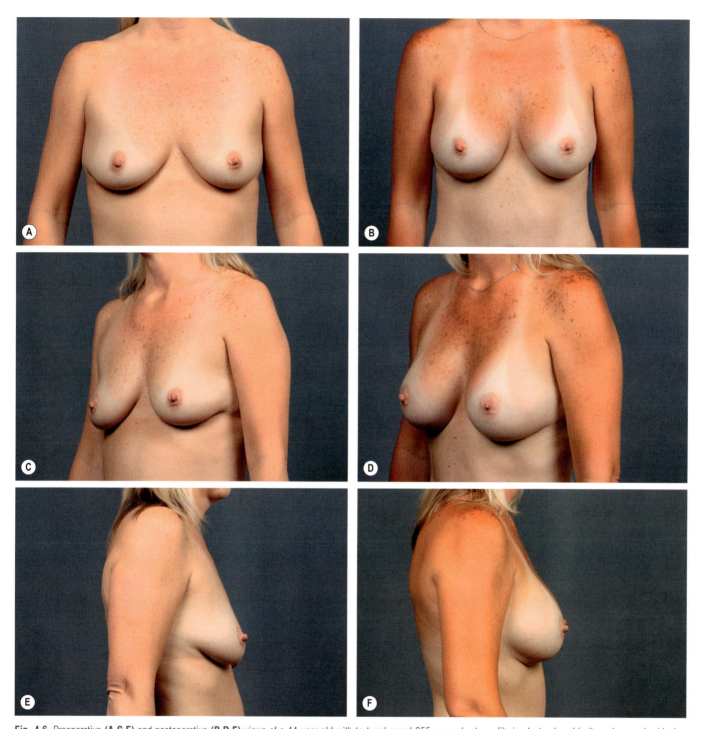

Fig. 4.6 Preoperative **(A,C,E)** and postoperative **(B,D,F)** views of a 44-year-old with textured round 355 cc moderate profile implants placed in the submuscular (dual plane 2) position to allow for adequate redraping of the pseudoptotic breast tissue over the implant.

based on the cohesiveness of the silicone gel within the implant. Silicone is a mixture of semi-inorganic morpolymeric molecules composed of varying length chains of polydimethyl siloxane monomers. The physical properties of silicone are quite variable depending on the average polymer chain length and the degree of cross-linking between the polymer chains. Silicone gels can be produced with varying viscosities by varying the length of the polymer chain or the amount of cross-linking. The

Allergan Natrelle implant and Mentor MemoryGel implants represent the fourth generation implants utilized since the early 1990s and FDA-approved for general use in 2006. The silicone gel in these implants is cohesive in nature with a cross-linked silicone gel, yet has a very soft feel. More recently, the term "cohesive" and "form-stable" have been used interchangeably to describe a newer generation of implants that are even more cohesive in nature with greater cross-linking, allowing the implants to maintain their shape in different positions and to resist the inherent deforming pressure and forces of the surrounding breast tissue. The greater cohesiveness of the silicone gel used in the implants has allowed not only more form-stable round implants but also the creation of implants with anatomic shape. The gel of the fifth generation implants is more cohesive and includes the Sientra HSC and Allergan's Natrelle Inspira cohesive round implants and the Sientra HSC+, Mentor MemoryShape and Allergan 410 cohesive silicone gel shaped implants. As form stability increases, so does the firmness of the implant. The Mentor MemoryShape implants are more form-stable than their Sientra HSC counterpart but less than Allergan's Style 410. Therefore, the Mentor MemoryShape would be considered softer than the Allergan 410 but firmer than the Sientra HSC. It is this balance between form stability and implant softness that characterizes each implant, and these attributes will ultimately contribute to implant performance and patient satisfaction.

Implant size

The selection of implant size is based both on the goals of the patient and the surgeon's assessment. Many approaches have been described including the biodimensional approach or the BodyLogic approach to implant selection. More elaborate systems such as the High-Five, as previously mentioned, can be used as well. In general, critical assessments in determining size include the dimensions of the breast, the compliance or stretch of the soft-tissue envelope and the desired volume for the resultant augmentation. As mentioned previously, the width of the breast is related to the width of the chest wall. It is critical to select an implant width that respects this width in order to maintain the normal landmarks such as the anterior axillary line and the appropriate cleavage and intermammary distance (see Fig. 3.11). Not respecting these landmarks may lead to an unnatural and deformed appearance. Size of implant is not only the width, but also the height and projection. In round implants, the width and height are the same, but in shaped implants they are sometimes different. The projection can vary within any one breast implant width and provide less or more volume while respecting the width dimension. The projection is determined in part by the compliance and potential laxity in the breast envelope, but also by the patient's desired look. A lower profile implant would provide less volume and a more natural look and is more appropriate when the breast envelope is tight. A higher projecting implant is used when breast soft-tissue laxity requires projection and volume to fill out the envelope and in patient's desire a more rounded, augmented look.

There is no doubt a patient's request for a particular breast size or shape greatly determines the dimensions of the breast implant utilized. In addition to physical assessment and a discussion with the patient, additional maneuvers may prove helpful including trying on some type of implant sizer or the use of a 4D imaging system to demonstrate for the patient the outcomes anticipated based on the implant selected.

Implant surface texture

The decision on whether to use a smooth or textured implant is really only applicable to round implants, as all anatomic shaped implants require texture to maintain their orientation and prevent rotation. In the past few decades when only saline and fourth generation round silicone implants were available in the United States, smooth surface devices were used in the vast majority of cases. For round devices, texture may impart some reduction in the capsular contracture rate and maintain its position within the breast pocket, especially with associated chest wall asymmetries or abnormalities. There is emerging evidence the texturing reduces the capsular contracture rates when placed subglandular/subfascial.[32,43-45] When placed submuscular, the smooth and textured devices have similar capsular contracture rates, although some recent data reveals a possible small protective effect of texture even in the submuscular position.[32,43] Recently, with greater choices of implants including shaped devices from all three manufacturers in the US, the use of texture devices has increased significantly. The textured surface creates a frictional interface between the implant surface and the capsule that tends to help the implant remain properly oriented.

Each manufacturer has a proprietary type of surface texture. The Mentor texture is created by pressing a thin sheet of polyurethane foam into a tacky thin sheet of silicone, imprinting the shell with a Siltex texture. This is the least aggressive texture and actual tissue ingrowth does not occur. The Mentor MemoryShape implant texture is more aggressive than the round MemoryGel implant. The Allergan 410 implant is referred to as BioCell. It is manufactured by adding salt crystals to the still tacky external surface of the implant shell and then covering the device with an additional thin layer of silicone. During the final phase, the thin external silicone layer is scrubbed away and the salt granules dissolve, leaving behind an open pore network of individual cells creating an aggressive type texture. This texture can actually create tissue ingrowth from the surrounding capsule. Sientra HSC and HSC+ implants have a TRUE Texture, which is created by a proprietary process and does not involve imprinting, soap-and-scrub technique or salt-loss, sugar-loss processing.

The main advantages of texture include providing stability of the implant with less movement and rotation and the added benefit of potentially reducing the incidence of capsular contracture, especially in the subglandular/subfascial plane. Texture has some distractors as well. With limited soft-tissue coverage, texture has shown a greater tendency to wrinkle and be more palpable compared to smooth devices. Texture has also been associated with late seromas and double capsules.[48,49] Texture can also create an implant that is less mobile and may actually remain too high as the breast slips off the implant (e.g. snoopy deformity). Recently, there has been a small incidence of anaplastic large cell lymphoma (ALCL) associated with breast implants. It has been reported that the ALCL seen on these capsules may have some association with the textured devices, although the data to date is still too preliminary to draw any definitive conclusions.[50] There has also been some early evidence that texture may be merely a passive potentiator and the real culprit may be a chronic immune response to a certain variety of bacteria.[51]

Implant shape

When considering implant shape and design, it is important to understand that dimensional analysis of the aesthetic breast reveals something more than simply a hemisphere or semicircle. Features include a gently sloping upper pole and a curved lower pole with the nipple areolar complex at the point of maximum projection. When selecting a breast implant, consideration must be given to the goals of the patient and the assessment by the surgeon to choose the implant that will provide the greatest chance for success.

A round breast implant has its point of maximal projection centrally with equal volumes distributed above and below this point. With round implants, implant selection is based on base width, projection and volume. There are typically three to four different projections for each implant, thus three to four different projections and volume for any given base width. This can be very helpful in accommodating different chest wall and breast shapes and achieving the desired look for the patient.

This is in contrast to the newer fifth generation shaped implants that typically have a flatter, sloping upper pole with the majority of the volume and projection distributed in the lower pole of the implant. Thus, the anatomically shaped implant will produce less convexity in the upper pole of the breast compared to a round implant for the same base width and volume. For anatomically shaped implants, implant selection is based on base width, projection, implant height and volume. Sientra,

Mentor and Allergan have each created a matrix of different shaped implants based on these characteristics. This provides the surgeon with a wide variety of shapes and volumes to use in creating the desired breast form. An anatomically shaped implant would be expected to achieve a more "natural" look with less convexity and rounding in the upper pole of the breast. With relative form stability of the gel and the greater volume and projection in the lower pole, some surgeons find shaped implants' ability to expand the lower pole helpful in correction of small amounts of ptosis and constricted breast deformity.

Treatment and surgical technique

The surgical treatment begins with patient markings made with the patient in the upright position which provides important landmarks during the procedure. Markings should at a minimum include a midline marking between the suprasternal notch and the xiphoid, the existing inframammary folds, and the proposed position of the new inframammary fold. After reviewing the plan, consent and postoperative instructions, the patient is taken to the operation room.

Patient positioning

Patients are placed on the operating room table in the supine position. The arms are secured either at the patient's side or outstretched on an arm-board, positioned at 45° to stabilize the patient in the upright position (Fig. 4.7). This allows access for the surgeon to stand and yet relaxes the pectoralis muscle, providing a more accurate assessment of the implant position and the redraping of the breast tissue overlying it. Placing

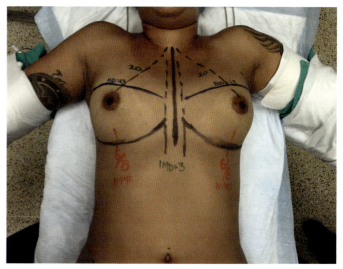

Fig. 4.7 The arms are secured to the armboard at 45° to allow appropriate evaluation of breast implant placement in the upright position.

Table 4.2 Breast local anesthetic formula

0.5% lidocaine plain	25 mL
0.5% lidocaine/1 : 200 000 epinephrine	25 mL
0.5% bupivacaine/1 : 200 000 epinephrine	25 mL
Injectable saline	25 mL
0.25% lidocaine, 0.125% bupivacaine, 1 : 400 000 epinephrine	100 mL

the arms by the patient's side is a useful alternative. Some surgeons position the patient with the arms outstretched at 90°, but this position can lead to misinterpretation of the breast–implant relationship due to breast elevation when placed in this position.

Infiltration of local anesthetic

Prior to surgical preparation, 50 mL of a local field block is injected of 0.25% lidocaine, 0.125% bupivacaine, 1 : 400 000 epinephrine (Table 4.2). The injection is placed in the dermis along the planned incision line, deep to the dermis along the inframammary fold, the medial pectoral border, the anterior axillary line and finally deep to the breast parenchyma in a fanning fashion throughout the area of planned pocket creation (Fig. 4.8). These injections provide not only assistance in operative hemostasis, but also in the management of postoperative pain. Alternatively, many surgeons opt not to inject any anesthetic agents prior to surgery.

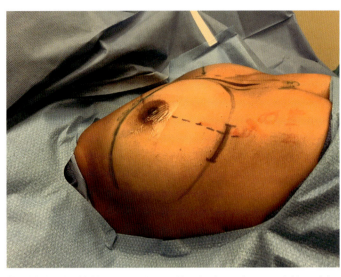

Fig. 4.9 Nipple shields are placed to provide a barrier against potential bacterial contamination.

Surgical prep and sterile

After local infiltration, nipple shields (created by placing a small piece of Tegaderm over each nipple areolar complex) provide a barrier against potential bacterial contamination[52] (Fig. 4.9). The patient is prepped with chlorhexidine or other alternatives and draped to provide a sterile field with the entire chest and bilateral breasts visible for assessment during the procedure. The sterile dressings must be secured to prevent disruption in the sterile field while placing the patient in the upright positon.

Inframammary approach

The inframammary incision is the most commonly used due to its direct access and visualization of the pocket with the least injury to surrounding structures.[55] After determining the inframammary fold position (either the native true fold position or the planned lowered position), a paramedian line is drawn through the center of the breast and bisects the newly drawn inframammary fold. The incision's medial extent begins 1 cm medial to the paramedian line and extends laterally for the appropriate distance as previously described (Fig. 4.10). A fiberoptic headlight is worn for visualization or a lighted retractor is used based on surgeon preference. The incision is made with a 15 blade through the skin to the mid-dermis. Dissection is then carried out with electrocautery through the skin and subcutaneous tissue beveling upward while rotating the breast off of the chest wall. Once dissection has been carried superiorly for 1 cm, the dissection is carried through the superficial Scarpa's fascia and towards the lateral pectoral border deep on the chest wall. This beveling maneuver preserves a small cuff of superficial fascia at the incision

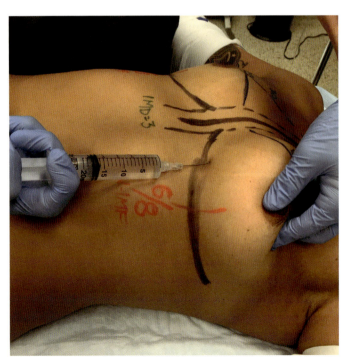

Fig. 4.8 Infiltration of local anesthetic

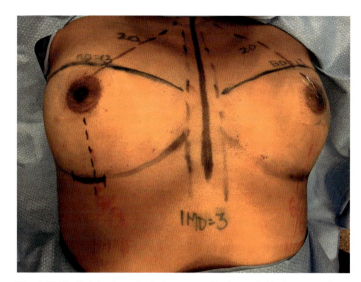

Fig. 4.10 The incision is made starting one centimeter medial to the paramedian line of the breast and extending laterally for the appropriate distance.

which insures the fold is not inadvertently lowered and also provides a cuff of fascia that will prove useful during closure (Fig. 4.11).

For subglandular pocket creation, dissection is carried out below the breast parenchyma but superficial to the pectoralis fascia and muscle. The pocket size is created to accommodate the implant selected for augmentation. If the implant is to be placed in the subfascial plane, the pocket is created deep to the pectoralis fascia and breast tissue, but superficial to the pectoralis muscle. This fascia becomes thicker and more obvious as dissection proceeds cephalad towards the clavicle. Medial intercostal vessels may be present and should be avoided or coagulated with insulated forceps in a prospective manner.

If the subpectoral or dual plane pocket is selected, the dissection initially proceeds to the lateral edge of the pectoralis major muscle. The lateral pectoral border is identified and fascia incised to expose the underlying muscle. Upward retraction of the breast tissue will usually elevate the lateral border allowing further dissection and placement of the retractor beneath the overlying pectoralis muscle (Fig. 4.12). It is an extremely important principle to never cut through the muscle if you cannot tent the muscle upward. Inability to elevate the muscle may indicate that the muscle fascia is extremely adherent, or more likely that the identified muscle is actually not the pectoralis, but rather the serratus, rectus or an intercostal muscle. Continuing the dissection through an intercostal could inadvertently penetrate the pleural space with a resultant pneumothorax. Once the edge of the pectoralis is safely elevated and the subpectoral space is identified, dissection is carried upward centrally to the superior extent of the pocket. Dissection is then carried laterally to identify the pectoralis minor and continued superficial to it until the lateral border of the pocket is reached. Dissection is then continued along the lateral border of the pocket, identifying and staying superficial to the serratus muscle until the inferior extent of the pocket at the inframammary fold is reached. Dissection should be performed bluntly along the lateral border to avoid injury to the lateral intercostal cutaneous nerves, especially the fourth intercostal which provides the primary innervation to the nipple areolar complex.

The muscle is then released along the planned inframammary fold, staying 1 cm superior to the fold to account for caudal muscle descent (Fig. 4.13). Dissection

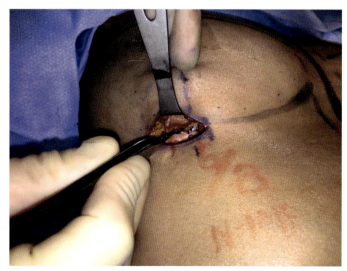

Fig. 4.11 Preservation of a small cuff of Scarpa's fascia during initial dissection avoids inadvertent lowering of the inframammary fold and assists in anchoring the fold during closure.

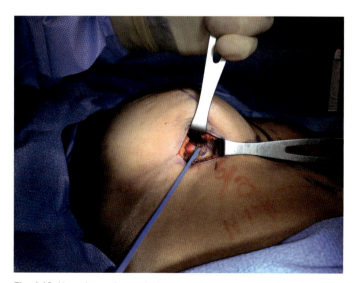

Fig. 4.12 Upward retraction on the breast tissue elevates the lateral border of the pectoralis muscle allowing further dissection and placement of the retractor under the muscle.

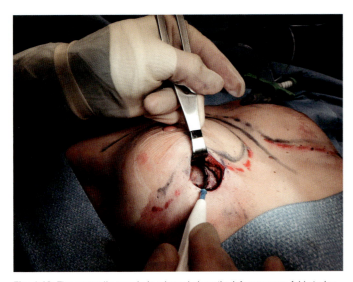

Fig. 4.13 The pectoralis muscle is released along the inframammary fold staying 1 cm superior to the fold to account for caudal muscle descent. Muscle release should end at the most caudal aspect of the medial muscle attachments and not extend superiorly along the sternum.

directly at the fold will often lead to a fold that is lower than planned as the muscle retracts inferiorly. In performing a dual-plane approach, great care should be taken to stop the dissection along the fold at the most medial extent along the sternum. Dissection should absolutely not be continued superiorly along the sternum as has been previously described. Preservation of the most caudal attachment of the pectoralis muscle along the sternum in a dual-plane approach is critical to minimize the chance of window-shading of the pectoralis, a phenomenon which often leads to medial implant exposure and unsightly animation deformities. The extent of the pocket is completed by defining the medial pectoral border by dividing the accessory slips of pectoralis muscle that insert along the ribs, preserving the main body of the muscle as it inserts along the sternum. Dividing these muscles with electrocautery and not depending on blunt dissection improves postoperative cleavage and maintains prospective hemostasis.

The final maneuver in the dual-plane approach is creating the subglandular pocket inferiorly. The levels of dual plane represent the amount of muscle released from the inferior breast tissue and resultant inferior subglandular pocket. Division of the inferior pectoralis muscle just above the inframammary fold during initial pocket dissection as was just described creates a dual plane level 1. The level of dual plane required varies and each surgery can be tailored to provide the optimal level based on soft-tissue requirements and implant selection. In general, creating a subglandular pocket inferiorly is required to either redrape relaxed or ptotic skin and breast tissue more accurately over the implant or for expansion and exposure of the lower pole, such as in a

tuberous or constricted breast. The levels of dual plane are a continuum and not fixed points. The release of the caudal edge of the muscle is performed incrementally, creating the least amount of release that will adequately address the lower pole (Fig. 4.14). When creating a dual plane to address the laxity of the lower pole, placement of a retractor into the breast pocket and elevating superiorly while rocking the breast tissue over the retractor will assist in assessing the effects of the implant on the skin and breast tissue once placed in the pocket. When a dual plane is created for expansion and exposure, the level will depend on the need to access the parenchyma for radial scoring. This usually requires at least a level 2 for complete access to the lower pole and often even a level 3 to expose the retro-areolar tissue.

If required, inframammary fold lowering must occur in the subglandular pocket as the attachments creating the fold are superficial to the deep pectoral fascia.[53] Thus, a subglandular/subfascial or dual-plane approach provide the necessary subglandular plane in the lower pole of the breast. Dissection deep to the deep pectoral fascia will likely result in maintenance of the fold structure resulting in a double bubble deformity.

Periareolar approach

Although used less often in the past few years, this incision initially described by Jenny in 1972 can be very useful for someone wanting to avoid a scar in the fold of the breast.[54,55] It is most inconspicuous when there is a distinct border and a marked color contrast between the areolar skin and surrounding breast skin.

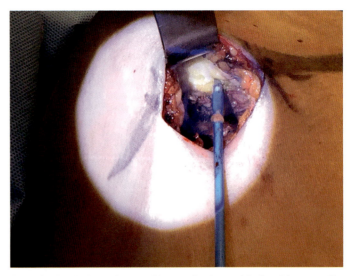

Fig. 4.14 The dual plane is created by exposing the caudal edge of the pectoralis muscle and incrementally releasing off the overlying breast tissue creating a subglandular pocket inferiorly. The dual plane levels are a continuum but a general guideline would include: level 1, the caudal edge of the muscle is present in the lower pole below the areola; level 2, the caudal edge is at the inferior areola; and level 3, the caudal edge is at the superior areola.

The periareolar incision can also allow for easy adjustments of the IMF and direct access to the parenchyma for scoring and release in constricted lower poles. Patients with smaller areolar complexes (<3 cm) also may be inappropriate due to difficulty in implant placement, especially with larger, textured or shaped implants as injury to the implant can occur while trying to place an implant through the longer breast tunnel associated with these incisions. There has also been concern with the potential contamination of the implant and breast pocket from transected lactiferous ducts, increased risk of nipple sensitivity changes, and the risk of hypopigmented scars in patients with darkly pigmented areola. The incision is made between 3 o'clock and 9 o'clock through the skin with a no. 15 blade precisely on the border between areola and adjacent breast skin. Dissection is carried through the inferior aspect of the breast directly through the breast tissue (transparenchymal) to the retroglandular plane until the lateral pectoralis border is identified. Care should be taken not to carry the dissection superiorly and inadvertently devascularize the nipple areolar complex. Dissection inferiorly in the subcutaneous plane down to the inframammary fold is preferred by some surgeons but may not be optimal in some patients as it can create significant distortion and stretch deformities in the lower pole of the breast. The lateral pectoral border is identified and the remainder of the dissection proceeds as described for the inframammary incision. If a constricted lower pole is present, the exposed parenchyma inferior to the dissection can be radial scored to allow for expansion and proper redraping of the tissue over the implant. A final check for hemostasis and pocket irrigation with antibiotic solution prior to implant placement is performed.

Implant placement

Once dissection is complete, the pocket is prepared for the implant. The pocket is irrigated with the Adam's solution of triple antibiotic solution (1 g cefazolin sodium, 50 000 units of bacitracin mixed in 500 mL of normal saline) or the modified Adam's solution which includes 50 cc of betadine (povidone-iodine) added to the formula.[56] It is the goal during the operation to achieve prospective hemostasis with minimal blood staining, however a final assessment is mandatory prior to implant placement. The implants are soaked in the irrigation solution prior to insertion. Gloves are changed and rinsed with the irrigation solution to remove any lint or powder.

The implant is then placed either manually or with the assistance of an insertion sleeve such as the Keller funnel[57] (Fig. 4.15). The opening of the funnel should be cut large enough to allow easy egress of the implant through the funnel. This can be easily confirmed by passing the implant with irrigation solution through the funnel prior to insertion. The implant orientation is then confirmed in the funnel and a maneuver of squeezing the implant through the funnel with pressure exerted on the back of the funnel allows the implant to slip into the breast pocket. These maneuvers provide a "no-touch" technique that has been associated with lower capsular contracture rates.[58] The funnel allows for easier implant placement with potentially smaller incision requirements compared to manual placement. It has proven especially helpful with textured implants, which can be much more challenging and require larger incisions compared to smooth implants.[31] Whereas many of the shaped implants can be placed with the funnel, the firmer and larger cohesive shaped implants may pose a challenge due to the lack of implant and gel flexibility and may not be appropriate for the funnel. Once the implant is in the pocket, a finger-assisted assessment and manipulation of the implant within the pocket is necessary to confirm its proper placement and assure appropriate redraping of the breast parenchyma over the implant. This maneuver is especially important with textured devices as these implants are less mobile and less likely to stretch the pocket and thus a distortion or wrinkling of the implant in a tight pocket may be permanent if not resolved prior to closure. Repeated removal and insertions of the implant should be avoided to minimize implant or incision damage, potential contamination and pocket overdissection. This is especially important with shaped implants as a stretched

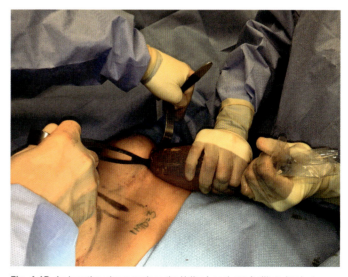

Fig. 4.15 An insertion sleeve such as the Keller funnel can facilitate implant placement. The implant should be oriented appropriately in the funnel prior to placement and the funnel opening must be adequate to allow a smooth and gentle passage of the implant.

pocket from overmanipulation could lead to implant rotation postoperatively.

Closure

Prior to incision closure, the patient should be placed in the upright position to assess implant position, fold position, symmetry and the adequacy of the dual plane (Fig. 4.16). Any additional adjustments of the dual plane can be accomplished after being placed back in the recumbent position by simply retracting the breast tissue superiorly off the implant, identifying the caudal edge of the muscle, and releasing it incrementally off the overlying breast tissue to the desired level. Reassessment in the upright position after appropriate adjustments is advisable to confirm position of implants and optimal relationship between the implant and the overlying breast tissue.

A significant advantage of the inframammary approach which is often underappreciated is the ability to accurately and effectively control the fold position during closure of the incision. The cuff of superficial Scarpa's fascia that was preserved during the initial incision is utilized to secure the fold during closure. In general, if the inframammary fold structure is well-developed and stable and has not been violated or lowered during the procedure, then re-approximation of the superficial fascia during closure is usually adequate. However, when the fold is unstable due to either inherent weakness in the fold structure or from disrupting it with fold lowering, closure should include

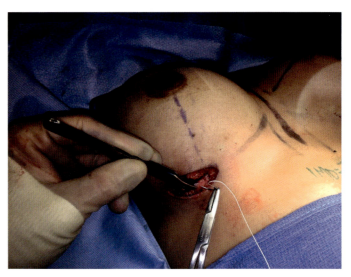

Fig. 4.17 When stabilization of the inframammary fold is required due to inherent weakness in the fold structure or secondary to fold lowering, closure requires incorporating deep fascial structures into the Scarpa's fascia closure to secure the fold position.

stabilization of the fold structure. This is accomplished by securing the caudal edge of the Scarpa's fascia present on the lower incisional edge to the underlying deep fascial structures with an absorbable suture such as 2-0 Vicryl or permanent suture (Fig. 4.17). This is usually done by simply incorporating the superficial and deep fascia together during closure, but can be also performed by first placing three sutures on the lower flap securing Scarpa's fascia to the underlying deep fascia followed by closure of the incision. Unique to both round and shaped textured devices, the implant must be seated accurately at the base of the breast pocket as it is less likely to settle in the breast pocket postoperatively as compared to smooth breast implants. Thus, special care must be taken during closure not to inadvertently injure the breast implants. The incision is closed in three layers: Scarpa's fascia superiorly to Scarpa's fascia (with or without deep fascia) inferiorly, deep dermis and subcuticular.

The periareolar incision lacks the ability to control the fold structure during closure. Closure includes closing the breast parenchyma deep to the incision, followed by deep dermal interrupted and a running subcuticular with absorbable sutures. A precise closure is required to achieve a well-healed camouflaged scar.

Transaxillary approach

Initially described by Hoehler in 1973 and later popularized by Bostwick and others, the transaxillary approach places the incision in the deep axilla and avoids a scar directly on the breast.[59] This dissection can be performed bluntly but visualization with the endoscope is preferred for controlled pocket dissection, precise muscle division

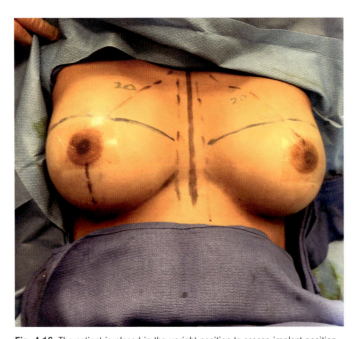

Fig. 4.16 The patient is placed in the upright position to assess implant position, fold position, symmetry and the adequacy of the dual plane and redraping of the breast tissue over the implant.

and prospective hemostasis. Any implant can be placed, but larger silicone implants and anatomically shaped implants can prove more difficult due to the long tunnel and limited access. An insertion sleeve can be very helpful in implant placement. With the patient's arms down to her side, the most anterior part of the axilla is marked and the incision should not extend anteriorly beyond this. The arm is then abducted 45° and a prominent axillary crease is identified, preferably high in the axilla. The incision length is the same as other approaches. The patient should be placed on the operating room table with the arms abducted 90°, but secured so that they can be adducted somewhat when the patient is placed in the upright position to check implant placement. The incision is made and the medial aspect of the incision is elevated. Superficial subcutaneous dissection carried out to the lateral border of the pectoralis major to prevent injury to the intercostobrachial nerve (sensation to the inner portion of the arm). The dissection is then carried under the pectoralis fascia (subfascial) or deep to the muscle (subpectoral) to create the implant pocket. It is very important to confirm the correct plane is entered before proceeding further.

When an endoscopically assisted transaxillary dissection is carried out, the endoscope is placed through the tunnel into the correct plane and the dissection continues under direct visualization with the use of a long insulated electrocautery instrument. Implant sizers are used after completion of the dissection to identify any areas that need final adjustments. After final confirmation in the upright position and pocket irrigation, the closure includes pectoralis fascia closure followed by a layered incisional closure.

Transumbilical

The transumbilical approach has the significant limitation of only allowing for augmentation with saline implants. During the moratorium when silicone implant use was significantly limited, saline augmentation was the predominant procedure and this approach was a viable option for patients. With the increased use of prefilled silicone implants and now anatomically shaped devices, this approach has much more limited applicability. Positioning and markings are identical to inframammary approach with an additional mark made from the umbilicus to the medial border of the areola bilaterally. An incision is made in the upper half of the umbilicus and an opening is made large enough to accommodate an index finger. An endotube is then passed along the rectus fascia along the drawn line up to the medial areola. The endotube should be carefully advanced in the subcutaneous tunnel continually palpating the tube and

placing upward pressure away from the abdominal and thoracic cavity. If the implant is being placed subglandular, then pressure is exerted upward at the IMF to stay in the subglandular plane. The tunnel ends up just cephalad to the nipple. Placement of the implant submuscular is possible with the use of special instrumentation to enter the fascial plane in a high lateral position. The tube can then be removed and an endoscope utilized to verify the correct pocket. Instrumentation is then removed from the tunnel and an expander is rolled up, placed through the incision and advanced up the tunnel through a subcutaneous "milking" technique with manual external pressure. The expander is filled with saline to 150% of the final volume of the planned implant. Some final pocket adjustments are made and the expander is removed through simple backward traction on the filler tube. The saline implant is then advanced into the breast pocket similar to the expander placement and filled to the desired final volume. The endoscope can then be reintroduced to confirm hemostats, valve patency and implant position. The patient is placed in the upright position to verify optimal implant positioning. The incision is closed with a single layer of absorbable suture and an abdominal binder placed for compression of the abdominal tunnels.

Postoperative management

The management of breast augmentation is quite variable amongst surgeons, but the type of device used can alter the postoperative protocols. In our practice, patients are given analgesics, muscle relaxant and antibiotics. Some surgeons advocate no narcotics and only anti-inflammatories postoperatively. The first postoperative appointment is usually 3–4 days after surgery. All patients are wrapped in an ace wrap for the first 24 hours followed by a sports bra to be worn 23 hours a day for the next 4 weeks. Early range of motion beginning in the recovery room is initiated for all patients that includes shoulder rolls in both directions as well as elevation of the arms outward to the sides and over the head. With smooth devices, implant massage begins postoperative day 4 and includes displacing the implant upward and downward in the pocket, crossing the arms and pulling the implants inward to create cleavage and downward pressure on the implants to stretch the lower pole. With textured implants, both round and shaped, limited arm movement other than range of motion is recommended for the first week. Implant massage is contraindicated as the textured surface can irritate the pocket and potentially create serous fluid around the implant. Likewise, the implants are placed in a controlled pocket with the implant positioned appropriately at the base of the pocket and displacement could lead to implant malposition or, in the case of shaped devices, rotation of the implant (see Fig. 3.13). The different types of texture available vary considerably in terms of texture aggressiveness and implant adherence, and the exact postoperative protocol and decision on drain placement should be based on those considerations. In primary breast augmentation, drains seem to offer very little benefit.

Patients are allowed to resume regular bras after 4 weeks, but should continue with a sports bra during bedtime for an additional 2–4 weeks to limit lateral implant movement during pocket formation. Normal activity resumes within a few days after surgery, but exercise and high impact activity should be delayed for 3–4 weeks. Whereas smooth implants often seem high initially and often require downward massage and/or the use of breast bands or bandeaus, textured devices that are appropriately seated in the base of the breast pocket should only occasionally require such maneuvers. Whereas smooth implants will seem more mobile and softer in the first few weeks after surgery compared to textured devices, the textured implants will soften with modest movement often present after 4–6 weeks. If a variety of smooth and textured (round and/or shaped) breast implants are being utilized within a practice, it is extremely important to communicate to ancillary staff the type of device placed with each patient in order to initiate the appropriate postoperative protocol as inappropriate instructions can lead to postoperative problems such as seromas, malposition and rotational deformities.

Postoperative follow-ups occur approximately at 3 days, 3 weeks, 3 months and one year postoperatively. Photographic documentation and critical evaluation of surgical outcomes is imperative. In our practice, every breast implant patient is placed on 400 IU of vitamin E to potentially reduce the incidence of capsular contracture. Whereas there is no evidence to the benefit of vitamin E in breast augmentation, there is encouraging data on the reduction of radiation-induced scarring in the treatment of radiation-induced fibrosis (RIF).[60]

Perioperative complications

Hematoma

The incidence of hematoma after a primary breast augmentation has ranged from 0.5–2.0%. The best prevention is achieving meticulous hemostasis intraoperatively.

Blind or blunt pocket dissection without surgery for hemostasis after should be avoided to limit the incidence of hematoma. Patients should likewise be counseled to avoid medications that increase bleeding or interfere with platelet function for at least two weeks prior to surgery (see Table 3.1). A hematoma is easily recognizable with a breast that is swollen, painful, bruised and exquisitely painful to palpation or often arm movement. Treatment includes reoperation with evacuation of the hematoma, hemostasis, pocket washout and drainage. Implant replacement is usually not necessary. A hematoma left untreated is discouraged as it can lead to prolonged healing, wound problems, delayed healing, infection and possible long-term issues of asymmetry and possible capsular contracture.[61]

Infection

Infection rates for primary breast augmentation can approach 2%.[62–64] It is well known the breast parenchyma and associated breast ducts harbor bacteria that can be introduced into the operative field or breast pocket.[52,65] Prevention is key and many operative maneuvers can assist in minimizing this possibility. Current recommendations are for skin preparation with chlorhexidine that covers most organisms including methicillin-resistant staphylococcus aureus (MRSA). Likewise, perioperative antibiotics and antibiotic pocket irrigation reduce implant contamination and possible infection. The standard treatment includes operative exploration, irrigation and debridement of the pocket with drainage. In most incidences, the implant is removed during this procedure and re-augmented six months later. There is the possibility of implant salvage with prolonged antibiotic therapy if the patient is clinically stable and the infection is limited, but failure of a salvage procedure would mandate implant removal.[66–68]

Sensation changes

Alterations in nipple sensitivity can manifest as either hypoesthesia or hyperesthesia and are often the result of traction injury, bruising, inflammation or possibly even injury to the lateral intercostal cutaneous nerve that enters the breast laterally on the deep surface just above the pectoral fascia. Although the major innervation is the fourth, there is some overlap from the anterior and lateral branches of the third and fifth intercostal nerves. There is evidence that nipple sensitivity changes are no more likely with a periareolar incision when compared to an inframammary incision.[69,70] The most common cause is aggressive pocket dissection laterally, especially with sharp dissection, with injury to the intercostal nerves.

Deflation and implant rupture

It is important to inform breast augmentation patients that breast implants do not last a lifetime. Implant rupture and failure of the shell is implant-style dependent. Any disruption of the outer shell of a saline implant leads to complete failure of the implant with the saline leaking out into surrounding tissue and is harmless. Saline implant failure can be associated trauma or a spontaneous leak that involves either fold fatigue on the shell of the implant or valve incompetence. Silicone implant rupture rates have been quite variable between devices and failures increase with the age of the implant. The fifth generation silicone gel implants have more cohesive gels and the silicone is less likely to egress from the implant shell leading to a much lower rupture rate than early fourth generation devices.[24,33,34,71,72] MRI imaging is currently the diagnostic technique of choice to discern a silicone implant rupture.

Capsular contracture

Capsular contracture remains the number one complications of breast augmentation with incidence ranging as high as 15–30% with the development of palpable and/or visible deformation of the periprosthetic capsule around the implant.[71–75] The development of a capsule around an implant is always present due to the unique foreign body reaction by the surrounding breast tissue. A periprosthetic capsular contracture that is clinically significant is characterized by excessive scar formation with shrinkage and often thickening of the capsule leading to firmness, distortion and displacement of the breast implant. Baker proposed a clinical classification system for capsular contractures that is still widely used today[76] (see Table 3.2). While there are many factors identified that seem to contribute to the incidence of capsular contracture, the exact etiology is not known. The hypertrophic scar theory proposes that myofibroblasts are stimulated in the capsule creating scar and contracture.[77] Irritants such as silicone gel, blood or seroma in the pocket may incite a contracture.[78–80] Also, stimulation and irritation from foreign body particles such as powder, lint or dust may also contribute.[81] The infection theory has been studied and appears currently to be the most cited explanation for capsular contracture development.[82–85] This theory entails a chronic subclinical infectious process located adjacent to the implant shell within a microscopic biofilm that is protective of the infectious process and inaccessible to cellular and humoral immune function to combat the inflammatory process. *Staphylococcus epidermidis, Propionibacterium,*

Enterobacter, Bacillus and other organisms have been implicated in this process.

Many techniques have been proposed to reduce the incidence of capsular contracture. With smooth implants, the concept of creating a large pocket with displacement exercises has been used to try and impede the development of a tightening capsule. The use of textured implants may have some protective properties as has been previously discussed in this chapter. Maneuvers to minimize tissue trauma, blood staining and seroma formation during pocket dissection have been employed as these may all contribute to capsular contracture formation. Periprosthetic fluid pockets generally resorb within the first week, and the use of topical antibiotic irrigation has been shown to decrease this rate.[86] Additionally, the use of an insertion sleeve (e.g., Keller funnel) for implant placement and placement of Tegaderm (nipple shield) over the nipple areolar complex have been employed to reduce bacterial contamination of the implant and potentially biofilm formation.[52,57] Pocket irrigation with antibiotic solutions has proven beneficial in reducing the incidence of capsular contracture. Whereas the original irrigation solutions contained betadine, some concerns over the use of betadine in the implant pocket and regulations imposed by the FDA led to the evaluation and popularization of a few different antibiotic combinations, including the "Adam's solution" of gentamycin 80 mg, bacitracin 50 000 units and cefazolin 1 g in 500 cc of normal saline, which have proved effective in reducing capsular contracture incidence.[56] Leukotriene receptor antagonists which are used to treat asthma, such as zafirlukast (Accolate) and montelukast (Singulair), have shown some benefit in reversing the clinical signs of capsular contracture but should be used with caution due to potentials side effects.[87,88] Box 4.2 summarizes some of the implant and surgical technique options that have been associated with lower capsular contractures.[32–36,43,45,46,52,56,57,89–94]

BOX 4.2 Items associated with reduced capsular contracture incidence

No-touch technique

Nipple shields

Pocket irrigation with triple antibiotics

Insertion sleeve

Submuscular implant pocket

Textured implants

Inframammary incision

Cohesive shaped implants

Implant malposition/rotation

Implant malposition is the second most common complication in most studies and is a rather broad category encompassing a wide range of complications. Malpositions include inferior malposition with disruption of the inframammary fold (double bubble) or inferior stretch deformity (bottoming out), lateral malposition, medial malposition (symmastia) and superior malposition which can often be associated with ptosis of the breast tissue off the implant (snoopy deformity). Most malpositions are preventable. Medial and lateral malpositions are most often the result of overdissection of the lateral pocket or over-release of the pectoralis sternal attachments, respectively. Inferior malposition is often due to mismanagement of the inframammary fold during lowering or use of implants larger than the lower pole can tolerate leading to stretch deformities. Superior malpositions are usually due to underdissection of the lower pole, inadequate dual plane if submuscular, inadequate lowering of the inframammary fold or the development of a capsular contracture. Another contributing factor to malposition is the effect of abnormal and/or asymmetric chest walls on the migration of the implants on the chest wall. The use of textured implants in this situation may help to reduce implant movement over time. Implant rotation is a complication only applicable to shaped devices and refers to the implant orientation becoming altered in the breast pocket. Because of this possibility, all shaped devices are textured to help maintain spatial orientation in the pocket. Creation of a controlled implant pocket that fits the implant accurately (hand-in-glove) is critical in minimizing this risk. Whereas it has been postulated that adherence of the textured implant to the surrounding capsule is required to prevent rotation, it appears that the frictional component of the textured devices positioned in a controlled pocket is adequate to minimize the risk of rotation.

Wrinkling/rippling

Adequate soft-tissue coverage takes priority in determining implant pocket location and minimizing the risk of wrinkling, rippling, visibility and/or palpability of the implant. Placement of the implant in the submuscular or dual-plane pocket provides the greatest coverage. Placement of an implant above the muscle requires at least a 2 cm upper pole pinch thickness. Even with adequate coverage, soft-tissue atrophy and lower pole thinning and stretching is possible. Wrinkling is more likely with inadequate or thin soft-tissue coverage, saline implants, textured implants and underfilled gel devices. Treatment of wrinkling may include implant exchange to the retropectoral position, implant exchange to an appropriate device with less wrinkling (e.g. saline to silicone, textured surface to smooth surface), fat grafting, and/or placement of a soft-tissue matrix.

Animation deformity

Implant distortion on muscular contracture is a phenomenon unique to implants placed in the submuscular position. It can be very noticeable and especially bothersome for patients who exercise or lift weights frequently. In one study, although mostly mild, 15% of patients were noted to have moderate or severe distortion on animation.[95] Placement of the implant in the subglandular/subfascial or subpectoral pocket is preventative and may be a preferable pocket for those patients at risk, but must be weighed against the benefits of subpectoral placement. If a severe animation deformity is present, correction may include conversion to preferably a subglandular/subfascial pocket or to a dual plane with or without acellular dermal matrix in patients who are not candidates for subglandular or subfascial placement.

Anaplastic large cell lymphoma

There has been over the past few years an increasing awareness and questions raised concerning reported cases of ALCL in women with breast implants (see also Chapter 12). To date, there have been nearly 200 cases, but this number continues to grow.[50] Initial presentation has included the development of a late periprosthetic fluid collection, a mass attached to the capsule, tumor erosion through the skin, lymph node involvement, or discovered during a revisional procedure. These have been associated with saline and silicone implants. Where the history of implants is known, most if not all are associated with having at least one textured implant in place as part of their history, the majority of these being of the "salt-loss" type of texturing. This observation suggests a probable chronic inflammatory cause, although the rarity of this lesion precludes any statistically certain causal relationship and is suggestive of a multifactorial inflammatory cause. As previously discussed, there is some early evidence that texture may be merely a passive potentiator and the real culprit may be a chronic immune response to a certain variety of bacteria.[51]

Conclusion

In any patient presenting with a late seroma one year or greater after implant surgery, evaluation should include image-guided fluid aspiration and appropriate fluid evaluation for culture, cell count and cytology.[96] All late seromas or capsular contractures associated with a mass should be evaluated and ALCL should be considered and ruled out. Even if idiopathic and not associated with infection or neoplastic process, surgical intervention is usually indicated and includes total capsulectomy with or without implant exchange. Appropriate staging is mandatory and dictates adjuvant treatment, including possibly chemotherapy, radiation therapy and/or high-dose stem cell infusion for local extracapsular involvement.

Disclosure

Dr. Calobrace has been a speaker for Mentor, Allergan and Sientra with no financial disclosure. He is also a stockowner and general partner of Strathspey Crown Advisory Board of which Alphaeon Corporation is a wholly-owned subsidiary.

Bonus content for this chapter can be found online at **http://www.expertconsult.com**

Table 4.1 Current approval status of gel breast implants in the United States.

Access the complete reference list online at **http://www.expertconsult.com**

28. Tebbetts JB, Adams WP. Five critical decisions in breast augmentation using five measurements in 5 minutes: the high five decision support process. *Plast Reconstr Surg.* 2005;116:2005–2016. *The authors describe their process of decision-making in breast augmentation that has evolved from the biodimensional and TEPID approach to breast assessment. This third generation is a process of breast assessment that prioritizes five critical decisions, identifies five key measurements, and completes all preoperative assessment and operative planning decisions in breast augmentation in 5 minutes or less.*

29. Adams WP. The process of breast augmentation: four sequential steps for optimizing outcomes for patients. *Plast Reconstr Surg.* 2008;122:1892–1900. *Optimizing patient outcomes in breast augmentation requires defining the overall process to allow for enhanced patient outcomes. The author describes a defined process of breast augmentation including structured patient education and informed consent; tissue-based preoperative planning consultation; refined surgical technique; and structured postoperative instructions, management, and follow-up.*

31. Calobrace MB, Kaufman DL, Gordon AE, et al. Evolving practices in augmentation operative techniques with Sientra HSC round implants. *Plast Reconstr Surg.* 2014;134(suppl 1):57S–67S.

34. Maxwell GP, Van Natta BW, Murphy DK, et al. Natrelle style 410 form-stable silicone breast implants: core study results at 6 years. *Aesthet Surg J.* 2012;32:709–717.

43. Stevens WG, Nahabedian MY, Calobrace MB, et al. Risk factor analysis for capsular contracture: a 5-year Sientra study analysis using round, smooth and textured implants for breast augmentation. *Plast Reconstr Surg.* 2013;132:1115–1123.

47. Tebbetts JB. Dual plane breast augmentation: optimizing implant-soft-tissue relationships in a wide range of breast types. *Plast Reconstr Surg.* 2001;107:1255–1272. *The author describes the indications and techniques for utilizing a dual-plane approach in breast augmentation. The submuscular pocket is adjusted to create variable amounts of subglandular only coverage in the lower pole. This dual-plane approach adjusts implant and soft-tissue relationships to optimize coverage and implant–soft tissue dynamics. Indications, operative techniques, results, and complications are reviewed for a series of patients.*

56. Adams WP, Rios JL, Smith S. Enhancing patient outcomes in aesthetic and reconstructive breast surgery using triple antibiotic breast irrigation: six-year prospective clinical study. *Plast Reconstr Surg.* 2006;118(suppl 7):46S–52S. *The authors demonstrate the clinical importance of incorporating triple antibiotic irrigation in breast augmentation procedures. This shows the incorporation of triple antibiotic solution irrigation is associated with a low capsular contracture rate compared to previously published reports, and its clinical efficacy supports previously published in vitro studies. The use of triple antibiotic irrigation is recommended in all aesthetic and reconstructive breast implant procedures and is cost effective.*

71. Spears S, Murphy D, Slicton A. Inamed silicone breast implant core study results at 6 years. *Plast Reconstr Surg.* 2007;120:8S–16S.

72. Cunningham B. The Mentor Core Study on silicone MemoryGel breast implants. *Plast Reconstr Surg.* 2007;120:19S–29S. *The authors provide an update on the post-approval study for Allergan's breast implants. The ongoing core study results demonstrate safety and effectiveness of the Natrelle smooth and textured silicone-filled round breast implants through six years of the 10 year study. The results reveal low rupture rates and significantly high patient satisfaction.*

96. Bengtson B, Brody GS, Brown MH, et al. Managing late periprosthetic fluid collections (seroma) in patients with breast implants: a consensus panel recommendation and review of the literature. *Plast Reconstr Surg.* 2011;128:1–7. *The authors review the development of late or delayed periprosthetic fluid collections post breast augmentation. A consensus report was created from a group of practicing plastic surgeons and device industry physicians concerning the management of this complication. Based on this collaboration, treatment recommendations and treatment algorithms were created to guide the management of these late-onset periprosthetic fluid collections.*

5

Breast augmentation with autologous fat grafting

Emmanuel Delay and Samia Guerid

 Access video lecture content for this chapter online at expertconsult.com

SYNOPSIS

- Breast augmentation with autologous fat grafting has been a controversial topic for the last thirty years. Based on our clinical and radiologic experience since 1998, we developed an efficient new technique to realize breast augmentation: lipomodeling.

- Our technique is efficient and safe and has become a standard procedure during breast reconstruction after cancer, correction of breast conservative treatment sequelae, breast and thorax malformations treatment, and aesthetic breast augmentation.

- Prior evaluation and accurate patient selection are mandatory. Ultrasound of the breast is performed on patients under 30 years of age, ultrasound and one mammography incidence between 30 and 40 years of age, and standard mammography and ultrasound over 40 years.

- In case of ACR 3, biopsy has to downstage the lesion to ACR 1 or 2, otherwise the procedure is contraindicated. Breast lipo-augmentation is only moderate unless done in multiple sessions, which is difficult in pure aesthetic surgery.

- Fat is harvested by means of a 3.5 mm cannula adapted to a syringe and centrifuged during 20 seconds at 3000 rpm. Fat transfer has then to be very accurate.

- Patient follow-up is done at 15 days, 3 months, and one year. At one year, a new radiologic evaluation is done by means of the same radiologic tools as preoperative work-up. In case of a new suspect lesion, biopsy is performed to obtain accurate diagnosis. No hematoma has been reported in our experience. Infection rate is very low (0.6%) and easily handled by pulling out some stitches, ice application, and antibiotic treatment.

- At the beginning of practice, some fat necrosis can be seen that becomes very rare through clinical experience. In 10% of cases, oil cysts are seen that can easily be managed by puncture at the follow-up visit.

Introduction

Transferring fat from areas where it is present in excess (abdomen, thighs) to the breast for aesthetic and reconstructive purposes is a surgical renewal. This approach has been considered since the very beginning of liposuction, particularly after the publication of Illouz's[1] and Fournier's[2] works. However, it remained controversial and never became widely used until the development of more precise tools and techniques. It was feared that autologous fat transfer would generate fat necrosis and calcifications which, at that time, were not readily assessable because of the limitations of available imaging modalities.

The American Society of Plastic and Reconstructive Surgeons had, in 1987 after a case presented by Bircoll,[3] advised to discontinue fat transfer surgery. Fat grafting procedures diminished significantly following this opinion (see Historical Perspective). In 1998, given the proven efficacy of fat transfer to the face demonstrated by Coleman[4,5] for facial rejuvenation or post-surgery reconstruction, we developed a research program aiming to evaluate the efficacy and safety of the procedure for thoraco-mammary reconstructions.

We adapted the technique for breast procedures, and we chose to name it "lipomodeling".[6,7] We assessed its efficacy and tolerance in patients and demonstrated the absence of significant clinical or radiological signs of adverse effects. Obtained results went largely beyond our hopes, and this technique has now a major role in breast plastic and aesthetic surgery.

The purpose of the present chapter is to present the evolution of ideas and the progress of knowledge about fat grafting to the breast, its applications, and to describe its indications and contraindications and precise technique. We will finally present clinical outcomes and results obtained with this technique for each clinical situation.

Access the Historical Perspective section online at
http://www.expertconsult.com

Basic science

Fat grafting technique is now very well described. Scientific research and surgical practice were able to show that each fat lobule has to be surrounded by vascularized tissue at a distance of 2 mm or less. The consequence of this observation is the grafting of fat spaghettis in a 3D grid where each tunnel has to be surrounded by recipient tissue with spaghetti of a diameter less than two millimeters. Spaghetti box concept is essential to understand to handle lipomodeling technique. It is actually possible to graft as much volume as can accept recipient tissue: while sticking to that rule, it is then possible to anticipate quantity of fat to be transferred and the number of sessions needed to achieve the planned result. With experience, it is important to learn how to scan the patient with hands and eyes and evaluate recipient tissues, which eases transfer precision.

Patient presentation

Lipomodeling of the breast and chest wall is a technique that nowadays has many indications. It has been of great help in reconstructive breast surgery. In aesthetic breast surgery and in selected cases, fat transfer can be used instead of implants (augmentation, mastopexy with a slight lack of fullness in the upper pole), and it can correct some defects of implant augmentations. The procedure is becoming a new gold standard to enhance breast aesthetic outcomes.

Poland syndrome

Correction of the breast and chest wall deformities of Poland syndrome is still today a challenge for plastic surgeons. Lipomodeling appears to be very useful in these cases. Breast rehabilitation with exclusive fat grafting leads to excellent outcomes with simple but repeated procedures[15,16,23,31,32] and very limited scarring

and donor site morbidity. The results are very interesting, and a breast almost identical to the opposite side can be achieved (Fig. 5.1). This technique appears to revolutionize the management of breast and chest wall deformities in Poland syndrome[15,16,23,24,31,32].

Pectus excavatum

Pectus excavatum is a complex deformity with hollowing of the anterior sternocostal wall. It usually has little or no impact on the respiratory function. In most cases the complaint is mainly morphological and aesthetic, with considerable deformity of the thorax, especially in severe or lateralized forms. Procedures involving modifications of bony and cartilaginous structures can be very invasive when done for aesthetic purpose. Fat transfer techniques give satisfactory correction for mild to moderate forms (Fig. 5.2),[15,16,23,24,33] or in association with a custom-made rigid implant (based on a 3D CT scan) in major forms.

Tuberous breasts

Tuberous breast is a deformity of the breast footprint, with onset at puberty when breast development begins. Various surgical approaches have been described, and a wide range of techniques has been published to obtain optimal results. Among them, lipomodeling[15,16,23,24,34] can correct the lack of volume (especially in unilateral cases) and improve base and shape of the breast (Fig. 5.3). It is a very useful adjunct in the treatment of tuberous breasts. The ideal indication is the unilateral hypoplastic tuberous breast (which usually requires two fat transfer sessions), associated with the lack of fullness of the upper pole. In cases of bilateral breast hypoplasia associated with tuberous deformity, implants remain the gold standard unless the clinical condition is associated with a lower body adiposity large enough to augment the two breasts efficiently. Lipomodeling can drastically enhance the results of these corrections by improving the décolleté area.

Asymmetric breasts

Asymmetry is a difficult problem, mostly when one breast has satisfactory fullness and perfect shape and the other is hypoplastic. Conventionally, implant augmentation in the underdeveloped breast is the standard procedure. While the initial result is usually good, asymmetry of shape and volume often reappears several years later, due to aging of the breasts. In this indication, lipomodeling yields a breast very similar to the normal breast,[15,16,23,24] and change over time is natural, in particular regarding ptosis. Depending on the degree of

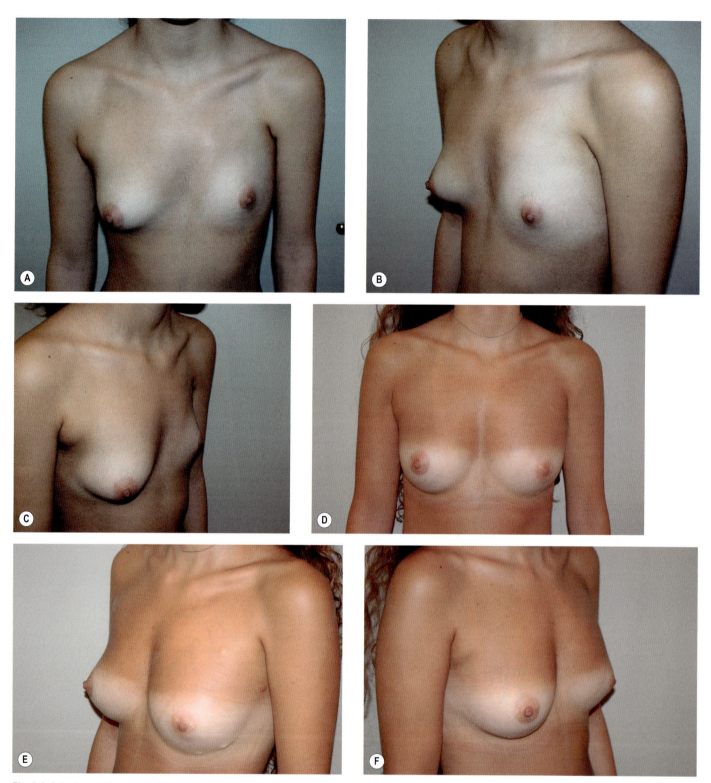

Fig. 5.1 Patient aged 16 years with Poland syndrome. Treatment of the deformity by 4 sessions of lipomodeling (157 mL, 286 mL, 272 mL during the 3rd session right breast lipomodeling 140 mL, 227 mL) at 3 to 6 months of interval. Result at 24 months after last session. (**A**) Preoperative view. (**B**) Preoperative oblique view. (**C**) Preoperative oblique view. (**D**) Postoperative view. (**E**) Postoperative oblique view. (**F**) Postoperative oblique view.

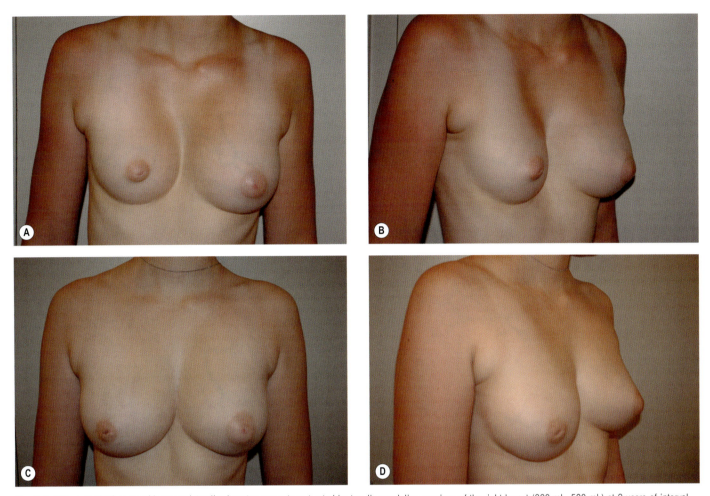

Fig. 5.2 Patient aged 16 years with severe lateralized pectus excavatum, treated by two lipomodeling sessions of the right breast (320 mL, 500 mL) at 2 years of interval. Result 1 year after second procedure. **(A)** Preoperative view. **(B)** Preoperative oblique view. **(C)** Postoperative view. **(D)** Postoperative oblique view.

asymmetry and hypoplasia, one or two fat transfer sessions will be needed for an optimal result (Fig. 5.4).

Bilateral breast augmentation

Lipomodeling in aesthetic surgery is developing fast. Our studies have shown that if lipomodeling is carried out according to the technique we described in this chapter, it does not generate any radiological images with differential diagnosis of breast malignancy or radiological follow-up problems, for breast imaging specialized radiologists. It is now accepted as a standard procedure for moderate or very moderate augmentation.

The indications of breast augmentation with fat grafting (lipoaugmentation) differ from those of implant augmentations. Lipoaugmentation is suitable for patients looking for a moderate or even very moderate increase of breast volume,[35] or who desire to recover the upper pole fullness they had before weight loss or pregnancy. The ideal patient is a young woman with a slim upper body and moderately small breasts,

and with sufficient localized adiposity of the lower body to allow for one or even two lipomodeling sessions (Fig. 5.5). In this indication, fat harvesting enhances the lower body contour and can be associated to standard liposuction to improve final result. After this procedure, we recommend a strict stability of patient's weight. Any change in weight might affect the breast volume and shape.

Composite breast augmentation

The first application of lipomodeling is primary breast augmentation in cases where the patient wishes to have a natural transition between thorax and implant or in skinny patients where an implant will inevitably be visible. The technique is the ideal complement to volume augmentation by implant as it allows for a perfect shape. Second application is as an option for correction, in secondary cases, of the imperfections due to implant augmentation. It enhances the décolleté area, improves tissue coverage of the implant, especially in the lower pole, reduces rippling in thin patients,

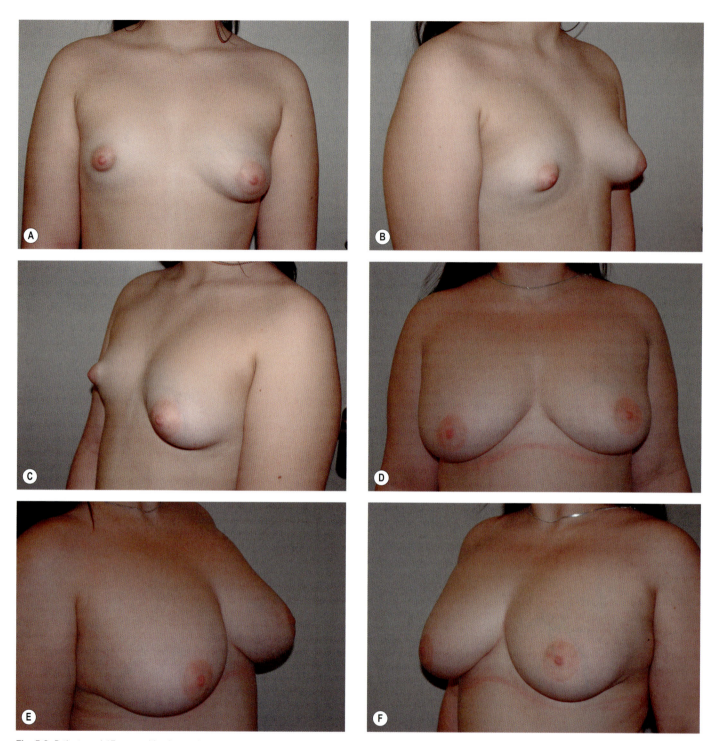

Fig. 5.3 Patient aged 17 years with tuberous breasts, treated by two lipomodeling sessions of the left breast (340 mL, 230 mL) and right lipomodeling (320 mL, 230 mL). Result 12 months after second procedure. (**A**) Preoperative view. (**B**) Preoperative oblique view. (**C**) Preoperative oblique view. (**D**) Postoperative view. (**E**) Postoperative oblique view. (**F**) Postoperative oblique view.

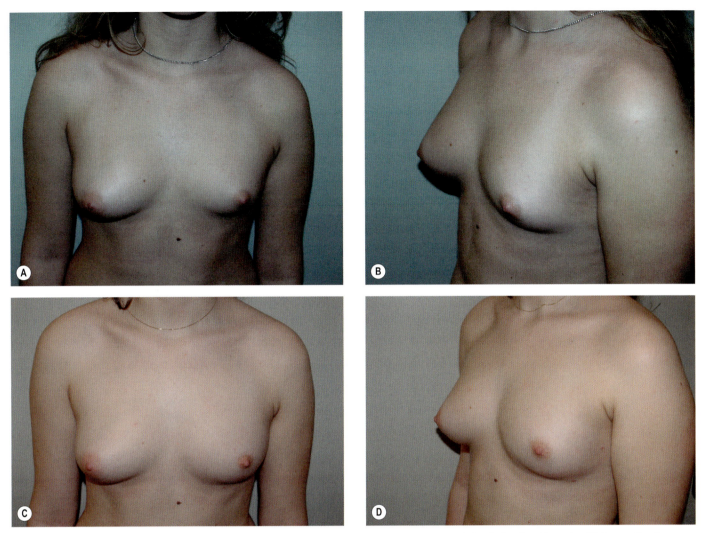

Fig. 5.4 Patient aged 19 years with breast asymmetry. Treatment by one lipomodeling session of the left breast (210 mL). Result at 12 months. (**A**) Preoperative view. (**B**) Preoperative oblique view. (**C**) Postoperative view. (**D**) Postoperative oblique view.

and reduces demarcation of the implant in the upper pole (Fig. 5.6). We also have a clinical impression that requires further scientific data, that complementary fat grafting might improve capsular contractures in moderate cases. In secondary implant changing, we usually recommend fat transfer with the previous implant in place. Once all the deformities are corrected, the implant is replaced, thus avoiding any risk of leaving a punctured implant.

The clinical results obtained with composite augmentation are so interesting that it seems to us that the technique could be, in the future, the new gold standard in breast implant augmentation.

Management of severe complications of breast aesthetic surgery

Breast reduction, breast augmentation, and mastopexy are commonly performed procedures in breast aesthetic surgery. The outcomes are most of the time satisfactory for the patient and the surgeon. In rare cases, complications can occur. In thin patients with smoking habits, exposure of an implant can result in implant withdrawal. Large breast reduction can result in fat and skin necrosis with subsequent breast deformity. Some of these patients are referred to our clinic for revision and secondary procedures. We find lipomodeling to be very useful in these cases. It efficiently enhances tissue thickness and improves tissue quality.

After implant complications with withdrawal, lipomodeling prepares the tissues to render the secondary augmentation safer. After complicated breast reductions, fat transfer can restore the suppleness of the breast while improving the quality of the suffering skin.

These complementary fat grafting procedures have reduced donor site morbidity while improving breast sequelae. We find them very useful in the management of these difficult patients with high expectations and risk of medico-legal issues for the previous surgeon.

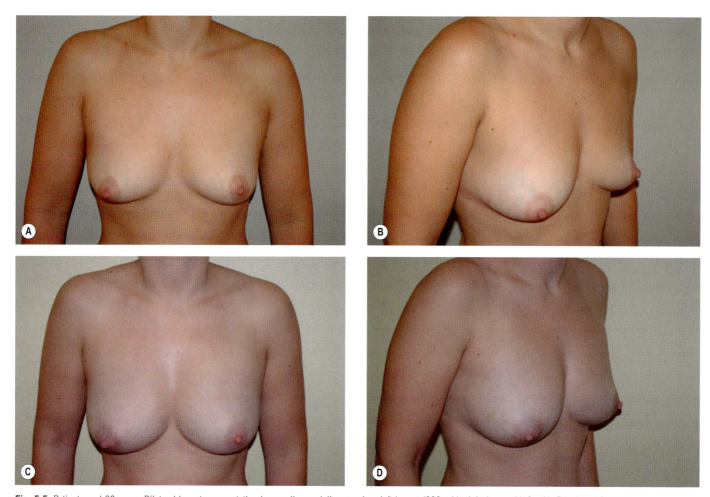

Fig. 5.5 Patient aged 30 years. Bilateral breast augmentation by one lipomodeling session: left breast (390 mL), right breast (410 mL). Result at 12 months. **(A)** Preoperative view. **(B)** Preoperative oblique view. **(C)** Postoperative view. **(D)** Postoperative oblique view.

Breast conservative treatment sequelae

Breast conservative treatment is an ideal indication for lipomodeling. Comprehensive examination of the breast is mandatory in order to determine which zones are to be fat grafted in order to obtain symmetry with the contralateral breast. Fasciotomies are necessary in this indication to allow for skin expansion under the scar. However, one has to be aware that irradiated breast is more prone to skin necrosis and fasciotomies have to be done sparingly. Patient information is very important in this setting because one has to exclude the risk of confusion with cancer recurrence and the patient has to be aware that at least two sessions are mandatory to achieve good results. The first session aims to enhance skin vascularization, and the second session allows volume gain and complete correction of the deformity (Fig. 5.7).

Patient selection

Very careful explanations of the procedure have to be given to the patients. The possibility of multiple fat grafting sessions has to be mentioned as well as

strict radiologic surveillance. In aesthetic indications, the information given to the patient is particularly thorough and extensive with especially elaborated comprehensive leaflets provided during preoperative consultations.[35,36] We have four different information leaflets: lipomodeling in breast reconstruction, lipomodeling for the correction of breast conservative treatment sequelae, lipomodeling for the correction of breast deformities, and aesthetic breast lipomodeling. The main feared risk is that a breast cancer may occur coincidentally with lipomodeling. In order to reduce this risk, imaging investigation (mammography and ultrasound) is carried out before lipomodeling by a specialized radiologist in order to ascertain the absence of any suspicious lesion. If there is any doubt, lipomodeling is delayed or contraindicated. The radiologist must give his agreement before the lipomodeling procedure and thereby becomes co-responsible of the follow-up.[37–40] The patient gives written consent to undergo the same investigations by the same radiologist one year after the procedure. If the radiologist observes a suspicious lesion on imaging at one year, micro-biopsy is systematically performed in order to establish a definitive diagnosis. Ultrasound is done under the age of 30,

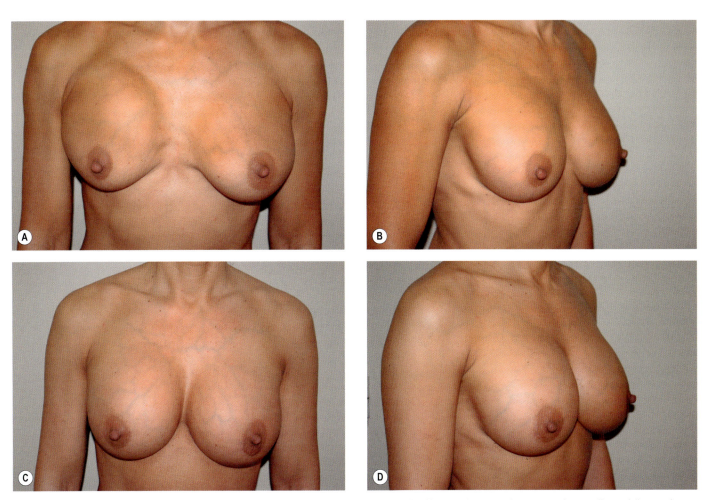

Fig. 5.6 Patient aged 47 years. Secondary case: bad result after previous breast implant augmentation. Treatment by composite augmentation: one lipomodeling session on the left breast (150 mL), right breast (165 mL), and bilateral implant changing during the same procedure. Result at 12 months. (A) Preoperative view. (B) Preoperative oblique view. (C) Postoperative view. (D) Postoperative oblique view.

ultrasound and one mammography incidence between 30 and 40 years of age, and mammography and ultrasound over 40 years. In case of ACR 3, biopsy has to downstage the lesion to ACR 1 or 2, otherwise the procedure is contraindicated.

Surgical technique

Preparation

Patients are informed of the operative technique and its potential risks and complications, and provided with an information leaflet with an information consent form to sign. The patient's weight should be stable at the time of the procedure, as the transferred fat retains the memory of its origins (if the patient loses weight after lipomodeling, she will lose some of the benefits of the procedure). Areas of the breast that require correction are identified and marked out on the upright standing patient (Fig. 5.8A).

The various adipose areas of the body are examined to identify fat deposits to be harvested. Generally, for reconstruction purposes, abdominal fat is used, as it is appreciated by the patients and harvesting in this area does not require a position change from the patient during the procedure. In breast aesthetic surgery, the trochanteric region (saddle bags) and the inside of the thighs and knees are preferred, according to patient choice. Future harvesting areas are outlined with a skin marker (Fig. 5.8B).

Anesthesia

Because of the important amounts of harvested fat, lipomodeling is performed under general anesthesia in the majority of patients. Conventional prophylactic antibiotics are usually given perioperatively, as we usually do in various plastic surgery procedures. No specific antibiotics are prescribed in the case of lipomodeling. Local anesthesia can only be used for minor revisions to correct any residual defect.

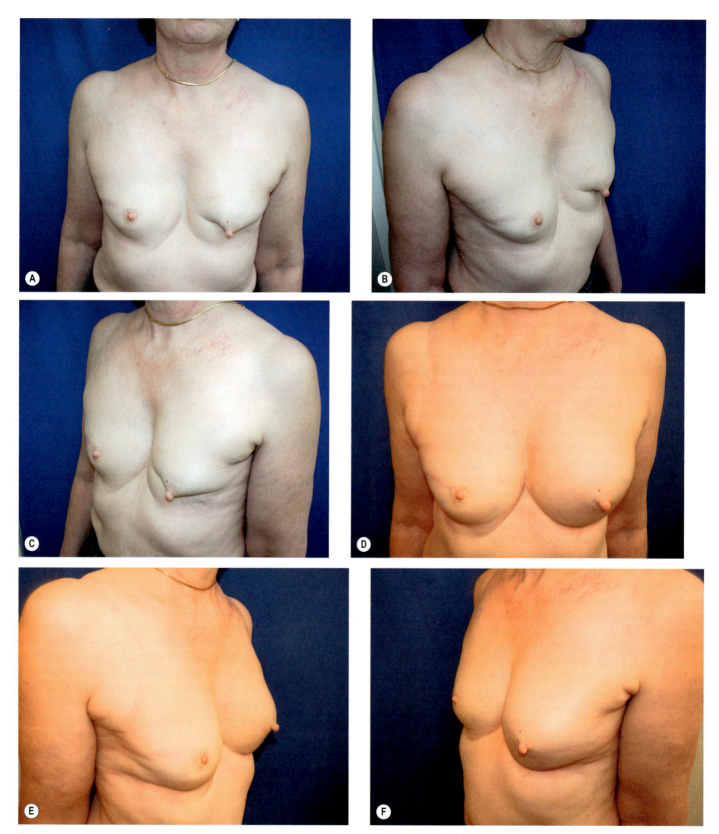

Fig. 5.7 Patient aged 58 years with severe breast conservative treatment sequelae and pectus excavatum, treated by two lipomodeling sessions of the left breast (324 mL, 270 mL) and right lipomodeling during the second session (130 mL). Result 12 months after second procedure. (**A**) Preoperative view. (**B**) Preoperative oblique view. (**C**) Preoperative oblique view. (**D**) Postoperative view. (**E**) Postoperative oblique view. (**F**) Postoperative oblique view.

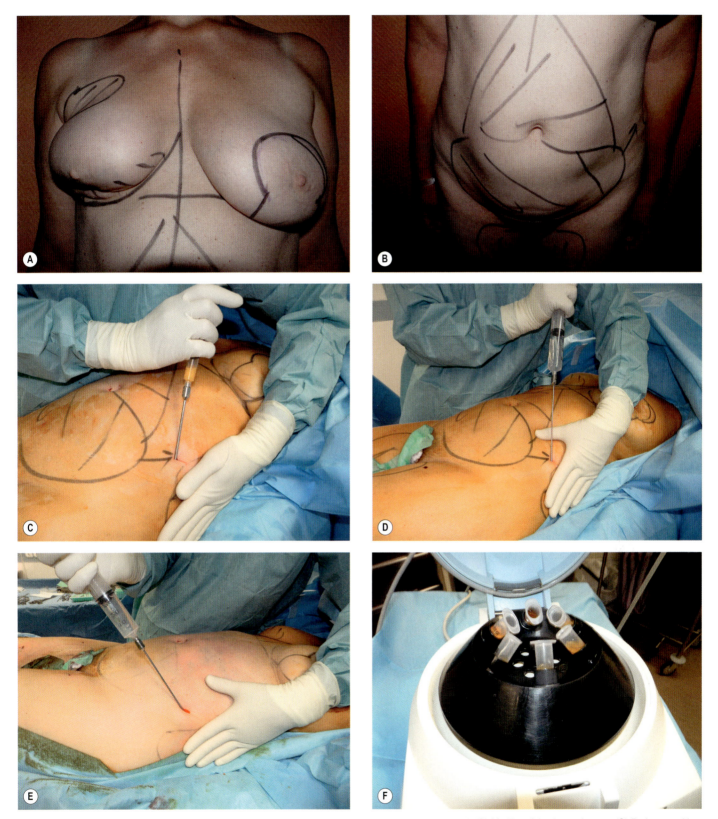

Fig. 5.8 Fat harvesting and preparation. (**A**) Marking of the recipient site (breast conservative treatment sequelae). (**B**) Marking of the donor site area. (**C**) Fat harvest with the harvesting cannula fitted directly on to the 10 mL Luer Lock syringe. (**D**) Infiltration with saline and epinephrine solution. (**E**) Infiltration of the donor site with ropivacaine. (**F**) Centrifugation of the syringes in batches of 6.

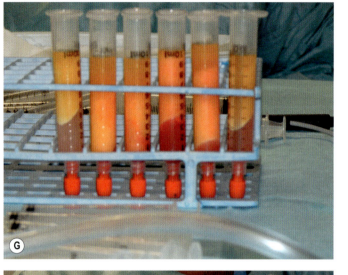
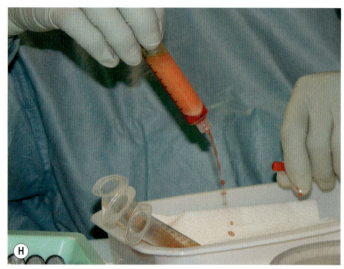
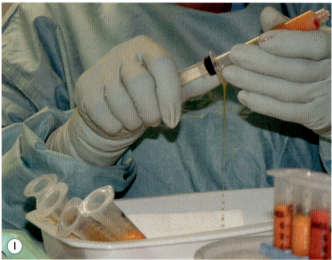
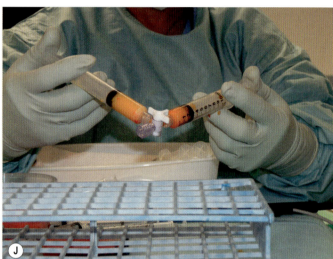

Fig. 5.8, cont'd (**G**) Centrifugation separates the fat into 3 layers. Only the middle layer of purified fat will be retained. (**H**) The bottom layer (serous fluid) is discarded by removing the cap. (**I**) The oily top layer is removed. (**J**) We prepare many 10 mL syringes containing pure fat.

Incisions

In the harvesting areas, incisions are made using a no. 15 blade. For abdominal harvesting, four incisions are made around the umbilicus, and a lateral incision on each side when lateral abdominal and supra-iliac fat is to be harvested. For the thighs, the patient is positioned in a ventral decubitus and an incision is made in each subgluteal fold. A complementary incision on the inside of the knees can be made for fat harvesting of this area. At the recipient site on the breast, punctiform incisions are done with an 18 G needle in previous scars when possible. In order to create a network of transfer tunnels, at least three incisions are needed, two of which are in the inframammary fold and one into the areola.

Fat harvesting

Recent studies on fat transfer have contributed to standardization of the technique of harvesting and injection and the reduction of any pitfalls at each stage. Meticulous work at each step enhances fat survival in the short, medium, and long term. A five holes cannula is used for harvesting. These cannulas have a blunt tip which can be inserted in a 4 mm incision made with a no. 15 blade. Harvesting is done with a 10 cc syringe, directly adapted to the cannula by means of a Luer Lock system (Fig. 5.8C). Subcutaneous infiltration with 500 cc of normal saline at 9% and 0.5 mg of epinephrine is done (Fig. 5.8D). Suction depression is moderate to minimize damage to the adipocytes. Too strong mechanical suction might have a harmful effect on adipocyte survival. Sufficient fat must be harvested to anticipate for the loss during centrifugation and the expected resorption after transfer.

If necessary, in order to obtain a perfect result at the donor sites, harvesting areas are finally smoothed with conventional liposuction using a 4 mm cannula. A solution of saline and ropivacaine is then infiltrated in the donor sites at the end of the harvesting in order to reduce pain after the procedure (Fig. 5.8E). The cutaneous incisions are closed with fine, fast absorbable sutures.

Fat preparation

During the harvesting process, the assistant prepares the syringes for centrifugation. They are sealed with a screw top and centrifuged in batches of six for 20 seconds at 3200 rpm (Fig. 5.8F).

Centrifugation separates the harvested fat into three layers (Fig. 5.8G):

- A layer at the top (oily fluid) containing chylomicrons and triglycerides resulting from cell lysis.
- A lower layer of blood remnants and serum, as well as the infiltration fluid especially if harvesting was done under local anesthesia.

- A middle layer of purified fat. This is the useful part which will be transferred. The other two layers are discarded, the lower layer simply by removing the cap (Fig. 5.8H) and the upper layer by pouring off the oil which covers the middle layer (Fig. 5.8I).

The team must be well organized so that fat preparation is carried out efficiently and rapidly. Using a three-way tap, the purified fat is grouped into 10 mL syringes, by transfer from one syringe to another, in order to obtain the required number of 10 cc syringes of pure fat (Fig. 5.8J).

Fat transfer

After fat preparation, 10 mL syringes of purified fat are ready for transfer. Fat is transferred directly to breast areas with the 10 mL syringes fitted with special disposable transfer cannulas of 2 mm diameter (Fig. 5.9A). These cannulas are longer and stronger than the ones

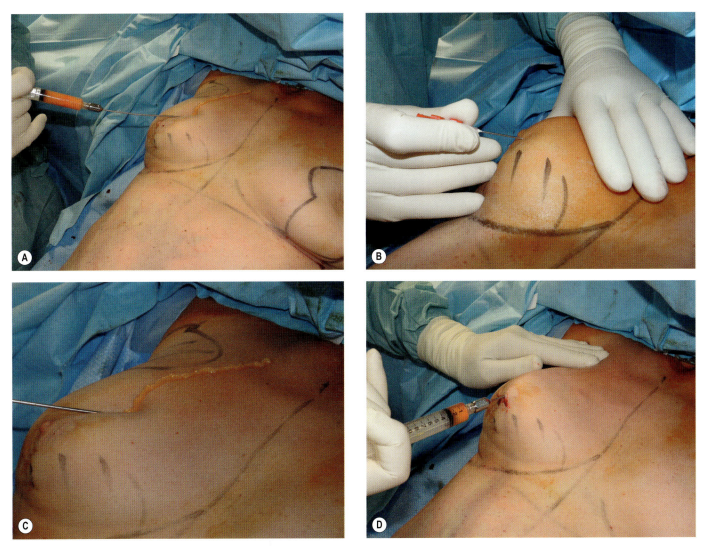

Fig. 5.9 Fat transfer. **(A)** Cannula designed for fat transfer in lipomodeling. **(B)** Incision in the breast with an 18-gauge trocar. **(C)** Demonstration of the principle of fat transfer: fat is transferred while the cannula is gently withdrawn, leaving a fine cylinder of fat resembling spaghetti. **(D)** Fat transfer into the breast.

used for facial fat grafting procedures because the recipient tissue is firmer and more fibrous. Incisions are made using an 18G trocar (Fig. 5.9B). This makes an adequate incision while limiting scarring. Several incisions are made in order to create a honeycomb of multiple microtunnels for fat transfer. Fat is grafted in small amounts, in the form of fine cylinders resembling spaghetti (Fig. 5.9C). Microtunnels must be created in many directions. Transfer is done from the deep to the superficial layer. Good spatial visualization is necessary to form a three-dimensional matrix and to avoid areas of fatty collections that would lead to fat necrosis. Each microtunnel must be designed to be surrounded by well-vascularized tissue (Fig. 5.9D). Fat is transferred under light pressure while gently withdrawing the cannula. It is necessary to overestimate the quantity of fat to be transferred when possible, anticipating the 20–30% expected fat resorption.

When the recipient tissues are saturated and cannot absorb further fat, it is useless to persist because of the risk of inducing areas of fat necrosis. Over-saturation of the recipient site with fat grafting must be avoided. Planning a supplementary session in a few months is preferred and leads to more steady results. Sutures are placed using very fine, fast absorbable suture material, and the breast is covered with an ordinary dry dressing for a few days.

Postoperative care

Harvesting sites

Pain in the harvested areas is the same as for standard liposuction procedures. Patients complain of moderate pain for 48 hours and can be treated with level 1 analgesics. We use an infiltration of diluted ropivacaine at the end of harvesting to control pain in these sites during the first 24 hours. At the end of the procedure, a compressive and elastic dressing is left in place for five days. Level 1 analgesics are prescribed for two weeks.

Bruising is very important and persists for three weeks. Postoperative edema resolves totally or almost totally in three months. To hasten resorption, we ask patients to massage their harvesting areas in a circular motion.

Breast

Bruising resolves in two weeks. Edema resulting from the procedure resolves in one month. During the first three postoperative months, 20–30% of the added volume is gradually lost. But because of the initial edema, the patient may have the impression that she has lost about 50% of her breast volume, as she sees the result the day after the procedure when the breast is already swollen.

Outcomes, prognosis, complications

Based on the first author's personal experience of 2500 procedures of reconstructive and aesthetic breast surgery, and with a 17-year follow-up for the first patients, reliable indications on long-term follow-up can be given.

Long-term clinical follow-up

All patients were clinically followed up and seen in consultation after 15 days, 3 months, and 1 year. Photographs were taken at each visit. A detailed follow-up protocol aimed to assess the quality of the result from the patient's and the surgeon's viewpoint, patient satisfaction, and any adverse effects or complications.

Results were considered very good or good in the majority of cases. Very few results were considered as moderately good and none as poor. As a matter of fact, if the result is insufficient, an extra lipomodeling session can be planned until optimal results are achieved. The percentage of good or very good results depends on the subpopulation studied in relation to the indication.

Long-term radiological follow-up

In 1998, when we developed this theme of research, the main fear concerning fat transfer in the breast was the risk that it would compromise imaging investigations. This fear had in fact led to the controversy of 1987 and its consequences, which we mentioned in the history part of this chapter. For this reason, we undertook to analyze the effect of fat transfer on breast imaging. We carried out three studies with imaging of breasts reconstructed by autologous latissimus dorsi flap and lipomodeling (mammography, ultrasound, MRI),[20] imaging of conserved breasts after lipomodeling (mammography, ultrasound, MRI),[30] and imaging of breasts with defects corrected by lipomodeling (asymmetry, tuberous breasts, Poland syndrome).

Our findings showed that if lipomodeling was carried out according to modern and standardized principles, it does not hinder correct breast imaging and follow up.

It is noteworthy that all the procedures were performed in a surgical team that has completed its learning curve and with specialized radiologists who are familiar with images potentially induced by fat transfer. These conditions are of fundamental importance to allow the use of fat transfer in aesthetic surgery. Imaging in the majority of reconstructed breasts was normal, with some images of oily cysts and fat necrosis. All the images observed were in favor of benign lesions easily distinguished from suspicious ones. Abnormal images were essentially oily cysts, occurring in 10–15% of cases.

The most complex situation concerned lipomodeling for the sequelae of conservative treatment. In this population, the fat necrosis aspect already develops in about 20% of patients following conservative partial mastectomy. Lipomodeling doubles this occurrence. It generates mainly oily cysts but sometimes more complex lesions of fat necrosis. Due to the spontaneous local carcinoma recurrence rate of about 1.5% per year, follow-up must be rigorous. We believe that this indication should be restricted to multidisciplinary teams working with radiologists who have perfect mastery of the subject.

Long-term oncological follow-up

Seventeen years of oncological follow-up have not revealed an increased risk of local recurrence after mastectomy or after conservative treatment. Further studies are needed to assess if, due to strict radiologic surveillance, the recurrence rate is even lower or any malignancy sooner discovered by these patients.

Clinical evaluation

The success rate is easy to evaluate by clinical examination, patient opinion, and comparison of the photographs taken at each consultation with earlier photographs. Twenty to 30% of the volume obtained with fat transfer is gradually lost. Volume is stable after 3 to 4 months and remains so if the patient maintains a steady weight. If the fat harvested is very oily, resorption may be higher, up to 40–50%, and may continue over a longer period of 5 to 6 months. If the patient loses weight, the volume of the transferred fat decreases and the result is a smaller breast with possible asymmetry. Therefore, it is important for the patient to understand that she must maintain a stable weight. Inversely, if she gains weight, breast volume increases. Very long-term evaluation (more than 10 years) confirms that volume remains stable. If breast asymmetry appears after weight loss or gain (for example after discontinuation of anti-hormonal treatments in adjuvant therapy of breast cancer), a complementary lipomodeling session can easily be performed at a later date. The technique can also be used in the other breast if asymmetry develops over time. This technique therefore offers flexibility and precision for long-term revision that is well appreciated by the patients.

Complications

At the harvesting sites, scars must be concealed as much as possible, generally in a fold or in the peri-umbilical region. No patients have complained of unaesthetic scars in a harvesting site. We had one case of irregularity in the supra-iliac region that required secondary correction by lipomodeling. The majority of patients are satisfied with the improvement of the donor sites. This secondary benefit probably contributes to the very high rate of satisfaction of the technique.[25] Irregularities at the donor sites may be due to uneven harvesting of the fat grafts, so harvesting is sometimes completed by standard liposuction to further improve the result and for greater patient satisfaction.

It is essential that this procedure should be carried out by experienced plastic surgeons who have completed their learning curve, as previous experience of cosmetic liposuction is valuable in these circumstances in order to limit the risk of complication and to give the patient the best possible cosmetic result. Local infection occurred in only one of the 2500. This was seen as redness around the umbilicus and was treated without difficulty by antibiotics and local application of ice, with no long-term consequences.

On the breasts, scars must be located in the submammary fold or in its axillary prolongation, or in the areolar region where scars are always of good quality. The presternal area should be avoided as there is increased risk of hypertrophic scarring, presenting as small red hypertrophic punctate scars. Incisions are usually invisible, since they are made with a trocar; they only measure 1.5 mm. Twelve infections occurred at the recipient site among the 2500 lipomodeling procedures of the breast and chest wall. They presented as redness of the breast. The suture at the recipient site was removed. An effusion of fat and pus was evacuated. Topical treatment, antibiotics, and the application of ice completely resolved the problem with no impact on the final result. It should be noted that we had one case of intraoperative pneumothorax (1 case in 2500 procedures), probably due to the transfer cannula piercing the pleura. Pneumothorax was revealed by oxygen desaturation during the procedure. A pleural drain was set, and oxygen saturation returned to normal with total recovery and no later consequences. To avoid this complication, projection of the areolar region should be improved via two incisions in the submammary fold, and not via the areolar region itself. We have had no case of fat embolism. There is a potential risk if fat is injected in a large vessel. Extreme caution is then mandatory in the subclavian area, in particular in the breast and chest wall deformities of Poland syndrome where subclavian vessels may lie lower than in normal anatomy. In 3% of cases, we observed focal clinical fat necrosis. The risk is higher during the surgeon's early experience (15% in the first 50 cases). In these cases, fat necrosis occurred in overtreated areas. When the recipient tissue is saturated with fat, the surgeon should not persist, as areas of fat necrosis may develop. Clinical signs of fat necrosis are typical: tender nodule, slightly sensitive but stable over time, then gradually decreasing. Any increase in size of a hard swelling, even in a reconstructed breast, should undergo micro-biopsy by a radiologist in order to rule out a malignant change.

Fat necrosis nodules are mainly seen in the early stages of the surgeons' learning curve and decrease as the experience increases, if they respect the principle of the 3D network and avoid fat oversaturation of the recipient site.

Secondary procedures

Multiple fat grafting sessions

As previously stated, another fat grafting session can be planned if the result is unsatisfactory. Ease of recovery and improvement of donor sites are strong positive arguments for the patient. Some associated procedures can also be done to enhance the results.

Liposuction of the inframammary area

In patients with a bulky inframammary area anterior to the inferior ribs, we perform a heavy liposuction (7–8 cm under the inframammary fold). This liposuction seems to enhance breast projection. It also enhances the inframammary fold definition while giving the impression of a complementary breast augmentation.

We use this tip in the setting of major breast reduction in overweight patients to improve the definition of the breast. It can also be used in tuberous breasts if possible and in exclusive lipomodeling breast augmentation to improve the final outcome.

The technique consists of a heavy liposuction, going from the deep to the superficial layers of the skin in the predefined area while insisting on the restoration of the inverted V resulting from the junction of the two inframammary folds and the intermammary valley. Because liposuction of this area is painful, we systematically infiltrate diluted ropivacaine at the end of the procedure.

Inframammary fold definition

In some cases of breast aesthetic surgery, the inframammary fold is ill defined or has been damaged by previous surgery. The wearing of a push-up bra enhances the fullness of the upper pole by displacing the mammary gland to the upper region while removing the necessary gland to define the inframammary fold from the lower pole. We consider the inframammary fold as the foundation of the breast. To create or recreate

the inframammary fold, we use a technique derived from our reconstructive experience in cases of latissimus dorsi with a low situated inframammary fold. We locate the desired level of the inframammary fold and mark it with a horizontal line on the midclavicular line. We draw a horizontal ellipse under this desired inframammary fold (5–6 cm width, and 2–3 cm height). The ellipse is de-epithelialized and the upper border of the ellipse is incised with the cautery to the thoracic wall.

Then the de-epithelialized flap is kept attached to the thoracic skin while undermining in the deep plane for 5 to 6 cm. This de-epithelialized flap is pulled up under the breast and fixed to the thoracic wall with no. 1 Vicryl sutures at the predefined position of the inframammary fold. The lower pole of the breast is undermined at the level of the pectoralis muscle, and then rolled to define the lower pole contour and sutured to the fixed inframammary fold. The main drawback of this technique is the resulting scar that is 6 cm long but most of the time hidden in the inframammary fold. The main advantage is the enhancement and efficient correction of the inframammary fold. In rare cases when this technique is associated to aesthetic lipomodeling augmentation of the breast, we start by fixating the inframammary fold then we do the fat transfer.

Fasciotomies

While transferring fat to the breasts, the plastic surgeon is often faced with fibrous strings or adhesion areas making the lipomodeling procedure difficult. The inferomedial area in tuberous breasts is the typical illustration. We developed the fasciotomy technique and had it published by one of our residents.[41,42] We recommend in these cases the use of an 18G trocard's tip to selectively rupture these strings and adhesions under local tension held on the skin by a double hook (Fig. 5.10A–C). Fasciotomies have to be done in different levels in order to obtain a mesh of fibrous tissue to allow for a full expansion of the skin envelope.[41,42] After mesh creation, a new moderate fat transfer is done to fill the newly created holes. Care must be taken not to undermine the area because fat grafting will not take if not in proper contact with the recipient site. Great care must also be taken, especially in young patients, not to do fasciotomies in the presternal region in order to avoid the formation of hypertrophic scars. Fasciotomies are a very powerful means to modify the shape of the breast and irregularities.

Thumb blocking technique

In order to lower the inframammary fold and to fix it in the right position, this maneuver is of utmost

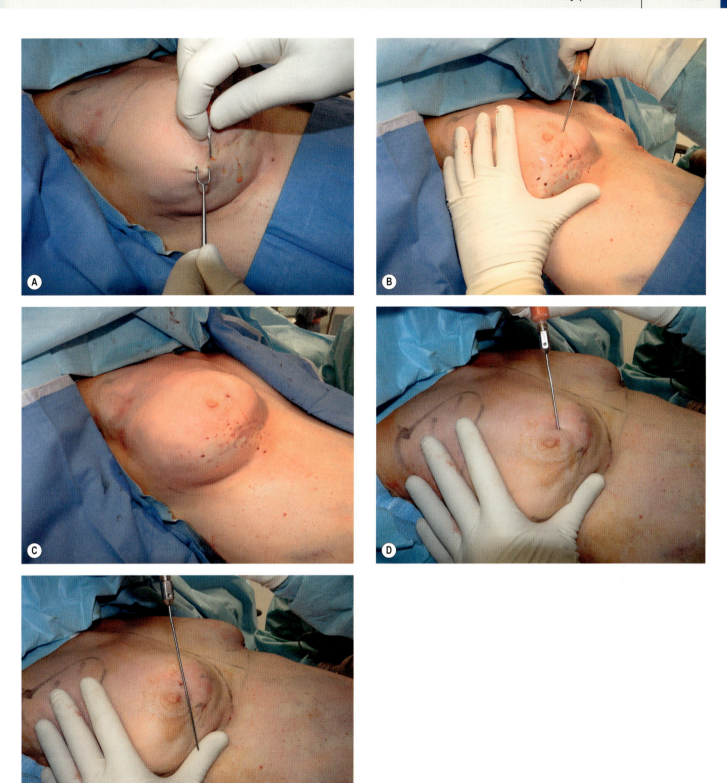

Fig. 5.10 Complementary procedures. (**A**) The "fasciotomies". (**B**) Complement of lipomodeling after fasciotomies. (**C**) Immediate result at the end of the procedure. (**D**) The "thumb blocking technique". (**E**) The "thumb blocking technique": the cannula is blocked by the upper part of the thumb.

importance. The surgeon has to open the first commissure of his hand at the exact place of the inframammary fold for the thumb and intermammary valley for the index. We call this technique the "thumb blocking technique" (TBT). Fat is then transferred with the tip of cannula coming up against the thumb or index finger (Fig. 5.10D,E). This technique will fix the boundaries of the breast while transferring fat only into the chosen breast base.

Conclusion

Lipomodeling is a huge step in plastic, reconstructive, and aesthetic surgery of the breast and represents one of the main surgical advances of the last twenty years.

In the setting of breast asymmetries and malformations, lipomodeling represents the ideal technique. Nowadays, it seems not desirable to treat an asymmetry by unilateral implant positioning. The vast majority of breast asymmetries should be treated by lipomodeling alone. Symmetry is then noteworthy and definitive if the patient stays weight stable. Application of lipomodeling to other thoraco-mammary malformations is now well described. In Poland syndrome, lipomodeling is a significant contribution and allows for a reconstruction of an unprecedented quality at the expense of interventions, with simple follow-ups and very little scar burden. Lipomodeling is also indicated to correct thoraco-mammary deformations of numerous unilateral and symmetric pectus excavatum. Fat grafting is a new therapeutic alternative for tuberous breasts correction, without implant, of associated breast asymmetries, especially when hypotrophy is unilateral. The technique can also be used for breast augmentation when desired augmentation is moderate. Our work has shown that radiologic breast surveillance can be safely performed after lipomodeling. Lastly, fat grafting has drastically changed the correction of breast conservative treatment corrections. The procedure can restore perfect symmetry in two sessions without the need of an implant or a flap.

🌐 Access the complete references list online at **http://www.expertconsult.com**

1. Illouz YG. *Body Sculpting by Lipoplasty*. Churchill Livingstone; 1989:504. *First comprehensive description of liposuction technique, representing a major step toward silhouette remodeling.*

13. Coleman SR. Facial recontouring with lipostructure. *Clin Plast Surg.* 1997;24:347–367. *Description of lipostructure technique allowing for long-term survival of fat grafting. This article was the new starting point of the fat grafting technique.*

16. Delay E. Lipomodeling of the reconstructed breast. In: Spear SE, ed. *Surgery of the Breast: Principles and Art.* 2nd ed. Philadelphia: Lippincott Williams and Wilkins; 2006:930–946. *A comprehensive chapter describing fat grafting technique and an important single operator series.*

20. Pierrefeu-Lagrange AC, Delay E, Guerin N, et al. Radiological evaluation of breasts reconstructed with lipomodeling [Article in French]. *Ann Chir Plast Esthet.* 2006;51:18–28. *This article reports a large series of follow-up patients after breast lipomodeling. Its conclusions show that breast lipomodeling does not hinder radiologic surveillance.*

31. Delay E, Sinna R, Chekaroua K, et al. Lipomodeling of Poland's syndrome: a new treatment of the thoracic deformity. *Aesthetic Plast Surg.* 2010;34:218–225. *Description of the technique in the setting of thoracic deformity. The article shows the method and gives precise information and preoperative evaluation to safely realize the procedure.*

34. Delay E, Sinna R, Ho Quoc C. Tuberous breast correction by fat grafting. *Aesthet Surg J.* 2013;33:522–528. *Article showing the evaluation and planning of fat grafting to correct tuberous breast deformity.*

35. Delay E, Sinna R, Delaporte T, et al. Patient information before aesthetic lipomodeling (lipoaugmentation): a French plastic surgeon's perspective. *Aesthet Surg J.* 2009;29:386–395. *Precise information given to the patient before undergoing breast lipoaugmentation. Might help plastic surgeons in writing their proper informed consent before the procedure.*

36. Delay E, Garson S, Tousssoun G, Sinna R. Fat injection to the breast: technique, results and indications based on 880 procedures over 10 years. *Aesthet Surg J.* 2009;29:360–376. *A single operator large retrospective study of fat injection to the breast in its different indications: reconstructive and aesthetic. Discussion of the techniques and its combination, the expected results, and the necessary follow-up of the patients.*

40. Veber M, Tourasse C, Toussoun G, et al. Radiographic findings after breast augmentation by autologous fat transfer. *Plast Reconstr Surg.* 2011;127:1289–1299. *A thorough description of the radiological imaging of breasts treated with fat grafting with typical benign calcifications and cysts. Any doubt on the images must be solved with complementary documentation, namely biopsy.*

41. Ho Quoc C, Sinna R, Gourari A, et al. Percutaneous fasciotomies and fat grafting: indications for breast surgery. *Aesthet Surg J.* 2013;33:995–1001. *Percutaneous fasciotomies are very important to enhance breast shape while performing fat grafting. Its indications and realization are described in this article.*

6

Mastopexy options and techniques

Robert Cohen

Access video and video lecture content for this chapter online at expertconsult.com

SYNOPSIS

- Breast ptosis presents in many forms and can be congenital in nature, or acquired due to causes such as aging, weight changes, and pregnancy.
- Patients with ptosis generally desire the same result – youthful and "perky" breasts. However, due to wide variations in breast volume and tissue quality, ultimate results vary with each patient, and as a result, preoperative management of expectations is critical.
- There are many surgical options that can be customized to patients' needs, but these generally address repositioning of the glandular tissue and nipple areolar complex and management of skin excess.
- Scar patterns include circumareolar, circumvertical (including J or L scar variations), and inverted-T patterns. Pedicles can be designed from all directions and are independent of the scar pattern.
- Ancillary procedures such as fat grafting, small volume tissue removal (direct or with liposuction), and mesh placement can be used to further improve aesthetic results.
- Complications can occur but can be minimized with careful patient selection, preoperative planning, and execution of surgery.

Introduction

Breast ptosis is one of the more common issues seen in plastic surgeons' offices, particularly those performing a significant amount of aesthetic breast surgery. Although ptotic breasts can be developmental and occur during breast growth at puberty, the image of drooping breasts elicits a sense of aging and loss of femininity for most patients. Beautifully shaped, "perky" breasts – regardless of size – are a symbol of youth and sexuality, and the lack of this trait can cause insecurity and self-esteem issues for many women.

It is important to keep the concept of ptosis separate from the issue of volume. Women can experience ptosis with breasts that (1) have volume deficiency; (2) have ideal volume for their personal sense of proportion; or (3) have volume excess as in the case of symptomatic macromastia. In the cases of volume deficiency, augmentation mastopexy is generally the best option, while in situations of symptomatic macromastia, breast reduction surgery offers the definitive correction.

The concept of augmentation mastopexy and breast reduction is addressed in other chapters, so this discussion will focus on the relatively narrow spectrum of women who have a relatively appropriate amount of breast volume, but are lacking the shape and position associated with a youthful and aesthetic breast. In these women, the primary treatment is rearrangement of the breast parenchyma combined with skin excision and re-draping. Possible small volume addition (via fat grafting) or small volume reduction (via direct tissue resection and/or liposuction) will also be discussed within the context of creating the best possible final breast shape and correcting preoperative asymmetry in women who otherwise have adequate volume. Augmentation mastopexy is only discussed in this chapter as it relates to correction ptosis due to tuberous breasts.

The focus of this chapter is on a practical overview of managing the patient who presents with breast ptosis (as opposed to breast volume issues) as the primary driver for surgery. This will include understanding the pathophysiology of ptosis, assessing the multiple variations of ptosis (including tuberous breasts), managing patient expectations based on their anatomic limitations, understanding and applying the appropriate surgical techniques, and preventing and/or managing possible complications. All patient photographs in this chapter are presented from the author's personal cases.

Breast tissue assessment

When assessing ptotic breasts, multiple tissue categories need to be evaluated and addressed. Thinking of the breast from superficial to deeper tissues, the surgeon must assess the skin thickness and elasticity; the thickness and relative proportion of subcutaneous fat; the density and consistency of breast parenchyma; the state of Cooper's ligaments; the prominence of the pectoralis major muscle and other chest wall musculature; and the nature of the bony base of the chest, including the sternum and ribcage. All of these tissue layers interact to create the final breast appearance, and each component and their interactions with one another must be assessed in order to provide each patient with the best surgical plan (Fig. 6.1).

The skin envelope can vary dramatically between patients. On one end of the spectrum are patients with thick, elastic skin with no evidence of striae. This skin type would more typically be seen in younger patients with developmental ptosis. On the other end of the spectrum are patients with thin skin, severe striae, and minimal elasticity; more commonly seen in multiparous patients and those who have undergone massive weight fluctuations. Loss of skin thickness and elasticity can be a significant contributor to breast ptosis. While the skin is only one part of what will ultimately support the results of a mastopexy, the thicker and more elastic the skin, the more favorable the ultimate outcome will be. This is something that must be addressed with patients preoperatively in order to manage expectations appropriately.

The amount and relative proportion of subcutaneous breast fat can vary dramatically between patients, and density of fat can also vary. These variables can have a significant impact on the ultimate result. In general, higher density of the soft tissues allows for a greater degree of control when reshaping the breast mound, as the tissues are less susceptible to gravitational distortion. A layer of fat padding under the skin can be very helpful in creating a smooth and natural final result, and can camouflage pre-existing irregularities in breast tissue, particularly in the case of fibrocystic breasts.

In many patients with a very high percentage of fat in the breasts (particularly soft, low density fat), it can be very difficult to maintain upper pole fullness, as the fat will tend to settle with gravity to the lower pole of the breast, creating a volume depleted or "scooped out" appearance of the upper breast. Additionally, softer fat has few fibrous elements that will hold a suture, so

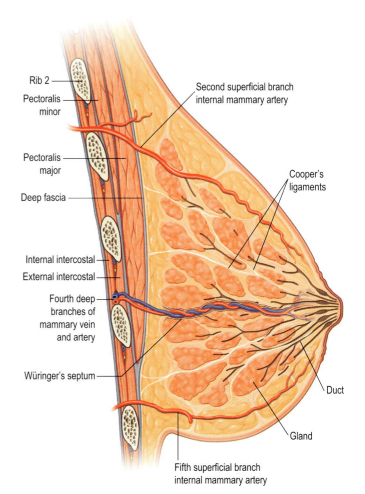

Fig. 6.1 Profile anatomic view of the hemisected human breast. The ligaments described by Sir Astley Cooper are clearly demonstrated to run from the posterior, or deep, breast fascia, which is intimately associated with the pectoralis major muscle fascia, to the anterior, or superficial, breast fascia, and insert into the dermis. The parenchyma, which is encapsulated within these fascial borders, changes with aging, implants, weight changes, and pregnancy. These types of parenchymal changes result in alterations to the integrity of Cooper's ligaments, the breast's fascial components, and the overlying skin and fat.

direct reshaping with sutures can be ineffective. As some degree of natural upper pole fullness is critical in creating a youthful and "perky" breast, patients with low density breasts should be advised of these anatomic issues before surgery and may need to consider upper pole volume augmentation with implants or fat grafting.

Breast glandular tissue, like breast fat, can vary widely in density and quality. Generally speaking, glandular tissue is firmer than fat and has more potential for reshaping and maintaining its shape over time. Mastopexy patients with a high proportion of dense glandular tissue can sometimes achieve a result that is comparable in appearance to an augmentation mastopexy. On the other extreme of the spectrum, it is also important to assess patients for fibrocystic changes, as these tissues can be more difficult to work with and can, in severe cases, result in irregular or "lumpy" appearing breasts if there is insufficient fat coverage to hide these irregularities.

Cooper's ligaments were discovered by Sir Astley Cooper and are ligaments that originate from the pectoralis fascia and penetrate through the breast parenchyma to the dermal layer. These ligaments can be very helpful in supporting the breasts in a youthful position. With time, gravity, changes from childbearing, and weight fluctuations, these ligaments can become attenuated and the breast as a whole can descend on the patient's chest. Although not much can be done directly by the surgeon to improve the strength of Cooper's ligaments, this discussion can further help patients understand why their breasts have changed over time and what the limitations of surgery are relative to these changes.

The size and shape of the pectoralis major muscles and bony architecture of the ribcage and sternum are not part of the breast anatomy *per se*, but these structures do have an indirect impact on the breast appearance and position. Ribcage asymmetry can affect breast projection and symmetry. The presence of a pectus excavatum or pectus carinatum can also impact the appearance of the intermammary region and affects the likelihood of medial or lateral migration of breast tissue, particularly in the supine position. Once again, these bony and muscular anatomic features are difficult to adjust without more aggressive surgery such as sternal remodeling; however, pointing these features out to patients preoperatively can be very helpful in managing patient's ultimate expectations.

Pathophysiology and classification of breast ptosis

As partially addressed in the above section on breast tissue considerations, there are multiple factors which can affect breast ptosis. In certain cases, ptosis of the breasts can be developmental due to naturally poor skin elasticity and weak Cooper's ligaments, often in conjunction with heavier, denser breast tissue. This can be further exacerbated in patients with naturally high inframammary folds, creating a pivot point around which the breast tissue can rotate. Other causes for ptosis can be situational, as in patients whose breast size has fluctuated due to pregnancies or weight changes, wherein the skin elasticity and ligamentous support becomes attenuated. Aging is also a significant issue, as the skin and soft tissue support naturally weakens over time. Finally, lifestyle choices can also affect the breasts. Patients who smoke or sustain significant sun damage

to the breasts, as well as women who rarely use bras or engage in frequent high impact exercise can accumulate more damage to the soft tissues of their breasts.

Once detailed tissue analysis of the breast tissues is completed by the surgeon, a classification of the type and degree of breast ptosis can be helpful in determining the best surgical course. Articles by Regnault and Brink help to divide ptotic breasts into predictable categories. Regnault[1] created the classification of breast ptosis used by most plastic surgeons today. His system is predicated on the relationship of the nipple to the inframammary fold (IMF). In mild, or Grade I ptosis, the nipple is situated within 1 cm of the inframammary fold and is above the lower pole of the breast. In moderate, or Grade II ptosis, the nipple is 1–3 cm below the inframammary fold but is still located above the lowest point of the breast. In severe, or grade III ptosis, the nipple is more than 3 cm below the inframammary fold and is situated at the lowest part of the breast (Fig. 6.2).

Brink[2] further included the categories of glandular ptosis, pseudoptosis, and parenchymal misdistribution (Table 6.1 & Fig. 6.3). Glandular ptosis is a specific variation of ptosis where the nipple remains situated above the lower pole of the breast, but the glandular tissue and nipple areolar complex begin to settle below the inframammary fold, creating a ptotic appearance. Pseudoptosis also involves glandular tissue descending below the inframammary fold; however, in this case, the nipple stays in a fixed position, leading to a progressively

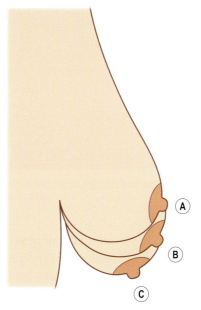

Fig. 6.2 Breast ptosis classification as described by Regnault. **(A)** Minimal ptosis: the nipple is at the level of, or just inferior to, the inframammary crease. **(B)** Moderate ptosis: the nipple is 1–3 cm below the inframammary crease. **(C)** Severe ptosis: the nipple is >3 cm below the inframammary crease. *(Redrawn from: Georgiade GS, Georgiade NG, Riefkohl R. Esthetic breast surgery. In: McCarthy JG, ed.* Plastic Surgery. *Philadelphia: WB Saunders; 1991:3839.)*

Table 6.1 Procedural specifics for forms of breast ptosis

	Inframammary fold position	Parenchymal position	Nipple areolar position	Nipple to fold distance	Clavicle to nipple distance	Clavicle to fold distance
True ptosis	Fixed normal	Fixed rotated	Low downward pointing	Unchanged normal	Elongated	Unchanged normal
Glandular ptosis Common	Mobile descended	Mobile descended	Low forward pointing	Elongated	Elongated	Elongated
Uncommon	Fixed normal	Mobile descended	Low relative to fold	Elongated	Normal to elongated	Unchanged
	Normal					Normal
Parenchymal	Fixed high	Fixed high maldistribution	Normal downward pointing	Short	Normal	Short
Pseudoptosis[a]	Variable, usually low[a]	Mobile re-descended	Surgically fixed	Elongated	Surgically fixed	Variable, usually elongated[a]

[a]Pseudoptosis is most common after corrective procedures for glandular ptosis where the fold has descended preoperatively.
(From Brink RR. Management of true ptosis of the breast. *Plast Reconstr Surg*. 1993;91:657.)

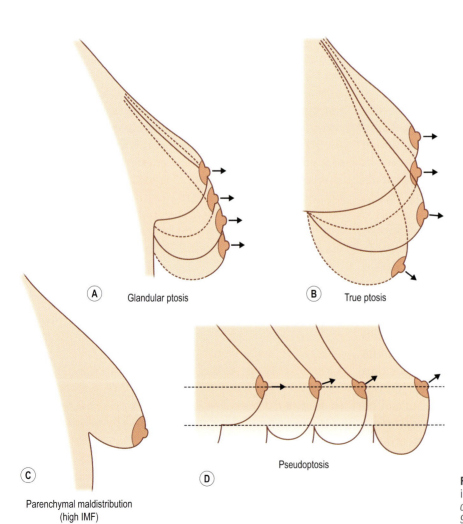

A Glandular ptosis

B True ptosis

C Parenchymal maldistribution (high IMF)

D Pseudoptosis

Fig. 6.3 (A–D) Different types of breast ptosis. IMF, inframammary fold. *(Redrawn after: Brink RR. Management of true ptosis of the breast.* Plast Reconstr Surg. *1993; 91:657–662.)*

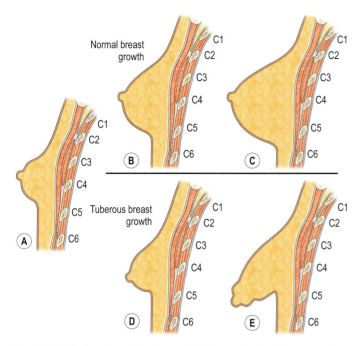

Fig. 6.4 (A–C) Normal breast development with forward and peripheral expansion. **(D, E)** Development of a tuberous breast, with limited peripheral expansion and exaggerated forward expansion. *(Redrawn from: Grolleau JL, Lanfrey E, Lavigne B, et al. Breast base anomalies: treatment strategy for tuberous breasts, minor deformities, and asymmetry. Plast Reconstr Surg. 1999; 104(7):2040–2048.)*

Table 6.2 von Heimburg's tuberous breast classification	
Class	**Anatomic features**
von Heimburg class I	Hypoplasia of lower medial quadrant
von Heimburg class II	Hypoplasia of both lower quadrants with adequate areolar skin
von Heimburg class III	Hypoplasia of both lower quadrants with limited areolar skin
von Heimburg class IV	Hypoplasia of all quadrants
(From von Heimburg D, et al. The tuberous breast deformity: classification and treatment. *Br J Plast Surg*. 1996;49:339–345. Reprinted with permission from The British Association of Plastic Surgeons.)	

oversized and protruding areolas (due to herniation of breast tissue), and conical or tubular breast shapes. Tuberous breasts occur on a spectrum and can also be very asymmetrical in nature.

The classification of tuberous breasts was further expanded by Grolleau[3] and von Heimburg.[4] Much crossover can be seen within these two classification systems (Figs. 6.4 & 6.5 and Table 6.2).

Initial patient assessment and management of expectations

Patients seeking mastopexy surgery will often present with an idea of how they wish to look after surgery. Many patients will bring in younger photos of themselves, show photos from plastic surgery website galleries, or present magazines with images of celebrities or models. Unfortunately, many of these patients do not fully understand the anatomic limitations they have, which can include weak and damaged skin, poor quality

longer nipple to IMF distance. Breasts with pseudoptosis are commonly referred to by surgeons as breasts that have "bottomed out".

The concept of parenchymal maldistribution in Brink's classification system refers to what is more commonly known as tuberous or constricted breasts, wherein abnormally tight tissues do not allow proper expansion of the breast during development, resulting in high inframammary folds, widely spaced cleavage,

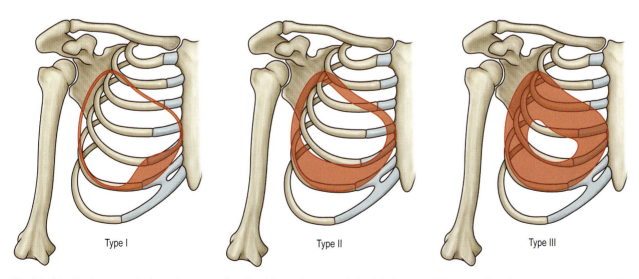

Fig. 6.5 Classification system for breast base anomalies. Type I breasts have hypoplasia of the lower medial quadrant. Type II breasts have hypoplasia of both lower quadrants. Type III breasts have hypoplasia of all four quadrants. *(Redrawn from: Grolleau JL, Lanfrey E, Lavigne B, et al. Breast base anomalies: treatment strategy for tuberous breasts, minor deformities, and asymmetry. Plast Reconstr Surg. 1999; 104(7):2040–2048.)*

or low density breast tissue, and pre-existing asymmetries. Aligning each patient's mental image of their ideal final result with a realistic and achievable result based on their actual anatomy is critical for surgical success.

Additionally, patients need to understand that the forces (such as gravity) and anatomic features (such as weak skin) that lead to ptosis in the first place will still be present, and that future maintenance with more surgery is highly likely. Frank discussions indicating that recurrent ptosis is "more a matter of when than if…" can be helpful to place patients in the right frame of mind. If they cannot accept the idea that mastopexy surgery is rarely a permanent correction, they should not be considered an appropriate candidate for surgery.

When assessing a patient for potential mastopexy surgery, one of the most important initial steps is to separate and analyze the components of ptosis and volume. Clearly, the ptotic component of the breast should be addressed surgically to create a more youthful and aesthetic shape. Breast volume needs to be assessed both as a distinct issue, and as it relates to the correction of ptosis. Specifically, most patients will have a sense of whether they have too little, too much, or the right amount of volume. If they are happy with their volume in bras, but do not like the shape of their breasts or skin laxity, they may be a good candidate for mastopexy only. If they are experiencing symptoms such as back or neck pain and feel that they are too large, they are likely candidates for a formal breast reduction, while other patients that desire more fullness may require simultaneous or staged breast augmentation or fat grafting.

Some of this evaluation can occur in the initial discussion, prior to the physical examination. Once the surgeon has a sense of a patient's satisfaction with their breast volume in bras, this must be reconciled with their actual anatomy during the physical exam. It is at this time that further recommendations based on the surgeon's understanding of each patient's unique anatomy should be made, to give the patient a realistic idea of what may be achieved with surgery. In many cases, what a patient wants with regard to size and shape may not be completely realistic. Their decisions need to be guided by a surgeon who can evaluate the many breast tissue variables and can synthesize options that will achieve the closest match between the patient's ideal result and a realistic result.

Decisions on the more extreme ends of the spectrum are generally easier to make. Patients with large, symptomatic breasts need a reduction in order to improve their physical symptoms and achieve a breast that is proportionate to their overall physique. Conversely, patients with significantly involuted breasts cannot

achieve a reasonable aesthetic appearance without volume around which the skin can be tightened, and these patients will usually need a breast augmentation. Patients in the middle of the spectrum are the ones who can be appropriate candidates for mastopexy only, but these patients can also be the most complicated with regard to preoperative discussions and choices.

As a general rule, performing a mastopexy without some type of augmentation creates the illusion of a smaller breast even if minimal tissue is removed. This is due to the fact that the breast tissue is compacted into a smaller area, and this compression effect will be more significant in patients with softer, lower density breast tissue. Furthermore, patients with a naturally wider breast base width diameter (BWD) or lower inframammary fold will also appear smaller than expected as the redistributed breast tissue will spread out over a larger surface area, providing less central projection and cleavage. The concept of the breast potentially appearing smaller must be addressed preoperatively, as for some patients this will be an unacceptable outcome. These patients will need to consider augmentation (for relatively larger volume increases) or possibly fat grafting (for relatively smaller volume increases).

Adding implants clearly adds additional risks and maintenance to breast surgery, although as demonstrated in recent studies,[5,6] the risks of adding augmentation to mastopexy are additive, not multiplicative. Regardless, patients need to weigh their final desired breast aesthetics with the ease and maintenance of their breasts over time. Once again, certain cases have more obvious courses of action than others.

An example of this can be derived from two of the author's patients. Both patients actively wished to avoid the use of breast implants, and both wished to have "perky" breasts. The first patient (Fig. 6.6A,B) had thick elastic skin and a large volume of firm glandular tissue. In this case, due to favorable volume and anatomy, a significant improvement with good upper pole aesthetics was expected, and the recommendation for mastopexy only was straightforward to make. A typical preoperative discussion regarding risks and expectations occurred.

In the second case (Fig. 6.6C,D), the patient had less favorable skin elasticity, lower density parenchyma, and less breast volume overall. There was potential for a fair degree of improvement with regard to ptosis; however, it was clear based on the preoperative anatomy that upper pole fullness would be suboptimal and the overall degree of change and improvement would be less dramatic than in the case of the first patient.

With this patient, a much longer preoperative discussion occurred, with a blunt explanation of what the

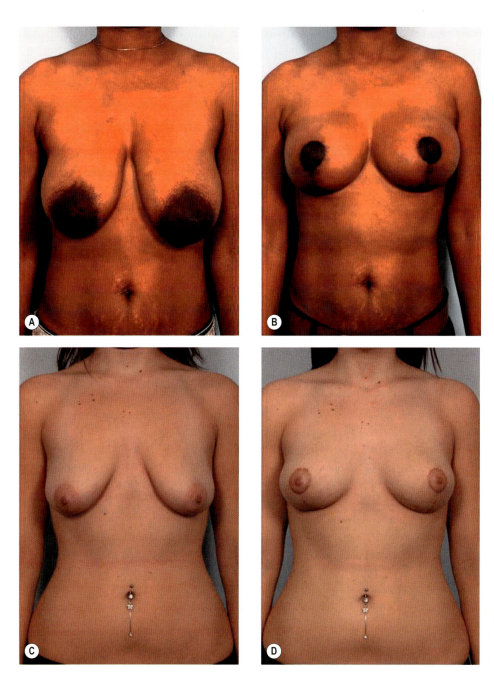

Fig. 6.6 (A–D) Pre- and postoperative photos of patients with **(A,B)** more favorable anatomy and **(C,D)** less favorable anatomy with regard to postoperative upper pole projection. Preoperative management of expectations should be customized to each patient's anatomic limitations.

expected upper pole shortcomings would be without simultaneous augmentation. Additionally, this patient was shown multiple examples of other patients with similar anatomy who underwent mastopexy only, so she could have a realistic idea of what to expect after her procedure. This in-depth process allowed her to weigh out the pros and cons of mastopexy only versus augmentation with mastopexy in her ultimate decision, thus enabling her to select which surgical route would best fit her lifestyle and sense of aesthetics.

This patient was very satisfied with her final results because they matched up with what she expected based on the presurgical discussions. Other patients might not

be happy with the relatively under-filled upper poles and would need to be steered towards implants prior to surgery. Of course, implants can be added or removed later, but no patient should be subjected to additional surgeries that could have been avoided with an appropriate preoperative discussion.

Once it is determined that a mastopexy, as opposed to a breast reduction or an augmentation mastopexy, is appropriate, further analysis and patient discussion regarding surgical technique, scar patterns, and ancillary procedures (such as lateral chest liposuction, small volume fat grafting, or small volume tissue removal for breast shaping and asymmetry correction) can be discussed. These discussions can be integrated into the larger discussion about general risks and complications.

Surgical decision-making

After the initial discussion and physical examination of the patient is completed, the surgeon can decide on the specific techniques that will be most appropriate for the patient. Some of these decisions will be extremely important to the patient (e.g., scar pattern), while others will seem less important to the patient but will be of major significance to the surgeon (e.g., pedicle orientation).

With regard to scars, many things that seem obvious to the surgeon may not be as clear to the patient. As an example, some patients will ask whether there will be any scar after surgery. They may think that plastic surgeons can perform scarless surgery or that scars will vanish over time. It is critical for patients to understand that there will be some type of permanent scar as a trade-off for the mastopexy. Furthermore, every patient needs to realize that while surgical technique and post-surgical management (such as massage, silicone sheeting, and other modalities) can directly affect the nature of the scars, a significant portion of how they heal will be based on their genetics.

With regard to the scar pattern, every patient wants the minimal amount of scars; however, it is important for them to understand that less scar is not a fair trade-off for residual ptosis or an unacceptable final breast shape. Therefore, it is necessary to explain that the type of scar pattern is largely determined by each patient's anatomy and the degree of ptosis. In some cases, a patient may be in a "gray area" between techniques (e.g., between a circumvertical and an inverted-T scar pattern). In these cases, the patient should go into surgery knowing that the larger scar pattern is a possibility, so they are not surprised or disappointed afterwards if that scar pattern is used. This will also allow the surgeon the greatest amount of flexibility in order to achieve the best overall result. Which specific technique should be applied to a given situation is discussed in detail later in the chapter.

Other presurgical considerations

As with any other aesthetic surgery, a thorough overall evaluation of the patient's mental and physical health should be completed prior to entering the operating room. Besides the standard general medical history, physical examination, and assessment for risks such as bleeding or clotting disorders, cardiopulmonary issues, etc., a few specific considerations should be given to the potential mastopexy patient. Management of expectations has been discussed at length, but it is also important to know if the patient has any history of body dysmorphia, eating disorders, or any other mental health issue that could affect ultimate satisfaction. A breast-specific history should also be taken to understand if the patient has a family or personal history of breast cancer or a history of surgery, injury, or radiation to the breasts. Patients should also be asked if their weight is stable or if they plan to have future pregnancies, as these changes could have a negative effect on the results. If they have had a recent pregnancy, especially in conjunction with breast feeding, they should wait until the breast size has stabilized and milk production has ceased. The spine and shoulders should be examined for scoliosis or other asymmetries, as these irregularities can impact postoperative breast asymmetry and should be pointed out to the patient. With regard to mammography, there is some variation in recommendations, but a preoperative screening at age 40 (or age 35 if there is a positive family history of breast cancer) is this author's practice.

Scars, pedicles, and ancillary procedures

There have been many techniques described to correct ptotic breasts, which differ in regard to final scar placement, pedicle orientation, management of the parenchyma, and the use of ancillary procedures. Scars include circumareolar techniques (popularized by Benelli,[7,8] and later modified by Spear and colleagues [9,10]); circumvertical techniques (popularized by Lassus,[11–14] Lejour,[15–18] and later modified by Hall-Findlay,[19,20] and Higdon and Grotting[21]); and inverted-T scar techniques (popularized by Wise and colleagues,[22,23] and later modified by McKissock,[24] Courtiss and Goldwyn,[25] and Marchac and Olarte).[26] Pedicles can come from any direction but are most commonly inferior, superomedial, superior, lateral, and central pedicles. Parenchymal management can include autoaugmentation and internal suturing (Rubin and Khachi[27]), internal mesh (Góes[28–30]), or a pectoralis muscle sling (Graf and Biggs[31]). Ancillary procedures include liposuction of the peripheral breast/chest to improve contouring, and fat grafting to the upper pole to improve volume in this region without the risks and maintenance of implants.

Many surgeons will incorporate components of different techniques to suit each patient's unique needs. It is important to note that the skin resection pattern and the vascular pedicle are generally independent of one another. The skin resection pattern should be chosen based on the degree of skin excess, while the pedicle can be chosen based on the location of the nipple on the breast.

In the previous edition of this textbook, Drs Higdon and Grotting wrote a beautiful and comprehensive chapter on mastopexy and the various historical and current techniques. Review of this chapter and reading the original journal articles referenced above is essential for the plastic surgeon who wishes to have in-depth knowledge of mastopexy techniques. Some of the more complex techniques (such as those involving multiple internal flaps or the use of mesh) have a relatively steep learning curve, and a step-by-step review of each one is beyond the scope of this current chapter.

For this volume, this author presents a relatively straightforward and somewhat universal marking, dissection, and reassembly process that uses concepts and techniques familiar to most surgeons currently performing some form of breast reduction and mastopexy surgery. The learning curve is relatively mild, and complications such as nipple necrosis, areolar distortion, and nipple areolar complex malposition are low.

Algorithm for technique selection

In the author's practice, in comparison to augmentation mastopexies and reduction mammoplasties (totaling >150 cases per year), mastopexy without augmentation or significant reduction is much less common, as the patient's aesthetic goals and anatomy must align closely for an acceptable final result that provides reasonable volume and a pleasing overall breast shape. Most patients in this category fit the profile of having a fairly significant amount of natural breast tissue (usually at least a C cup) and enough ptosis (generally Regnault grade II or III) to warrant the surgery and the resulting scars. Most patients who are candidates for mastopexy only have enough breast density to create aesthetic upper breast fullness. However, patients with less firm tissues are still candidates, as long as they understand that their tissues will limit the degree of upper poles fullness despite the correction of their nipple position and lower pole ptosis. Skin elasticity and thickness for mastopexy patients can vary widely, and once again, these variations must be discussed with patients for the best management of expectations.

Although the author frequently uses a version of circumareolar tightening in appropriate augmentation mastopexy and tuberous breast correction patients (discussed in more detail later in this chapter), this technique is rarely used in pure mastopexy patients due to the flattening effect of this technique and the inherent limitations with regard to superior repositioning of the nipples and tightening the skin of the lower poles without distorting the areolas or lower breasts. (The exception to this would be patients with large, dense, conical breasts with mild ptosis, wherein a flattening effect would be aesthetically beneficial. [Video 6.1 ▶]).

Bearing the above in mind, the majority of patients appropriate for mastopexy without augmentation will have grade II or III ptosis, which will benefit from circumvertical skin resection, which tightens the lower pole, raises the IMF, and increases breast projection. An inframammary skin resection (inverted-T scar) can be added in patients with significant lower pole skin excess and poor skin elasticity, where lower pole skin overlap would still be present after a circumvertical resection. In "gray area" cases, a circumvertical skin resection is planned and tailor-tacked during surgery, and if excess lower pole skin is still present, the patient can easily be converted to an inverted-T scar, on the table.

In terms of pedicle orientation, the author has found the superomedial and superior pedicles to be most useful. In the majority of patients, a superomedial pedicle represents a shorter distance to the nipple than an inferior pedicle. Additionally, this leaves the base of the pedicle in the area of the breast where fullness is most needed, and allows the pedicle to be suspended from above as opposed to being pushed up from below, which is the case with inferior pedicles. If the distance from the skin resection to the nipple is very short – making any rotation of the pedicle difficult – a superiorly based pedicle is used by the author.

With regard to ancillary procedures, in cases where patients wish to be modestly fuller in the upper pole, but do not wish to have implants, the author offers fat grafting (if appropriate harvest sites are available). Biologic materials such as resorbable mesh or ADM can also be offered in patients with particularly soft breast tissue and weak skin. These reinforcement materials can act as an internal support bra and be sutured to the pectoralis fascia. In patients with wide, poorly-defined breasts, lateral chest liposuction is offered as a means of sculpting the outer curve of the breast and providing more definition between the breast and the lateral chest.

Marking technique

Proper preoperative breast markings are critical in performing mastopexy surgery. The markings guide the surgeon with regard to symmetry and nipple placement, and allow for intraoperative adjustment as needed, without losing sight of important anatomic landmarks. Appropriate markings will also alert surgeons to possible tilting of the torso and reduce the risk of asymmetrical nipple placement when the patient is examined in the seated position.

The following is a description of the author's preferred marking technique. The patient is marked in the standing position with shoulders relaxed. The sternal notch is marked with a "V", and a midline is drawn down to the umbilicus (Fig. 6.7A). After this, a measuring tape is draped around the patient's neck to assist marking the patient's breast meridians (Fig. 6.7B). Keep in mind, these lines bisect the breast, but they may not intersect the nipples if the nipples are medially or laterally situated. These marks are continued down the breasts to include the lower poles, and then continued down on to the abdomen.

The inframammary folds (IMF) are marked (Fig. 6.7C), and if a significant fold asymmetry is present, it should be noted for adjustment during surgery. A large caliper is then used to transpose the inframammary fold onto the breast on each side, and these marks are re-measured from the low point of the sternal "V" marking to ensure symmetry (Fig. 6.7D,E).

Each breast is rotated medially and laterally, and with each rotation, a line is drawn as a plumb line from the transposed IMF mark on the breast to the meridian line which had previously been drawn on the abdomen (Fig. 6.7F,G). These two new lines represent the extent of safe

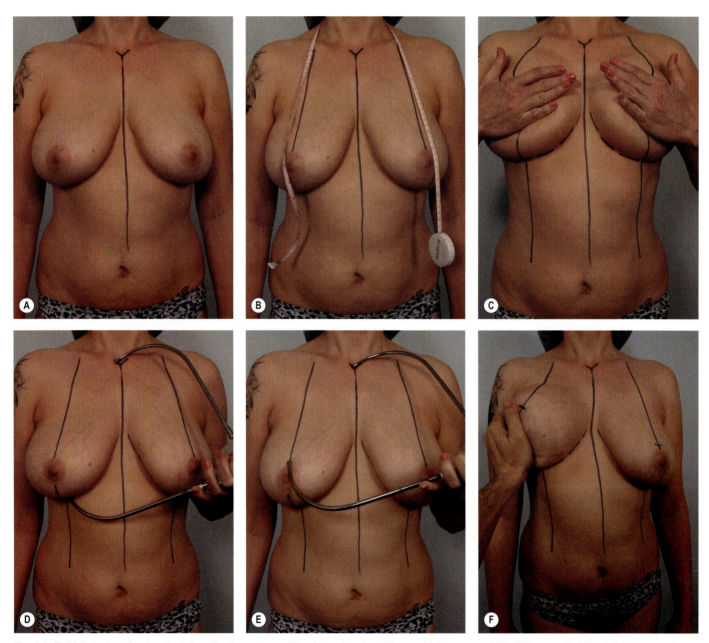

Fig. 6.7 (A–L) Author's preferred method of marking for mastopexy. The midline, breast meridians, and inframammary folds (IMF) are marked. The IMF is transposed on the breast, and the breast is rotated medially and laterally to determine the amount of skin resection. The vertical limbs are measured at 7 cm, and the areas for skin undermining (in the case of vertical mastopexy) or skin resection (for inverted-T scar mastopexy) are marked, leaving approximately 3 cm of skin from the bottom of the skin resection to the IMF.

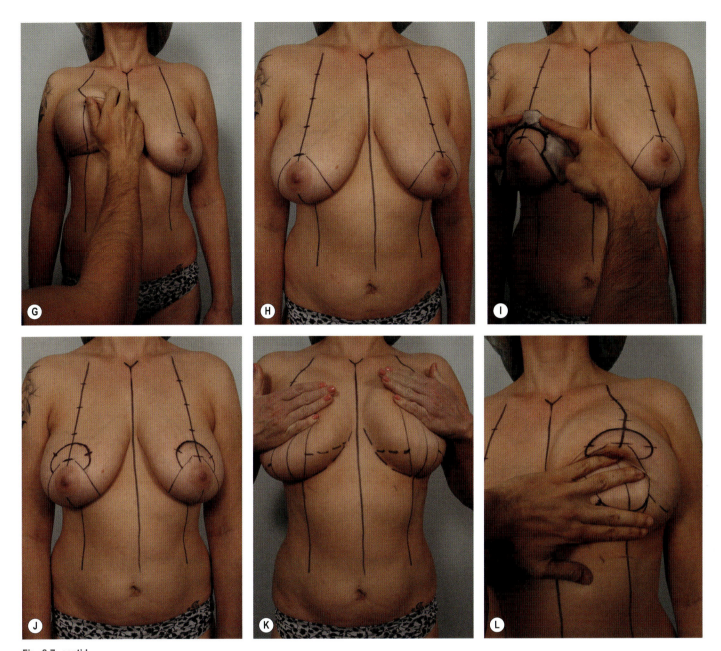

Fig. 6.7, cont'd

skin resection. Marks at 5 cm increments are drawn up the meridian lines from the transposed IMF marking to allow other points of reference in case intraoperative adjustments are made (Fig. 6.7H). A pre-made template with a keyhole of 42 mm (or 38–40 mm in patients with smaller areolas) is centered on the transposed IMF mark. The template is opened and matched to the medial and lateral rotation plumb lines (Fig. 6.7I,J). This template can be easily created using two layers of foam tape on top of each other and then placed sticky side to sticky side for a total of four layers, with a 42 mm hole cut in the center, split up the 6 o'clock position and with cross-hatches drawn at the 3 o'clock, 12 o'clock, and 9 o'clock positions.

Marks are made 7 cm below the bottom of the keyhole (Fig. 6.7K). In cases where a circumvertical is planned (Grade I, most Grade II, and rarely Grade III ptosis), dashed lines are extended medially and laterally and connected with the IMF markings. Another mark is made 2 finger-widths (approximately 3 cm) up from the IMF, which becomes the lowest point of skin resection (Fig. 6.7L). The parenchyma between the IMF and the marks 7 cm down from the keyhole is later undermined and either resected or, more commonly, sutured up to the pedicle to create more fullness. In cases where an inverted-T scar skin resection is planned, the skin between these markings is removed, and the underlying parenchyma handled in the same way as noted above.

Finally, the pedicle is marked. Generally, this is a superomedial or superior pedicle, although in many cases, the entire area within the skin resection pattern with the exception of the nipple areolar complex is simply de-epithelialized to maximize volume and blood supply.

Circumvertical mastopexy with the option of inverted-T scar conversion

After administering preoperative intravenous antibiotics, the patient is brought to the operating room and the following is the author's preferred procedure. With the patient prepped and draped in the supine position under general anesthesia, one or both breasts can be quickly tailor-tacked at the proposed incisions, and the patient examined in the seated position to ensure proper skin resection. There will be mild lower breast distortion given that no dissection has yet occurred, but this maneuver will confirm that the markings are not excessively aggressive. With more experience, this maneuver can quickly be done by pinching the skin together manually, or skipped altogether, depending on the surgeon's confidence in the markings.

Next, the central breast is placed on maximum stretch by the surgical assistant, and the areola is marked (usually with a 42 mm cookie-cutter) and scored with a 15-blade scalpel. The previously made markings for the mastopexy are scored with a scalpel (Fig. 6.8A). If a circumvertical skin resection is planned, the medial and lateral areas of skin undermining (marked with a "U" in the photos) are injected with approximately 10 cc per breast of local anesthetic containing epinephrine to minimize bleeding (Fig. 6.8B). Then the pedicle (in large breasts), or the entire area within the markings (in smaller breasts), is de-epithelialized with a 10-blade scalpel (Fig. 6.8C). Electrocautery is then used for hemostasis and to contract the dermis (Fig. 6.8D).

The lower dermis is released (Fig. 6.8E), and a 10-blade scalpel on a flat handle is placed parallel to the skin and used in progressively advancing circular movements to undermine the skin in the inferomedial and inferolateral breast areas, leaving a few millimeters of subcutaneous fat to maintain blood supply and smoothness (Fig. 6.8F). After this, electrocautery is carefully used for hemostasis of this undermined skin.

Next, a lateral flap of 1.5–2 cm thickness is developed down to the level of the chest wall, and the areas of parenchyma below the undermined inferomedial and inferolateral skin flaps skin are dissected off the chest wall leaving a thin layer of fat down on the fascia to maximize lymphatic drainage and create a gliding plane

after healing (Fig. 6.8G). The parenchyma from the undermined areas is usually maintained for maximum volume and sutured to the main pedicle with 3.0 Vicryl suture (Fig. 6.8H). In cases where a small reduction is preferred, this undermined tissue is resected and sent to pathology for evaluation. Regardless, the tissue should be dissected out from the lower breast in order to re-establish a sharp, higher inframammary fold.

At this point in the surgery, the pedicle is superomedially or superiorly based, but unlike a breast reduction, this "pedicle" essentially represents all of the breast tissue besides the tissue connected to the lateral skin flap. If dense, white glandular tissue is present, the author usually leaves a thin (0.5–1 cm thick) layer of this as part of the lateral flap, to help maintain a smooth, firm contour of the lateral breast and to provide extra soft tissue support.

The lower half of the pedicle is undermined at the level of the chest wall, and the pedicle (again, representing the majority of the breast tissue) is rotated in a superomedial direction or shifted in a superior direction, and sutured at its deep lateral and inferior border to the chest wall using 3.0 PDS suture (polydioxanone suture) (Fig. 6.8I). This stabilizes the tissue in a higher position during the healing process and elevates the new inframammary fold. Care must be taken not to over elevate the tissue as this can cause a distortion and over-rotation of the lower pole of the breast. The suture points are usually 1–1.5 cm above the original IMF.

Once the dissection and stabilization of the parenchyma in its new position is completed, the skin is temporarily tailor-tacked with a stapler (Fig. 6.8J) and checked with the patient in the seated position. Based on the appearance of the breast, small adjustments in the pedicle position and the amount of skin resection can be made. Also, the lower breast skin excess can be evaluated, and if significant skin-on-skin contact is still present, the patient can be converted to an inverted-T scar pattern by simply resecting the undermined skin of the inferomedial and inferolateral breasts.

This is also an excellent time for the circulator to take a front view photo, which shows one breast essentially completed (except for final suturing), while the other breast is in its original state (Fig. 6.8K). This photo can be a very dramatic visual tool for patients to understand the true degree of correction the surgery created.

The patient is returned to the supine position, and attention is turned to the left breast where the same procedure is performed with considerations made for asymmetry correction. If an inverted-T scar pattern was necessary on the right breast, this type of skin resection

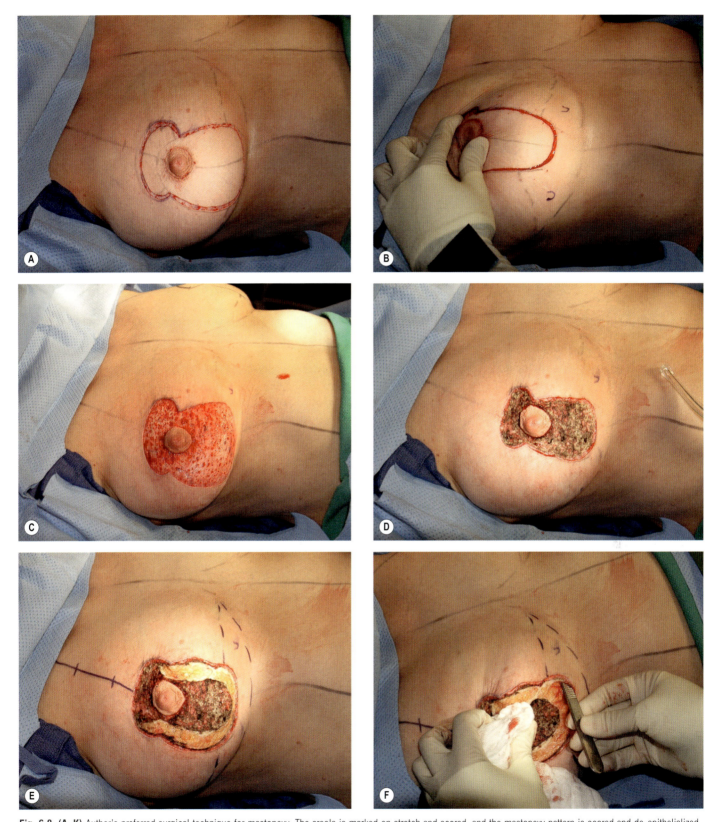

Fig. 6.8 (A–K) Author's preferred surgical technique for mastopexy. The areola is marked on stretch and scored, and the mastopexy pattern is scored and de-epithelialized. The skin is cauterized and released, leaving a superomedial or superior pedicle. Inferomedial and inferolateral flap undermining is performed, and a lateral flap of approximately 1.5–2 cm thickness is developed to the chest wall. The pedicle is consolidated with 3.0 Vicryl and then elevated and sutured approximately 1–1.5 cm above the original inframammory fold with 3.0 PDS. Layered closure is performed, and a photograph is taken to compare the repaired breast with the original anatomy.

Continued

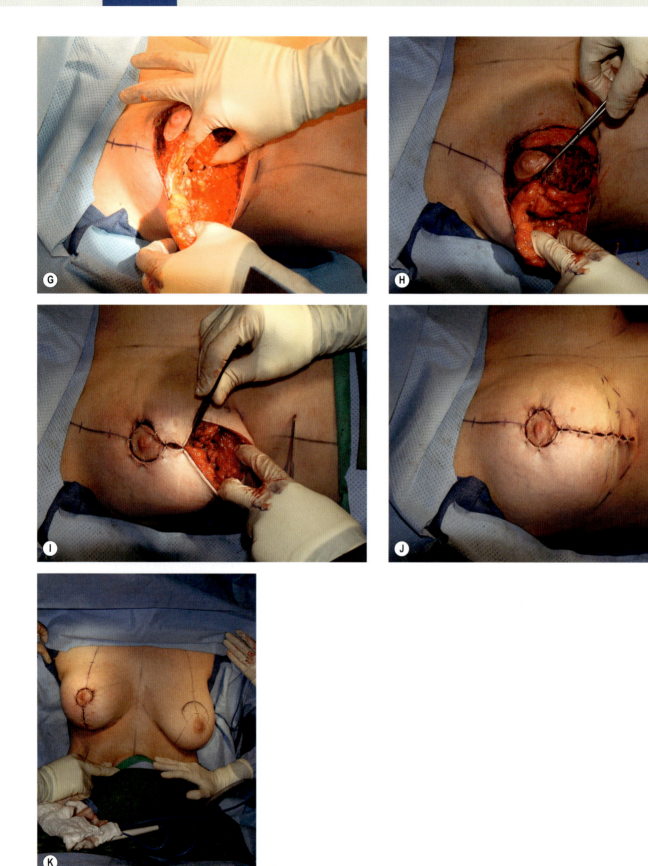

Fig. 6.8, cont'd

can be performed immediately on the left, skipping the skin-undermining maneuvers.

Once the left breast dissection is completed, it is tailor-tacked as well, and the patient is carefully checked in the supine and seated position for good shape, size, and symmetry. Staples are then removed after a marking pen is used to make cross-hatches on the vertical to ensure that proper orientation between the medial and lateral flaps is maintained during closure.

If reasonably strong breast tissue or superficial fascia is present, parenchymal pillar sutures can be placed with 3.0 PDS in interrupted fashion for additional deep support. If a more extensive circumvertical resection was performed, a single 10-French hubless Blake drain on each side is an option to help the undermined tissue adhere down to the chest wall. If a smaller circumvertical resection or an inverted-T scar resection was performed, no drains are used. Prior to closure, the wounds are irrigated with saline, final hemostasis is ensured, and quarter-percent bupivacaine with epinephrine is generally infiltrated for early postoperative analgesia. In appropriate patients with very weak tissues, additional support such as a re-absorbable mesh can be used as an internal bra to offload weight from the skin. The support mesh is used in a similar orientation to a real bra and is sutured just below and lateral to where the parenchyma was sutured to the pectoralis fascia.

Final closure is performed in layers of running suture to minimize knots and the risk of spitting sutures. First, a 3.0 PDS suture is used at the bottom of the areolar keyhole with the knot and suture tail buried deeply. This suture is used in running whip-stitch fashion to reapproximate the deep dermis down to the inframammary crease and is run back up the vertical incision and then around the areola for deep dermal support. The same technique is applied to the inframammary incision if such an incision was used. Any de-epithelialized dermis between the suture bites is invaginated and fuses to itself over time. An equivalent strength barbed suture (2.0 PDO) can also serve this purpose. The areolas are checked for good shape and symmetry, and a cookie-cutter can be used at this point for further areolar shape and diameter refinements. After the deep closure, the skin is run closed with a 4.0 Monocryl in subcuticular fashion.

In appropriate patients where increased upper pole fullness without implants is desired and recommended, fat grafting is performed. Liposuction of areas such as the flanks and thighs can be performed, the fat processed, and then re-injected into the subcutaneous space of the upper poles with a small, blunt fat grafting cannula.

Although there were concerns in the 1980s with oncologic issues after fat grafting to the breasts,[32] these issues have since been re-examined, and the technique of fat grafting to breasts is now a common adjunctive procedure in both aesthetic and reconstructive surgery.[33]

With the technique of fat grafting, a volume deficient upper breast pole can generally be filled in a more direct and effective way than can be achieved with a mastopexy alone (Fig. 6.9). Additionally, this provides a lower maintenance option than breast augmentation with implants, and is particularly beneficial in larger breasted patients where only a modest amount of volume (approximately 100–300 cc) per breast is needed.

The primary limitation for fat grafting is the presence of sufficient donor site fat and the patient's willingness to accept additional surgical sites. Patients must understand that there is somewhat less predictability with regard to volume increase than there would be with an implant; however, this is the trade-off for lower maintenance associated with a totally autologous procedure.

Besides eliminating implant complications such as capsular contracture and implant malposition, fat grafting allows preferential volumetric filling in the areas where that volume is needed most. Additionally, by embedding fat in the subcutaneous tissues of the upper breast, there is less direct force on the lower pole of the breast than there would be with an implant, potentially reducing the risk of a lower pole stretch deformity.

In other patients who need removal of lateral chest fat for reshaping purposes, tumescent can be placed and careful deep lateral chest liposuction can be performed to better contour the breasts.

Once closure is completed, the incisions are cleaned and dried, and mastisol and Steri-Strips are applied. The patient is placed in a gently compressive surgical bra, extubated, and sent to the post-anesthesia care unit (PACU) for recovery. Patients are sent home the same day of surgery, and pain is usually mild and easily controlled with oral medications.

Tuberous breast correction

Tuberous breasts, as noted in the section on breast anatomy, are generally defined by constricted lower poles, a wide intermammary distance, conical breast shapes, oversized and protruding areolas, and an excess of herniated, retroareolar breast tissue combined with a general paucity of breast tissue. In order to create an aesthetic breast in a tuberous breast patient, a reversal of all these problems must be achieved. In essence: high inframammary folds with constricted lower breast tissue need to be released and expanded. Oversized and protruding areolas with herniated breast tissue need to

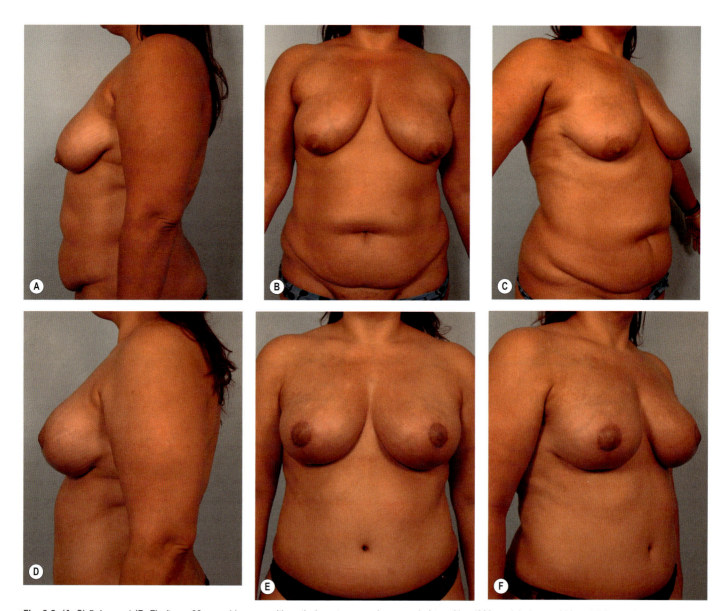

Fig. 6.9 (A–C) Before and **(D–F)** after, a 39-year-old woman with vertical mastopexy and upper pole fat grafting (300 cc right breast; 200 cc left breast due to preoperative asymmetry), liposuction of flanks, and full abdominoplasty.

be corrected by reducing the areolar diameter, forcing the retroareolar tissue back into the main breast mound (sometimes requiring tissue resection). Finally, undersized and widely-spaced breasts generally require correction with augmentation.

For correction of tuberous breasts, the author's procedure starts with a thorough evaluation of the breast anatomy as noted above. Of key importance is the patient's ideal breast base width diameter, as this will determine the proper width of the implants. The true base width of the chest in a tuberous breast patient is almost always wider than the breast base width of the constricted breast, and it is on the true chest width that the implant width is selected. The author also generally prefers highly cohesive textured implants to allow for greater stability, lower capsular contracture rates,[34] and

greater resistance against implant compression. When form stable anatomic implants are an option, these can potentially provide other benefits due to their resistance to compression and ability to create preferential lower pole expansion.

For most of these cases, the author performs a periareolar approach, as this allows the minimum amount of scarring in the lower pole of the breast where expansion is needed the most. This also eliminates concerns about IMF incision placement, where less lower pole expansion than expected preoperatively may be an issue. Although IMF approaches have shown lower rates of capsular contracture, this benefit is reduced for tuberous breast patients because aggressive scoring of the lower breast and tissue resection is often necessary, which exposes the implant to glandular tissue and possible bacteria residing in the milk ducts. The author often uses a superior periareolar approach in these cases to maximize the distance of unscarred lower breast for tissue expansion, and to reduce the chance of lower areolar scar tethering or distortion with flexion of the pectoralis muscles. Prior to making a periareolar incision on the true areolar edge, a 40–42 mm cookie-cutter is used to mark the areola on maximum stretch, and this is lightly scored for the later circumareolar mastopexy.

Once the main incision for implant placement is made (usually a superior periareolar incision on the true upper edge of the areola) and dissection is continued down to the chest wall, the author generally performs a dual-plane 3 retropectoral dissection as described by Tebbits.[35] This offers the benefits of upper pole submuscular coverage for a more natural slope and lower capsular contracture rate, while the majority of the lower half of the breast is subglandular, allowing for maximum tissue expansion.

The lower pole parenchyma is usually very tight, and fibrous tissue bands are often identified. These bands and areas of dense, tight tissue are radially scored with electrocautery to release them and allow maximum expansion. Criss-cross scoring can be used carefully in more severe cases. Caution should be taken not to score the breast tissue too close to the skin, as this can cause visible skin irregularities or issues with blood supply. It is helpful to guide the degree of scoring by using implant sizers. Bands of tightness which are not obvious without tension become much more apparent to internal digital palpation when a sizer is in the breast pocket. Periodically checking the patient in the seated position is also helpful to ensure the most aesthetic roundness of the lower pole and to assess for persistent irregularities.

In many cases, a disproportionate amount on glandular tissue will be seen in the retroareolar area, which contributes to the oversized and protruding areolar appearance. It can be helpful to resect some of this tissue, leaving an even thickness of glandular tissue that is consistent with the remainder of the breast mound. Any resected breast tissue should be sent to pathology for analysis.

Once a precise pocket has been created, the lower pole scored, the inframammary crease lowered as needed to create an optimal nipple to IMF distance (based on the implant width), and the excess tissue resected (if needed), the pockets are irrigated with a triple antibiotic solution as described by Adams et al.[36] and the implants placed with a funnel device to minimize contamination of the implant shell and limit trauma to the gel. If textured implants are used, they are manually adjusted to seat them in the lowest position of the pocket.

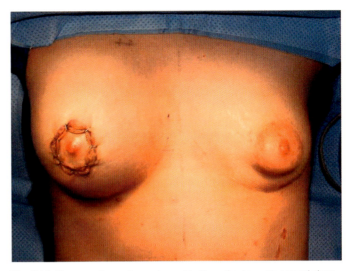

Fig. 6.10 Circumareolar mastopexy is used by the author to create a round shape out of a naturally "pointy" breast, and is also used to reduce the appearance of a "double-bubble" caused by a naturally high inframammory fold.

Deep closure is performed in layers with 3.0 Vicryl, and at this time, attention is turned towards the circumareolar mastopexy. This portion of the procedure serves multiple functions. First of all, it reduces areolar size and protrusion. Second, if the outer oval of resection is shifted in a relatively superior position to the inner areolar incision, it will shift the areolas into a higher position on the breast (usually 2–2.5 cm maximum). Third, with aggressive lowering of the IMF, which is generally needed with tuberous breasts, the old crease can create a "double-bubble" appearance. The circumareolar mastopexy will tighten the breast skin around the implant, which redistributes the tissue and helps to reduce the appearance of the crease (Fig. 6.10). Finally, circumareolar mastopexies have a flattening effect on the breast, which helps to create a rounder, more aesthetic appearance in a conical shaped tuberous breast (Fig. 6.11A–D).

With regard to the author's specific circumareolar mastopexy technique, a multilayer approach is performed. The area for skin resection is marked with the vertical distance approximately 1 cm longer than the transverse distance to avoid an oval final shape (Fig. 6.12A). (Please note the measurements in centimeters are written on the patient's skin for demonstration purposes.) Then, the area of skin resection is de-epithelialized (Fig. 6.12B), and cautery is used for hemostasis and to shrink the dermis (Fig. 6.12C). 3.0 PDS suture is used in running whip-stitch fashion to imbricate the dermis to take tension off the final closure (Fig. 6.12D). A deep subcuticular style placement of 3.0 Prolene is then placed to stabilize the diameter of the areola (Fig. 6.12E), and skin closure is completed with 4.0 Monocryl (Fig. 6.12F).

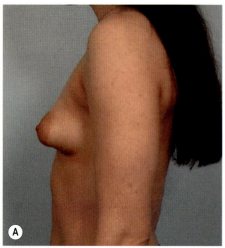 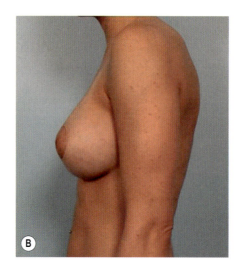 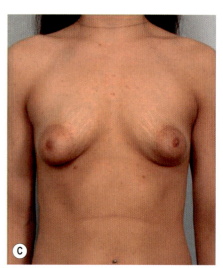

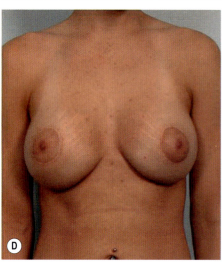

Fig. 6.11 (A–D) Preoperative and postoperative views of a tuberous breast correction that utilized the author's preferred technique of breast augmentation, radial scoring, small volume retroareolar glandular tissue resection, and circumareolar mastopexies.

Postoperative care for mastopexy patients

The following is the author's preferred postoperative care procedure. After surgery, the patient is encouraged to perform early ambulation and deep breathing exercises. A gentle range of motion exercises are also encouraged, but the patient is asked to avoid strenuous activity or lifting more than a few pounds. If drains are placed, they are usually removed once outputs are <25 cc per day. Light, non-impact exercise can be resumed at 4 weeks, and easing into a full exercise routine can be started 6 weeks after surgery. The patient is kept in a soft, non-underwire bra after surgery and can use ice for comfort as needed. Underwire bras can be resumed at 4–6 months, if comfortable.

Risks and complications

The risk of a major complication with mastopexy, if performed judiciously, is fairly low. An extensive form

including all foreseeable risks should be read and signed by the patient after a discussion with her surgeon and an opportunity to ask any final questions. There are a few risks more common to mastopexy surgery, which should be discussed in more detail with patients. These are noted below.

Scarring

As discussed earlier, acquisition of new scars on the breasts is the primary trade-off for mastopexy surgery. In some cases, genetics, excessive skin tension, or spitting sutures can exacerbate the degree of scar thickness or scar spreading. Patients must understand that suboptimal scarring is a possibility and should be prepared for this issue. Thankfully, scarring can often be reduced with steroid injections, silicone sheeting, scar massage, time, and newer wound dressings designed to reduce skin tension at the scar sites.

Wound healing issues

Small wounds can be common along the incisions (most often near the lower portion of the vertical scar or at the

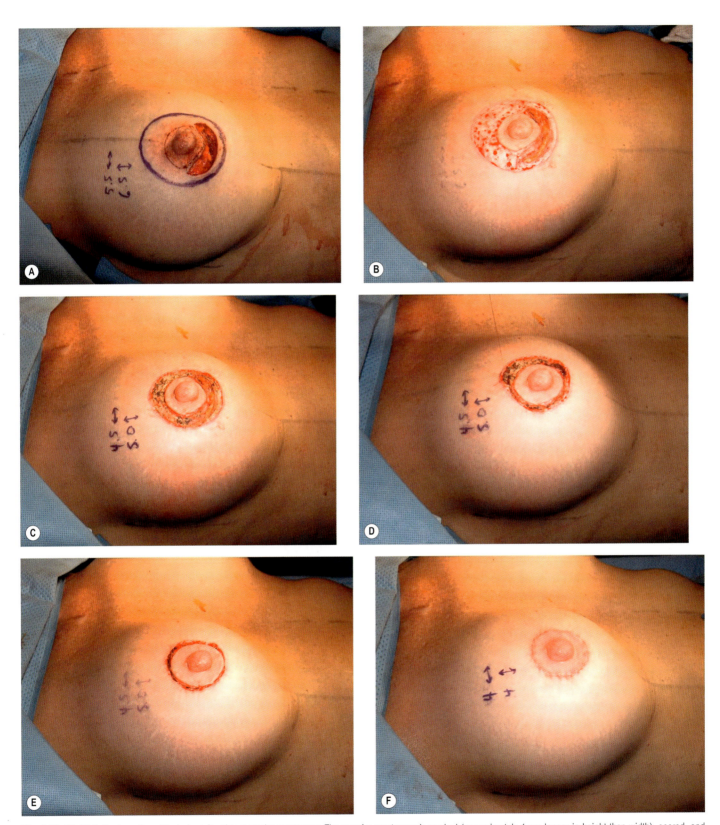

Fig. 6.12 (A–F) Author's preferred technique for circumareolar mastopexy. The area for mastopexy is marked (approximately 1 cm longer in height than width), scored, and de-epithelialized, and cautery is used for hemostasis and to contract the dermis. Imbrication of the dermis is performed with 3.0 PDS suture in deep running fashion. Stabilization is further secured with 3.0 Prolene in deep "subcuticular" fashion. True subcuticular closure is then performed with 4.0 Monocryl.

junction of the vertical and the areolar incisions, or the vertical and inframammary incisions when applicable). Wounds most commonly appear between weeks 3 and 6, unless there is an early issue due to poor blood supply. Reducing suture burdens (particularly suture knots), resecting appropriate amounts of skin, reducing tension to surface wound closure via deep and long-lasting sutures, being cautious about operating on patients with medical conditions that affect wound healing (such as diabetes), and strictly avoiding patients that are active smokers can all help to reduce wounds. Most wounds are small and will heal with dressing changes over time. Occasionally, revision surgery is necessary. Large wounds are uncommon, but can be challenging to heal, and may require adjunctive measures such as hyperbaric oxygen therapy.

Tissue necrosis

Tissue necrosis, including loss of a nipple areolar complex or a skin flap, is an extremely rare but terrible complication. Proper patient selection (healthy, non-smoking, etc.) is the first step in avoiding this problem. Leaving thick lateral flaps and a broad-based pedicle also helps to reduce the risk of this problem. If ischemia is noted on the table, options include releasing the skin and re-checking the pedicle to ensure there is no kinking in the blood supply. If the nipple is clearly de-vascularized, an option is to convert to a free nipple graft. This is a reasonable maneuver within the first 12 h. Other options during this time period and after 12 h include suture release to reduce tension, use of nitropaste or leeches (in the case of venous congestion), antibiotics, and possible hyperbaric oxygen. If a nipple is lost, it is important to wait for the tissue to demarcate, and nipple reconstruction techniques and tattooing can be utilized to improve the final aesthetics.

Asymmetry

Some degree of postsurgical asymmetry is to be expected after surgery, and patients undergoing mastopexy need to understand this. Areola size, position, and shape can vary mildly, and breasts can be affected by different starting volumes and base widths. Breasts can also settle differently over time with different degrees of recurrent ptosis. In the case of more noticeable asymmetry, skin adjustments can often be made under local anesthesia. While this may not totally correct the asymmetry, patients are generally happy with significant improvements.

Recurrent ptosis

As stated earlier, some degree of recurrent ptosis over time is more a matter of "when" than "if". The factors that caused ptosis in the first place (such as weak skin or attenuated Cooper's ligaments) will remain after surgery. As with asymmetry issues, recurrent ptosis can be improved but may require re-tightening via the patient's old incisions.

Nipple malposition

Significant nipple malposition can generally be avoided with careful planning and proper preoperative marking. Nipples should generally be situated on the center of the breast near the point of maximum projection. This usually coincides with the point of the IMF transposition on the breast, but it may be somewhat higher or lower. Making reference marks preoperatively, tailor-tacking the breasts, and examining patients in the seated position is important because it can allow on-table adjustments if the nipples are clearly too low or too high. If nipple malposition is noted after surgery, the scar tissue should be given time to mature and adjustments can be made. Re-elevation of low nipples generally requires repeating a circumvertical skin resection and closure. Lowering of areolas in the case of an excessively long nipple to IMF distance can be performed by taking out a transverse segment of skin from the lower breast in the inframammary region. If even further lowering is needed, tissue expansion of the upper breast or transposition of the nipple might be necessary; however, this can create unacceptable scars of the upper breast. Because of these issues, it is better to err on the side of under-elevating the nipple as opposed to over-elevating it when performing a mastopexy.

Dissatisfaction with shape and size

Once again, as noted earlier, mastopexy surgery is relatively limited by the patient's tissues and pre-existing volume, and as a result, extensive preoperative selection and management of patient expectations is critical for success. The most common disappointment will be due to a suboptimal degree of upper pole fullness. If this is an issue for a patient, options include fat grafting to the upper poles or placement of implants. Hopefully, if proper preoperative discussions were held, the patient will know this was a possibility and will be somewhat prepared for such an ancillary procedure if necessary.

Conclusion

Mastopexy surgery can be a highly satisfying surgery for patients with a relatively easy recovery and less required maintenance than augmentation mastopexy. Unlike augmentation mastopexy, the surgeon has much less control of the breast volume and upper pole fullness and they are fairly limited by the patient's preoperative anatomy and volume. Consequently, great care in patient selection and management of expectations should be taken prior to performing this surgery. Although many techniques are available, it is possible to apply a relatively low number of straightforward surgical techniques to correct an array of breast ptosis problems. Complications can occur but are generally rare and relatively minor when proper preoperative planning and intraoperative execution is performed.

Access the complete reference list online at **http://www.expertconsult.com**

1. Regnault P. Breast ptosis. Definition and treatment. *Clin Plast Surg.* 1976;3:193–203. *This paper established the standard system for assessing and classifying various types of breast ptosis.*

3. Grolleau JL, Lanfrey E, Lavigne B, et al. Breast base anomalies: treatment strategy for tuberous breasts, minor deformities, and asymmetry. *Plast Reconstr Surg.* 1999;104:2040–2048. *This publication further expanded concepts of tuberous breast assessment and management proposed by von Heimberg, et al.*

4. von Heimburg D, Exner K, Kruft S, et al. The tuberous breast deformity: classification and treatment. *Br J Plast Surg.* 1996;49:339–345. *This publication established the standard for assessing and managing tuberous breasts.*

7. Benelli L. A new periareolar mammaplasty: the "round block" technique. *Aesthetic Plast Surg.* 1990;14:93–100. *This paper established the basis for multiple future circumareolar mastopexy techniques, giving particular consideration to the propensity for scar spread and areolar stretching when a permanent suture is not used.*

17. Lejour M. Vertical mammaplasty for breast reduction and mastopexy. In: Spear SL, ed. *Surgery of the Breast: Principles and Art.* Philadelphia: Lippincott-Raven; 1998:73. *This chapter expands on the concept of vertical breast reduction and mastopexy with a focus on techniques.*

19. Hall-Findlay EJ. A simplified vertical reduction mammaplasty: shortening the learning curve. *Plast Reconstr Surg.* 1999;104:748–763. *This paper simplified and explained the techniques behind vertical mastopexy procedures.*

20. Hall-Findlay EJ. Pedicles in vertical breast reduction and mastopexy. *Clin Plast Surg.* 2002;29:379–391. *This publication discussed the various pedicle options that could be paired with the vertical breast reduction and mastopexy skin resection technique.*

21. Higdon K, Grotting JC. Mastopexy. In: Neligan PC (ed), Grotting JC (vol. ed). *Plastic Surgery.* Vol. 5. 3rd ed. Edinburgh: Elsevier Saunders; 2013:119–151. *This book chapter is a comprehensive overview of breast lift techniques and is the inspiration and basis for this current chapter.*

33. Coleman SR, Saboeiro AP. Fat grafting to the breast revisited: safety and efficacy. *Plast Reconstr Surg.* 2007;119:775–785. *This publication is the seminal article providing basis for modern breast reduction and mastopexy techniques.*

7

One- and two-stage considerations for augmentation mastopexy

Emily C. Hartmann, Michelle A. Spring, and W. Grant Stevens

 Access video content for this chapter online at expertconsult.com

SYNOPSIS

- Augmentation mastopexy is a particularly challenging procedure, as the surgery has multiple opposing goals – to increase the volume of a breast, change the shape, and simultaneously decrease the skin envelope.
- Successful outcomes in augmentation mastopexy, one- or two-stage, can be expected with proper planning, technique, and patient education.
- Patient selection is of utmost importance given the range of patients and pathologies in need of augmentation mastopexy (e.g., massive weight loss patients, the constricted breast, or severe ptosis).
- Preoperative planning, markings, and surgical technique are discussed in detail for both single stage and two-stage approaches. The author provides a step-by-step approach.
- Postoperative management can be crucial to ensure the best possible outcome.
- This chapter focuses on common indications and patient selection for one- and two-stage augmentation mastopexy, techniques for safe and effective procedures, challenges of the combined procedure, postoperative care, as well as potential complications, outcomes, and secondary procedures.
- A review of outcomes in the literature is examined. Knowledge of key complications is critical to stave them off during surgical planning, and in order to recognize them postoperatively should a patient experience a complication. Treatment for these complications is discussed.
- Secondary procedures may be necessary to correct implant malposition, inframammary fold (IMF) asymmetries, scar revisions, or nipple position asymmetries.

 Access the Historical Perspective section online at
http://www.expertconsult.com

Introduction

In 2014, the number of mastopexies had increased from 1997, by 568.5%, and similarly, the number of breast augmentations increased by 183.4%, according to the ASAPS national statistical data.[1] As these cases increase, there is also likely to be an increase in patients who would benefit from both an increase in breast volume as well as lift. Whether these procedures are performed simultaneously or in a staged approach has been the subject of some debate over the years.[2]

One-stage augmentation mastopexy was initially described more than 50 years ago by Regnault and Gonzalez-Ulloa[3,4] although many plastic surgeons prefer a two-stage approach to the ptotic and deflated breast. Simultaneous breast augmentation and mastopexy is, however, gaining traction[2,3,5–20] but is often considered to be one of the most difficult cosmetic breast surgeries. The challenge is in the fact that the surgery has multiple opposing goals – to increase the volume of a breast, change the shape, and simultaneously decrease the skin envelope. Successful outcomes in augmentation mastopexy, one- or two-stage, can be expected with proper planning, technique, and patient education. This chapter focuses on common indications and patient selection for one- and two-stage augmentation mastopexy, techniques for safe and effective procedures, challenges of the combined procedure, postoperative care, as well as potential complications, outcomes, and secondary procedures.

Basic science/disease process

Breast anatomy

As with any operative technique, anatomy is the foundation of success. Vascular anatomy is of particular importance in breast surgery in order to preserve blood flow to the nipple areolar complex. The nipples form an equilateral triangle with the sternal notch and are located at the level of the 4th rib, approximately 9–10 cm from the midline.[25] The breast parenchyma extends horizontally from the sternum to the anterior axillary line and vertically from the level of the 2nd or 3rd rib to the inframammary fold, and with variable axillary extension as the Tail of Spence.[26]

The support system of the breast is comprised of fascial layers and Cooper's ligaments, which together give rise to overall breast shape and integrity against gravity. The superficial fascial layer lies between the dermis and breast parenchyma. The deep layer lies on the pectoralis fascia. The relationship of the deep fascia and the retromammary space allows the breast tissue to move on the chest wall.[26]

Ligamentous suspension consists of Cooper's ligaments and the horizontal septum. Loss of elastic fibers within these structures in the course of aging may contribute to a loss of their supporting function and of the firm shape of the breast. Cooper's ligaments provide suspensory support and connect the superficial fascia and skin to the deep fascia. The horizontal septum emerges from the pectoralis fascia at the level of the 5th rib, which divides the gland into cranial and caudal portions. This septum carries the weight of the breast and prevents descent of its base. The horizontal septum also carries the main neurovascular bundles supplying the breast, which run along this septum and guide the vascular supply to the nipple.[26,27]

Breast vascular supply

Blood supply to the nipple areolar complex is of great importance in augmentation mastopexy surgery. Multiple arteries supply the breast, all of which overlap and lead to variability of tissue perfusion. The dominant arterial sources are the internal mammary artery perforators (Fig. 7.1). These perforators traverse the anterior thoracic wall just lateral to the sternum and course through the medial pectoralis major muscle. They can be encountered directly when dissecting the medial subpectoral pocket. Specifically, the 2nd–4th internal mammary perforators are the main blood supply for a superior or superomedial pedicle. Several in-depth articles are available for vascular anatomy of the breast.[28–32]

Subpectoral placement of the breast implants does not disrupt the musculocutaneous perforators and is less likely to interfere with blood supply. On the contrary, if the implant is placed in the subglandular plane and significant tissue undermining is performed, the

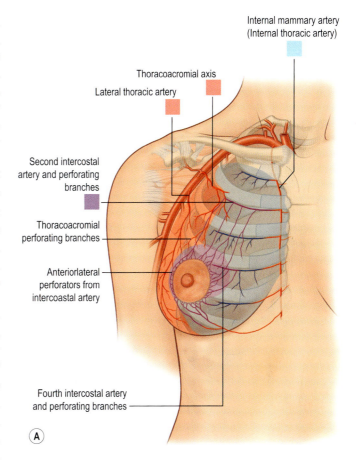

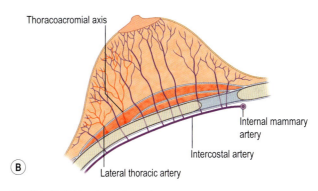

Fig. 7.1 (A,B) Breast vascular anatomy.

blood supply could be severely compromised. Vascular supply to the tissue can also be compromised if the implant size is too large and too much tension is placed on the skin edges, leading to tissue necrosis.

Definition and classification of ptosis

In the hypomastia patient, the diagnosis of breast ptosis is critical in the decision-making algorithm to determine the type of mastopexy necessary when combined with an augmentation. Regnault (Fig. 7.2) is the most well-known classification system for breast ptosis and it is

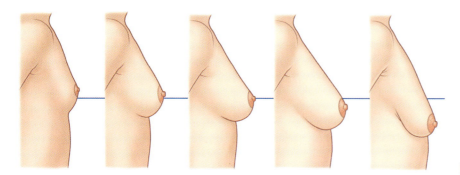

Fig. 7.2 Regnault classification of ptosis.

defined by the location of the nipple to the inframammary fold.[25] Other classification schemes are essentially modifications of this system based on skin elasticity, glandular volume, and parenchymal distribution.[33,34]

Diagnosis and patient presentation

In the case of augmentation mastopexy, it is the rare patient that presents knowing exactly what they need to achieve their desired appearance. The surgeon must often use lay terminology and also astutely pick up on body language and hand motions to fully understand the patient's desires. Patients generally fall into two categories when they present for aesthetic breast surgery. One group is the smaller-breasted patient who seeks augmentation and does not recognize they have a certain degree of ptosis. The second group is the patient requesting a breast lift but also wants fuller breasts that can only be achieved with an additional augmentation. These patients present a particular challenge because they may not have emotionally accepted the idea of using an implant and will require extra time to process this.

In general, patients requiring augmentation mastopexy are often older than patients desiring enlargement with implants. Factors such as weight loss, pregnancy, and breast feeding are often at play and their sequelae of increased tissue laxity, parenchyma loss, striae, and nipple ptosis require a mastopexy to create an aesthetic breast shape. In the initial consultation, it is very important to distinguish the tuberous-breasted patient, which can present additional challenges that are not within the scope of this chapter.

Patient selection and indications for augmentation mastopexy

Once the desired size and shape have been established, the surgeon can then select the appropriate mastopexy incision (Fig. 7.3) through which an implant may be

placed, to shape the breast into an aesthetically pleasing result. It is a balance of all factors to create an aesthetically pleasing breast contour with an appropriately positioned nipple areolar complex, upper pole fullness, tightening of the loose skin envelope, breast symmetry, and increased breast volume.

Pseudoptosis

In this case, the nipple is in the ideal location but the lower pole breast tissue is ptotic. The "smile" mastopexy may be employed if the tissue needs to be reduced in the vertical plane only, and the "sailboat" mastopexy if both the vertical and the horizontal planes must be reduced. The pseudoptotic breast can also be addressed with a dual-plane augmentation, which would allow the breast tissue to lift and create more upper pole fullness.[35]

Grade 1 ptosis

These patients require no more than 2 cm of nipple movement and can be addressed with a "crescent" or "circumareolar" mastopexy. Circumareolar mastopexies have higher rates of revisions and patient dissatisfaction,[7] and the authors avoid them unless less than 2 cm of lift is needed. In terms of acceptable scarring, the authors generally use the circumareolar incision, even though some surgeons report success with the crescent mastopexy.[7,36–39]

Grade 2 ptosis

These patients generally require 3–4 cm of nipple elevation. The circumvertical "owl" mastopexy is utilized if they only require a reduction in the horizontal plane. A triangular base of skin known as the "owl with feet" is sometimes made to decrease the vertical plane and shorten the nipple to IMF distance.

Grade 3 ptosis

Patients requiring more than 4 cm of nipple elevation will benefit from a wise pattern mastopexy. This category often includes the massive weight loss patients who deserve special annotation for their unique features and underlying protoplasm. Patients often present with medialization of the nipple areolar complex and extension to a lateral chest roll.[40] Several techniques utilizing a variety of parenchymal flaps exist to create volume and stability to the breast,[41–45] though long-term durability of these flaps remains to be proven.

Implant selection

The base width provides a general guide for implant selection, however skin envelope laxity and parenchyma volume should be taken into consideration. The use of sizers in the operating room with tailor-tacking can help guide the surgeon in choosing the correct implant size. For those who need a mathematical approach to determine ideal breast implant shape and volume, the Tebbetts' method is helpful.[46] Planning excessively large implants at the same time as a mastopexy may create more postoperative complications given the opposing forces on the tissues.

The type of implant shape and profile determines the distribution of fill within the breast. The authors primarily use silicone implants and avoid saline implants, which lead to deflations, more complaints about implant visibility and palpability, and higher revision rates.[5,8,9,47]

The incidence of capsular contracture, implant palpability, and excess upper pole fullness is diminished with subpectoral implant placement, though subpectoral placement is associated with more postoperative pain and muscle flexion deformity when compared with subglandular positioning.[48,49] It is also known that mammography is also more accurate with subpectoral placement.[50,51]

One or two stages

The decision to stage or combine is based on the clinical scenario, surgeon's experience and the patient's choice. The authors believe this decision should not be based primarily on a concern for increased risk to the patient and a review of the single-stage augmentation mastopexy patients showed a revision rate and return to the operating room of 16.9% compared with 100% of staged patients requiring a second operation. Additionally data compared favorably with previously reported revision rates for breast augmentation or mastopexy alone.[7] There are, however, cases in which staging the procedure is the safest option. Women with high risk for wound-healing complications, such as diabetics, smokers, and immunocompromised patients, are not good candidates for a combined augmentation mastopexy.[8,22,52,53]

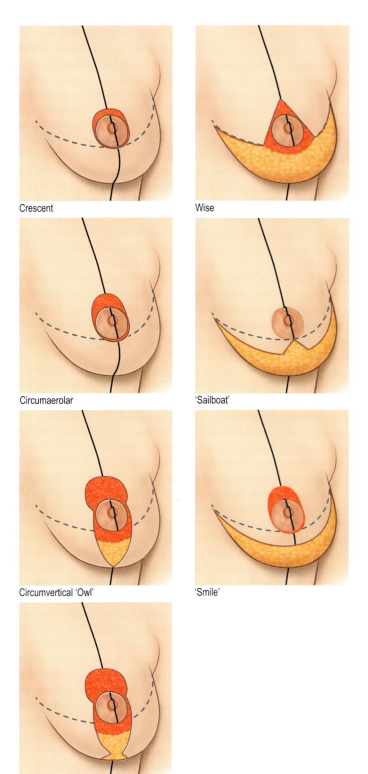

Crescent

Wise

Circumaerolar

'Sailboat'

Circumvertical 'Owl'

'Smile'

'Owl with feet'

Fig. 7.3 Types of mastopexy incisions. (Redrawn after Spring MA, Macias LH, Nadeau M, Stevens WG. Secondary augmentation-mastopexy: indications, preferred practices, and the treatment of complications. Aesthetic Surgery Journal 2014;34(7):1018–1040.)

Should the surgery be staged, many surgeons will proceed with the mastopexy first and then follow with an augmentation no earlier than 3 months postoperatively. This allows for tissue related revisions at the time of the second procedure if necessary. Placing the implant first helps to stretch out the soft tissue and would not necessarily be the wrong choice. In making your decision of whether to perform the mastopexy or the augmentation first, it is important to consider the fact that the patient may not return for the second procedure. In this scenario, a decision must be made as to which would be preferable – an augmented ptotic breast or a lifted but hypovoluminous breast. The answer varies from patient to patient.

Preoperative preparation

To ensure efficiency, repeatability, and reliability, it is crucial to establish a preoperative checklist for every patient. Managing patient expectations and well-documented informed consent are important components of preoperative preparation, as mastopexy surgery is a frequent source of litigation in plastic surgery.[54,55] The main checklist items should be:

1. Review patient history and discuss pertinent medical clearances – labs may need to be drawn in accordance with the patient's age and history;
2. An information pack for the patient detailing the day prior to surgery (skin preps, NPO status, medications to avoid, etc.), when to arrive for surgery, directions to get there, details of aftercare, name of the person to be contacted, and postoperative follow-up appointments;
3. Prescriptions for medications to be started after surgery;
4. Consents (surgical, photo release, arbitration agreements, anesthesia, etc.);
5. Last but not least, preoperative photos should be taken.

With regard to mammogram status, the use of "routine" mammograms prior to breast surgery should be avoided. This is in accordance with the American Board of Internal Medicine and recognized by the American Society of Plastic Surgeons. Patients should undergo annual screening mammograms for patients of specific age groups and additional screening is not necessary unless there are concerning aspects of the patient's history or physical exam which require further investigation.[56]

The preoperative visit is also an opportunity for patients to review their desires with their surgeon. Photo documentation also provides an opportunity to point out asymmetries and specific anatomic details the patients may not recognize as well as the ability to review scar placement. The patient will also then have the opportunity to point out areas she would like changed and to what degree (upper pole fullness, areolar size, etc.). Having these discussions preoperatively will hopefully avoid the surprised and sometimes unhappy patient. Mild implant palpability or rippling when patients bend over is usually the consequence of having breast implants, particularly in thin patients or those without substantial breast tissue. Patients may consider it a complication when they feel the implant edge laterally if they are not forewarned of this.

The adage often used is that breasts are "sisters and not twins", when reminding the patient that no two sides of the body are mirror images of each other. Additionally, breast implants are not designed to be lifetime devices, and the patient should be informed that she may need additional surgery on her breasts in the future, as well as the FDA recommendation for surveillance of silicone breast implants.

Treatment/surgical technique

Patient markings

The patient is always marked in the preoperative holding area just prior to surgery – "proper planning precludes poor performance". As the tissues are manipulated and the patient reviews their wants, the surgeon can essentially perform the surgery in his/her mind, well before an actual incision is made.

The midline and sternal notch are first marked. The meridian of each breast is then marked to look for symmetry of each breast. A measurement of the meridian to the midline marking is taken to assess any differences. The inframammary fold (IMF) is then marked, extending to the midline. A breast caliper is Dr. Stevens' preferred tool to measure the dimensions of the breast. The base diameter is noted, which will determine the approximate implant selected. The sternal notch to IMF distance is used to mark the new nipple site on the meridian. The new areola is then drawn with the superior edge 2 cm above the nipple mark and made circular. This will be confirmed on the operating table with the nipple marker. The limbs are then drawn based on how much horizontal dimension needs to be reduced. If a reduction in the vertical dimension is required based on the nipple to fold distance, then the "feet" component may be added. Once the patient is lying on the table, all marks are re-measured and re-drawn. The length of the vertical limb is determined by the cup size the patient would like to be (Table 7.1 and Video 7.1 ▶).

Table 7.1 Vertical limb length based on desired cup size

Desired cup size	Vertical limb length (cm)
B cup	5
C cup	6
D cup	7
DD cup	8

Setting the stage

All patients are given a dose of preoperative antibiotics and lower extremity sequential compression devices are placed. The authors generally perform these in an outpatient surgery center for low risk patients and patients can recover at home with a caregiver unless combined with another procedure when it is recommended that they recover at an aftercare facility. The patient is placed on the table in a position suitable for hip sitting up multiple times during the procedure, with the arms abducted and secured to the arm boards. Preoperative photographs of the patient taken at the time of their prior appointment are taped to the wall for easy reference during surgery. This is helpful due to the change in appearance of the breasts with the patient supine. Patients are encouraged to select photos of model breasts that they would like to resemble, from a book provided in the clinic. These are also placed on the wall for reference. Lastly, headlights are worn if a lighted retractor is not used during pocket creation.

Step-by-step technique

1. The marked incisions are infiltrated with 1% lidocaine and 1:100 000 epinephrine solution prior to skin prep. The skin is then prepped with betadine or chlorhexidine/alcohol. The field is then draped.
2. The first step is to re-measure and mark the incisions to reaffirm symmetry and cleanness of the cuts. *It is critical to remember that one can always take more and to start as minimal as possible when first getting comfortable with this procedure.*
3. The areola is marked with a 42 mm ring (unless smaller or larger is determined by patient/surgeon preference) (Fig. 7.4).
4. The mastopexy incisions are then made and de-epithelialization commences. The skin inferior to the areola may be removed full thickness (Fig. 7.4). *At this point if tissue is to be resected for symmetry or to reduce the breasts slightly, tissue may be excised from the lateral sides of the vertical opening.* This technique involves skin excision as the initial step. It should be altered slightly if the surgeon is just getting comfortable with augmentation mastopexies or if the case is particularly difficult due to asymmetries or unusual anatomy. In these cases, *it is prudent to start with implant placement and then tailor-tacking of the mastopexy markings to ensure enough skin is left for closure and the surgeon is satisfied with the aesthetics.* Only after the surgeon has performed a number of them and determined that the markings consistently do not need adjustments should he/she proceed with the skin excision first without tailor-tacking.

5. The nipple areolar complex (NAC) is freed using a U incision and then a suture is used to attach the 12 o'clock position of the NAC to the new midline incision. This maneuver tacks the NAC out of the way to allow the parenchyma to be pulled around inferiorly (Fig. 7.5).
6. The implant pocket is created through the vertical incision, unless a circumareolar incision is planned. *The advantage of a vertical incision is that a 1–2 cm cuff-off tissue is maintained inferiorly, which protects the implant should the T-junction breakdown.* The dissection is carried down to the pectoralis major muscle edge, releasing the inferior and inferomedial fibers of the pectoralis major muscle to allow for ideal position of the implant. It is at this time that a variable degree of dual-plane may be created depending on the patient's needs (Fig. 7.6).
7. Meticulous hemostasis is achieved.
8. Sizers are placed into the pocket to assess for proper position, pocket size, and adequate release of the pectoralis muscle. The parenchyma can be closed with temporary sutures to appropriately emulate the soft tissue position over the implant.
9. Tailor-tacking of the mastopexy incisions is performed to determine implant size as well as degree of skin excision. The inferior pole of the breast should be flat on profile rather than a gentle curve. This is because over time, the implant will descend and the soft tissue will stretch and lead to a natural appearing lower pole. If the lower pole already looks good at the time of surgery, it will result in too much laxity over time as the skin stretches due to the weight of the implant.
10. The pockets are irrigated with triple antibiotic solution followed by betadine that is rinsed out thoroughly, and once the implants are placed, the deep tissue is closed completely. Fig. 7.7 shows the implant in position.
11. The vertical midline tissue is brought together with a running locking 3-0 Vicryl suture starting

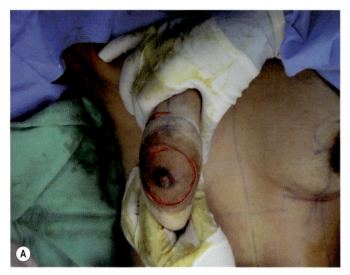

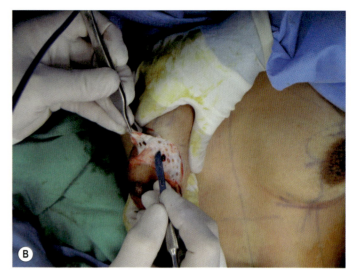

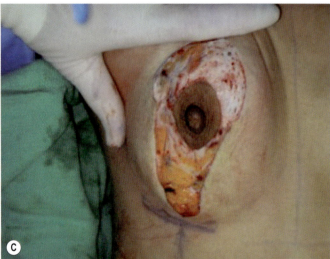

Fig. 7.4 (A) Periareolar and mastopexy lines are incised. **(B)** The skin around the areola is de-epithelialized. **(C)** A full thickness skin excision is made inferior to the areola.

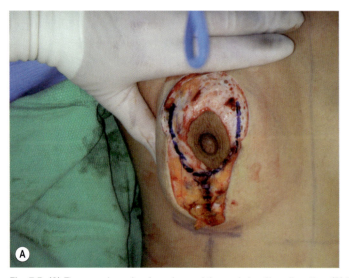

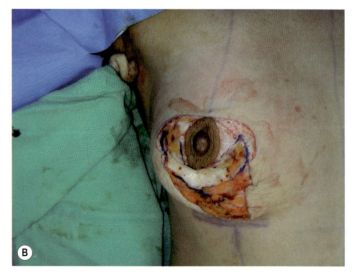

Fig. 7.5 (A) The parenchyma is released around the areola in a U configuration. **(B)** The release of the parenchyma allows the NAC to be moved superiorly and is secured at the 12 o'clock position. This allows the NAC to be moved out of the way during pocket formation as well as an easier closure.

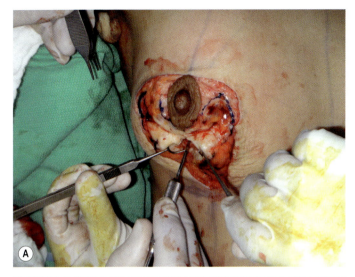

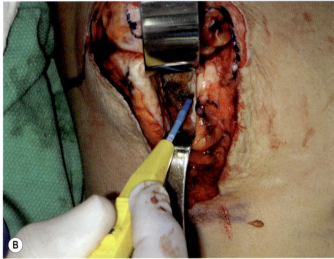

Fig. 7.6 (A) Pocket creation via a vertical incision. **(B)** The edge of the pectoralis major muscle is found and the appropriate pocket is created for implant insertion.

inferiorly and deep and heading in the superior direction. Once the suture reaches just underneath the NAC it is brought more superficial to proceeds inferiorly until it meets the T-junction. This method approximates the deep tissue in preparation for skin closure (Fig. 7.8).

12. Very limited undermining is performed in order to bring the skin edges together (Fig. 7.9).

13. The skin edges are closed with 3-0 Monocryl interrupted deep dermal sutures and a running 3-0 Monocryl. The areola is inset with a 4-0 Monocryl interrupted deep dermal and a running 4-0 Monocryl.

14. Upon inset of the NAC, if it does not appear perfectly round or shows a teardrop deformity it should be addressed on the table (Fig. 7.10). The nipple marker should be used and skin excised.

Special considerations

Borderline ptosis

Patients with borderline ptosis require less than 2 cm of nipple areolar complex elevation and thus often benefit from a circumareolar mastopexy (Figs. 7.9 & 7.10). A non-absorbable interlocking wagon-wheel or purse-string suture is placed in the deep dermis with the knot buried deeply (Figs. 7.11 & 7.12). There are some nuances to be aware of with this technique:

1. Avoid a tight purse-string suture that can cause vascular compromise to the nipple as the areolar skin is pulled taught.

2. There is often mild pleating of the skin that resolves postoperatively.

3. Scar and areolar widening can occur postoperatively, but the permanent help reduce this consequence.

4. With significant skin excision, the breast can also appear flattened.

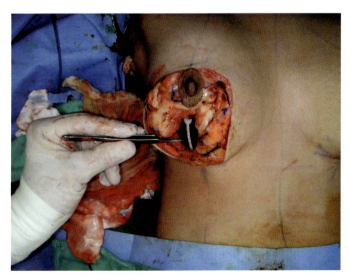

Fig. 7.7 The implant is shown sitting in the pocket. Here an anatomic implant was placed and the white line indicates orientation of the implant.

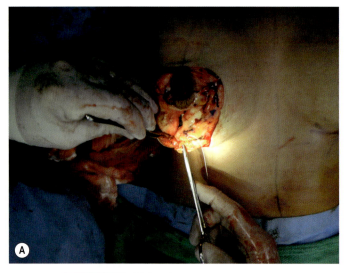

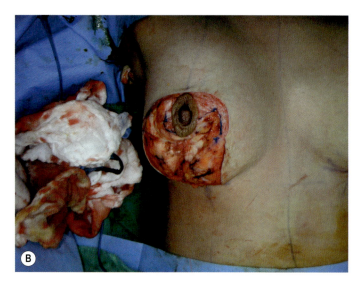

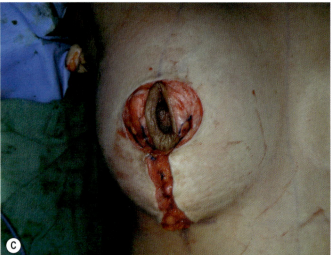

Fig. 7.8 (A–C) Pocket closure begins with a running suture starting the deep inferior parenchyma heading up toward the NAC, then transitions more superficial and then runs back down inferiorly in a locking fashion.

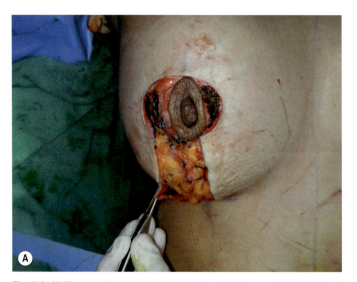

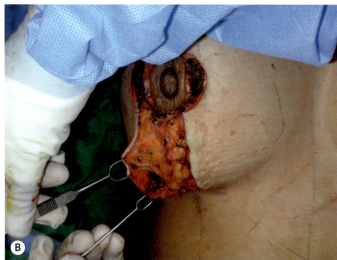

Fig. 7.9 (A,B) Limited flap undermining is performed just enough to take the tension off the skin and allow for closure.

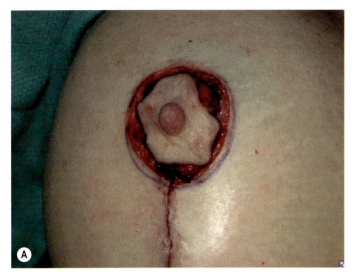

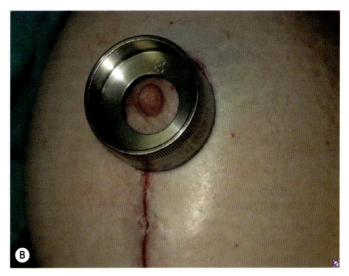

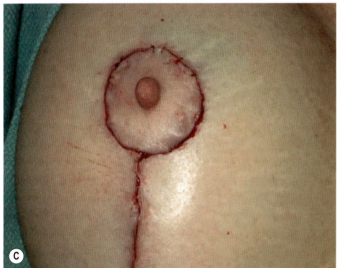

Fig. 7.10 (A–C) Nipple areolar complex adjustments. If a perfectly circular areola does not shape up once the skin is brought together then final adjustments can be made with the areolar marker and fine scissors or scalpel. It is best to address these issues on the table. The junction with the vertical incision should be perpendicular; otherwise a teardrop deformity will occur.

Pseudoptosis

Patients with pseudoptosis may have adequate nipple position and areolar size. Mild pseudoptosis can often be corrected with an augmentation alone, however, in the face of heavy pseudoptotic glandular tissue, the authors find that a more pleasing breast shape is created by performing a mastopexy to elevate the parenchyma and excise redundant skin (Fig. 7.13). This situation can be treated with only a sailboat or smile mastopexy, although most patients benefit from slight repositioning of the areolas.

The constricted breast

Constricted breast deformity can have a profound impact on postoperative shape and it is estimated that over 80% of women who present for breast augmentation have some form of constriction.[57] Anatomic shaped implants can be useful in this patient population, as the form stable silicone helps to differentially put pressure on the lower pole of the breast. Intraoperative release of inferior and inferior-medial parenchymal bands and tight tissue can create a more rounded lower pole. They are better candidates for a circumareolar mastopexy, given their lack of horizontal excess, to reduce enlarged areolas and limit breast tissue herniation. They may also benefit from a subglandular implant pocket,[58] however, the authors believe aggressive scoring of the inferior pole parenchymal bands and a subpectoral pocket can achieve a good result.

Breast asymmetry

Those with significant breast asymmetry can be treated by reduction in parenchyma on the larger side or with different size implants. When debating between placing the same size implants or trying to correct a slight size asymmetry, the authors find that patients are most satisfied if postoperative asymmetry corresponds with what they are used to – i.e., if the patient's right breast is

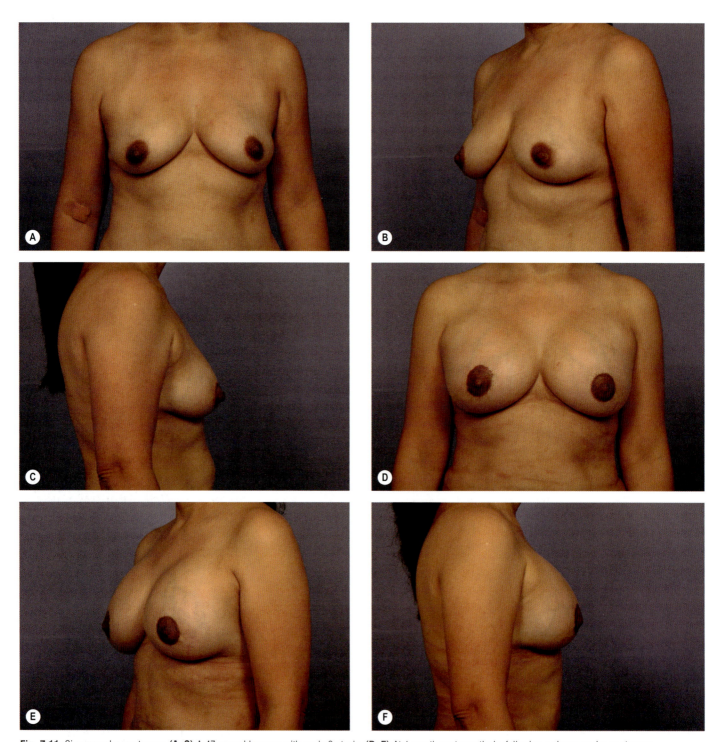

Fig. 7.11 Circumareolar mastopexy. **(A–C)** A 47-year-old woman with grade 2 ptosis. **(D–F)** At 1 month postoperatively, following a circumareolar mastopexy augmentation. Of note, the implants are appear in a high position, however, gravity will slowly bring them down into an ideal position over the next several months. It is important to educate patients about this anticipated change.

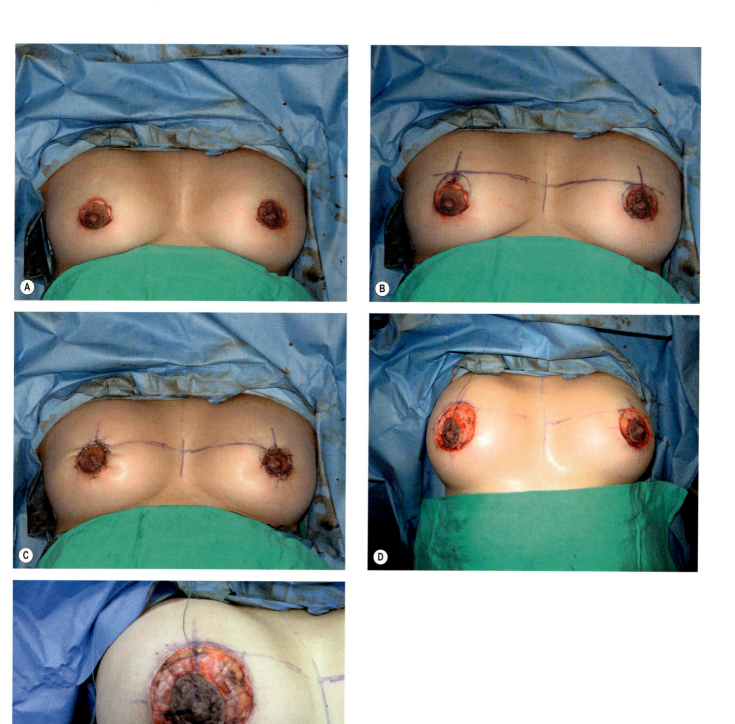

Fig. 7.12 Intraoperative view of circumareolar mastopexy. **(A)** The areola is partially inset evenly prior to marking for the lift. **(B)** The nipple and areola position is determined and re-marked using the appropriate-sized cookie-cutter.
(C) The areolar incision is made. **(D)** The circumareolar skin is de-epithelialized.
(E) A wagon-wheel closure is performed using a permanent suture, and the skin is then closed using a running subcuticular suture.

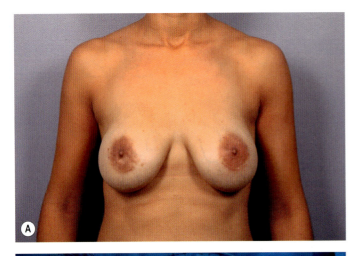

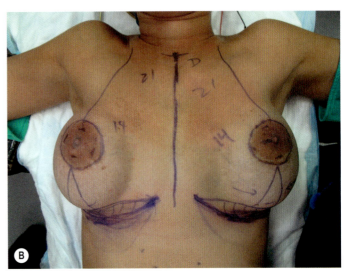

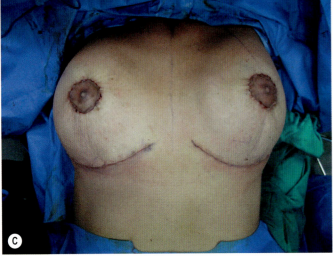

Fig. 7.13 (A) This woman presented with widened areola and pseudoptosis following breast augmentation 6 years previously. Intraoperatively, she was marked for a "sailboat" mastopexy to reduce both vertical and horizontal excess, as well as circumareolar excision of the widened areola. **(B)** She underwent removal of her old implants with capsulotomies and replacement with 547 cc silicone devices. Once the implants were placed, the vertical component of the mastopexy was not necessary and **(C)** she underwent a "smile" mastopexy to reduce the vertical excess.

slightly larger preoperatively, and placing a bigger implant on the contralateral side leads to a slightly larger left breast, patients will not tolerate this as well as using the same size implants and accepting the fact that they will have asymmetry based on their native breast tissue.

Postoperative care

The following is the senior author's (W.G.S) postoperative regime. This is not to be seen as absolute but rather an example of what has been found to work in one practice setting.

Postoperative care is of the utmost importance to ensure a stable recovery period and to create consistent protocols for nursing staff to follow. Patient education as to what to expect postoperatively is also critical and should be started at the preoperative appointment.

Patients are given an information pack that details medications to avoid pre- as well as postoperatively. Unless allergic, patients are given the following postoperative medications: a narcotic with acetaminophen

for pain control; a benzodiazepine as an anxiolytic and to lessen muscle spasms; and 7 days of postoperative antibiotics. According to the Surgical Care Improvement Project,[59] antibiotics are not recommended after 24 h postoperatively and each physician must decide which protocol works best in their practice. Patients are also given Arnica Montana oral tabs and topical cream that serve as a homeopathic treatment for bruising and swelling. Scientific studies of Arnica have been equivocal.[60] A randomized-control study showed that it decreased edema in rhinoplasty patients when compared with placebo,[61] which countered an earlier placebo-controlled study showing no difference from placebo in post-laser ecchymosis.[62] In the author's experience, the benefits of Arnica outweigh the risks.

Immediately following closure of the incisions, the wounds are dressed with Xeroform, thick, soft cotton padding, and wrapped with a Kerlix roll and ace wrap or bias-cut cotton wrap. The configuration should create a halter-top type appearance with tape placed at the front V to avoid rubbing on the neck. As stated previously, drains are rarely used, however, if they are present, they are safety-pinned to the outside of the wrap. Patients are discharged home with a caregiver if they are not having another combined surgery.

Patients are then seen on POD No. 1, where their dressings are removed completely, the incisions are cleaned gently with dilute hydrogen peroxide and saline. Steri-Strips are applied and the patient is placed in a surgical bra. Prior to bra placement, a thick layer of Arnica cream, again evidence is equivocal,[60] is applied on the entire breast bilaterally "like spreading cream cheese on a bagel". The patient is instructed to apply the cream daily for 2 weeks after showering. Scar therapy with silicone gel begins at approximately 3–4 weeks following surgery. The patient is allowed to wear an underwired bra at 6 weeks. Standard follow-up, including photos, proceeds at 1 week, 2 weeks, 1 month, 3 months, 6 months, and at 1 year. Patients are then asked to return every year for photos.

The authors routinely use textured implants and thus do not implement a massage protocol, however, if smooth implants are used, patients are encouraged to do gentle implant mobility exercises starting within the first week of surgery.

If the implant appears to be too high or there is significant upper pole swelling it may be possible to apply a bandeau (either an ace wrap or a commercial product designed for this use) around the top of the implant for downward pressure to be maintained. The patient should wear this constantly and the pressure "should feel like a hug", to avoid applying it too tightly.

Additional maneuvers may be implemented in an effort to maximize the aesthetic outcome. The authors have utilized the "shoelace cast", as designed by Dr. Dan Mills of Laguna Beach, in patients who need correction of mild IMF asymmetries or double bubbles. This technique is effective and easy to implement when following Dr. Mills' outlined protocol.[63]

Postoperative reassurance for the patient is important, since this implant settling can occur at different rates for each patient. It is reassuring to the surgeon to recall that when the patient was in the operating room the pockets were symmetric and the implants were in good position.

Patients often ask about returning to their normal activity, which includes work and exercise routine. The first 2 weeks are a critical time to keep seromas and hematomas at bay. The implant should be properly immobilized in a surgical bra at all times (except when showering); arm movement should be limited to avoid implant motion underneath the pectoralis major muscle; and blood pressure should not be elevated. The patient is asked to refrain from heavy arm activity (unless they are a secondary mastopexy and already had an implant)

for 2 weeks and gently work up to their normal activity until they are 6 weeks postoperative.

Returning to work depends heavily on what the patient does for a living. If it is a desk job with minimal activity, they may return to work as early as 1 week; however, 2 weeks is recommended before returning to a job with more physical activity. With regard to an exercise routine it is recommended that they start gently walking around the house for the first few days after surgery and then progress to walking around the block over the next 2 weeks. They should be cautioned not to raise their blood pressure and heart rate in the first 2 weeks, to stave off hematoma or seroma formation. At 2 weeks postoperatively, they may start light workouts such as the elliptical or stationary bike and slowly progress to their full workouts at 6 weeks.

Complications and secondary procedures

An exhaustive description of complications related to implants or mastopexy is outside the scope of this chapter. Instead it will touch on common complications following augmentation mastopexy as reported in the literature.[6,11,13,23,64–66]

Immediate complications

Hematoma

Hematomas are a known complication of breast surgery and can occur despite meticulous hemostasis. The pooled hematoma rate for combined augmentation mastopexy is 1.37%.[23] Some authors condone that direct visualization and cauterization of vessels rather than blunt dissection can help avoid the occurrence of hematomas.[67] They should be drained promptly to not only avoid excess pressure on the tissues and subsequent ischemia but because blood collections can increase the risk for both infection and capsular contracture.[68]

Infection

Infection of the soft tissues must be treated aggressively with antibiotics and frequent follow-up to avoid wound breakdown and involvement of the implant. Sequelae following implant infection include the immediate removal of the implant as well as long-term consequences such as capsular contracture.[69] The "no touch" technique[70] has been adopted for implant handling, which has greatly decreased the incidence of infection.[71] Intraoperative techniques such as: re-prepping the chest; changing gloves; avoiding multiple people handling the implants; placing an occlusive dressing over the nipple;[72,73] utilizing a "no-touch" technique; irrigating the pocket with antibiotic solution[74] or Betadine solution and rinse;[75] and avoiding powdered gloves, have all been utilized to help reduce risk. The pooled risk of infection following simultaneous augmentation mastopexy is 2% (ranging from 0% to 14% in the current literature).[23]

Soft tissue concerns

Nipple ischemia following breast lift can be transient and has minimal consequences. Reported rates of moderate or prolonged nipple ischemia following breast surgery are 5–11% and full thickness ischemia/necrosis occurs in approximately 0.5–7.3% of all cases of cosmetic, oncologic, or reconstructive breast surgery.[76,77] A working knowledge of treatment algorithms is essential to maximize the salvage of nipple tissue.[76] It is important to obtain any history of previous breast surgeries, and consider nipple blood supply when performing simultaneous augmentation mastopexy. Skin necrosis or breakdown can occur most commonly at the T-zone of an anchor type mastopexy. Careful tissue handling, closure without excessive tension, excision of traumatized tissue, and minimal undermining should all be utilized to minimize soft tissue-related complications.

Delayed complications

Implant-related

We know that saline implants tend to ripple more than silicone implants.[78] Rippling can worsen over time as pressure from the implants thin the tissue. Methods for correction include: exchanging textured shells to smooth; saline to gel-filled implants; moving the implant from a subglandular to subpectoral pocket; creating a completely new pocket in the subfascial or subcapsular plane; utilizing acellular dermal matrix to provide more implant coverage; or placing fat grafts to add additional support and volume to the area.

Implant malposition is usually apparent early and may be a result of faulty or asymmetric pocket dissection or incomplete release of the pectoralis major muscle. In these cases, revisions require either further dissection, plication of an overly dissected pocket, or the creation of new pockets for the implants.[15,16]

Animation deformity is caused by implant motion with flexion of the chest muscles. This is even more pronounced in thin patients who lack breast parenchyma volume. Over-dissection of the pectoralis major muscle from the medial insertion to the sternum can also result in increased distortion. Correction of this deformity can be done by suturing the pectoralis major muscle to the

chest wall and moving the implant to a subglandular pocket.[79]

Tissue-related

Pseudoptosis can be due to the relatively thin inferior pole skin and tissue stretching under the weight of the implants or actual violation of the inframammary fold and displacement of the implants inferiorly. As described above, the authors strive to create a flattened lower pole at the time of surgery to allow for postoperative stretch. Conservative dissection of the IMF is also important and one should not violate the IMF unless necessary. If the IMF needs to be lowered, tacking sutures may be necessary to reinforce the fascia and prevent dropping of the implant.

Capsular contracture is a common reason for revision of breast augmentation, with or without mastopexy.[80] The etiology of capsular contracture is an enigmatic phenomenon evident by the litany of studies.[49,75,81–84] Factors contributing to capsular contracture include infection and bacterial contamination,[81] subglandular pocket placement,[49] periareolar approach[85] presumably due to more bacterial contamination from the ductal tissue,[18] and smooth implants.[3,4,8,17,19,80] Hematoma formation has also been correlated with capsular contracture[68,86] and the use of drains is associated with a higher prevalence of capsular contracture.[81]

Nipple malposition, either too high or too low, is due to either placement error during initial marking or secondary changes as the implant shifted and tissue laxity set. Nipple position marking is covered in the "patient marking" section above. It is important to remember that it is far easier to raise a nipple than to lower one. Conservative elevation is therefore encouraged if one is concerned the nipple placement is too high. In addition to nipple malposition there can also be areolar shape distortions. A mosque-pattern areola design is often used, however, this does not guarantee a symmetric circular areola. The authors advise taking care of this problem on the table when a non-circular shape is noted. This irregularity will only get worse with time.

A double-bubble deformity is caused by one of two problems. The first is ptosis of glandular tissue drooping over an implant. This occurs when the breast tissue projects over and hangs below the more superiorly located implant. Perhaps the mastopexy was not tight enough and too much glandular tissue was left behind, or the pectoralis major muscle was not released enough inferiorly causing the implant to remain high. Repositioning or resizing the implant may be necessary, and a revision of the mastopexy should be considered. Second, a double-bubble deformity may occur if a persistent inframammary crease occurs when the pocket is dissected inferiorly to accommodate a large implant or purposefully lower an asymmetric crease or a constricted lower pole. Over time, this may improve as pressure from the implant stretches the skin. Correction includes a shoelace cast,[63] placing smaller implants and plicating the IMF versus creating a neosubpectoral pocket with capsular reinforcement of the fold. If the breast implant position is correct, fat grafting can be used to camouflage the contour depression.

Outcomes

A large meta-analysis by Khavanin *et al.* was recently published which examined 23 single stage, augmentation mastopexy review articles.[23] The total pooled complication rate was 13.1% with the most common complication being recurrent ptosis (5.2%), followed by poor scarring (3.7%). Capsular contracture rates were 3.0% and tissue-related asymmetry was 2.9%. Infection, hematoma, and seroma rates were less than 2% each. Reoperation rates were 10.7%. The pool of articles displayed extreme heterogeneity and despite inherent drawbacks from a meta-analysis, this meta-analysis remains a good outcomes resource.

The authors recently published a review of 615 consecutive one-stage mastopexy augmentations,[7] Silicone implants were placed in 79%, and textured implants were used in 92% of cases. The average volume of the implants was 323 cc. In total, 93% of implants were placed in a submuscular pocket. The five most common complications were: poor scarring (5.7%); wound healing issues (2.9%); implant deflation (2.6%); areolar asymmetry (1.9%); and capsular contracture (1.6%). Over the period of the study, 16.9% of patients underwent some kind of revision procedure. Tissue-related complications were looked at separately, and poor scarring was the most common indication, with circumareolar mastopexies leading to a statistically higher rate of revision. This finding is consistent with other studies.[6,87]

Access the complete reference list online at **http://www.expertconsult.com**

2. Nahai F, Fisher J, Maxwell PG, et al. Augmentation mastopexy: to stage or not. *Aesthet Surg J.* 2007;27:297–305. *A panel discussion from breast surgery experts with clinical examples of augmentation mastopexy challenges.*

6. Calobrace MB, Herdt DR, Cothron KJ. Simultaneous augmentation/mastopexy: a retrospective 5-year review of 332 consecutive cases. *Plast Reconstr Surg.* 2013;131:145–156. *The authors describe their large experience with combined augmentation mastopexy procedures, resulting in a 20 percent reoperation rate in primary combined procedures and a 30 percent reoperation rate in secondary combined procedures.*

7. Stevens WG, Macias LH, Spring M, et al. One-stage augmentation mastopexy: a review of 1192 simultaneous breast augmentation and mastopexy procedures in 615 consecutive patients. *Aesthet Surg J.* 2014;34:723–732. *A single-center review of 615 consecutive patients that underwent one-stage augmentation mastopexy with demographic and surgical descriptions, clinical examples and complication statistics.*

8. Stevens WG, Freeman ME, Stoker DA, et al. One-stage mastopexy with breast augmentation: a review of 321 patients. *Plast Reconstr Surg.* 2007;120:1674–1679. *A retrospective review of 321 consecutive patients who underwent one-stage augmentation mastopxy. The review includes information about patient demographics, operative technique, postoperative results, complications and revision rates.*

11. Spear SL, Pelletiere CV, Menon N. One-stage augmentation combined with mastopexy: aesthetic results and patient satisfaction. *Aesthetic Plast Surg.* 2004;28:259–267. *A retrospective chart review of 34 patients who underwent one staged augmentation mastopexy. An aesthetic rating scale survey was conducted, showing that on average patients were satisfied with their result.*

15. Parsa AA, Jackowe DJ, Parsa FD. A new algorithm for breast mastopexy/augmentation. *Plast Reconstr Surg.* 2010;125:75e–77e. *The authors have devised an algorithm for augmentation mastopexy based on the degree of breast ptosis. In addition they suggest a classification of "breast nadir" rather than nipple position to classify ptosis.*

52. Spear SL, Dayan JH, Clemens MW. Augmentation mastopexy. *Clin Plast Surg.* 2009;36:105–115.

64. Spear SL, Low M, Ducic I. Revision augmentation mastopexy: indications, operations, and outcomes. *Ann Plast Surg.* 2003; 51:540–546. *An 8-year retrospective review of 20 patients who underwent revision augmentation mastopexy. Capsular contracture and recurrent ptosis were the most common indications for revision.*

65. Spear SL, Boehmler JH 4th, Clemens MW. Augmentation/mastopexy: a 3-year review of a single surgeon's practice. *Plast Reconstr Surg.* 2006;118:136S–151S. *A retrospective study of 166 patients who underwent primary and secondary augmentation and primary and secondary augmentation/mastopexy. They found that primary augmentation/mastopexy has a significantly higher complication rate than primary augmentation. Secondary augmentation/mastopexy has higher revision and complication rates as well.*

83. Barnsley GP, Sigurdson LJ, Barnsley SE. Textured surface breast implants in the prevention of capsular contracture among breast augmentation patients: a meta-analysis of randomized controlled trials. *Plast Reconstr Surg.* 2006;117:2182–2190. *A meta analysis of 11 trials which demonstrate a decreased capsular contracture rate with textured implants vs smooth.*

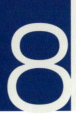

Secondary aesthetic breast surgery

Scott L. Spear[†] and Benjamin J. Brown

SYNOPSIS

- The best intervention is to prevent secondary deformities through thoughtful planning and careful and principled techniques.
- "Re-operation" is defined here as any subsequent surgery on a previously operated breast, including non-aesthetic procedures such as a lumpectomy.
- Scarring, tissue atrophy, and altered blood supply make secondary aesthetic breast surgery more challenging than primary aesthetic breast surgery, and therefore, these revisionary procedures carry a higher risk of complications and patient disappointment.
- Reasons for early revisionary breast surgery are deformities that arise shortly after the initial operation, such as implant malposition, early capsular contracture, double-bubble deformity, and Snoopy-nose deformity.
- Reasons for late revisionary surgery include deformities, such as breast ptosis, implant rupture, size change, and late capsular contracture.

Introduction

Despite our best efforts, there are many complications that can occur after aesthetic breast surgery. The best intervention is to prevent these secondary deformities through thoughtful planning and careful and principled techniques (covered elsewhere). The focus of this chapter is on revisionary surgery after prior breast augmentation, mastopexy, and augmentation-mastopexy. The authors believe in making the distinction between re-operation and revision. "Re-operation" is defined here as any subsequent surgery on a previously operated breast, including non-aesthetic procedures such as a lumpectomy. In this chapter, "revision" refers to

procedures performed with the goal of correcting a deformity caused by prior aesthetic breast surgery. Scarring, tissue atrophy, and altered blood supply make secondary aesthetic breast surgery more challenging than primary aesthetic breast surgery, and therefore, these revisionary procedures carry a higher risk of complications and patient disappointment.[1] Careful analysis and planning, however, can set the stage for and improve the likelihood of a good outcome and a satisfied patient.

"Early" revisionary surgery is defined here as an operation performed within 12 months of the index aesthetic procedure. Reasons for early revisionary breast surgery are deformities that arise shortly after the initial operation such as implant malposition, early capsular contracture, double-bubble deformity, and Snoopy-nose deformity. Late revisionary surgery is performed to correct deformities that develop after 1 year. These deformities are less likely to be technique- or judgment-related and may actually be inevitable and not necessarily preventable. Reasons for late revisionary surgery include deformities such as breast ptosis, implant rupture, size change, and late capsular contracture.

Revisionary surgery after breast augmentation

Gabriel *et al*. followed 1800 patients after primary breast augmentation and found a re-operative rate of 12% at 5 years.[2] Allergan 10-year data on fourth generation smooth round silicone implants found a 10-year re-operation rate of 36.1% (Table 8.1).[3]

Table 8.1 Adverse outcomes at 10 years post-implantation with Allergan Natrelle silicone gel-filled breast implants.

	(%)
Rupture	10.1
Capsular contracture (III or IV)	19.1
Re-operation for any reason	36.1

Early complications

Implant malposition refers to an implant that is located beyond the ideal borders of an aesthetic appearing breast. Implant malposition can be superior, inferior, medial (symmastia), and/or lateral. Some of the most common causes of implant malposition include over-dissection of the pocket beyond the ideal medial, lateral, and inferior breast footprint. Inadequate lower pole dual-plane release, hematoma, and/or an excessively large or wide implant can also result in implant malposition. Inferior implant malposition is usually caused by over-dissection inferiorly and disruption of the inframammary fold. Medial implant malposition is usually caused by over-dissection medially as well as using an excessively wide implant. Lateral implant malposition is the most commonly observed implant malposition. Lateral implant malposition is usually caused by over-dissection of the pocket laterally, which can be further exacerbated by the convexity of the chest wall and compressive forces generated by the pectoralis major muscle. Superior implant malposition is most commonly seen following transaxillary and periareolar breast augmentation due to inadequate lower pocket release or dissection.

The treatment for implant malposition involves recreating an implant pocket of appropriate shape, location, and size. For lateral implant malposition, the pocket must be moved medially. This is usually accomplished by shifting the lateral breast border more medially and, if indicated, performing a medial capsulotomy as well. The lateral border of the pocket can be reconstructed in a number of ways, including a capsulorrhaphy, as described by Spear and Little in 1988, whereby the implant capsular tissue is incised and repaired with sutures to reduce the size of the pocket (Fig. 8.1).[4,5] Medial implant malposition, often termed "symmastia", is a more difficult problem to solve because it is typically associated with the separation of pre-sternal tissues from the sternum. Reconstructing these attachments requires a strong and durable repair because the implant acts like a wedge and will often re-open the undesired space if left in the same tissue plane. For this reason, the authors' preferred technique for the correction of symmastia is a site change, including converting subglandular to subpectoral, subpectoral to subglandular, or creation of a neosubpectoral pocket (Fig. 8.2).[6] This new pocket, dissected just superficial to the previous aberrant subpectoral plane, allows the implant to sit on the repair and act as a buttress reinforcing the repair, rather than as a wedge trying to disrupt the repair. Capsular flaps, as described by Bengtson et al. in 1993, is another useful technique to alter the pocket.[7,8] Capsular flaps can be used to create vascularized slings to alter the implant pocket. Unlike a simple capsulorrhaphy, the use of capsular flaps can give the surgeon more freedom to place the suture line in a more advantageous location to reduce the ability of the device to disrupt the repair (Fig. 8.3).

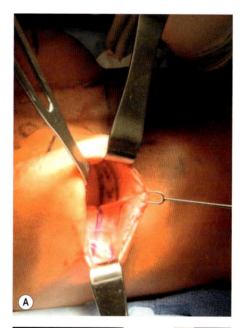

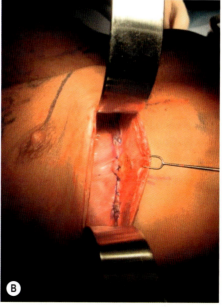

Fig. 8.1 (A,B) Capsulorrhaphy to modify pocket. The implant capsular tissue is incised and repaired with sutures to reduce the size of the pocket. (Case courtesy of Scott Spear, MD.)

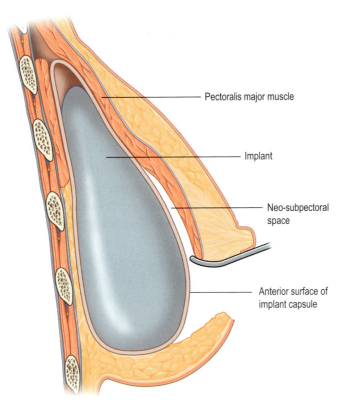

Fig. 8.2 Neo-subpectoral pocket. The neo-subpectoral plane is shown located between the anterior surface of the anterior implant capsule and the posterior surfaces of the pectoralis major muscle superiorly and breast parenchyma inferiorly. Correction of symmastia is a site change including converting subglandular to subpectoral, subpectoral to subglandular, or creation of a neo-subpectoral pocket. *(Redrawn after Spear SL. Surgery of the Breast: Principles and Art, 3, Illustrated. Philadelphia: Lippincott Williams & Wilkins; 2010:1479.)*

Labels on figure:
- Pectoralis major muscle
- Implant
- Neo-subpectoral space
- Anterior surface of implant capsule

The authors most commonly utilize capsular flaps or the neo-subpectoral pocket for treating inferior implant malposition. For superior implant malposition, the authors have found that isolated inferior capsulotomy is insufficient to treat the problem and the preferred technique for treating superior implant malposition is the dual-plane conversion, as described by Spear *et al.* in 2003 (Fig. 8.4).[9] Acellular dermal matrices (ADM) can be used to reinforce a capsulotomy, capsulorrhaphy, capsular flap, or anywhere there is a paucity of stout tissue (Fig. 8.5).[10,11] An additional benefit of ADM are their application when the "reconstructive technique" is used to support the weight of the implant by off-loading the skin and glandular tissue by supporting and covering the implant with ADM and pectoralis major muscle (Fig. 8.6).[10] Although the cost of ADM is significant, its cost is less than the cost of additional operations, not to mention the time spent recovering. For cases of inferior and lateral implant malposition, some surgeons advocate a pocket change to the subglandular pocket to remove the compressive force of the pectoralis major muscle that squeezes the implant inferiorly and laterally; however, if the implant is in a dual-plane position,

then the inferior and lateral portions of the pocket are already subglandular and so would need additional repair of some sort. It is possible that once a repair has been performed, a textured device may be less prone to recurrent malposition, but there is no known evidence that would substantiate that belief.

Nipple areolar complex (NAC) malposition refers to an unaesthetic location of the NAC after breast augmentation. NAC malposition is often not caused by breast augmentation but rather accentuated and made apparent by it. All women have some degree of nipple asymmetry, and therefore it is wise for the plastic surgeon to point this out preoperatively. NAC malposition caused by breast augmentation is usually related to implant malposition, the treatment of which is described above. If NAC malposition is due to unrecognized ptosis, it can be treated by subsequent mastopexy, which is described elsewhere in this text.

A scar tissue capsule inevitably forms around all breast implants. Capsular contracture refers to the symptomatic and pathologic contracture of this otherwise non-problematic scar capsule. Capsular contracture is a poorly understood process but is thought to be an exaggerated foreign body response that, if severe enough, can produce hard, deformed, and painful breasts.[12] The

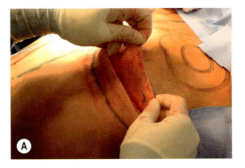

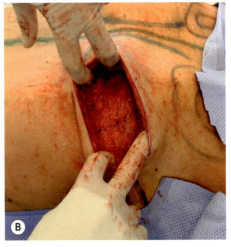

Fig. 8.3 (A,B) Capsular flaps can give the surgeon more freedom to place the suture line in a more advantageous location to reduce the ability of the device to disrupt the repair. *(Case courtesy of Ben Brown, MD.)*

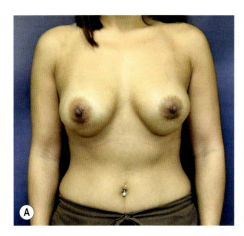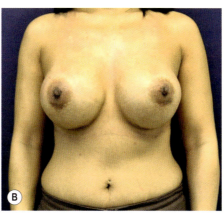

Fig. 8.4 (A,B) Converting an existing implant pocket to a dual-plane pocket. Our preferred technique for treating superior implant malposition and double-bubble deformity is the dual-plane conversion. *(Case courtesy of Ben Brown, MD.)*

grading system for capsular contracture around breast implants was defined by Baker in 1977 and modified by Spear for reconstructive cases in 1995.[13,14] Early capsular contracture refers to capsular contracture that occurs within 1 year of implant placement. For early capsular contracture, the authors recommend aggressive management, similar to how one might treat a periprosthetic infection. This includes a total capsulectomy, systemic antibiotics, creation of a virgin pocket, and placement of a new device. The use of an ADM has also shown promise in preventing capsular contracture.[10]

Visible rippling is the result of implants deforming to a "more" anatomic shape beneath an inadequate soft-tissue envelope. As gravity shifts the saline or gel from the superior portion of the device to the inferior portion of the device, the superior portion becomes relatively "under-filled" and the redundant superior shell subsequently ripples. Treatment options for visible rippling include increasing the soft-tissue coverage and decreasing the rippling of the actual device. Options to improve soft-tissue coverage include upper pole pectoralis muscle coverage as a dual-plane conversion (Fig. 8.4) if the device was in a subglandular plane. Fat grafting or placement of an onlay or supporting ADM can also be used to improve soft-tissue coverage. Options to decrease device rippling include exchange for an implant with a higher fill ratio or the use of a more highly cohesive silicone gel implant.

A double-bubble deformity is the presence of a constricting band or fold in the inferior pole of the breast

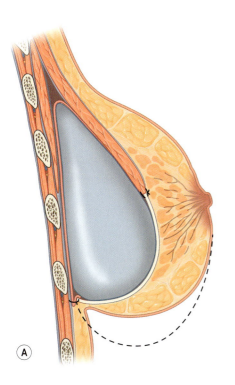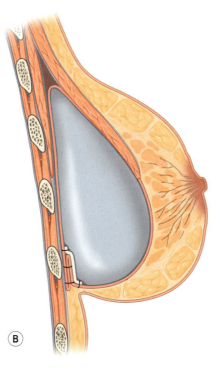

Fig. 8.5 Gutter technique. Acellular dermal matrices can be used to reinforce a capsulotomy, capsulorrhaphy, capsular flap, or anywhere there is a paucity of stout tissue. *(Redrawn after Spear SL, Seruya M, Clemens MW, Teitelbaum S, & Nahabedian MY. Acellular dermal matrix for the treatment and prevention of implant-associated breast deformities.* Plastic and Reconstructive Surgery. *2001; 127(3):1047–58. doi:10.1097/PRS.0b013e31820436af.)*

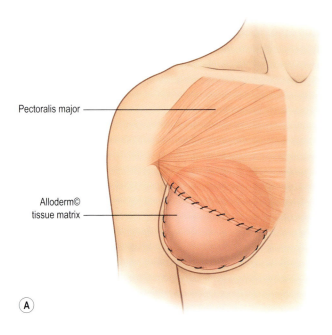

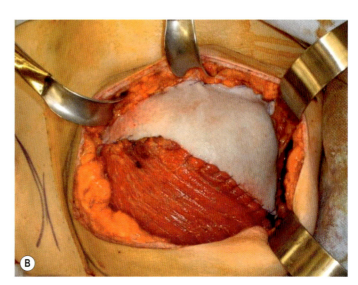

Pectoralis major

Alloderm©
tissue matrix

Ⓐ

Ⓑ

Fig. 8.6 (A,B) Moving the pectoralis major muscle into a more anatomic position by freeing its superficial surface from the overlying breast and anchoring the muscle with an overlapping sheet of acellular dermal matrices (ADM) to the inferior and lateral breast folds similar to the ADM-assisted reconstruction technique. *(Case courtesy of Scott Spear, MD.)*

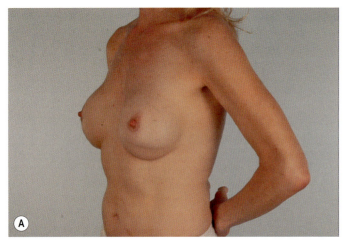

Ⓐ

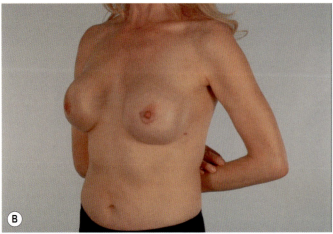

Ⓑ

Fig. 8.7 (A,B) A double-bubble deformity is the presence of a constricting band or fold in the inferior pole of the breast that creates the appearance of two folds. *(Case courtesy of Scott Spear, MD.)*

that creates the appearance of two folds (Fig. 8.7). This constricting band is usually the native IMF that remains apparent above the illusion of a new fold created by an inferior implant malposition. It can also be the result of incomplete detachment of the lower border of the pectoralis major muscle associated with a submuscular pocket dissection. Another cause of the double-bubble deformity is failure to obliterate the native IMF during intentional placement of the implant inferior to the native IMF, as in cases of tuberous breast deformity. Treatment options for double-bubble deformity include raising the IMF to its native position as described above, fat grafting, or obliterating the fold utilizing a dual-plane conversion.[15,16] The dual-plane conversion will ensure sufficient freedom of the pectoralis major muscle from the native IMF and lysis of any dermal attachments.

A "Snoopy" deformity refers to ptotic glandular tissue that appears to be "falling" of the implant. Milder cases can be treated by conversion to a dual-plane II or III, which would allow the pectoralis major muscle and overlying glandular tissue to "window-shade" or "ascend" up over the device (Fig. 8.8).[17] More severe cases of a Snoopy-nose deformity may require a mastopexy to treat the ptotic glandular tissue. A Baker grade III or IV capsular contracture can create the appearance of a Snoopy deformity with relative ptosis of the breast as the breast implant is deformed into a more spherical shape and shifted superiorly. For these patients, treatment of the capsular contracture is most appropriate.

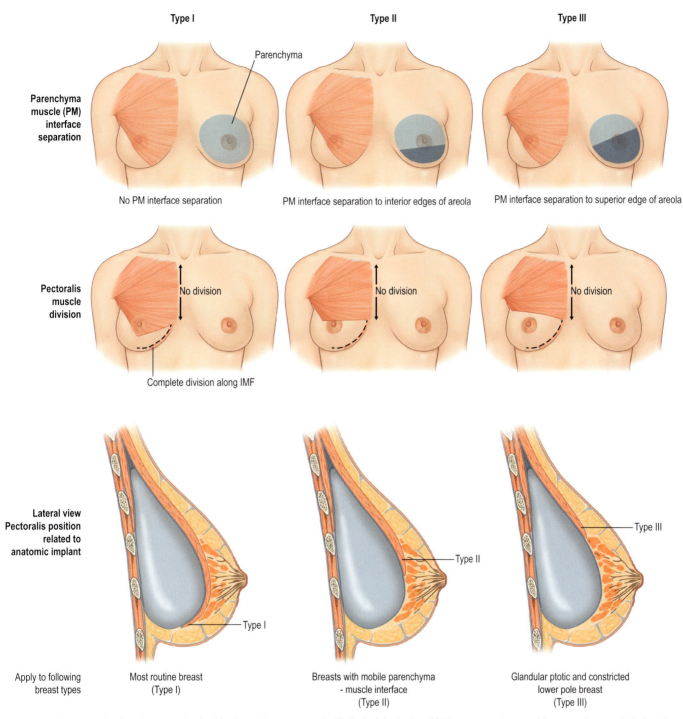

Type I

Type II

Type III

Parenchyma muscle (PM) interface separation

Parenchyma

No PM interface separation

PM interface separation to interior edges of areola

PM interface separation to superior edge of areola

Pectoralis muscle division

No division

No division

No division

Complete division along IMF

Lateral view Pectoralis position related to anatomic implant

Type I

Type II

Type III

Apply to following breast types

Most routine breast (Type I)

Breasts with mobile parenchyma - muscle interface (Type II)

Glandular ptotic and constricted lower pole breast (Type III)

Fig. 8.8 A "Snoopy" deformity refers to ptotic glandular tissue that appears to be "falling" of the implant. Milder cases can be treated by conversion to a dual-plane II or III, which would allow the pectoralis major muscle and overlying glandular tissue to "window-shade" or "ascend" up over the device. *(Redrawn after Tebbetts JB. Dual-plane breast augmentation: Optimizing implant-soft-tissue relationships in a wide range of breast types.* Plastic and Reconstructive Surgery. *2001; 107(5):1255–72.)*

Animation deformity refers to visible distortion of the breast implant shape or position secondary to contractions of the overlying pectoralis major muscle. This may be made more apparent as a result of inadequate soft-tissue coverage over the pectoralis major muscle. It may also be related to how the subpectoral or submuscular dissection is performed as well as the extent of muscle development in a given patient. In reality, there is likely more than one form of animation deformity, including ironically, either under or overly aggressive muscle release. One variety is likely due to excessive detachment of the pectoralis major muscle from its sternal origin, resulting in muscle fibers that "window-shade" excessively superiorly and also may make the dislocated muscle appear more bulky. Fortunately, animation deformity is quite rare in correctly performed dual-plane breast augmentations and is usually only seen in competitive bodybuilders.[18] Inadequate release of the lower edge of the pectoralis major, intended or inadvertent dissection behind the pectoralis minor muscle, or subserratus dissection may all contribute to some variation of animation deformity. The treatment of animation deformity is difficult and, in most cases, unpredictable. The most predictable form of correction is achieved by replacing the implant in a pre-pectoral position and replacing the muscle(s) back on the chest wall as anatomically as possible.[18] Other, much less reliable, options include fat grafting to camouflage the deformity or moving the pectoralis major muscle into a more anatomic position by freeing its superficial surface from the overlying breast and anchoring the muscle with an overlapping sheet of ADM to the inferior and lateral breast folds similar to the ADM-assisted reconstruction technique (Fig. 8.6). The ADM in this maneuver acts like a fascial attachment, which may help the muscle from "window-shading" superiorly while also creating an interface to promote the gliding of the soft-tissue over the surface of the muscle and implant. It is worth emphasizing again that pre-pectoral repositioning is by far the most reliable approach to address this challenging problem.

Late complications

Some amount of breast ptosis is an inevitable component of aging and may be exacerbated by breast augmentation due to the increased forces on the tissues from the weight of the implant. The treatment for breast ptosis with or without an implant is a mastopexy, which is described elsewhere in this text.

Late capsular contracture appears to be more related to the natural history of breast implants and less related to perioperative factors such as contamination and inflammation. Therefore, the authors take a less aggressive approach to late capsular contracture than early capsular contracture. Treatment of late capsular contracture includes total or sub-total capsulectomy and placement of a new device.

Rupture refers to a disruption of the implant shell that allows the silicone gel to escape the shell and leak into the implant pocket and more rarely into the surrounding tissues. The longer an implant is in place, the more likely it is to rupture.[3] Most cases of rupture are silent, especially with highly cohesive gel implants.[19] Symptoms such as palpable lumps, skin changes, and axillary adenopathy are usually only present in cases of extracapsular spread of silicone. MRI currently remains the gold standard for diagnosing implant rupture,[20] although it is expected that, for reasons of convenience, comfort, safety, and cost, ultrasound will eventual become the best option. The treatment for silicone gel implant rupture is when possible a total capsulectomy without disruption of the capsule, in order to contain and remove the silicone gel. When this is not possible, the authors recommend removing as much silicone as possible by a combination of wiping, irrigating, and cleaning with Shur-Clens, a useful solvent in which silicone is soluble.

Late seroma has been defined by the Dr. Spear as a clinically symptomatic seroma that develops at least 12 months after the most recent breast implant surgery.[21] The majority of late seromas are idiopathic, without clear evidence of infection or malignancy. However, late seromas must be taken seriously given the remote but ominous possibility of breast implant-associated anaplastic large cell lymphoma (BI-ALCL). The incidence of BI-ALCL with textured implants is thought to be between 1:30 000 and 1:300 000, with as many as 5% of those patients afflicted by ALCL dying from the disease.[22] At the time of writing, it remains unclear whether there were any documented cases of BI-ALCL with smooth devices. In the published review of Dr. Spear's practice, the average interval from the patient's most recent breast surgery to late seroma onset was 4.7 years and 96% of these patients had a textured device. Ultrasound-guided therapeutic aspiration with culture and cytology is a rational first step, as this was successful in 56% of the time. If this resolves the problem, nothing further needs to be done. Indications for capsulectomy and placement of a new smooth device include a thick capsule, an abnormal mass within the capsule, evidence of infection or inflammation, and failure of a prior percutaneous drainage procedure.[21]

Stretch deformity refers to an increase in the nipple to IMF distance, with maintenance of the native IMF. If an increased nipple to fold distance is due to disruption of the native IMF – this deformity would be more appropriately classified as inferior implant malposition. Lower pole stretch deformity can occur in any breast but most commonly occurs in patients with excessively large implants. The weight of these devices place excessive stress on the soft-tissues of the lower pole of the breast leading to atrophy of breast tissue and expansion of the lower pole skin. After determining that the native IMF is intact and the deformity is, in fact, a lower pole stretch deformity – treatment options include some form of mastopexy or skin reduction procedure (Fig. 8.9) to remove the excess lower pole skin, exchange for a smaller device, and possible reinforcement of the lower pole of the breast with ADM using the reconstructive technique (Fig. 8.6).[23,24]

Impending implant extrusion refers to severe atrophy of breast tissue, such that the device is nearly exposed.

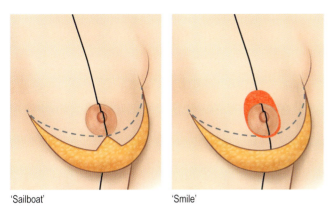

'Sailboat'   'Smile'

Fig. 8.9 Stretch deformity refers to an increase in the nipple to inframammory fold (IMF) distance with maintenance of the native IMF. If an increased nipple to fold distance is due to disruption of the native IMF – this deformity would be more appropriately classified as inferior implant malposition. Lower pole stretch deformity can occur in any breast but most commonly occurs in patients with excessively large implants.

As long as there is no actual exposure and the device pocket is not contaminated, treatment options include device removal without replacement or exchange for a smaller device with ADM reinforcement using the reconstructive technique, muscle flaps, anterior capsular rotation flaps, or posterior capsular flaps (Fig. 8.3).[23,24] Nipple ptosis and excess lower pole skin may be addressed with mastopexy techniques.

Women who underwent breast augmentation earlier in life may wish to have smaller breasts later in life. For the vast majority of women who want to keep their breast implants, one option is exchanging the existing implants with smaller implants. However, the implant pocket and skin envelope may need a reduction in size to aesthetically accommodate a smaller implant. What may initially seem like a rather simple operation, exchanging large implants for smaller implants may become a deceptively complicated procedure as it is a mastopexy on a previously operated augmented breast. The blood supply to the NAC has been necessarily and significantly altered in the previously augmented breast. This is made more significant as the breast tissue typically becomes atrophic after years of supporting an implant (Fig. 8.10). The blood supply to the nipple and breast skin is also altered and becomes more dependent on the collateral circulation rather than the normal deep circulation. One option to reduce the risk of complications in these patients is staging the operation so that the capsule and skin are not operated on simultaneously. The key, however, to safely operating on these patients is to recognize and respect the compromised blood supply. To help unweight the skin flaps and support the implant, one can utilize an ADM to internally support the device, thereby offloading the breast tissue (Fig. 8.7). For women who wish to have smaller breasts and live without implants, simply removing the implants and doing nothing else may be sufficient, while for others, this will leave the breasts deflated and "aged" in appearance. A mastopexy can help in this situation; however, this needs to be performed very cautiously with minimal undermining in order to preserve the tenuous blood supply to the nipple as well as the rest of the breast (Fig. 8.11)

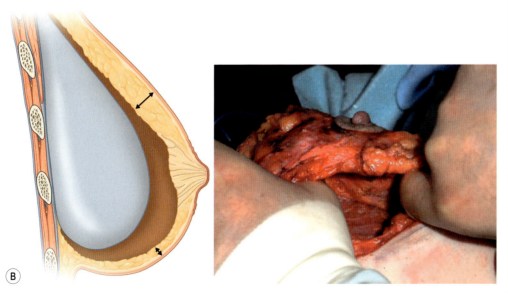

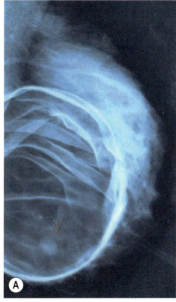

Fig. 8.10 (A,B) Exchanging existing implants with smaller implants. The implant pocket and skin envelope may need a reduction in size to aesthetically accommodate a smaller implant. What may initially seem like a rather simple operation may become a deceptively complicated procedure as it involves mastopexy on a previously operated augmented breast. (Reproduced with permission from Spear SL. Surgery of the Breast: Principles and Art, 3, Illustrated. Philadelphia: Lippincott Williams & Wilkins; 2010: 1542.)

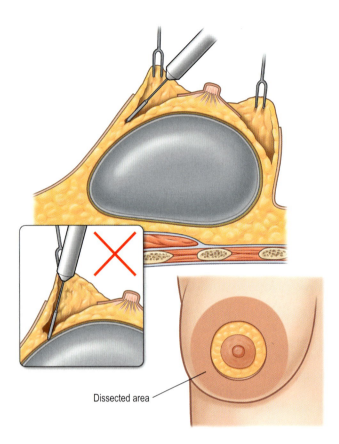

Fig. 8.11 Some patients may wish to have smaller breasts and live without implants. Simply removing the implants and doing nothing else may be sufficient, while for others this will leave the breasts deflated and "aged" in appearance. A mastopexy can help in this situation; however, this needs to be performed very cautiously with minimal undermining in order to preserve the tenuous blood supply to the nipple as well as the rest of the breast.

For those women who wish to have their implants removed but retain some semblance of their augmented volume, one option to consider is the use of fat grafting as described by Spear, or fat grafting with pre-expansion as described by Del Vecchio (Fig. 8.12).[1,25]

Breast enlargement from weight gain and or pregnancies may cause some women to request removal of their breast implants to achieve smaller and lighter breasts. Many techniques exist depending on the current breast size, volume of the implants, and patient goals. One option is implant removal with a small to moderate amount of fat grafting. Mastopexy may be necessary to reduce the size of the breast envelope, with or without fat grafting. A breast reduction may be an appropriate solution for patients who have excess breast tissue after implant removal and wish to be significantly smaller in size.

Revisionary surgery after mastopexy

NAC malposition after mastopexy refers to an NAC that is too high, too low, or to the right or left of the breast meridian. Mallucci and Branford performed a morphometric analysis of breasts and found that breasts with an upper pole to lower pole ratio of 45:55 universally scored the highest.[26] Therefore, for the purposes of this discussion, the "ideal" nipple position would be on the breast meridian with a slightly fuller lower pole. An NAC that is only a couple of centimeters too high can sometimes be corrected with a mastopexy limited to the lower pole of the breast by simply shortening the nipple to IMF distance, assuming that the sternal notch to nipple distance is not too short (Fig. 8.8). Correction of an NAC that is too low after mastopexy involves a repeat or revision mastopexy to elevate the NAC to the appropriate location. Interestingly, Dr. Spear has found that vertical limbs of the WISE pattern form an upright "V" in revision mastopexies and reductions, whereas primary mastopexies and reductions generally have vertical limbs that form an inverted or upside-down "V".[27] The authors caution against techniques that involve lowering the IMF to correct an NAC that is too low.[28] Although lowering the IMF can create the appropriate upper pole to lower pole ratio without actually moving the NAC, these techniques risk creating a double-bubble deformity and women generally do not like their breast mounds positioned low on their chests. Because most mastopexy techniques leave a scar round the areola, one must be vigilant in revision mastopexies to maintain continuity between the NAC and the underlying glandular pedicle (Fig. 8.11). For cases of more severe NAC malposition

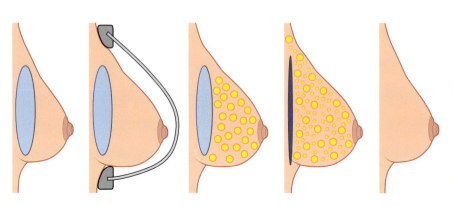

Fig. 8.12 Some patients may wish to have their implants removed but retain some semblance of their augmented volume. One option to consider is the use of fat grafting as described by Spear or fat grafting with pre-expansion as described by Del Vecchio. *(Redrawn after Del Vecchio, DA, Bucky, LP, Breast augmentation using preexpansion and autologous fat transplantation: A clinical radiographic study. Plastic and Reconstructive Surgery. 2011;127(6):2441–50. doi:10.1097/PRS.0b013e3182050a64.)*

not correctable with mastopexy techniques, one may consider performing transposition flaps or composite nipple grafting.[29,30]

Under-correction of glandular ptosis following mastopexy refers to breasts that have the NAC appropriately placed at the IMF but have excess skin and breast tissue hanging below the IMF. To the untrained eye, these breasts can appear to have superior NAC malposition due to the excess lower pole tissue. Treatment of this deformity is revision mastopexy, typically utilizing a sailboat or smile mastopexy pattern (Fig. 8.10).

Over-resection of tissue in a mastopexy can leave patients dissatisfied with the size of their breasts after surgery. In a series of 61 patients, Weichman *et al.* showed that mastopexy alone may result in an average decrease in one brassiere cup size.[31] Preoperatively, patients should be advised accordingly. For the rare patient who after a mastopexy wishes to have a larger breast size, treatment options include augmentation with implants or augmentation with fat grafting.

Necrosis of the nipple areolar complex, although rare, is one of the most feared complications in aesthetic breast surgery. Should it occur, NAC reconstruction becomes more complex than skin sparing mastectomy cases because of the compromised tissue and scar burden at the location of the former and future NAC. The areola can be reconstructed with full-thickness skin grafting. Dr. Spear recently utilized Integra Dermal Regeneration Template (Integra LifeSciences, Plainsboro, NJ) followed by skin grafting (Fig. 8.13) to reconstruct the areola. Nipple reconstruction using local flaps is a poor solution in these patients given the compromised tissue and scar burden; for this reason the authors recommend composite nipple grafting if the contralateral donor nipple can afford it.[30] If nipple sharing is not an option, tattooing with artistic shading can create the illusion of a 3D nipple.[32]

Revisionary surgery after augmentation-mastopexy

Deformities after augmentation-mastopexy include those resulting from the implant, those associated with the soft-tissue envelope, and those associated with the interaction between an altered soft-tissue envelope and the device within. For an explanation of implant-related problems and their solutions, refer to the "Revisionary surgery after breast augmentation" section above. For an explanation of soft tissue–related deformities and their solutions, refer to the "Revisionary surgery after mastopexy" section above. The remainder of this section focuses on special considerations

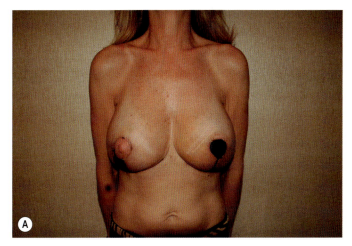

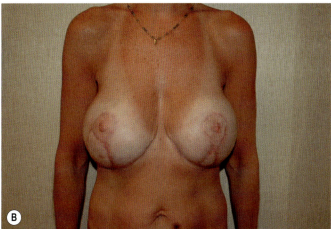

Fig. 8.13 Necrosis of the nipple areolar complex, although rare is one of the most feared complications in aesthetic breast surgery. The authors were recently referred a patient who suffered necrosis following an augmentation-mastopexy. The eschar was excised, and Integra Dermal Regeneration Template (Integra LifeSciences, Plainsboro, NJ) was utilized followed by skin grafting to reconstruct the areola. *(Case courtesy of Scott Spear, MD.)*

in augmentation-mastopexy due to the interaction between an altered soft-tissue envelope and the device within.

The most important consideration in both primary and revision augmentation mastopexy is maintenance of an adequate blood supply to the NAC. Losee *et al.* reported that secondary breast reductions can be safely performed with a different pedicle than the primary breast reduction.[33] The authors maintain NAC perfusion in both primary and secondary augmentation-mastopexy by utilizing a superior glandular pedicle, even when an inferior pedicle had been used previously. This pedicle is maintained by performing little to no undermining superiorly between 3 and 9 o'clock. Using this technique, the NAC is translated superiorly, while its pedicle is theoretically imbricated beneath the skin closure; however, in practice this "imbrication" is not apparent and has not, in our experience, created any subsequent skin tethering or irregularities.

The risk of implant exposure following augmentation-mastopexy can be reduced by planning the operation such that the glandular incision to create the implant pocket is not confluent with a T-junction at skin closure. When certain that a vertical scar will be necessary, the authors prefer to perform the augmentation first through a vertical incision located between the two vertical limbs of the planned mastopexy. The authors recommend de-epithelializing a centimeter or so around this vertical incision to allow future multi-layer closure, including a dermal layer, over the device. Once the devices are in place and the vertical parenchymal incisions are closed, the skin is tailor-tacked using the preoperative markings as a guide. The mastopexy markings are adjusted as deemed appropriate, and the skin within the markings is de-epithelialized. Next, the dermis along the markings is incised full thickness with the Bovie on cut, just enough to release it without injuring the subdermal plexus. No flaps are created. Full-thickness dermal scoring usually allows the skin to close and evert nicely without any tethering or contour deformities. If undermining is necessary, it should be done judiciously, no more than 1–2 cm, in a very superficial plane under the dermis so as to not compromise the glandular pedicle perfusing the NAC (Fig. 8.12).

Periareolar deformities are most common after periareolar mastopexy techniques. Patients find periareolar mastopexy techniques appealing because they avoid vertical and inframammary scars on the breast. Unfortunately, the power and control offered by periareolar techniques are very limited. Not surprisingly, patient satisfaction after periareolar techniques is lower than with other more powerful mastopexy techniques.[34] Most periareolar deformities arise when plastic surgeons push the limits of a periareolar mastopexy in the hope that it will correct more severe cases of ptosis. The authors recommend limiting the use of periareolar mastopexy techniques for the treatment of large areolas and minimal degrees of NAC ptosis, no more than 2 cm. Unsightly periareolar scars around the areola are unfortunately common due to excessive tension at the time of purse-string closure of the large outer aperture to the smaller inner aperture around the remaining areola. Spear *et al.* have published guidelines for the use of periareolar mastopexy to help reduce such complications.[35] The use of a scar blocking stitch placed in a wagon-wheel fashion around the areola, as described by Hammond *et al.*, is a technique used by many to help prevent unsightly scars around the areola (Fig. 8.14).[36] In most cases, treatment of periareolar deformities involves performing a circumvertical mastopexy. The addition of the vertical limbs provides the plastic surgeon with much more power and control to reposition the NAC

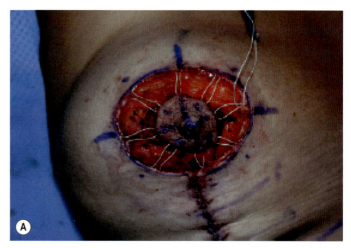

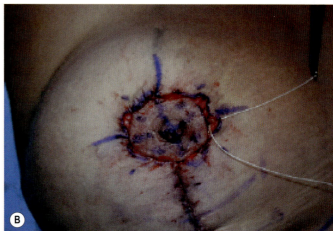

Fig. 8.14 (A,B) The use of a scar blocking stitch placed in a wagon-wheel fashion around the areola, as described by Hammond, is a technique used by many to help prevent unsightly scars around the areola. *(Reproduced with permission from Hammond DC, Khuthaila DK, & Kim J. The interlocking gore-tex suture for control of areolar diameter and shape.* Plastic and Reconstructive Surgery. *2007;119(3):804–9. doi:10.1097/01.prs.0000251998.50345.e9.)*

and reshape the breast. In cases of periareolar deformities, the addition of vertical limbs to the mastopexy pattern allows the outer aperture to be designed nearly the same size as the new areola, thereby reducing the tension at closure and improving the resultant scar.

Conclusion

Armed with an understanding of the various problems that can occur following cosmetic breast surgery, the astute plastic surgeon can take measures to help prevent their occurrence. When treating patients with an unsatisfactory result following cosmetic breast surgery, remember that scarring, tissue atrophy, and altered blood supply make secondary aesthetic breast surgery more challenging than primary aesthetic breast surgery. These revisionary procedures deserve thoughtful planning, sufficient OR time, and meticulous execution.

Access the complete reference list online at   **http://www.expertconsult.com**

6. Spear SL, Dayan JH, Bogue D, et al. The "neosubpectoral" pocket for the correction of symmastia. *Plast Reconstr Surg.* 2009;124:695–703. *The neosubpectoral pocket is a useful and effective technique for correction of symmastia. By placing the implant into a new tissue plane, it serves a buttress to help maintain closure of the former implant pocket.*

9. Spear SL, Carter ME, Ganz JC. The correction of capsular contracture by conversion to "dual-plane" positioning: technique and outcomes. *Plast Reconstr Surg.* 2003;112:456–466. *Capsular contracture is a common problem that frequently presents with superior implant malposition. Anterior/inferior capsulectomy with conversion to a dual-plane pocket is an effective and reliable technique to treat this problem.*

10. Spear SL, Seruya M, Clemens MW, et al. Acellular dermal matrix for the treatment and prevention of implant-associated breast deformities. *Plast Reconstr Surg.* 2011;127:1047–1058. *This article summarizes the many uses of ADM in secondary aesthetic breast surgery. We often counsel patients that although the use of ADM is an added cost, it is generally less than the cost of yet another revisionary procedure.*

17. Tebbetts JB. Dual plane breast augmentation: optimizing implant-soft-tissue relationships in a wide range of breast types. *Plast Reconstr Surg.* 2001;107:1255–1272. *This is the seminal article on the "dual-plane" technique for breast augmentation.*

21. Spear SL, Rottman SJ, Glicksman C, et al. Late seromas after breast implants: theory and practice. *Plast Reconstr Surg.* 2012;130:423–435. *Late seromas can be the sign of a more serious problem, and therefore all plastic surgeons should understand how to manage these patients.*

22. Clemens MW, Butler CE, Hunt KK, et al. Breast implant-associated anaplastic large cell lymphoma: staging, disease progression, and management strategies. *Plast Reconstr Surg.* 2015;135:1184. *Breast implant-associated ALCL is very rare. Because breast implants are so common, every plastic surgeon should be aware of the current guidelines regarding the evaluation and management of breast implant-associated ALCL.*

23. Spring MA, Macias LH, Nadeau M, et al. Secondary augmentation-mastopexy: indications, preferred practices, and the treatment of complications. *Aesthet Surg J.* 2014;34:1018–1040. *Excellent article that reviews Dr. Grant Steven's experience with secondary breast augmentation-mastopexy.*

26. Mallucci P, Branford OA. Population analysis of the perfect breast: a morphometric analysis. *Plast Reconstr Surg.* 2014;134:436–447. *This article objectively and geometrically describes the "ideal" nipple position.*

35. Spear SL, Giese SY, Ducic I. Concentric mastopexy revisited. *Plast Reconstr Surg.* 2001;107:1294–1300. *This article is a concise overview of the periareolar mastopexy. It describes its limitations and pitfalls as well as how to plan, mark, and execute the procedure.*

36. Hammond DC, Khuthaila DK, Kim J. The interlocking Gore-Tex suture for control of areolar diameter and shape. *Plast Reconstr Surg.* 2007;119:804–809. *The interlocking Gore-Tex suture is one of the greatest contributions to breast surgery in the past decade. This technique does an excellent job insetting areolae and maintaining their size over time.*

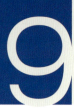

Reduction mammaplasty with inverted-T techniques

Maurice Y. Nahabedian

 Access video lecture content for this chapter online at expertconsult.com

SYNOPSIS

- The inverted-T technique for reduction mammaplasty is diverse and can be applied for the majority of women seeking reduction mammaplasty.
- Patient selection is a critical aspect with regard to the type of pedicle selected for transposition of the nipple areolar complex.
- The bipedicle techniques were among the first described and have been performed less frequently in favor of the unipedicle methods.
- The inferior pedicle reduction mammaplasty utilizing the inverted-T design is the most commonly utilized technique.
- The medial pedicle technique incorporates the dominant internal mammary perforators as its primary blood supply and may be useful for women with moderate to severe mammary hypertrophy.
- The central mound technique incorporates the 4th intercostal artery to perfuse the nipple areolar complex and is useful for mild to moderate volume reduction mammaplasty.
- Complications following inverted-T reduction mammaplasty are infrequent and include delayed healing at the trifurcation, loss of nipple areolar sensation, fat necrosis, and complex scar.

 Access the Historical Perspective section online at
http://www.expertconsult.com

Introduction

The evolution of reduction mammaplasty over the past century can be characterized as innovative, imaginative, and diverse. It is estimated that over 50 variations and techniques for reduction mammaplasty have been described. These variations are based on skin pattern design, as well as pedicle selection for transposition of the nipple areolar complex. Skin patterns have varied from short scar to long scar techniques and nipple transposition techniques have varied from free graft to dermal pedicles to dermo-parenchymal pedicles with orientations that can be anywhere along a 360° circle. All of these approaches have demonstrated success in certain situations. The debate as to whether one technique for reduction mammaplasty would be sufficient for all types of patients and breasts has been abandoned for all intent and purposes. It is accepted that individualized options for reduction mammaplasty are preferred and will usually generate optimal outcomes.

An important concept with reduction mammaplasty is differentiating the "cosmetic" reduction mammaplasty from the "functional" reduction mammaplasty. There is an overlap between these two because all reduction mammaplasty procedures are aesthetic in concept and design. The principles governing cosmetic versus functional reduction mammaplasty are important to differentiate for a variety of reasons that include patient expectations, surgical technique, and insurance reimbursement. The purely cosmetic patient is usually one that has mild to moderate mammary hypertrophy that typically requires a minimal reduction defined as less than 300 g. These patients usually are not symptomatic or debilitated by the size of their breasts and are primarily concerned with shape and contour and often wish to minimize scar. It is recognized, however, that there are situations in which a thin and petite woman with relative mammary hypertrophy would functionally benefit from a reduction that was less than 300 g. There is a another subset of patients with moderate to severe mammary hypertrophy who are symptomatic and plagued with back pain, intertrigo, and postural changes and who are primarily interested in relieving symptoms, secondarily interested in improving aesthetics, and are less concerned with the amount and location of the scars. These patients typically require a functional reduction mammaplasty. These differences are important to differentiate because whether the patient pays for the operation or has it paid for by a third party will vary based on patient characteristics, amount of breast tissue removed, type of insurance, as well as state or country of residence.

Breast anatomy

Reduction mammaplasty requires a specific understanding of breast anatomy with an emphasis on the parenchymal architecture, vascularity, and innervation. Although breast anatomy is covered in a previous chapter, the salient aspects will be reviewed here. The vascularity to the breast is diverse and includes the perforating branches of the internal mammary and the lateral thoracic artery and vein. Many anatomic studies allude to the internal mammary perforators as the dominant blood supply to the breast. Other sources include the intercostal and thoracoacromial vessels. Most pedicles are designed to capture one or several sources of blood supply to the nipple areolar complex.

The vascularity to the nipple areolar complex is derived primarily from the subdermal plexus of vessels that are supplied by the internal mammary and lateral thoracic perforators (Fig. 9.1 ⊕). The intercostal vessels are also contributors with the 4th intercostal being the primary deep source (Fig. 9.2). Within the breast, along the 4th intercostal space, is a horizontal structure known as Wuringer's septum.[5,6] This contains the 4th intercostal artery and vein that can maintain vascularity to the nipple areolar complex. This becomes especially important in the event that the peripheral subdermal plexus is violated resulting in reduced blood supply to the nipple areolar complex.

Fig. 9.1 appears online only.

The innervation to the breast and the nipple areolar complex is through the 2–6 intercostal nerves. Preservation of sensation to the nipple areolar complex is best achieved by understanding the neural pathways within the breast that lead to the nipple areolar complex. In a cadaveric study, Schlenz demonstrated that the 3–5 lateral and anterior intercostal nerves innervated the nipple areolar complex.[7] The course of the anterior nerve was more superficial in the majority of cases, whereas the lateral intercostal traversed more deeply within the pectoral fascia in the majority of cadavers.

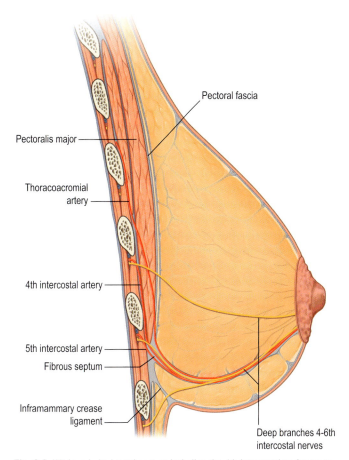

Fig. 9.2 Würinger's horizontal septum including the 4th intercostal perforator to the nipple areolar complex. (Reproduced with permission from Würinger E, Mader N, Posch E, Holle J. Nerves and vessels supplying ligamentous suspension of the mammary gland. Plast Reconstr Surg 1998;101:1486.)

The implication is that sensation is more likely preserved by minimizing the amount of medial dissection and by preserving the deep central mound along the 4th intercostal segment.

The inverted-T skin pattern

The inverted-T pattern has undergone several modifications over the years. The original pattern described by Robert Wise was based on the manufacturing process for a woman's brassiere taking into account the somewhat conical shape of the breast. A skin pattern was delineated that had relationships to the chest circumference, angulation of the chest wall, and the breast size. The classic inverted-T pattern had vertical and horizontal limbs with a keyhole pattern at the upper apex for insetting of the nipple areolar complex. A variation of this method, shown below, has been adopted by the author and has provided consistent and reproducible results.

Markings

The typical markings for the inverted-T incision are as follows (Fig. 9.3 ⊕). The sternal midline is delineated. The breast meridian is delineated bilaterally bisecting the midline of the breast. Any pre-existing asymmetry of the nipple areolar complex will be corrected during the operation in order to center the nipple along the breast meridian and to ensure that the distance from the sternal midline to the nipple will be equal on both sides. The inframammary fold is delineated bilaterally. The ideal nipple position is marked and based on the level of the inframammary fold. This may be done with calipers or freehand. The vertical limbs of the inverted-T pattern are delineated with a length that ranges from 8 to 9 cm. This will vary based on the volume of the breast. The angle of the apex is usually 60° and can be narrowed or widened based on the base width of the breast. For breasts with a wide base width, the angle can be increased to 70° and that will facilitate narrowing of the breast. For breasts with a normal to narrow base width, the angle is reduced to 50°. Although the keyhole pattern is described with the original description, the authors prefer not to delineate the keyhole at the time of the original markings but rather wait for completion of the reduction mammaplasty to accurately place the nipple areolar complex. The horizontal component of the inverted-T pattern is then marked and extends from the inferior point of both vertical limbs to the lateral and medial limits of the inframammary fold. The horizontal incision should never cross the sternal midline and should be tailored laterally to eliminate any dog-ear and to follow the desired lateral mammary fold to optimize contouring and appearance.

Fig. 9.3 appears online only.

The primary reasons for using the inverted-T technique are numerous. The resections are accurate because the incisions permit wide exposure of the parenchyma with precise resection of glandular tissue. The technique has proven useful for breasts of all sizes; however, it is especially useful for breasts that will require at least 300 g resections. The naturally ptotic breast almost always conceals the horizontal scar. The complication profile is similar with the inverted-T technique to the other short scar techniques. Finally, the breast appearance upon completion of the operation is usually excellent and is not as dependent upon breast remodeling and scar contracture when compared with the short scar techniques.

Patient selection

Patient selection begins with a thorough history and physical examination. Common complaints include back pain, neck pain, postural changes, bra-strap indentations, and/or intertrigo. Comorbidities such as diabetes mellitus, hypertension, and cardiac disease are asked about. Other important considerations include inquiries on whether the breast size restricts activities in daily living and whether dieting and prior weight loss has been effective in reducing breast volume. These are important when considering insurance preauthorization for reduction mammaplasty because it will reinforce the functional importance of performing a reduction mammaplasty. Women over the age of 35 are encouraged to obtain a mammogram. On examination, an assessment of volume and symmetry is made. Important measurements include the sternal notch to nipple, inframammary fold, base width, and nipple to sternum distances.

There is a thorough review of the risks and benefits. Patients are told that their symptoms may improve, but it is not a guarantee. Risks include but are not limited to bleeding; infection; scar; fat necrosis; inability to adequately nurse following childbirth; altered sensation of the nipple areolar complex; delayed healing; poor cosmetic result; partial or total nipple areolar necrosis; and further surgery. Incisional patterns and pedicle techniques are reviewed with each patient. In general, the authors' preference is to select the inverted-T for resections that are estimated to be greater than 300 g. Short scar techniques are usually performed for reduction weight that is estimated to be less than 300 g. Pedicle techniques are usually based on the distance that the nipple areolar complex will be elevated from the natural position of the nipple areolar complex on the breast.

The following algorithm is the authors preferred approach for pedicle selection and is based on nipple elevation in centimeters (Box 9.1). The central mound or superomedial pedicle is considered when nipple elevation is <6 cm, a medial pedicle is considered when nipple elevation is > 6 cm, and the inferior pedicle is selected when the length of the proposed inferior pedicle is less than the medial pedicle. Free nipple graft is considered when the pedicle length exceeds the perfusion capacity of the vascularity to the nipple areolar complex. This is usually the case for severe mammary hypertrophy with resection volumes in excess of 2000 g/breast.

BOX 9.1 Skin pattern and pedicle selection

- <6 cm of nipple elevation – central mound or superomedial pedicle
- >6 cm of nipple elevation – medial or inferior pedicle
- <300 g resection – short scar technique
- >300 g resection – inverted-T technique

Treatment/surgical technique

The bipedicle technique

There are two bipedicle techniques for reduction mammaplasty that incorporate the inverted-T incision pattern. These are the horizontal bipedicle also known as the Strombeck, and the vertical bipedicle also known as the McKissock, named after the surgeons that described them.[8,9,10] The horizontal bipedicle technique was initially described in 1960 with the intent of improving the vascularity to the nipple areolar complex. A schematic illustration of this technique is illustrated in Fig. 9.4. Prior to the description, upper pole resections of the breast that tended to disrupt the vascularity of the nipple areolar complex were common. The benefit of the bipedicle technique was that it included perforators from the medial and lateral segments of the breast, thus preserving the vascularity. In a review of 100 patients following the Strombeck repair, late complications included wide scars in 51%; loss of nipple sensation in 27%; and nipple inversion in 18%. Patient satisfaction was achieved in 96%.

Paul McKissock initially described the vertical bipedicle technique for reduction mammaplasty in 1972 (Fig. 9.5). The impetus for this technique was that many of the previous techniques were plagued by skin or nipple areolar necrosis, loss of sensation, and irregular contour. The vertically oriented bipedicle flap was thought to minimize some of these shortcomings. Simplification of this vertical bipedicle ultimately led to the development of the inferior pedicle technique that was later described by Robbins in 1977.[11] For a while thereafter there was controversy as to whether vertical bipedicle was superior, equivalent, or inferior to the inferior pedicle technique. Two groups of patients were later studied to discern any differences. Ramon's study[12] evaluating 27 patients following the McKissock repair and 24 patients following the inferior pedicle repair demonstrated good to excellent aesthetic outcomes in both. The subjective evaluations of the patients and the surgeons were also found to correlate without any significant differences.

Thus, with our improved understanding of the vascularity and innervation of the breast these bipedicle techniques have largely been replaced by the unipedicle techniques described throughout the remainder of the chapter. Although not commonly performed, these bipedicle methods have established a foundation for the pedicle techniques that are commonly used today.

Inferior pedicle technique

The inferior pedicle technique for nipple areolar transposition with the inverted-T skin pattern was one of the first techniques described in the modern era of reduction mammoplasty.[11,13,14] As mentioned, it represents an

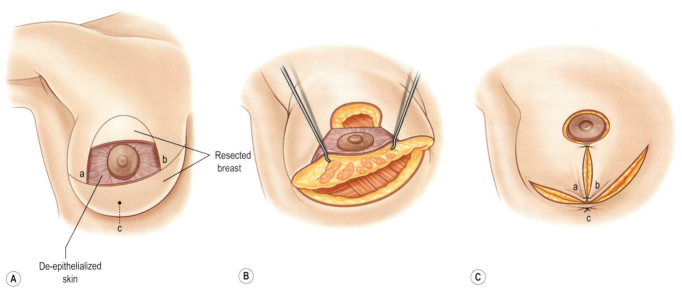

Fig. 9.4 Strombeck horizontal bipedicle technique. **(A)** The creation of a horizontal bipedicle allows for resection of parenchyma above and below the pedicle. The image depicts the de-epithelialized horizontal bipedicle shown in pink on either side of the nipple areolar complex. The solid semilunar line above the horizontal bipedicle and the parenchyma below the horizontal bipedicle will be resected. Point 'a', the confluence of the horizontal and vertical incisions of the lateral breast; point 'b', the medial breast analog; point 'c', the point along the inframammary fold incision at the breast meridian. **(B)** The breast after superior and inferior parenchymal resection, creating a horizontal bipedicle to carry the nipple areolar complex, before inset and closure. **(C)** Inset of the nipple areolar complex into the area of superior parenchymal resection. The skin of the remaining breast after resection is brought together to cone the breast and allow for final closure. This is accomplished by suturing in an inverted-T type closure the tip of the lateral breast skin flap (point 'a') to that of the medial breast skin flap (point 'b') and finally to point 'c' on the inframammary fold. Inframammary fold, periareolar, and vertical incision final sutures complete the closure. *(Redrawn after Lickstein LH, Shestak KC. The conceptual evolution of modern reduction mammoplasty. Operat Tech Plast Reconstr Surg. 1999;6:88–96.)*

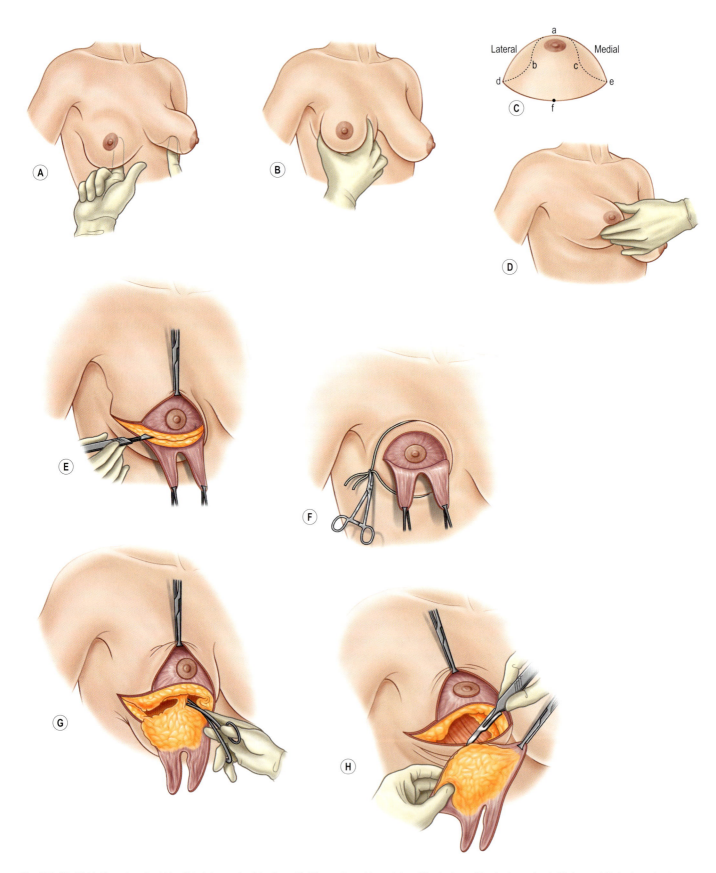

Fig. 9.5 **(A–N)** McKissock vertical bipedicled dermoglandular flap with Wise-pattern skin excision. **(A)** nipple position is determined; **(B)** base width is determined; **(C)** breast markings outlined; **(D)** medial and lateral breast excursion determined; **(E)** inferior de-epithelization; **(F)** peripheral constriction band; **(G)** lower pole excision; **(H)** lower pole parenchymal excision; **(I)** central parenchymal excision; **(J)** excision pattern; **(K)** excision completed; **(L)** glandular repositioning and reshaping; **(M)** skin closure; **(N)** skin closed. *(Redrawn after Lickstein LH, Shestak KC. The conceptual evolution of modern reduction mammoplasty. Operat Tech Plast Reconstr Surg. 1999;6:88–96.)*

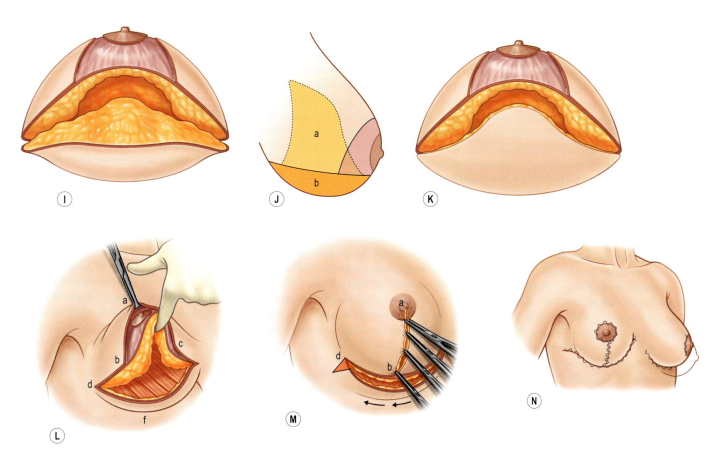

Fig. 9.5, cont'd

evolution from the vertical bipedicle technique described by McKissock. The vascularity to the nipple areolar complex is derived from the subdermal plexus from the intercostal and internal mammary perforators that are included with the inferior pedicle (Fig. 9.6). An important consideration with the inferior pedicle technique is the length to width ratio of the pedicle. This may range from as low as 1.5:1 and as high as 4:1. Although no optimal ratio has been established, it is generally agreed that ratios exceeding 2:1 may be associated with increased morbidity. It is always important to assess the arterial and venous bleeding from the distal edge of the flap. When absent, conversion to a free nipple graft is considered. Fluorescent angiography can assist with this decision. Figs. 9.7 and 9.8 illustrate the technique in a schematic format.

Markings

The patient is marked in the upright position. Important breast measurements include the sternal notch to nipple distance, nipple to inframammary fold distance, and the base diameter of the breast. The sternal midline, breast meridian, and the inframammary fold are marked bilaterally. The new position of the nipple areolar complex is marked and correlates to the level of the inframammary fold along the breast meridian. The distance from the sternal notch to the desired nipple areolar complex will vary but typically ranges from 22 to 27 cm. An inverted-T pattern is delineated and based on the location of the desired nipple areolar complex. The inferior pedicle is

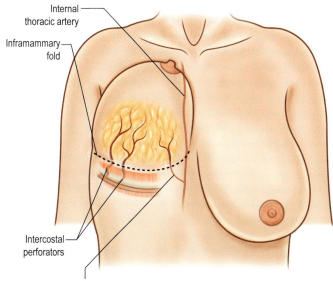

Fig. 9.6 Blood supply of the inferior pedicle.

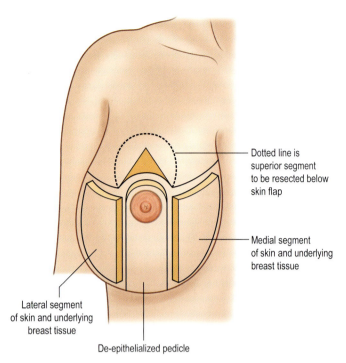

Dotted line is superior segment to be resected below skin flap

Medial segment of skin and underlying breast tissue

Lateral segment of skin and underlying breast tissue

De-epithelialized pedicle

Fig. 9.7 Outline of the three segments to be resected: the medial, lateral, and superior.

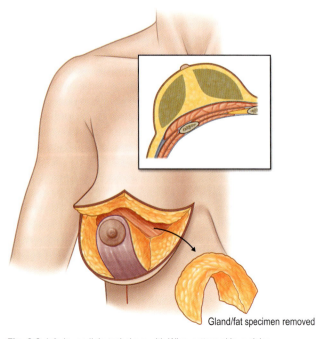

Gland/fat specimen removed

Fig. 9.8 Inferior pedicle technique with Wise-pattern skin excision.

delineated in the operating room with the patient in the supine position. The base of the inferior pedicle typically ranges from 6 to 10 cm and is dependent upon the base diameter of the breast. The inferior pedicle is usually centered along the inferior breast meridian and always includes a cuff of tissue measuring 1 cm around the areola to preserve the vascular plexus supplying the nipple areolar plexus.

Surgical technique

The patient is transported to the operating room, placed in the supine position, usually under general endotracheal anesthesia. The arms are usually positioned at approximately 60° of abduction, although they may be placed along the trunk as well. Pneumatic compression devices are applied, and intravenous antibiotics are administered. The preoperative markings are redelineated. The nipple areolar complex is inscribed with a 42 or 45 mm cookie-cutter. A scalpel is used to incise the epidermis of the nipple areolar complex and the inferior pedicle. The inferior pedicle is de-epithelialized preserving the subdermal plexus. The remaining inverted-T incisions are created. Medial and lateral dermoglandular wedge excisions are performed taking care not to narrow the base of the inferior pedicle. The nipple areolar complex is maintained on a dermo-parenchymal inferior pedicle of tissue that includes chest wall perforators. The perfusion of the nipple areolar complex is assessed based on arterial and venous bleeding from the cut edges. The upper breast skin flaps are undermined to the pectoral surface and contoured by excision of additional fat and parenchyma to better contour the upper pole of the breast. The excised tissues are weighed. The wounds are irrigated with an antibiotic solution, and hemostasis is achieved using electrocautery. A trifurcation suture is applied at the T-junction, and the skin is temporarily closed using staples. The patient is sat up to approximately 45°, and the contour, volume, and symmetry are assessed. A tailor-tack approach is used laterally to improve contour and to better define the lateral mammary fold. A scalpel and electrocautery is used to excise the excess skin. The operative field is inspected for hemostasis and irrigated with an antibiotic solution. The inferior pedicle and nipple areolar complex are inspected for bleeding and tissue viability. The pedicle is oriented such that the nipple areolar complex is at the apex of the vertical limbs. A closed suction drain is placed through the lateral incision and secured. Layered skin closure is completed using absorbable monofilament sutures. A cookie-cutter is used to delineate the new site of the nipple areolar complex. The base of the areola is positioned at 5–6 cm from the inframammary fold along the breast meridian. Following the incision, the nipple areolar complex is exteriorized and sutured. Steri-Strips and iodoform gauze are applied over the incisions followed by dry gauze and Tegaderm. A soft compression bra is applied. Fig. 9.9 illustrates a patient following reduction mammaplasty using an inverted-T approach and an inferior pedicle.

Outcomes

The inferior pedicle and inverted-T techniques have demonstrated success since its description in the 1970s. Complications are infrequent and seem to correlate to volume of resection. Large resections exceeding 1000 g/breast have been demonstrated to have an increased rate of incisional dehiscence and clinical infection. Other morbidities such as hematoma, seroma, nipple necrosis, fat necrosis, and cyst formation are independent of resection volume. Tobacco use is an independent predictor of complications and unrelated to resection volume. Factors such as necrosis of the nipple areolar complex are dependent on a variety of factors that include the base width and length of the inferior pedicle as well as the presence of intercostal perforators. Most studies report an incidence for nipple areolar necrosis at 2%. Delayed healing at the trifurcation point is usually related to tension along the incisions. Wound infection is also related to a variety of factors that include the amount of thermal injury, length of the operation,

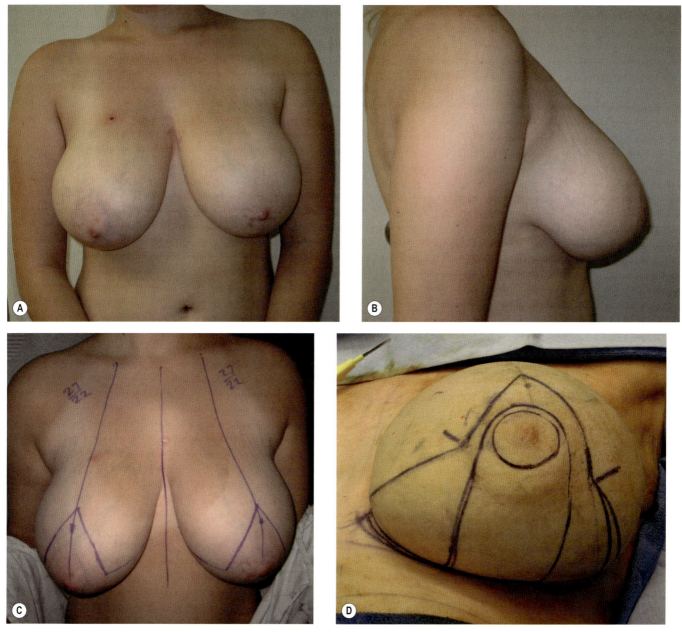

Fig. 9.9 **(A)** Preoperative image of a patient scheduled for an inverted-T reduction mammaplasty using an inferior pedicle. **(B)** Right lateral view. **(C)** Inverted-T pattern is delineated. The sternal notch to nipple distance is 27 cm, and the new nipple position will be at 22 cm. **(D)** The inferior pedicle is delineated. *Continued*

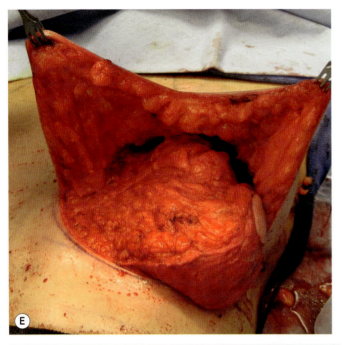

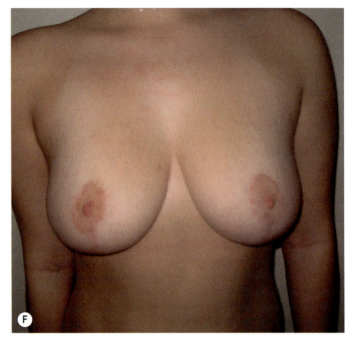

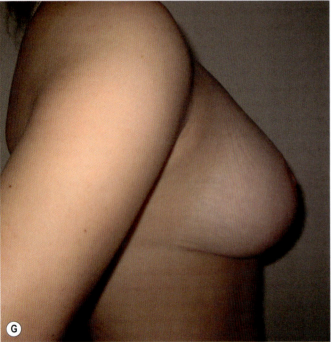

Fig. 9.9, cont'd **(E)** The inferior pedicle is created, and the upper skin flaps are elevated and undermined. **(F)** A 1-year postoperative view is demonstrated. **(G)** A right lateral view is depicted.

desiccation of the exposed tissues, and insufficient antibiotic prophylaxis. Fat necrosis is related to poor tissue perfusion, thermal injury, infection, elevated parenchymal pressures following closure, and improper surgical technique. Sensory changes to the nipple areolar complex may be secondary to transection of the intercostal innervation between the 2nd and 6th intercostal segments. It is estimated that approximately 10% of women will experience some degree of permanent sensory alteration.

The medial pedicle

The medial pedicle technique is this author's preferred technique for large volume resections that exceed 600 g with a nipple areolar complex that will be elevated at least 6 cm.[15,16] The benefits of the medial pedicle are listed in Box 9.2. The medial pedicle derives its blood supply from the internal mammary perforators and its innervation from the anterior branches of the intercostal nerves. The internal mammary artery and vein have

improved hemostasis. A 42–45 mm cookie-cutter is used to inscribe the nipple areolar complex. The epidermis is incised to the level of the mid-dermal layer. The medial pedicle is de-epithelialized leaving the nipple areolar complex intact. The inverted-T pattern is incised. Dermoglandular wedge excisions are performed primarily along the inferior and lateral aspect of the breast. The medial pedicle is defined as a dermoglandular pedicle leaving the pectoral and intercostal vascular perforators attached. The pedicle is thinned laterally as needed

been demonstrated to be the dominant blood supply in 70% of patients.[17] Innervation of the nipple areolar complex is derived primarily from the anterior and lateral 4th, 5th, and 6th intercostal nerves.[18,19] The medial pedicle design permits inclusion of the dominant medial and chest wall perforators, a wider arc of rotation, and added flexibility in placement and positioning the nipple areolar complex. The medial pedicle has demonstrated success and provided excellent breast shape, projection, and contour in the majority of patients.

Markings

The inverted-T pattern is delineated with the patient standing (see Fig. 9.3). The nipple areolar complex is circumscribed with a 42 or 45 mm cookie-cutter. The medial pedicle is delineated on the operating room table with the patient supine (Fig. 9.10). The base of the medial pedicle is along the medial axis of the breast and inverted-T pattern. The midpoint of the medial vertical limb of the inverted-T is marked. A marking pen is used to delineate the medial pedicle coursing around the nipple areolar complex including a 1 cm cuff around the edge of the areola. The marking is extended to the upper horizontal limb completing the pedicle design. The base of the pedicle typically ranges from 6 to 11 cm and the length of the pedicle ranges from 10 to 19 cm. The distal aspect of the medial pedicle is delineated with a 1 cm margin around the nipple areolar complex to preserve the vascular plexus.

Surgical technique

Following transport to the operating room, the patient is placed in the supine position under general anesthesia. Pneumatic compression garments are placed on both lower extremities. A urinary catheter is usually not necessary. Intravenous antibiotics are administered. A cephalosporin is usually given; however, additional prophylactic coverage for anaerobic organisms is sometimes considered. Local anesthetic agents with epinephrine can be considered prior to the incisions for

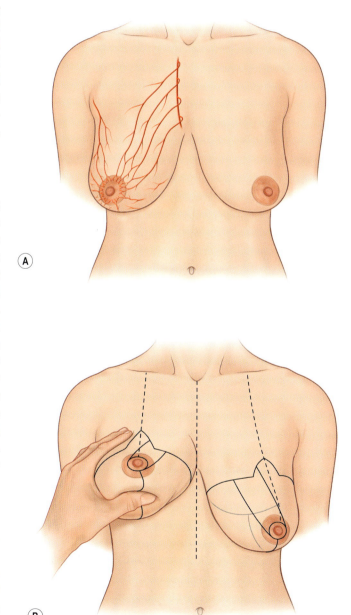

(A)

(B)

Fig. 9.10 Schematic illustrations of the medial pedicle and its blood supply and orientation. (Redrawn after Nahabedian MY, McGibbon BM, and Manson PN. Medial pedicle reduction mammaplasty for severe mammary hypertrophy. Plastic and Reconstructive Surgery. 2000;105:896–904.)

to reduce bulk. Distal pedicle bleeding is assessed to ensure perfusion of the nipple areolar complex. Absence of bleeding usually dictates conversion to a free nipple graft. The breast skin flaps are elevated with a thickness that correlates to the interface of the parenchyma and the subcutaneous tissue. A temporary trifurcation suture is placed approximating the inferior corner of the medial and lateral vertical limbs of the inverted-T pattern to a predetermined point on the inferior horizontal incision (Fig. 9.11). A dog-ear is avoided medially by ensuring equal length. Skin adjustments are made laterally using a tailor-tack approach. The nipple areolar complex is rotated superiorly towards the apex of the vertical limbs. Twisting or kinking of the pedicle is avoided. The skin edges are temporarily stapled and the patient

positioned to approximately 60° to assess breast symmetry, fullness, and nipple position. The nipple areolar complex is exteriorized such that the length from the inferior aspect of the nipple areolar complex is 5–6 cm from the horizontal incision. A single drain is placed, and the incisions are closed with interrupted dermal and continuous subcuticular sutures. Fig. 9.12 illustrates a patient following reduction mammaplasty using an inverted-T pattern and a medial pedicle.

Outcomes

Patient outcomes following inverted-T reduction mammaplasty using a medial pedicle have been favorable.[16,20,21,22] Nahabedian *et al.* studied a series of 45 breasts with severe mammary hypertrophy and demonstrated viability of the nipple areolar complex in 44/44 breasts and retained sensation in 42/44 breasts.[15] Loss of sensation was related to pedicle length rather than the weight of tissue excised, as resections of 2500 g did not result in sensory loss. Mean resection volume was 1627 g on the left and 1580 g on the right. One woman required a free nipple graft that had a resection volume of 2530 g and a pedicle length of 18 cm. Patient satisfaction was assessed using a non-validated questionnaire demonstrating 100% satisfaction with nipple projection and 22/23 patients satisfied with breast shape.

Abramson *et al.* reviewed a series of 88 consecutive patients that had reduction mammaplasty using an inverted-T approach and a medial pedicle.[16] The overall complication rate was 6.8% and included hematoma, partial nipple necrosis, incisional dehiscence, and fat necrosis. Bottoming out of the breast was minimized using this technique. At the 1-year follow-up, the nipple to inframammary fold distance increased 11% when the resection volume was between 500 and 1200 g/breast and 34% when greater than 1200 g/breast.

Sensation and viability studies of the nipple areolar complex have also demonstrated favorable results using the inverted-T approach and the medial pedicle.[21,22] In a study comparing 41 medial and 31 inferior pedicle techniques, sensory retention was demonstrated in 68 of 79 breasts (86%) using a medial pedicle and in 50 of 54 breasts (92%) using an inferior pedicle. Viability of the nipple areolar complex was demonstrated in 74 of 79 breasts (94%) using a medial pedicle and in 53 of 54 breasts (98%) using an inferior pedicle. Mean resection volume for the medial pedicle cohort was 1490 g (range, 930–2910 g) and 720 g (range, 400–1580 g) for the inferior pedicle cohort. Nipple areolar sensation using a pressure specified sensory device was studied in eight women following inferior pedicle reduction mammaplasty and in nine women following medial

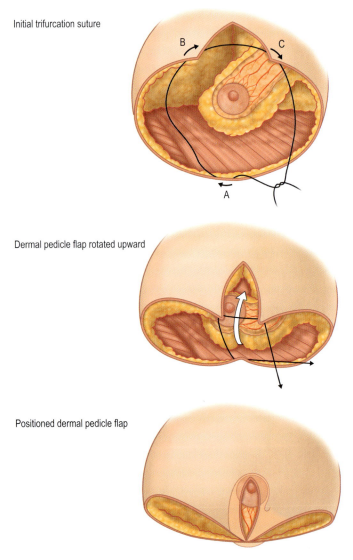

Initial trifurcation suture

Dermal pedicle flap rotated upward

Positioned dermal pedicle flap

Fig. 9.11 Schematic illustrations following glandular excision and the trifurcation suture. *(Redrawn after Nahabedian MY, McGibbon BM, and Manson PN. Medial pedicle reduction mammaplasty for severe mammary hypertrophy. Plastic and Reconstructive Surgery. 2000;105:896–904.)*

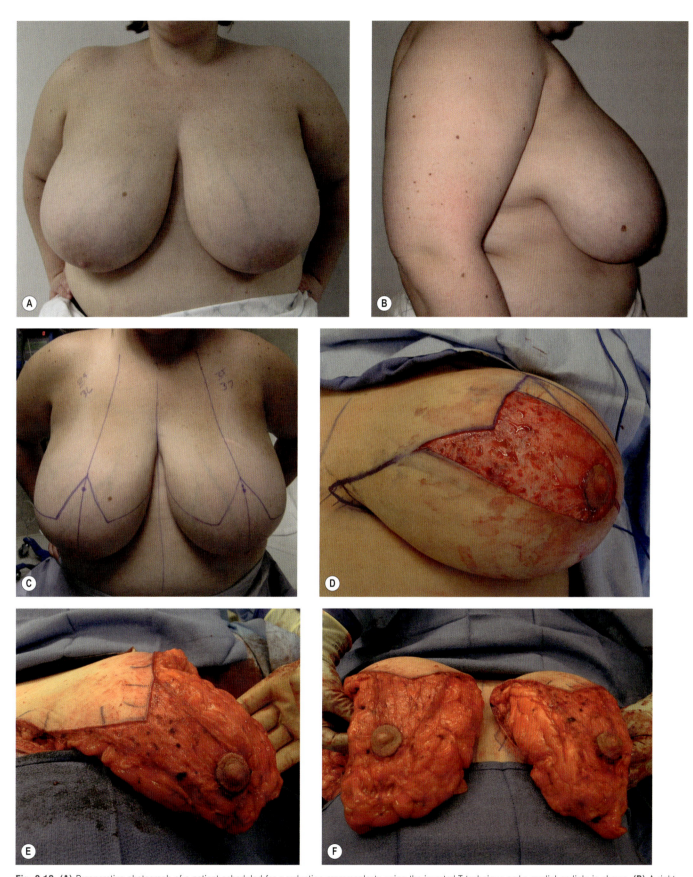

Fig. 9.12 (A) Preoperative photograph of a patient scheduled for a reduction mammaplasty using the inverted-T technique and a medial pedicle is shown. **(B)** A right lateral view is depicted. **(C)** The inverted-T is delineated. **(D)** The medial pedicle is delineated and de-epithelialized. **(E)** The glandular resection is completed and the medial pedicle is isolated. **(F)** The bilateral medial pedicles are depicted.

Continued

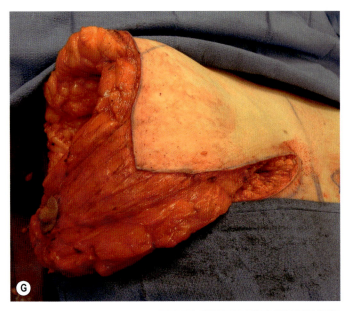

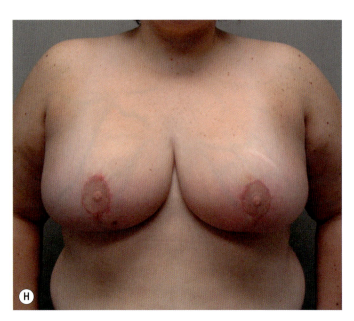

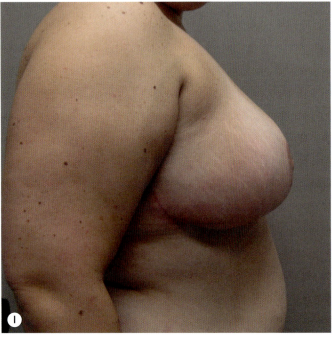

Fig. 9.12, cont'd (G) The medial pedicle is rotated towards the apex of the breast. **(H)** A postoperative photograph at 3 months is depicted following a reduction mammaplasty using an inverted-T pattern and a medial pedicle. **(I)** A right lateral view is shown.

pedicle reduction mammaplasty. When comparing the two techniques, there were no significant differences in postoperative sensory outcomes, despite significantly greater reduction volumes using the medial pedicle technique (mean of 1.7 kg vs 1.1 kg). In addition, the amount of breast tissue removed did not correlate with postoperative sensory outcomes.

Superomedial pedicle technique

Orlando and Guthrie originally described the superomedial reduction mammaplasty technique using the inverted-T in 1975.[23,24,25] Early studies focused on the nipple areolar complex and demonstrated viability in 100% of patients and retention of sensitivity in 83–92%

of patients. The length of nipple transposition ranged from 4 to 15 cm, with a median of 8 cm. The weight of breast tissue excised ranged from 210–1850 g per breast. It was subsequently opined that the superomedial pedicle technique was suitable for breasts of moderate volume rather than large volume. Fig. 9.13 illustrates the basic markings and technique of the superomedial pedicle.

Markings

With the patient standing, an inverted-T pattern is delineated as previously described. The desired position of the nipple areolar complex serves as the focal point of the pattern. With the patient in the supine

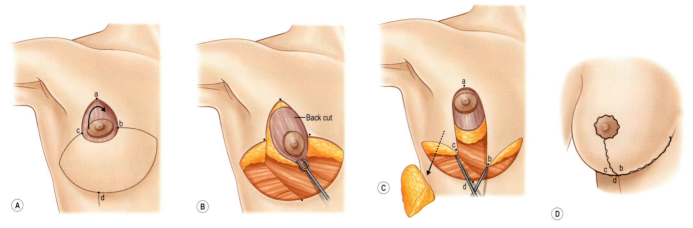

Fig. 9.13 (A–D) Superomedial pedicle with Wise-pattern skin closure. (**A**) Skin markings; (**B**) inferior parenchymal resection; (**C**) lateral parenchymal resection and trifurcation suture; (**D**) skin closure.

position, the superomedial pedicle is delineated. Although similar in design to the medial pedicle, there are differences in orientation. The superior limb of the pedicle is oriented in a true vertical position, whereas the medial limb is oriented approximately 45° off the vertical. The pattern extends around the nipple areolar complex with a 5–10 mm peripheral zone to preserve the integrity of the subdermal plexus.

Surgical technique

Local anesthetic agents with epinephrine are considered prior to the incisions for improved hemostasis. A 42–45 mm cookie-cutter is used to inscribe the nipple areolar complex. The epidermis is incised to the level of the mid-dermal layer. The superomedial pedicle is de-epithelialized. The inverted-T markings are incised. Dermoglandular wedge excisions are performed and based inferiorly and laterally. The superomedial pedicle is usually maintained on its dermo-parenchymal attachments such that the chest wall perforators are included. This maneuver increases the likelihood of adequate perfusion to the nipple areolar complex. The superomedial pedicle is then repositioned such that the nipple areolar complex is at the apex of the vertical limbs. Because of the vertical limb, rotation may be compromised and some degree of folding of the de-epithelialized pedicle may occur. A back-cut on the inferior limb may augment the degree of rotation to minimize any tension on the pedicle. Parenchymal suturing can be considered for optimal shaping and contour but may not be necessary. A trifurcation suture is placed to ensure tension free closure of the inverted-T incision. Irrigation is performed, and hemostasis is ensured followed by closed suction drain placement. The skin is closed in layers with absorbable sutures. Fig. 9.14 illustrates a patient following superomedial reduction mammaplasty using an inverted-T technique.

Outcomes

Davison *et al.* have reviewed their 6-year experience with the superomedial pedicle in 215 patients.[26] The incisional patterns included 30 circumvertical; 43 circumvertical with short transverse scar; 133 inverted-T; and nine free nipple grafts with an inverted-T. The selected incisional pattern correlated with resection volume. The mean weights were 688 g/breast following circumvertical reduction; 1137 g/breast following circumvertical reduction with a short transverse scar; 1184 g/breast following inverted-T reduction; and 1929 g/breast following free nipple graft using an inverted-T pattern. The overall complication rate using an inverted-T approach was 18% and included seroma (3.7%); hematoma (3.7%); delayed healing (0.75%); cellulitis (1.5%); altered nipple sensation (0.75%); superficial necrosis (1.5%); and complex scar (1.5%). There were no cases of total nipple loss. The advantages of the superomedial pedicle included superior vascularity; shorter pedicle length; less de-epithelialization; favorable arc of rotation; no need to use parenchymal suturing techniques; providing superomedial fullness; and reduced incidence of bottoming-out.

Lugo *et al.* studied the efficacy of the superomedial medical technique for women with severe mammary hypertrophy defined as greater than 1000 g per breast. A total of 200 patients met the criteria for analysis. Mean resection volume was 1277 g on the right and 1283 g on the left. Mean nipple areolar transposition was 11.25 cm on the right and 11.4 cm on the left. Partial nipple necrosis occurred in 10.5%, and 98% of patients reported normal sensation of the nipple areolar complex.[27] Altuntas *et al.* have demonstrated that the position of the nipple areolar complex did change over time following superomedial reduction mammaplasty using an inverted-T pattern with a descent of 1.61 cm on the right breast and 1.79 cm on left breast at a mean follow-up of 15 months. The length from the nipple areolar complex to the inframammary fold increased by 3.31 cm and 3.59 cm on the right and left breast, respectively. These changes were related more to descent of the lower pole rather than upward migration of the nipple areolar complex.[28]

Central mound technique

Balch described the central mound technique for reduction mammaplasty in 1981.[29] The rationale for this technique was that the vascularity of the nipple areolar complex would not depend on a dermal pedicle but instead on the deep parenchymal vascularity. The original description included resection of medial and lateral pillars with the benefit of less bottoming out that was sometimes seen with inferior pedicle techniques. Hester reported his experience with the central mound technique in 65 patients. The vascularity was predominantly from the perforating branches from the lateral thoracic artery, intercostal, internal mammary, and thoracoacromial vessels with the pectoralis major muscle as the foundation. The benefit of this technique was that it could be used for small and large reductions, pedicle length issues were avoided, and postoperative breast

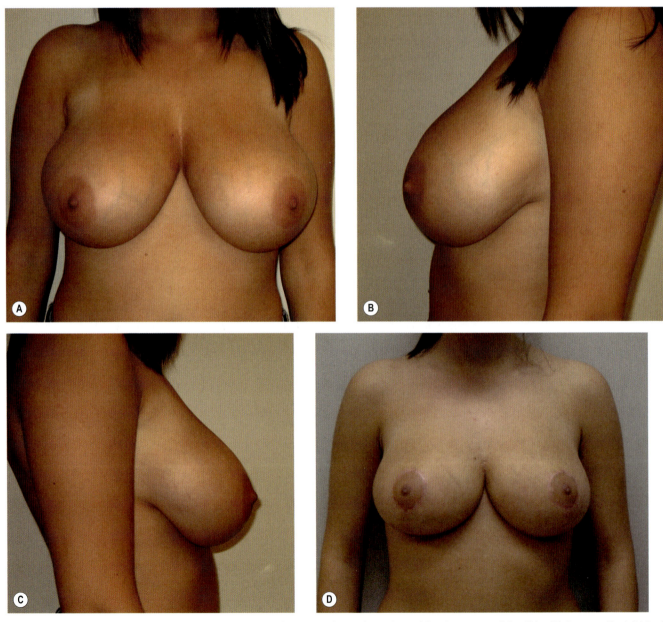

Fig. 9.14 **(A)** A preoperative image of a patient scheduled for reduction mammaplasty using an inverted-T and a superomedial pedicle. **(B)** A preoperative left lateral view is depicted. **(C)** A preoperative right lateral view is depicted. **(D)** A postoperative photograph at 6 months is depicted following reduction mammaplasty using the inverted-T technique and a superomedial pedicle.

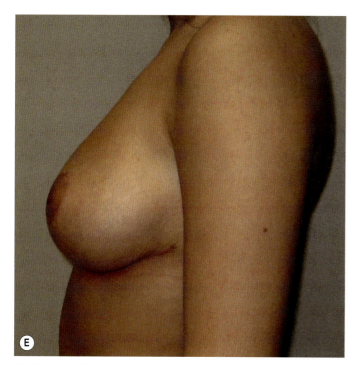 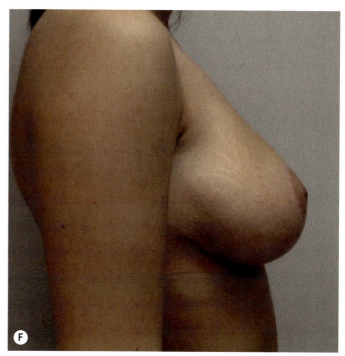

Fig. 9.14, cont'd **(E)** A postoperative left lateral view. **(F)** A postoperative right lateral view.

projection and contour was optimized. Fig. 9.15 illustrates the central mound technique.

The central mound technique is very different than the traditional pedicle orientations for transposition of the nipple areolar complex. The primary vascularity of the central mound is derived from the intercostal perforators and secondarily through the vessels supplying the breast. Wuringer in 1998 described the horizontal fibrous septum of the breast.[5] The significance of this septum is that it essentially bisects the breast into a cephalad and caudal half and includes a significant contribution of the vascularity and innervation to the breast parenchyma and nipple areolar complex. It includes dominant vascular contributions from the thoracoacromial, internal mammary, lateral mammary, and intercostal vessels, as well as innervation from the anterior and lateral divisions of the 2nd–4th intercostal nerves. The central mound technique preserves this septum and provides excellent vascularity and innervation to the nipple areolar complex.

The central mound is typically performed in women in need of small to moderate reduction mammaplasty, with resection volumes ranging from 200–600 g with nipple elevation less than 6 cm. The central mound becomes less effective for severe mammary hypertrophy or when the nipple areolar complex requires more elevation because of the potential risk to the horizontal septum and vascularity.

Markings

The usual breast landmarks including the sternal notch, midclavicular point, sternal midline, breast meridian, nipple areolar complex, and inframammary fold are marked and delineated with the patient in the upright position. The inverted-T pattern is drawn as previously described. The central mound is marked with the patient supine. In the majority of cases, the actual position of the nipple areolar complex lies within the boundaries of the vertical limbs or just below it. The inferior border of the central mound extends around the nipple areolar complex forming a triangle with the inferior point of the vertical limbs.

Surgical technique

Following transport to the operating room, the patient is placed under general anesthesia; however, sedation and local anesthesia can also be considered. Pneumatic compression devices are applied, and intravenous antibiotics are administered. Local anesthetics agents are sometimes used. The nipple areolar complex is delineated with a 42–45 mm cookie-cutter then incised. The central mound outline is incised then de-epithelialized using heavy surgical scissors or a scalpel. The inverted-T pattern is incised. Dermoglandular wedge excisions are performed inferiorly and laterally. Inferiorly, it is important not to undermine the breast because of

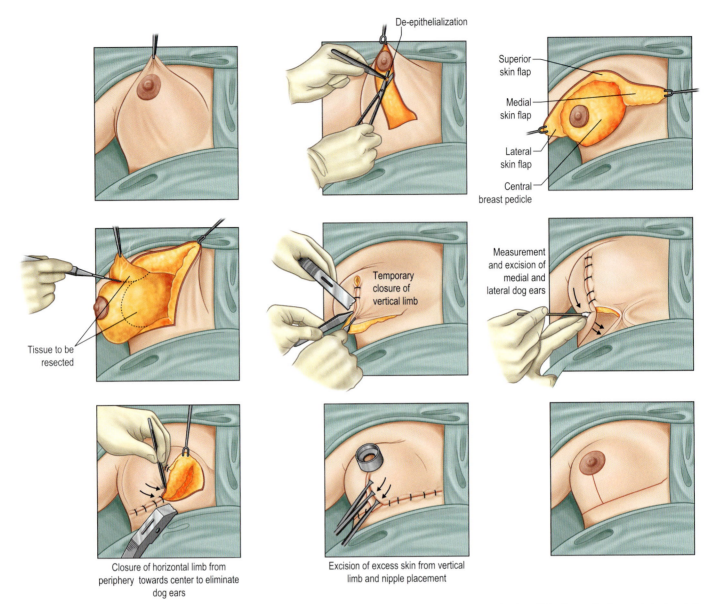

Fig. 9.15 Central mound technique popularized by Hester. *(Redrawn from Hester TR Jr, Bostwick J III, Miller L. Breast reduction utilizing the maximally vascularized central pedicle.* Plast Reconstr Surg. *1985;76:890–900.)*

possible damage to the horizontal septum. Sometimes this septum and intercostal vessels can be visualized and protected. The excision should always be directed toward the inframammary fold. An inferior wedge is excised extending from the inferomedial to inferolateral breast. The lateral resection can be more aggressive because the vascularity to the nipple areolar complex is based on the chest wall perforators. The parenchymal resection extends to the level of the subcutaneous fat. The subdermal plexus is preserved and protected. This dissection is sometimes performed using sharp dissection techniques to avoid thermal injury. The wound is irrigated, and hemostasis is ensured. A temporary trifurcation suture is placed, and the remaining incisions are temporarily stapled. The patient is sat upright to approximately 45° to assess volume and contour symmetry. Lateral adjustments using a tailor-tacking approach are sometimes necessary. A closed suction drain is placed along the inferior aspect of the breast. The ideal location for the nipple areolar complex is determined and delineated with the appropriate cookie-cutter. The incision is created, and the nipple areolar complex is exteriorized and sutured using absorbable dermal and subcuticular placement. The remaining incisions are closed in the same fashion. Surgical dressings and a soft compression bra are applied. Fig. 9.16 illustrates a patient having a central mound reduction mammaplasty using an inverted-T pattern.

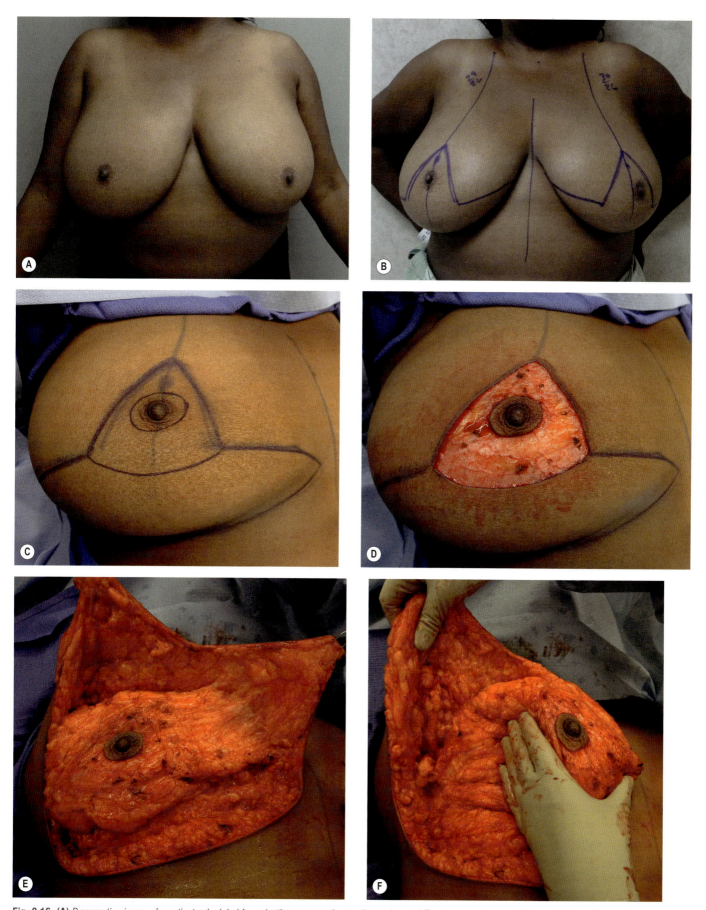

Fig. 9.16 **(A)** Preoperative image of a patient scheduled for reduction mammaplasty using an inverted-T and a central mound. **(B)** Inverted-T markings with measurements. **(C)** Central mound markings. **(D)** Central mound de-epithelialized. **(E)** Central mound created with elevated skin flaps. **(F)** Central mound with lateral excision.

Continued

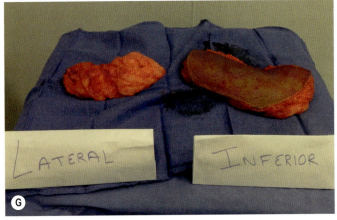

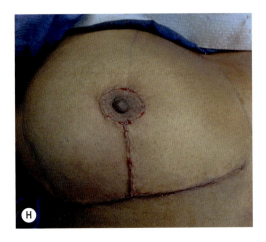

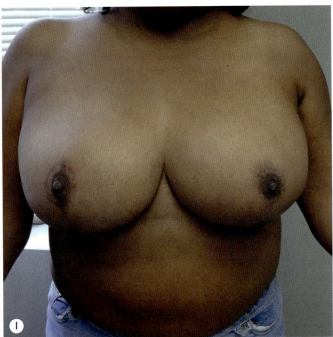

Fig. 9.16, cont'd (G) The inferior and lateral excisions are depicted. (H) Immediate closure following central mound reduction mammoplasty. (I) A 1-year postoperative photograph following central mound reduction mammoplasty.

Special circumstances

Reduction mammaplasty and radiation therapy

The management of localized breast cancer is often performed with lumpectomy and postoperative radiation therapy. This is sometimes performed in the setting of moderate to severe mammary hypertrophy. Performing a reduction mammaplasty following radiation therapy can pose additional challenges because of the soft tissue changes following radiation.[30] Complications such as delayed healing, fat necrosis, incisional dehiscence, and nipple necrosis may be more common because of diminished fibroblast activity, decreased soft-tissue elasticity, fat atrophy, and changes to the microcirculation. Modification in patient selection and surgical technique are therefore necessary to minimize the occurrence of these adverse events.

Patients that present with a mild to moderate degree of radiation damage are usually considered for reduction mammaplasty when indicated; however, patients with severe radiation damage are usually discouraged from proceeding because of the increased likelihood of complications. Tobacco use and poorly-controlled diabetes mellitus should be considered absolute contraindications for reduction mammaplasty, regardless of the degree of radiation damage. Specific maneuvers for reduction in this setting include designing skin flaps with shorter, wider, and broader pedicles. Undermining of the breast parenchyma is usually avoided in favor of wedge resections. Pedicle selection should be based on the previous incision location. If the previous lumpectomy was performed in the lower pole of the breast, then an inferior pedicle should not be used in the breast reduction. The pedicle should be remote from the lumpectomy site. Breast amputation techniques with free nipple grafting are also considered for these patients.

Fig. 9.17 illustrates a patient following medial pedicle reduction mammaplasty using an inverted-T pattern.

Outcomes following reduction mammaplasty in the setting of prior radiation are mixed, but all demonstrate increased complications compared with the non-radiated patients. In the author's series of 12 patients, mean age was 49.5 years and the mean BMI was 29. Most women were a D to a DD cup. There was one smoker in the cohort and 11 non-smokers. The mean time from completion of radiation therapy and reduction mammaplasty was 2.5 years. All women had an inverted-T pattern using a variety of pedicles that included the inferior, medial, central mound, superomedial, superolateral, and McKissock. Mean resection weight was 623 g (range, 141–1139 g). Minor complications included delayed healing at the trifurcation junction in three patients, infection in one patient, and breast skin necrosis in one patient. All were managed with local wound care. Major complications occurred in one patient and included infection, delayed healing, as well as skin and fat necrosis. This patient required surgical debridement and a latissimus dorsi flap.

Reduction mammaplasty and breast asymmetry

Breast asymmetry can manifest in a variety of ways in women with mammary hypertrophy and includes unilateral or bilateral enlargement, nipple areolar asymmetry, asymmetries in the breast footprint, or following breast biopsy or excision procedures. Reduction mammaplasty in women with breast asymmetry is managed using a combination of variables including measuring the differences, assessing the contour and position of the nipple areolar complex, planning the correction, and differentially excising skin and parenchyma. This is commonly performed using the inverted-T skin pattern with transposition of the nipple areolar complex on a vascularized pedicle or as a graft.

One of the more challenging asymmetry situations to manage is when the breast footprint dramatically different. A patient with breast asymmetry due to a significant difference in the position of the inframammary fold is shown in Fig. 9.18. On examination, the distance from the sternal notch to nipple areolar complex was similar at 30 and 32 cm; however, there was a 5 cm difference in the position of the inframammary fold. This made fitting into a brassiere difficult and uncomfortable. Correction of this type of deformity is facilitated using the inverted-T technique because the right and left patterns can be delineated to accommodate the difference. On the right breast, the horizontal limb of the inverted-T pattern was positioned 5 cm above the inframammary fold. Following the glandular resection, the soft tissues

between the inframammary fold and the incisional edge are defatted and the skin flap is repositioned on the chest wall such that the cut edge will form the new inframammary fold. Following parenchymal rearrangement and temporary skin closure, the patient is sat up to approximately 45° to assess symmetry.

The management of parenchymal and nipple areolar complex asymmetry is simplified using an inverted-T pattern. With parenchymal asymmetry, differences in shape and contour are analyzed. Most patients will be larger on one side versus the other. With severe mammary hypertrophy, pedicle selection is based on length and arc of rotation. Medial pedicles are usually selected because of their relatively short length and favorable arc of rotation. However, inferior pedicles are selected when the nipple areolar complex is at the lowest point of the breast because its short length will minimize the bottoming out phenomena. Parenchymal resection is performed systematically but focused on the inferior and lateral aspects of the breast. The specimens are accurately weighed for both breasts. Adjustments are made based on the visual assessment of breast contour and symmetry as well as the difference in weight. When there are asymmetries of the nipple areolar complex, adjustments are made by equalizing the distance from the sternal notch to the desired position. The breast meridian is delineated based on the width of the breast and desired location of the nipple areolar complex. Symmetry is confirmed by ensuring equal distance from the midsternum to the desired nipple areolar complex.

Secondary reduction mammaplasty

Some patients following reduction mammaplasty may require a second reduction mammaplasty, usually because of weight gain.[31] Secondary reduction mammaplasty can pose challenges because of the scars, disruption of the primary blood supply, and uncertainty regarding the previous reduction mammaplasty technique. The primary concern with secondary reduction mammaplasty is nipple areolar necrosis and fat necrosis. Questions regarding whether it is safe to use the same pedicle or another pedicle as well as the optimal timing for secondary reduction have generated discussion. Many surgeons have opined that both options are viable because of the revascularization of the breast parenchyma, skin, and the nipple areolar complex. However, the predictability of the revascularization pattern is compromised. It is therefore important to have an understanding of the normal, and to some extent the reconfigured, vascularity of the breast. It is also important to ensure that adequate time has elapsed before embarking on the secondary procedure.

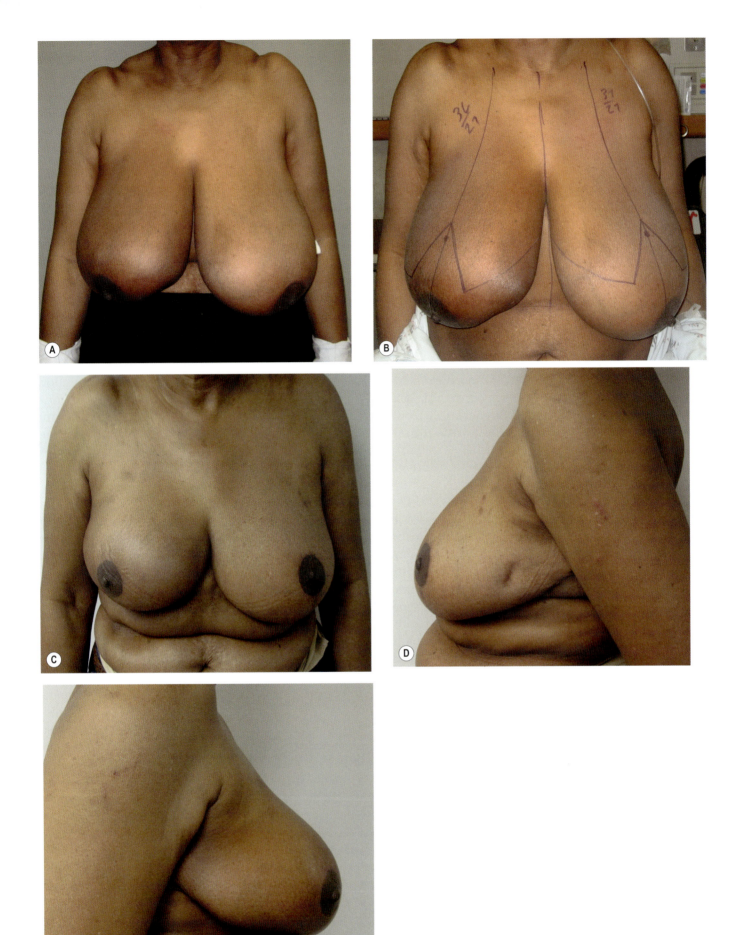

Fig. 9.17 (A) Preoperative photograph of a woman with mammary hypertrophy and right breast radiation. **(B)** Inverted-T markings and breast measurements. **(C)** A 3-year postoperative image following reduction mammoplasty. **(D)** Left lateral view. **(E)** Right lateral view.

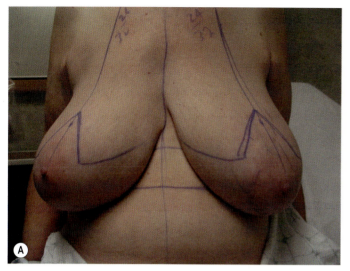

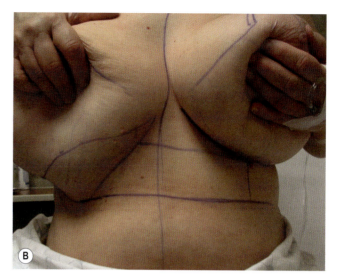

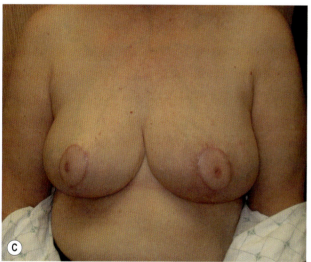

Fig. 9.18 (A) Preoperative photograph of a woman with breast asymmetry. **(B)** Footprint asymmetry is noted with discrepancy of the right inframammary fold. **(C)** A 1-year postoperative photograph following correction of asymmetry and reduction mammaplasty.

Perhaps the safest method for secondary reduction mammaplasty would be liposuction. This technique can be safely performed without any detailed knowledge of the vascularity. Although effective for volume reduction, there may be minimal effect in skin envelope change. Some degree of skin tightening and contracture may occur, but this is unpredictable. A second option would be a wedge excision of the previous scars and underlying parenchyma. Parenchymal undermining is avoided; therefore, there is minimal disruption of the underlying vascularity to the nipple areolar complex. When the surgeon has knowledge of the prior type of pedicle technique, then the reduction can proceed using that same pedicle with greater certainty that the vascularity will be maintained. However, a new pedicle can also be considered. In these situations, it may be prudent to use a dermoparenchymal pedicle and incorporate the dominant intercostal perforators that have been described. In the event that there are questions regarding the tissue or nipple areolar complex perfusion, fluorescent angiography techniques can be used. In the event of no blood flow to the nipple areolar complex, free graft techniques are recommended.

Postoperative care

The postoperative care following reduction mammaplasty using the inverted-T pattern is routine. Immediately following completion of the procedure, the incisions are infiltrated with a longer acting local anesthetic. Steri-Strips, Xeroform strips, dry gauze, and a clear adhesive are applied. The nipple areolar complex is visible through the clear adhesive. A chlorhexidine patch is placed over the drain site until the drain is removed. A soft compressive surgical brassiere is applied making sure that excessive pressure is avoided. In the event that the nipple areolar complex becomes mottled or congested, it is recommended that sutures be removed and the patient return to the operating room for exploration. Patients are usually discharged home on the day of surgery with narcotics and a few days of oral antibiotics.

The patients usually return to the office on either postoperative day 1 or 2 to remove the dressings and usually to remove the drain. It is unusual to require prolonged drain care unless the output is unusually high, exceeding 50 cc/24 h, without a progressively diminishing output. The patients are permitted to shower 24 h following drain removal or on postoperative day 3 if the drain is still in place. The patients are instructed to wear the soft bra continuously and to avoid wearing any underwired bra for 2 months. When everything is proceeding as expected, patients are usually seen 7–10 days later for re-evaluation. In the event that there is any incisional dehiscence or small ulceration, local wound care measures are implemented using a silver sulfadiazine ointment. Patients are instructed to avoid strenuous activities such as heavy lifting or running for 1 month. Subsequent follow-up appointments are scheduled for 6 weeks and 6 months. All patients are instructed to obtain a mammogram 6 months following the operation, as this will be the new baseline for future mammograms.

Complications

The complications following mastectomy with the inverted-T technique have been discussed throughout the chapter. They include, but are not limited to, bleeding; infection; scar; asymmetry; hematoma; seroma; delayed healing; nipple areolar necrosis; T-junction necrosis/delayed healing; inability to breast-feed; loss of nipple sensitivity; fat necrosis; contour abnormality; asymmetry; and further surgery.[32] Despite these untoward events, reduction mammaplasty remains an operation that is commonly performed with high patient satisfaction. Complications rates vary and range from 10% to 20%. Complications have been correlated with increasing breast size and volume of resection. Figs. 9.19–9.23 illustrate some of the common complications following reduction mammaplasty.

Conclusion

The inverted-T method has proven to be a diverse and versatile method for achieving excellent outcomes with reduction mammaplasty. Its diversity is exemplified by the variety of orientations that the pedicles can assume. Outcomes have been consistent and reliable for a wide variety of breast shapes, volumes, and contours. The inverted-T has a strong safety profile with a complication profile that is similar to all methods of performing reduction mammaplasty. It is easy to teach and to learn and should be in the armamentarium of all plastic surgeons.

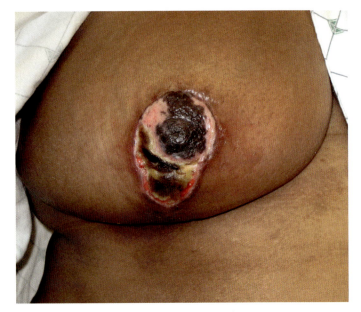

Fig. 9.19 Delayed healing of the nipple areolar complex.

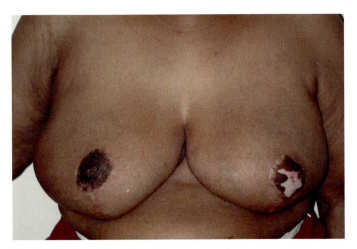

Fig. 9.20 Depigmentation of the nipple areolar complex.

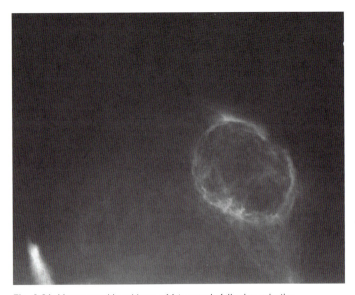

Fig. 9.21 Mammographic evidence of fat necrosis following reduction mammaplasty.

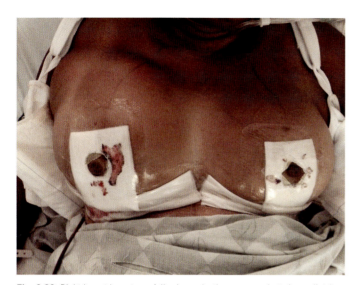

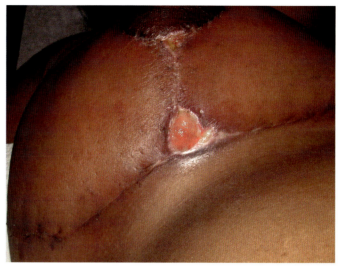

Fig. 9.22 Right breast hematoma following reduction mammaplasty immediately postoperative.

Fig. 9.23 Delayed healing at the T-junction.

🌐 Access the complete reference list online at **http://www.expertconsult.com**

5. Wuringer E, Mader N, Posch E, et al. Nerves and vessels supplying ligamentous suspension of the mammary gland. *Plast Reconstr Surg.* 1998;101:1486–1493. *This cadaveric study of 28 breasts demonstrated two structures, the fibrous sling and the vascular and nervous membranes attached to it. These were consistent anatomic findings and determined to be the principal source of vascularity and innervation to the nipple areolar complex.*

7. Schlenz I, Kuzbari R, Gruber H, et al. The sensitivity of the nipple-areola complex: an anatomic study. *Plast Reconstr Surg.* 2000;105:905–909. *This cadaveric study of 28 female breasts demonstrated that the lateral and anterior cutaneous branches of the 3rd, 4th, and 5th intercostal nerves innervated the nipple areolar complex. The anterior cutaneous branches coursed superficially within the subcutaneous tissue terminating at the medial areolar border.*

15. Nahabedian MY, McGibbon BM, Manson PN. Medial pedicle reduction mammaplasty for severe mammary hypertrophy. *Plast Reconstr Surg.* 2000;105:896–904. *The use of a medial pedicle for severe mammary hypertrophy was studied in 23 women. The medial pedicle successfully transposed the nipple areola complex in 44 of 45 breasts (98%). Mean change in nipple position was 17.1 cm, and mean weight of tissue removed was 1604 g per breast.*

21. Mofid MM, Dellon AL, Elias JJ, et al. Quantitation of breast sensibility following reduction mammaplasty: a comparison of inferior and medial pedicle techniques. *Plast Reconstr Surg.* 2002;109:2283–2288. *A total of 34 women following inferior and medial pedicle reduction mammaplasty were studied using computer-assisted neurosensory testing to generate normal breast sensation data and to compare sensory outcomes between the two pedicles. No significant differences in postoperative sensory outcomes were demonstrated. In addition, the amount of breast tissue removed did not correlate with postoperative sensory outcomes.*

26. Davison SP, Mesbahi AN, Ducic I, et al. The versatility of the superomedial pedicle with various skin reduction patterns. *Plast*

Reconstr Surg. 2007;120:1466–1476. *This study reviewed 279 breast reductions using the superomedial pedicle. No patient had nipple loss, and the overall complication rate was 18%. The authors concluded that the superomedial dermoglandular pedicle is a safe and reliable technique for reduction mammaplasty.*

28. Altuntas ZK, Kamburoglu HO, Yavuz N, et al. Long-term changes in nipple-areolar complex position and inferior pole length in superomedial pedicle inverted T scar reduction mammaplasty. *Aesthetic Plast Surg.* 2015;39:325–330. *This retrospective study reviewed 48 women following superomedial reduction mammaplasty. The authors demonstrated that the new nipple areolar complex position descends over time. The authors advocate that the NAC be placed 1.5–1.75 cm below the most projected area of the breast after final shaping so that in the long term, the nipple areolar complex would be at the proper position.*

30. Spear SL, Rao S, Patel KM, et al. Reduction mammaplasty and mastopexy in previously irradiated breasts. *Aesthet Surg J.* 2014;34:74–78. *The authors review their experience with 12 reduction mammaplasty operations in patients that had been previously radiated. Average specimen weight was 623 g. Four patients (22%) experienced five minor complications, and one patient had a major complication requiring flap reconstruction. Proper patient selection is critical when considering reduction mammaplasty in previously radiated patients.*

32. Cunningham BL, Gear AJ, Kerrigan CL, et al. Analysis of breast reduction complications derived from the BRAVO study. *Plast Reconstr Surg.* 2005;115:1597–1604. *Data from 179 patients was reviewed from the Breast Reduction Assessment: Value and Outcomes (BRAVO) study. The overall complication rate was 43% (77 patients). Conclusions included resection weight correlated with increased risk of complications; delayed healing correlated with resection weight and inversely with increasing age and anesthesia times; vertical incisions may be associated with higher complications; and complications had no negative effect on improvement in Short Form-36.*

10

Reduction mammaplasty with short scar techniques

Frank Lista, Ryan E. Austin, and Jamil Ahmad

▶ Access video content for this chapter online at expertconsult.com

SYNOPSIS

- Reduction mammaplasty is one of the most commonly performed plastic surgery procedures.
- Short scar techniques aim to improve symptomatic mammary hypertrophy while enhancing the long-term shape of the breasts with minimal scarring.
- Commonly described short scar techniques include periareolar scar, short scar periareolar inferior pedicle reduction (SPAIR), vertical scar, L-short scar, and no vertical (horizontal only) scar.

Access the Historical Perspective section online at
http://www.expertconsult.com

Introduction

Reduction mammaplasty continues to be one of the most commonly performed procedures in plastic surgery. In 2014, the American Society for Aesthetic Plastic Surgery reported that over 114 000 breast reductions were performed, and these figures remain relatively constant year-to-year.[1] The goals of reduction mammaplasty are three-fold: (i) improvement in the physical symptoms associated with mammary hypertrophy, (ii) improvement in the appearance of the breast, and (iii) long-lasting results. However, traditional reduction mammaplasty techniques (i.e., inverted-T or Wise pattern scar) add significant scar burden to the breast.

Short scar reduction mammaplasty techniques were developed to improve long-term projection of the breasts while minimizing the scar burden associated with other breast reduction techniques. In recent years, short scar reduction techniques have become increasingly popular, as reflected in the surveys of board-certified plastic surgeons from the American Society for Aesthetic Plastic Surgery (2002),[2] the American Society of Plastic Surgeons (2006),[3] and the Canadian Society of Plastic Surgeons (2008).[4] As more plastic surgeons are trained in the use of short scar techniques, adoption of such procedures into clinical practice will likely continue to grow.

Since 1989, we have exclusively performed our modified vertical scar reduction mammoplasty technique for patients requiring breast reduction. As our practice demographic evolved, we saw younger women presenting for reduction mammaplasty who were not only interested in relief of their symptoms secondary to mammary hypertrophy, but were also concerned with the amount of scarring that resulted from the procedure and the long-term appearance of their breasts.

Many variations of short scar reduction mammaplasty techniques have been described. This chapter will present an overview of some of the commonly described short scar techniques, with a focus on our vertical scar reduction mammaplasty technique.

Key points

- Patients presenting with ≥2 symptoms of mammary hypertrophy (upper back, neck, shoulder, or arm pain; arm numbness; rashes; and bra strap grooves) are more likely to significantly improve following reduction mammoplasty.
- Postoperative breast size will likely remain larger using short scar techniques in comparison to

inverted-T scar techniques, and may be unsuitable for patients who desire a small postoperative breast size but have significant mammary hypertrophy.

- A higher rate of complication has consistently been reported in active smokers and obese individuals. Consideration must be given before performing an elective operation on these higher-risk patients.
- Markings for vertical scar reduction mammaplasty, particularly the new position of the nipple areolar complex (NAC), are different from inverted-T scar reduction mammaplasty techniques.

Basic science/disease process

Blood supply of the nipple areolar complex

The most critical aspect of repositioning the NAC is ensuring adequate blood supply. While nearly any pedicle can and has been employed in short scar reduction techniques, the two most commonly utilized pedicles are superior and superomedial. A closer study of the blood supply to the NAC provides a better understanding of why the selection of a superior or superomedial pedicle provides a reliable blood supply for transposition of the NAC.

Since Manchot (1889)[51] first described the blood supply to the breast, many varying observations of the vascular anatomy have been made. More recently, van Deventer[52] performed anatomical studies on 15 female cadavers in an attempt to further clarify the blood supply to the NAC. This study found that in all breasts, the NAC received a blood supply medially or superiorly from one or more branches of the internal thoracic artery, most commonly the third (47.5%) or second (25.0%) intercostal perforators.[52] In 13 of 27 breasts, the NAC did not receive any blood supply from superiorly. Contributions from the lateral thoracic artery, posterior intercostal arteries, and axillary artery were variable; however, there were abundant anastomoses between these varying blood supplies around the NAC. From this study, van Deventer et al.[53] concluded that the NAC generally has a dual blood supply, inferomedially from the internal thoracic intercostal artery system and superolaterally from the lateral thoracic artery and other minor contributors, with the most reliable blood supply arising from the internal thoracic artery.

Michelle le Roux et al.[54] examining the neurovascular anatomy in 11 female cadaveric breasts reported that the arterial supply to the superomedial pedicle originated from a single dominant vessel while the venous drainage was through an extensive branching network. Along with intercostal nerve branches innervating the

pedicle, the blood supply coursed through the pedicle in a superficial plane. They concluded that thinning of the superficial aspect of the superomedial pedicle could lead to vascular compromise or denervation of the NAC, and instead recommended resection be done from the deep surface or the base of the pedicle if needed.

Based on these studies, we believe that a superior pedicle may have either an axial or random blood supply while a superomedial pedicle is more likely to have an axial blood supply, which further supports the safety of the partial thickness superior or superomedial pedicle design that we use in our technique.

Reducing and reshaping the breast

The goals of reduction mammaplasty procedures include the ability to effectively reduce breast size to achieve symptomatic relief, while transposing the NAC to a more aesthetically pleasing position on the breast and reshaping the remaining breast parenchyma. One common criticism of vertical scar techniques is that at the completion of the procedure, the breast mound has a distorted appearance with characteristic flattening of the inferior pole and exaggerated superior pole fullness. However, in the early postoperative period, the breast settles into the shape that resembles the long-term appearance.[55–57]

Three-dimensional imaging of breasts following vertical scar reduction mammaplasty has given us a better understanding of how the breast changes over time. Eder et al.[55] showed that edema following vertical scar reduction mammaplasty is resolved by 3 months postoperatively, and that further contour changes in the breast are complete by 9 months postoperatively. In 2008 we reported our results at long-term follow-up, showing that pseudoptosis does not occur, attesting to the maintenance of breast shape and projection following this procedure (Fig. 10.1).[58] We also found that, compared with preoperative skin markings, the NAC was located significantly higher (approximately 1.3 cm) at both early and long-term follow-up (Fig. 10.2).[58] We attribute the superior movement of the NAC to excision of central and inferior pole breast tissue, which unweights the remaining breast tissue including the NAC, allowing for elastic recoil of the superior pole skin. The excision of the inferior pole parenchyma also directly helps to prevent pseudoptosis by removing this weight from the inferior pole. Further, suturing of the medial and lateral pillars produces coning of the breast, which not only pushes the NAC superiorly but also redistributes skin laxity in the breast to avoid inferior displacement of the NAC.[58] At 4 years, the distance from

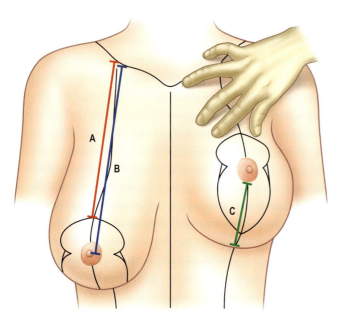

Fig. 10.1 Studying the fate of nipple areolar complex (NAC) position and inferior pole length following vertical scar reduction mammaplasty. **(A)** The shortest distance between the inferior edge of the clavicle and planned postoperative position of the superior border of the NAC. **(B)** The shortest distance between the inferior edge of the clavicle and the nipple. **(C)** The distance between the inframammary crease and the inferior border of the NAC. *(Adapted with permission from: Ahmad J, Lista F. Vertical scar reduction mammaplasty: the fate of NAC position and inferior pole length.* Plast Reconstr Surg. *Apr 2008;121(4):1084–1091.)*

the inframammary crease to the inferior border of the NAC was significantly shorter, confirming that pseudoptosis does not occur after our technique for vertical scar reduction mammaplasty.[58]

Diagnosis/patient presentation

Women presenting for reduction mammaplasty are a diverse patient population, ranging greatly in age, body habitus, and breast size. Patient goals in seeking reduction mammaplasty range from purely functional to purely aesthetic, with most patients falling on a spectrum between the two. However, this remains an important distinction to make preoperatively, given that in our healthcare system, reduction mammaplasty is an insurance-covered procedure that requires preapproval to ensure medical necessity.

With mammary hypertrophy, breast size or body mass index (BMI) does not correlate with subjective physical symptoms. Studies have not found a direct correlation between preoperative breast size and the severity of preoperative symptoms.[59,60] Symptomatic mammary hypertrophy can have a detrimental effect on quality-of-life. Studies have shown that the impact of symptomatic mammary hypertrophy on a woman's

quality-of-life is similar to individuals living with moderate angina, renal transplant, or osteoarthritis of the knee.[60–62]

Kerrigan *et al.*[63] reported an evidence-based definition of medical necessity for breast reduction in an effort to establish clear, practical, and objective criteria that could be applied by physicians to help differentiate women seeking breast reduction primarily for symptom relief vs. aesthetic improvement. They identified seven symptoms specific to breast hypertrophy: upper back pain, neck pain, shoulder pain, arm pain, arm numbness, rashes, and bra strap grooves. Results of this study established that women reporting at least two of seven physical symptoms all or most of the time improved to a significantly greater extent than women reporting less than two symptoms all or most of the time. Their data suggested that women reporting at least one of seven physical symptoms might also report greater improvement than those with no symptoms all or most of the time. We have found this definition of medical necessity useful in evaluating patients that will benefit most from breast reduction.

Patient selection

Selecting individuals who are suitable candidates for short scar reduction mammaplasty techniques is important, as these procedures are not suitable for all patients or breast shapes. However, in our experience, short scar techniques are versatile procedures that can be widely adapted to the majority of patients seeking reduction mammaplasty.

The major criticism of short scar reduction mammaplasty techniques is that these procedures limit the amount of breast volume reduction that can be achieved. However, when thinking about short scar reduction mammaplasty, we suggest physicians conceptually separate the two main aspects of the procedure: skin excision and parenchymal resection. Short scar reduction techniques, by their nature, limit the amount of skin excision possible when compared to traditional techniques. Much more skin excision will be possible with an L-short scar than with a periareolar scar.

However, we believe that the amount of parenchymal resection possible with short scar techniques, the vertical scar in particular, is greater than previously suggested.[64] In our 2006 review of 250 consecutive patients who underwent vertical scar reduction mammaplasty, the average weight of tissue excised was 526 g, with the largest excision exceeding 2000 g.[49] The safety and feasibility of larger volume reductions using the vertical scar,[65–68] SPAIR,[69] and L-short scar[29] techniques have all been well documented in the literature.

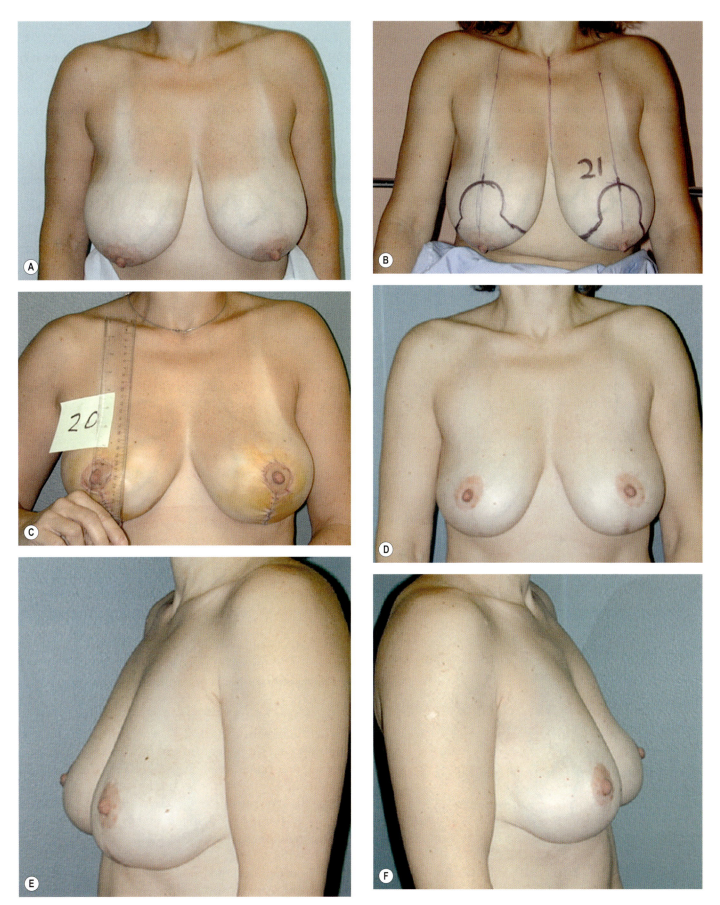

Fig. 10.2 **(A)** A 38-year-old woman underwent vertical scar reduction by mammaplasty using bilateral superior pedicles. From the right breast, 375 g was excised and 325 g from the left. **(B)** Preoperatively, the distance from the inferior edge of the clavicle to the level of the planned postoperative position of the superior border of the nipple aveolar complex (NAC) was 21 cm. **(C)** At 5 days postoperatively, the distance from the inferior edge of the clavicle to the superior border of the NAC is 20 cm, resulting in a difference of 1 cm. **(D,E,F)** At 4 years follow-up, the distance from the inframammary crease to the inferior border of the NAC was unchanged. *(From: Ahmad J, Lista F. Vertical scar reduction mammaplasty: the fate of NAC position and inferior pole length.* Plast Reconstr Surg. *2008 Apr;121(4):1084–1091.)*

While it is possible to perform this technique on patients with extremely large breasts, it is important for these patients to realize that their postoperative breast size will likely remain larger when compared to other traditional techniques because of the amount of skin preserved with a vertical scar technique. In patients with severe mammary hypertrophy desiring a very small postoperative breast size, this technique is not suitable. Along with other authors,[40,45] we recommend learning this technique by initially operating on patients with mild to moderate hypertrophy and good skin quality. As more experience is gained, one can progress to performing this technique on patients with greater degrees of mammary hypertrophy and poorer skin quality.

Patient characteristics and complications

Patient selection plays an important role in preventing and minimizing postoperative complications. In our 2006 review of complications in 250 consecutive breast reductions, there was a statistically significant difference between groups for BMI, with complications occurring less frequently in patients of normal weight (BMI: 18.5–25.0 kg/m^2),[49] a finding which is supported by other studies.[70–78] Associations between smoking and complications in reduction mammaplasty have also been reported, in particular, wound healing/dehiscence and wound infection.[75,77–80] A study by Bikhchandani et al.[81] found that wound related complications occurred in 35% of smokers and that smokers had a 2–3 times higher risk of developing a complication.

In our practice, we do not perform this procedure on patients with a BMI >35.0 kg/m^2 or on active smokers. Patients presenting for breast reduction with a BMI >35 kg/m^2 are advised to lose weight prior to undergoing this procedure. Smokers are instructed to quit smoking for at least 4 weeks preoperatively and 4 weeks postoperatively to decrease their risk for complications.[82,83]

Treatment/surgical technique

Vertical scar reduction mammaplasty

We routinely perform vertical scar reduction mammaplasty as a day surgery procedure. The average operating time is less than 70 min.[49] Multiple authors have shown that there is no increased risk of complications following breast reduction as a day surgery procedure.[72,84–87] In addition, Buenaventura et al.[86] estimated between $1500 and $2500 US dollars were saved when breast reduction surgery was performed as a day surgery

procedure as opposed to requiring inpatient admission, while Nelson et al.[4] reported an estimated cost savings of $873 Canadian dollars.

The American Society of Plastic Surgeons' Patient Safety Committee provides an overview of perioperative steps that should be completed to ensure appropriate patient selection for the ambulatory surgery setting.[88] In addition, guidelines for perioperative cardiovascular evaluation,[89,90] prevention of pulmonary complications[91,92] and venous thromboembolism prophylaxis[93,94] are also available.

Below is a description of the planning and surgical technique for our vertical scar reduction mammaplasty.

Skin marking

The patient is marked preoperatively in a standing position, with arms relaxed at the sides. The midline of the chest and the inframammary creases are marked (Fig. 10.3). The central axis of the breast is drawn by extending a straight line from the midpoint of the clavicle, typically located 7–8 cm from the midline, through the nipple to intersect with the inframammary crease. One hand is inserted behind the breast to the level of the inframammary crease, and this point is projected anteriorly onto the breast and marked (point A). Point A represents the superior border of the new NAC. This point is transposed onto the contralateral breast instead of using the contralateral inframammary crease, as asymmetry in inframammary crease height can result in asymmetry of the NAC position postoperatively.

The inferior limit of the planned skin excision is marked (point B) 2–4 cm above the inframammary crease, depending on the size of the reduction. This distance is shorter in smaller reductions (less inframammary crease movement) and longer in larger reductions (greater inframammary crease movement). The inframammary crease moves superiorly after vertical scar breast reduction, which accounts for the extension of the vertical scar onto the chest wall in earlier techniques. Limiting the inferior end of the vertical scar to a point above the inframammary crease prevents this problem.

A mosque dome pattern is used in this technique. The roof of the mosque dome is drawn by extending curved lines from point A to points C and D, which form the border of the new NAC. The roof is drawn such that when points C and D are brought together and the breast is coned, the roof will form a circle. The vertical limbs of the mosque dome pattern are drawn by extending curved lines from point B to points C and D, thus forming the margins of the planned skin excision. Blocking triangles should be drawn at points C and D, toward the central axis of the breast, to prevent a teardrop

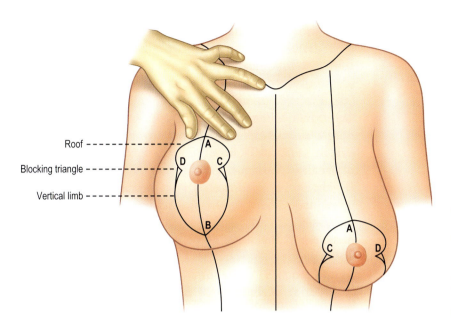

Roof ------
Blocking triangle ------
Vertical limb ------

Fig. 10.3 Mosque dome skin marking pattern. Point A is at the level of the anterior projection of the inframammary crease on the breast. Point A will be the new location of the superior border of the areola. Point B is the inferior limit of the skin excision. Point B is 2–4 cm above the inframammary crease along the central axis of the breast. Blocking triangles are extended from points C and D. *(Adapted with permission from: Lista F, Ahmad J. Vertical scar reduction mammaplasty: 15-year experience including a review of 250 consecutive cases.* Plast Reconstr Surg. *2006 Jun;117(7):2152–2165.)*

deformity of the areola. The inferior extent of the skin resection is marked in the shape of a 'V' instead of a 'U' as described in other techniques, as we feel that this allows for easier skin closure and helps to prevent dog-ear formation at the inferior extent of the vertical scar.[45,49]

The areas where liposuction will be performed at the axillary area and along the lateral chest wall are marked. The new NAC and pedicle selection and marking are performed after induction of anesthesia.

> **Tips**
>
> In cases of asymmetric vertical scar breast reduction (>100 g difference), Point A on the larger side should be marked 1–2 cm lower than on the smaller side to account for differential unweighting of the breasts.

Anesthesia and positioning

We perform breast reduction surgery under general anesthesia. The patient is in the supine position with both shoulders abducted to 90° to allow for liposuction of the tail of the breast and lateral chest wall. We do not sit the patient up during surgery with this technique, as the breast mound has a distorted appearance with characteristic flattening of the inferior pole and exaggerated superior pole fullness. Instead, we assess the patient for symmetry of shape and volume in the supine position. In addition, we do not utilize tacking sutures from the breast parenchyma to the pectoralis fascia, as these sutures can cause unwanted tethering of the

breast. We achieve shaping of the breast using other techniques.

Infiltration

A small incision is made superior to point B, between the vertical limbs, through the skin that will later be excised. Infiltration is performed just deep to the skin vertical limb incision lines, as well as within the breast parenchyma. Each breast is infiltrated with 500 mL of a solution composed of 1000 mL of Ringer's lactate solution, 40 mL of 2% lidocaine, and 1 mL of 1:1000 epinephrine. The lateral chest wall is also infiltrated at this time in preparation for later liposuction.

Selection of the pedicle

In the supine position, a tourniquet is applied to the breast to keep the skin taut. The NAC is outlined using a metal washer, 45 mm in diameter, centered over the nipple. At this point we select the type of pedicle to be used to transpose the new NAC (Fig. 10.4). If any part of the new areola lies superior to a line joining the blocking triangles (points C and D), a superior dermoglandular pedicle is used; if all of the new areola lies inferior to this line, a superomedial dermoglandular pedicle is used (Fig. 10.5). This rule limits pedicle length and helps to avoid vascular compromise of the NAC. The superior pedicle is drawn from the blocking triangles inferiorly, leaving a 2.5 cm border around the NAC. The superomedial pedicle is drawn with a base extending from the midpoint of the mosque dome roof to the medial blocking triangle. A 2.5 cm border is left around the NAC. The base of the superomedial pedicle should be wide

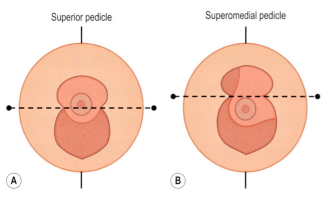

Fig. 10.4 Approach for pedicle selection. A superior pedicle is used if any part of the new areola lies superior to a line joining the blocking triangles **(A)**, and a superomedial pedicle if all of the areola lies inferior to this line **(B)**.

enough to maintain a pedicle width-to-length ratio of no less than 1:2 to preserve its blood supply but should be narrow enough to allow easy rotation and insetting of the NAC into the roof of the mosque dome.

In our experience, the superior pedicle is the most commonly employed, while the superomedial pedicle is reserved for cases of mammary hypertrophy with greater degrees of ptosis when the NAC must be transposed a greater distance. The axial blood supply to the superomedial pedicle is more reliable in these cases. In cases where the NAC is situated too medially, a superolateral pedicle may be required to allow for adequate rotation and insetting.

Tips

If any part of the new areola lies superior to a line joining the blocking triangles, a superior dermoglandular pedicle is used; if all of the new areola lies inferior to this line, a superomedial dermoglandular pedicle is used

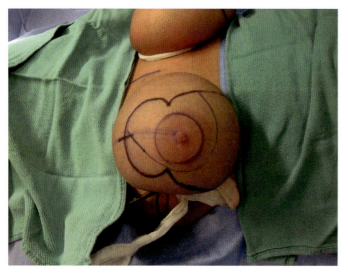

Fig. 10.5 Mosque dome skin marking pattern with superomedial pedicle.

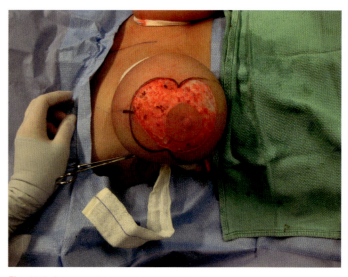

Fig. 10.6 Superomedial pedicle de-epithelialized.

De-epithelialization

Leaving the breast tourniquet in place will facilitate de-epithelialization of the dermoglandular pedicle by increasing skin tension over the breast. Prior to de-epithelialization, the NAC and the pedicle are marked, as explained previously. To prevent damage to the blood vessels travelling superficial through the pedicle, it is important to leave the deep dermis intact when de-epithelializing as opposed to removing the skin full thickness (Fig. 10.6).

Excision of breast tissue

Surgical excision of skin, fat, and breast parenchyma is performed en bloc, as outlined by the preoperative skin markings. Modification of these markings intraoperatively is not necessary. We find that the following sequence of steps is helpful in maximizing the efficiency of the excision while ensuring adequate volume reduction. Begin by incising around the borders of the dermoglandular pedicle to a depth of 2.5 cm. A dermoglandular flap containing the NAC is then raised at a thickness of 2.5 cm. It is important to maintain this 2.5 cm thickness under the NAC so as not to disrupt its neurovascular supply.

The medial parenchymal pillar is developed by incising the medial vertical limb straight down through skin, fat, and breast parenchyma to a level just superficial to the pectoralis fascia. This will leave move breast parenchyma medially, which contributes to more medial breast fullness and a better final breast shape (Fig. 10.7). The lateral parenchymal pillar is developed in a manner similar to the dermoglandular pedicle. An incision through the lateral vertical limb is carried through skin, fat, and parenchyma to a depth of 2.5 cm. Dissection is

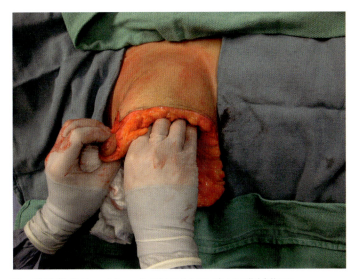

Fig. 10.7 Medial breast tissue is left intact preserving medial fullness.

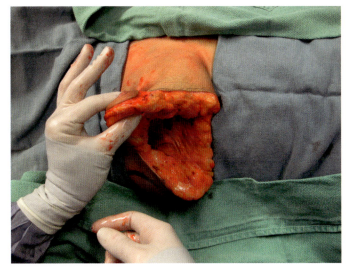

Fig. 10.9 Partial thickness superomedial pedicle is 2.5 cm thick.

then carried laterally while maintaining this 2.5 cm depth. The lateral dissection will not be completed at this point.

At the inferior extent of the skin excision, the lateral and medial vertical limbs are joined in the shape of a 'V' as previously explained. At this point the lateral and medial parenchymal dissections can be joined and carried down to the chest wall. The inferior extent of the resection specimen should be lifted off the pectoralis fascia from inferior to superior, taking care to leave a layer of breast tissue over the pectoralis fascia to prevent bleeding and postoperative pain. At this time the lateral flap dissection can be completed by continuing to develop the 2.5 cm thick flap until the lateral border of the breast is reached (Fig. 10.8).

Once the parenchyma is incised and freed from its deeper attachments, inferiorly directed retraction on the tissue to be excised will allow for a more extensive resection of breast tissue, particularly in the superolateral quadrant. While maintaining inferiorly directed tension on the tissue to be excised, the superior flap is developed by continuing the 2.5 cm thick flap from under the dermoglandular pedicle (Fig. 10.9). The dissection is completed by curving deep, towards the pectoralis fascia, at the superior margin of the breast (Fig. 10.10). After excision is complete, the medial, superior, and lateral skin flaps should feel even in thickness and smooth (Fig. 10.11).

The tissue between the inferior edge of the vertical wound and the inframammary crease is thinned to prevent a dog-ear from forming (Fig. 10.12). The skin is typically left about 0.5 mm thick, and a layer of fat should be left on the deep fascia to prevent the skin tethering down to the fascia. We have not found it necessary to perform any excisional modification of the skin in this region to control dog-ear formation.

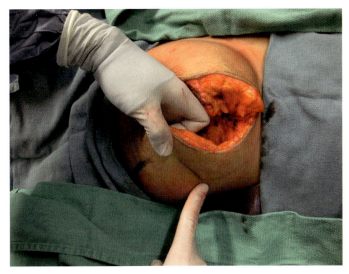

Fig. 10.8 Extent of lateral excision.

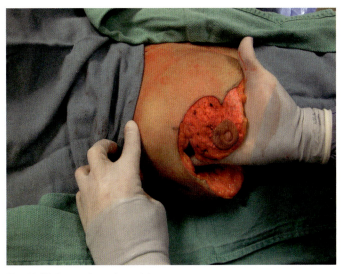

Fig. 10.10 Extent of superior excision.

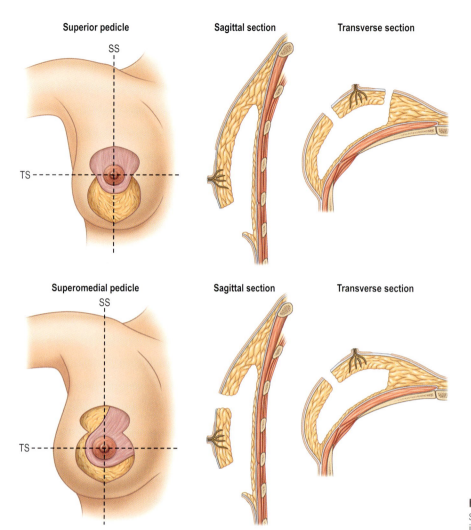

Superior pedicle   Sagittal section   Transverse section

Superomedial pedicle   Sagittal section   Transverse section

Fig. 10.11 Extent of breast tissue excision using a superior pedicle **(A)** and superomedial pedicle **(B)** shown in sagittal (SS) and transverse sections (TS)

> ### Tips
>
> Maintaining a 2.5 cm flap thickness throughout the superior and lateral flaps is important, as over-resection can lead to contour irregularities while under-resection can result in an inadequate volume reduction of the breast, by as much as 100–300 g per side.

Liposuction

Given the utility of liposuction for both breast volume reduction and contouring of the lateral chest wall, we now use liposuction in all cases. In particular, liposuction of the lateral thoracic compartment helps to shape the lateral breast border.

Liposuction is performed using a 4 mm, three-hole, blunt cannula for volume reduction of the axillary area of the breast and contouring of the lateral chest wall. Liposuction is performed following parenchymal excision because it is very difficult to accurately assess the composition of the breast preoperatively by clinical

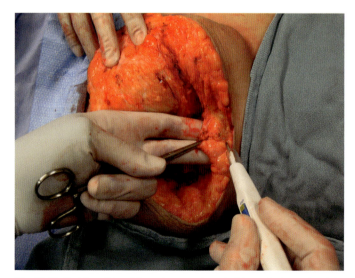

Fig. 10.12 Excision of breast tissue between the end of the vertical wound and the inframammary crease to prevent a dog-ear from forming.

examination. In excessively fatty breasts, liposuction can also be performed on the superior half of the breast for volume reduction. Access to these areas is through the medial and lateral pillars created by the surgical excision.

Breast shaping

Shaping of the breast in the vertical scar reduction is largely achieved by reapproximating the medial and lateral parenchymal pillars using inverted #1 Vicryl sutures (Ethicon, Inc., Somerville, NJ) placed through the breast capsule (Fig. 10.13). These parenchymal pillar sutures may contribute to improved long-term projection of the breasts by preventing pseudoptosis or "bottoming out" of the breast. Typically, two parenchymal pillar sutures are required. Temporary skin staples are used to close the vertical wound while suturing the skin.

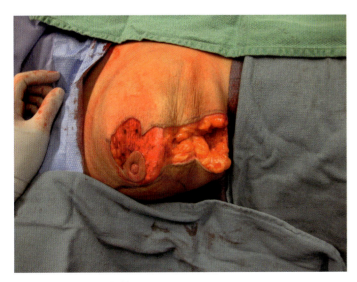

Fig. 10.13 Parenchymal pillar sutures.

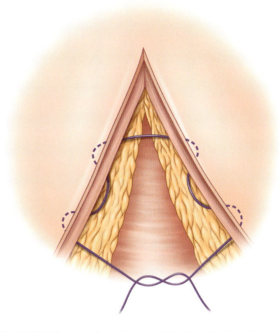

Fig. 10.14 A four-point box stitch is used to gather the skin of the vertical wound.

Wound closure

All layers of wound closure are performed using a 3-0 Monocryl plus suture (Ethicon, Inc., Somerville, NJ). To begin, the NAC is advanced or rotated into position, depending on the pedicle orientation, and inset prior to closure of the vertical scar. If there is any tension during insetting of the NAC, a small superficial incision through the dermis may be required extending superiorly from the blocking triangles to facilitate insetting. The NAC is inset with inverted deep dermal sutures at the 3, 6, 9, and 12 o'clock positions and closed using a running subcuticular suture.

Next, a four-point box suture is used to gather the skin of the vertical wound (Fig. 10.14). Starting at the inferior apex of the vertical scar and working towards the areola, sequential box sutures allow for selective gathering of the vertical wound, thereby preventing dog-ear formation and providing control over the length of the vertical scar. The distance between the box suture points on the same side of the vertical wound should be 15–25 mm to create a powerful gathering effect, and all of these sutures should be buried. It is important to begin each additional four-point box suture immediately adjacent to the previous one to avoid gaping. Skin within 2 cm of the areola is not gathered to prevent distortion of the areola. The remainder of the wound is closed with simple inverted deep dermal sutures.

After gathering of the skin, there may be gaping of the horizontal pleats caused by the box sutures along the vertical wound (Fig. 10.15). These are corrected

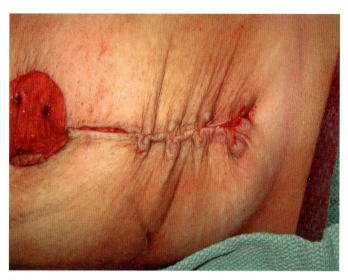
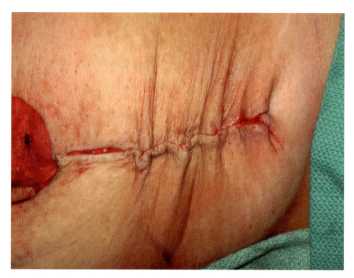

Fig. 10.15 The vertical wound has been gathered using four-point box stitches resulting in gaping of the gathered wound edges. The gaping of the horizontal pleats has been corrected using inverted deep dermal sutures.

using an inverted deep dermal suture. Correction of horizontal pleats is essential because they do not settle with time and lead to small horizontal scars within the larger vertical scar. Skin staples are used along the vertical wound for final closure along the length of the vertical scar (Fig. 10.16).

Using box sutures, the skin can be gathered several centimeters so that the vertical scar measures 8 cm or less. However, in some cases a longer vertical scar is acceptable. Cutaneous wrinkling of the vertical scar associated with gathering of the skin will disappear by 6 months postoperatively.[95]

We do not routinely use drains in conjunction with reduction mammaplasty procedures, a practice supported by evidence in the literature.[96–99] Wrye *et al.*[97] reported that performing reduction mammaplasty without the use of closed suction drainage does not increase complications and is preferred by patients.

> **Tips**
>
> Lassus[39] measured the distance between the inferior border of the areola and the inframammary crease in young women with aesthetically pleasing breasts and found measurements ranging from 4.5 to 10 cm. Hall-Findlay[45] has shown results where this distance postoperatively was up to 12 cm. Along with other authors,[44] in our experience the length of the vertical scar does not increase over time after vertical scar reduction mammaplasty.[58] Though some suggest gathering of the vertical incision does not impact the long-term length of the vertical scar,[100] we feel this is a critical step in our vertical scar reduction mammaplasty technique.

Dressings and wound care

Each breast is injected with 10 mL of 0.5% bupivacaine with 1:200000 epinephrine for postoperative pain relief. The wounds are dressed with paraffin gauze, followed by dry gauze, and finally by abdominal pads. These are held in place by a surgical bra.

Postoperative care

Patients should wear a bra at all times for 4 weeks following surgery. On postoperative day 1, they are instructed to shower and wash their wounds with soap and water and dress them with dry gauze. Patients are seen on postoperative day 5, at which point skin staples are removed and replaced with Steri-Strips (3M, St. Paul, MN). We typically see patients again at 1 month and 3 months postoperatively. Patients may return to their normal level of activity 3 weeks postoperatively and can begin physically demanding activity 1 month following surgery.

Fig. 10.16 The nipple areolar complex has been inset and skin staples are used along the vertical wound for final closure.

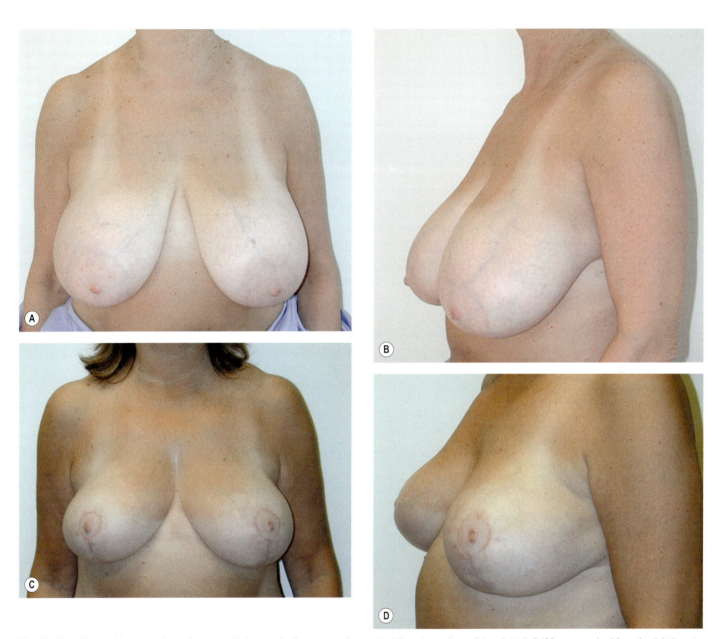

Fig. 10.17 A 19-year-old woman who underwent vertical scar reduction mammaplasty using bilateral superior pedicles. A total of 420 g was excised from the right breast and 400 g from the left; 50 mL was liposuctioned from the right breast and 100 mL from the left. Results 3 months postoperatively are shown.

Outcomes, prognosis, and complications

As previously mentioned, the primary goals of reduction mammaplasty are three fold: (i) improvement in the physical symptoms associated with mammary hypertrophy, (ii) improvement in the appearance of the breast, and (iii) long-lasting results. Short scar reduction mammaplasty techniques, vertical scar procedures in particular, meet all of these criteria (Fig. 10.17). Several studies have shown that following short scar reduction procedures, patients have high levels of satisfaction[101–103] and significant improvements in both macromastia-related symptoms and quality-of-life.[59,66,104] These results have been shown to persist over time.[58,103]

With younger patients presenting for reduction mammaplasty, the ability to breast-feed following surgery may be an increasing concern. Rates of lactation reported in the literature are 60–80% for superior pedicle techniques[105–108] and 48–65% for medial pedicle techniques,[105,106,109] which are not significantly different from breast-feeding rates in patients who have not had breast surgery. In our practice, we emphasize to patients preoperatively that breast-feeding is a complex process, and that even patients who have not have breast reduction surgery can have difficulty breast-feeding.

Reported complication rates for short scar reduction mammaplasty procedures are highly variable, ranging from 3% to 25%.[59,66,67,110,111] Commonly reported complications include superficial wound dehiscence (0–14.3%), hypertrophic scarring (0–8.8%), seroma (0–17%), hema-

Table 10.2 Complications following short scar reduction mammaplasty	
Early complications	**Late complications**
Bleeding/hematoma	Over-resection/under-resection
Seroma	Asymmetry
Infection (cellulitis, abscess)	Contour irregularities
Wound dehiscence	Pseudoptosis
Fat necrosis	Hypertrophic scar
NAC vascular compromise/ necrosis	NAC malposition/shape
Skin vascular compromise/ necrosis	NAC widening (periareolar scar/SPAIR)
Altered nipple sensation	Permanent suture infection/ extrusion
	Inability to lactate

NAC, nipple areolar complex; SPAIR, short scar periareolar inferior pedicle reduction.

toma (0–8.6%), infection (0–8.3%), altered nipple sensation (0–11%), and fat necrosis (0.8–6.2%) (Table 10.2).[49,66,67,110,112,113] Though instances of NAC necrosis have been reported, we have not experienced any cases of partial or total nipple necrosis using our vertical scar technique. Rates of revision surgery following vertical scar reduction mammaplasty range from 2% to 8%, with the most common indication being scar revision.[67,112,114] Studies comparing complication rates in vertical scar and inverted-T scar pattern reduction mammaplasty have not demonstrated consistent results on the relative rate of complications between these procedures.[110,112,115]

In 2006, we reviewed 250 consecutive cases of vertical scar reduction mammaplasty and found our complication rate was 5.6%.[49] The most common complications were superficial wound dehiscence (2.2%), hematoma (1.2%), fat necrosis (0.8%), and seroma (0.4%).[49] Our analysis found no statistically significant difference between groups (i.e., complication vs. no complication) in regard to pedicle selection (p=0.662) and use of liposuction (p=0.831).[49] Although our review found no association between complications and amount of reduction (p=0.107), other studies have reported higher complication rates with larger resection specimens.[78,79]

The following are some problems encountered after vertical scar reduction mammaplasty and how they can be prevented.

Wound dehiscence

Superficial wound dehiscence was the most frequent complication in our review of 250 consecutive cases, occurring in 2.2% of breasts. The area where this occurs is typically in the middle portion of the vertical wound, as this is the area under greatest tension. Although other

authors[42,45] have described using a continuous intradermal suture to gather the skin of the vertical wound, this may be a source of wound healing problems due to constriction of the blood supply to the skin edges. To mitigate these factors, our use of the four-point box suture gathers the skin of the vertical wound effectively while causing less skin edge ischemia. Staples provide further approximation of the skin edges without causing additional ischemia.

Under-resection

Short scar reduction mammaplasty techniques have been criticized because it can be difficult, for those who normally perform inferior pedicle/inverted-T scar reduction mammaplasty techniques, to assess the adequacy of the reduction.[116] At the end of the operation, there is exaggerated superior pole fullness, inferior pole flatness, and indrawing of the nipple with which one must become familiar. Although vertical scar techniques have a characteristically unusual appearance on the operating room table at the end of the procedure, they invariably give a much more aesthetically pleasing result postoperatively.

While learning this technique, there is a tendency for under-resection due to inadequate tissue resection laterally and superiorly. However, with the straightforward design of the excision in our technique, increased reduction can be safely achieved by excising breast tissue laterally to the anterior axillary line and superiorly deep to the pedicle, if necessary. Provided that the thickness of the pedicle and skin flaps is 2.5 cm, it is possible to resect more tissue without compromising the blood supply of the pedicle or breast skin.

Secondary procedures

Patients may present for consideration of repeated breast reduction for many reasons including inadequate breast volume reduction, breast and NAC asymmetries, and recurrent symptomatic mammary hypertrophy. These patients should be assessed in a manner similar to patients presenting for primary reduction mammaplasty consultation; however, additional attention must be given to (i) scars on the breast, (ii) areas of parenchymal excess, and (iii) the patient's goals for the procedure.

One of the major concerns regarding repeated breast reduction is the blood supply of the NAC, particularly in cases where the original dermoglandular pedicle design is unknown. To date, there have been 3 reported cases of complete NAC necrosis, 2 cases of partial necrosis, and 2 cases of ischemia/epidermolysis.[117] In 2012, we reported our experience performing a modified technique for vertical scar breast reduction in 25 patients who had undergone previous breast reduction; since then, we have used this approach in over 40 patients. To date, we have had no cases of either partial or total necrosis of the NAC. In our experience, repeated breast reduction using our modified technique for vertical scar breast reduction technique is a safe procedure even when the initial breast reduction technique is unknown.[50,117]

In cases of repeated breast reduction, our technique is similar to that outlined above; however, the following modifications are used when determining the optimal pedicle selection:

1. If the NAC is in an ideal position preoperatively: only a vertically oriented, inferior wedge excision is performed; or

2. If superior transposition of the NAC is required: a partial-thickness, superior pedicle with careful de-epithelialization preserving the deep dermis is performed (Fig. 10.18).

This strategy for pedicle selection combined with a vertically oriented, inferior wedge excision limiting the amount of undermining of breast tissue helps to maintain blood supply to the remaining breast tissue. Additionally, liposuction is an important adjunct to achieve volume reduction while limiting the amount of dissection during repeated breast reduction and is used in all cases.

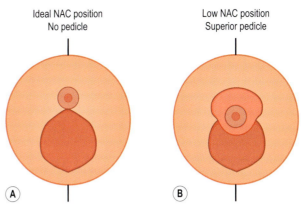

Fig. 10.18 Approach for pedicle selection in repeated breast reduction. **(A)** If nipple areolar complex (NAC) is in an adequate position, an inferior wedge resection with no pedicle is selected. **(B)** If the NAC is low and requires transposition, a superior pedicle is used. *(Adapted with permission from: Ahmad J, McIsaac SM, Lista F. Does knowledge of the initial technique affect outcomes after repeated breast reduction? Plast Reconstr Surg. 2012 Jan;129(1):11–8.)*

Conclusion

In over 20 years experience of more than 3000 patients, we have found our method of vertical scar reduction mammaplasty to be a versatile technique that can produce reliable results in most patients. While it is possible to perform this technique on patients with large breasts, it must be noted that the postoperative breast size will likely remain larger in comparison to other traditional breast reduction techniques. In patients with significant mammary hypertrophy desiring a small postoperative breast size, this technique may be unsuitable. Overall, vertical scar reduction mammaplasty results in a more projected breast with a narrower base, preservation of superomedial breast fullness, minimal scar burden, and long-lasting breast shape, which are the *sine quibus non* of aesthetic breast surgery.

🌐 Access the complete reference list online at **http://www.expertconsult.com**

12. Hammond DC, Khuthaila DK, Kim J. The interlocking Gore-Tex suture for control of areolar diameter and shape. *Plast Reconstr Surg.* 2007;119(3):804–809.

17. Hammond DC. The short scar periareolar inferior pedicle reduction (SPAIR) mammaplasty. *Semin Plast Surg.* 2004;18(3):231–243.

30. Chiari Júnior A. The L short-scar mammaplasty: a new approach. *Plast Reconstr Surg.* 1992;90(2):233–246.

37. Lalonde DH, Lalonde J, French R. The no vertical scar breast reduction: a minor variation that allows you to remove vertical scar portion of the inferior pedicle wise pattern T scar. *Aesthetic Plast Surg.* 2003;27(5):335–344.

47. Hall-Findlay EJ. Pedicles in vertical breast reduction and mastopexy. *Clin Plast Surg.* 2002;29(3):379–391. *A succinct review of various breast reduction techniques and the pedicles that are used to transpose the NAC. Dr. Hall-Findlay describes in detail her technique for vertical scar reduction mammaplasty.*

49. Lista F, Ahmad J. Vertical scar reduction mammaplasty: 15-year experience including a review of 250 consecutive cases. *Plast Reconstr Surg.* 2006;117(7):2152–2165. *We describe our technique for vertical scar reduction mammaplasty using a superior or medial pedicle. We performed a review of 250 consecutive patients including an analysis of complications. Technical considerations are discussed in detail, and a review of previously described techniques of vertical scar reduction mammaplasty is included.*

53. van Deventer PV, Page BJ, Graewe FR. The safety of pedicles in breast reduction and mastopexy procedures. *Aesthetic Plast Surg.* 2008;32(2):307–312.

58. Ahmad J, Lista F. Vertical scar reduction mammaplasty: the fate of nipple–areola complex position and inferior pole length. *Plast Reconstr Surg.* 2008;121(4):1084–1091. *We report on the early and long-term fate of the NAC position and inferior pole length. Compared with preoperative skin markings, the NAC was located significantly higher at both early and long-term follow-up. Based on these findings, we adjusted their skin marking technique so that the superior border of the NAC is marked at the level of the inframammary crease. We also observed that at 4 years, the distance from the inframammary crease to the inferior border of the NAC was significantly shorter, and pseudoptosis did not occur after vertical scar reduction mammaplasty.*

63. Kerrigan CL, Collins ED, Kim HM, et al. Reduction mammaplasty: defining medical necessity. *Med Decis Making.* 2002;22(3):208–217. *An evidence-based definition of the medical necessity for breast reduction is described in an effort to establish clear, practical, objective, and fair criteria that could be applied by physicians to help differentiate women seeking breast reduction for symptom relief versus aesthetic improvement.*

117. Ahmad J, McIsaac SM, Lista F. Does knowledge of the initial technique affect outcomes after repeated breast reduction? *Plast Reconstr Surg.* 2012;129(1):11–18. *We report our modified technique for vertical scar reduction mammaplasty used in patients presenting for repeated breast reduction. This approach was used safely in patients regardless of whether or not the previous pedicle was known.*

11

Gynecomastia surgery

Charles M. Malata and Kai Yuen Wong

 Access video content for this chapter online at expertconsult.com

SYNOPSIS

- Gynecomastia is the benign enlargement of male breast tissue. It is a common condition and can be associated with significant psychological morbidity. The mainstay of treatment is surgery.
- When surgery is indicated, the aim is to restore a normal looking male chest contour with minimal scarring whilst maintaining the viability of the nipple areolar complex.
- A wide range of surgical techniques have been described for gynecomastia treatment including various forms of liposuction, open glandular excision, skin reduction, and combinations of these.
- Liposuction has now become established as the prime modality in the surgical treatment of gynecomastia, either alone or in combination with other techniques.
- This chapter outlines the salient features and principles of the main surgical techniques. We propose an evidence-based approach to achieving predictable and safe results. An algorithm to facilitate surgical success is presented.

 Access the Historical Perspective section online at
http://www.expertconsult.com

Introduction

Gynecomastia, or abnormal breast tissue enlargement in men, is the most common breast pathology amongst males. It has a reported prevalence of 30–70% depending on age group,[1–3] and the condition can pose a significant psychological challenge to the patients.[4,5] Most cases, especially those occurring during adolescence, are benign and self-limiting. The majority of patients presenting for surgical treatment have already had a medical cause excluded by the referring physician or have not responded to drug therapy. Severe breast enlargement or lesser degrees of gynecomastia may be directly referred for surgery on account of severe emotional or psychological distress. The aim of treatment is restoration of a normal male chest contour while minimizing the evidence of surgery and protecting the nipple areolar complex.

There is a plethora of described techniques for the surgical management of enlarged male breasts. In contrast there are few reports on an integrated surgical approach in general and the roles of different treatment modalities in particular.[6–9] Although excisional techniques have traditionally been the accepted standard, liposuction has now become established as the prime surgical modality either alone or in combination with more invasive methods. More recently, other minimally invasive surgical techniques have been described, but their roles have yet to be established. Gynecomastia patients may constitute a challenging group with respect to satisfaction postoperatively.[10] The many surgical options and their inter-relationship are therefore outlined here with a guide to technique selection and optimization of outcomes.

Basic science

Gynecomastia is thought to primarily result from an increased estrogen to androgen ratio since estrogens stimulate breast tissue while androgens antagonize its effects.[16,17] This hormonal imbalance may therefore arise from an absolute or relative excess of estrogens, or an absolute decrease of androgen levels or their action (Table 11.1). Interestingly, a recent review identified 49

Table 11.1 Classification of the causes of gynecomastia		
Idiopathic		
Physiological	Neonatal, pubertal, aging	
Pathological	Congenital	Klinefelter's, anorchia, hermaphroditism, androgen resistance syndromes, enzyme defects of testosterone synthesis, increased peripheral tissue aromatase
	Endocrine	Castration, mumps, Cushing's syndrome, congenital adrenal hyperplasia, adrenocorticotropic hormone deficiency, hyperthyroidism, hypothyroidism, panhypopituitarism, hyperprolactinemia
	Tumors	Testicular (choriocarcinoma, Sertoli and Leydig cell tumors); adrenal (adenoma, carcinoma); pituitary adenoma; breast carcinoma; tumors that secrete human chorionic gonadotrophin (lung, liver, kidney, stomach, and lymphopoietic)
	Drugs	Hormones (estrogens, androgens, gonadotrophins); anti-androgens (cimetidine, spironolactone, digitalis, progesterone, cyproterone, flutamide); stimulators of prolactin (phenothiazines, reserpine, hydroxyzine); drugs of abuse (marijuana, heroin, methadone, amphetamines); anti-tuberculosis drugs (isoniazid, ethionamide, thiacetazone)
	Metabolic	Thyrotoxicosis (altered testosterone/estrogen binding); renal failure (acquired testes failure); cirrhosis (increased substrate for peripheral aromatization); starvation (same as cirrhosis); alcoholism
	Other	Human immunodeficiency virus, chest wall trauma, cystic fibrosis, physiological stress

medications reported to be associated with gynecomastia where, in the majority of cases, hormonal imbalance could not explain the breast enlargement.[18]

Etiologically gynecomastia can be physiological or pathological in nature. The former may occur during three different age groups. In the neonate, gynecomastia is attributed to high levels of maternal estrogen during pregnancy. During puberty, up to 65% of boys may have gynecomastia, but this usually resolves in 75% of cases within 2 years of onset.[19] Gynecomastia is also very common in older men with a reported prevalence of 72% in the hospitalized male population aged 50–69 years.[20] Proposed mechanisms for this include enhanced peripheral aromatization secondary to increased total body fat, and decreased levels of androgens associated with aging.[16,21–23] Older men are also more likely to be taking medications, which may themselves cause gynecomastia.[18]

Diagnosis/patient presentation

A thorough history is important to determine the underlying cause of gynecomastia (Table 11.1) and rule out breast cancer and other tumors. On the other hand, it should be noted that around 25% of gynecomastia cases may be idiopathic.[24] Salient points include patient age, onset and duration of breast enlargement, symptoms of associated pain, recent weight change, and a systems review with particular attention to possible endocrine and liver abnormalities. Medications and recreational drug use need to ascertained as they may cause 10–20% of gynecomastia cases.[18,24,25] It is also important to explore the psychological and social effects of gynecomastia as social embarrassment is the most

common presenting complaint in those seeking surgical treatment.

On physical examination, gynecomastia is usually bilateral and felt as glandular tissue under the nipple areolar complex and extends to a variable size in all directions. It needs to be differentiated from pseudogynecomastia or lipomastia, which is adipose tissue hypertrophy without glandular proliferation. Breast cancer is uncommon and accounts for less than 1% of malignancies in men in the UK and USA.[26,27] It typically presents unilaterally and is felt as a hard mass located outside the nipple areolar complex. As part of the systems review, physical examination should include assessment of secondary sexual development and the thyroid, as well as looking for signs of chronic kidney or liver disease. When examining the genitalia, it is also important to look for any testicular masses or atrophy. Liver enlargement may sometimes be encountered.

Laboratory tests (Box 11.1) are tailored according to the clinical findings. Extensive work-up is rarely indicated and often does not influence treatment.[28] Biochemical assessment includes tests for liver, kidney, and thyroid function; and serum levels of testosterone, prolactin, follicle-stimulating hormone, and luteinizing hormone. Additional tests may be necessary in cases of recent or symptomatic gynecomastia to rule out tumors.[2] For example, serum levels of estrogens, human chorionic gonadotrophin (hCG), dehydroepiandrosterone (DHEA), and urinary 17-ketosteroids.

Routine mammography and breast ultrasonography with or without biopsy is not routinely recommended unless breast cancer is suspected[29–33] or the patient presents with unilateral breast enlargement. Similarly, testicular ultrasonography or abdominal computer tomography may be performed if a testicular or adrenal

- Laboratory tests:
  - Testosterone
  - Estrogen±β-human chorionic gonadotrophin
  - Prolactin, follicle-stimulating hormone, and luteinizing hormone
  - Urea and electrolytes
  - Liver function tests
  - Thyroid function tests (thyroxine and thyroid-stimulating hormone)
  - ±Dehydroepiandrosterone or urinary 17-ketosteroids
- Radiological examination:
  - Breast ultrasound scan
  - Mammogram
  - ±Abdominal computer tomography scan
  - ±Testicular ultrasound scan
- ±Core or fine-needle biopsy

- Persistent enlargement after puberty (>2 years) and exclusion of medical causes
- Inadequate response to medical treatment
- Severe breast enlargement
- Significant asymmetry or unilateral condition
- Severe psychosocial effects or morbidity
- Patient request
- Post massive weight loss
- Specific clinical conditions:
  - Drug induced – prostate cancer treatment
  - Drug induced – anabolic steroid use or cannabis use (as unlikely to respond to medical therapy or resolve spontaneously)

Treatment/surgical technique

Medical management

Most cases of gynecomastia do not require treatment as they are benign and self-limiting.[19,37,38] Weight loss should be recommended for male patients with pseudogynecomastia in the first instance. Specific treatment should be directed at addressing any identified underlying cause (see Table 11.1).

Medical therapies essentially focus on correcting the imbalance of androgens and estrogens.[28,39,40] Anti-estrogens such as tamoxifen are often used as a first-line medication, including men with prostate cancer[41–44] and persistent pubertal gynecomastia.[45–47] Other medications include testosterone, danazol (gonadotrophin inhibitor), and aromatase inhibitors such as testolactone. The evidence base for medical therapies is limited by the difficulty in differentiating treatment effects from spontaneous resolution of gynecomastia.[48,49] Furthermore, medications are probably most effective during the active, proliferative phase of gynecomastia. In patients with long-standing gynecomastia of over 1 year, medical treatment is often ineffective as the breast glandular tissue progresses to irreversible dense fibrosis and hyalinization.[2,24,35,38] Such cases should be considered for surgical treatment.

Radiation treatment has been used prophylactically in older men with prostate cancer treated by anti-androgens.[50–52] Conversely, it is not recommended for the treatment of pubertal gynecomastia due to the increased lifetime risk of breast cancer, albeit very small.

When treatment is indicated, most patients do not need a trial of medical therapies and are best managed with surgery, which is the mainstay modality (see Table 11.2).

mass is suspected based on clinical findings and investigations.

Patient selection

Various clinical and histological classifications have been suggested for gynecomastia.[6,7,34,35] Simon *et al.*'s classification[36] is the most practical as it takes into account not only the size of the breast but also the amount of redundant skin (Table 11.2). The boundaries between the categories are, however, not well defined, leading to subjectivity and interobserver variability. Therefore, in our practice we classify gynecomastia into two clinical groups:[6] small to moderate size with no or minimal skin excess (Simon's grades I and IIA), and moderate to large size with moderate to marked skin excess (Simon's grades IIB and III). This facilitates choice of treatment modality as will be discussed in the following section. The indications for gynecomastia surgery are summarized in Box 11.2.

Table 11.2 **Simon *et al.*'s classification of gynecomastia**			
		Breast enlargement	Skin excess
I		Small	No
II	A	Moderate	No
	B		Yes
III		Marked	Yes
(Adapted from Simon BE, Hoffman S, Kahn S. Classification and surgical correction of gynecomastia. *Plast Reconstr Surg.* 1973;51:48–52.)			

Surgical management

Well-established surgical techniques for gynecomastia treatment include various forms of liposuction, open glandular excision, skin reduction, and combinations of these. Liposuction is now the prime surgical technique as it is minimally invasive, improves contouring by feathering the peripheries, and is frequently successful as a single modality.[6,9,53,54]

Various forms of liposuction have been described including conventional, power-assisted, ultrasound-assisted, laser-assisted, and vibration amplification of sound energy at resonance (VASER)-assisted.[32–36] The most common types used are conventional and ultrasound-assisted liposuction. The salient features of the main available surgical modalities are outlined below.

Anesthesia and infiltration

We perform all surgery under general anesthesia as day cases (ambulatory care setting) except when skin reduction is planned, in elderly prostate cancer patients, when it is envisaged that a drain may be required (which is rare except for very large gynecomastia), and in patients with underlying medical problems or those travelling from a long distance away. All have preoperative photographic documentation of their breasts by professional medical photographers. All patients receive perioperative broad-spectrum antibiotic prophylaxis at general anesthetic induction (see Table 11.2).

Patients are marked preoperatively in the upright sitting position highlighting the inframammary fold, breast boundaries, planned stab-incision sites, and concentric topography-type marks centered on the most prominent portion of the breast (Fig. 11.1). The breast tissue is infiltrated through a stab incision in the lateral inframammary crease using a superwet (near-tumescent) technique. The wetting solution consists of Ringer's lactate containing 1 mL of 1 in 1000 solution of adrenaline (1 mg) and 30 mL of 1% lignocaine (300 mg) per liter.

Conventional liposuction

Conventional liposuction, also referred to as "traditional liposuction" or "suction-assisted lipectomy" (SAL) was introduced by Yves Illouz in the 1970s with a series of over 3000 cases[12] of body contouring at different sites. It is useful for diffuse breast enlargement of soft to moderately firm consistency[28,53,55–57] (Fig. 11.2). However, residual subareolar tissue is a frequently encountered complication with this technique.[6,8,54] This persistent tissue is often uncomfortable leading to patient requests for further surgery. Additionally, SAL is not suitable for severe cases or in breasts with primarily fibrous tissue[7]

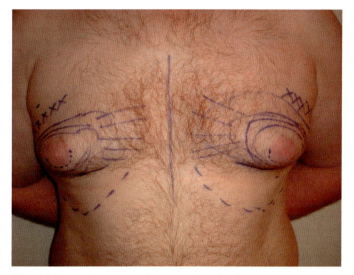

Fig. 11.1 Preoperative marking of gynecomastia patient in upright position. Concentric topography-type marks are centered on the most prominent portion of the breast. The dots around the nipple areolar complex mark the inferior periareolar incision for potential intraoperative conversion to open excision. The straight lines indicate areas of tapering of the liposuction in the areas adjacent to the breast tissue while the crosses mark the areas not to be "violated" during the liposuction procedure. The interrupted lines illustrate the inferior extent of the liposuction to allow successful skin redraping.

and can be associated with intraoperative conversion to open excision in up to 39% of cases.[54] It can be effective in soft breasts even if large, but good skin quality is important for later contraction and avoiding the need for skin resection. Liposuction allows the achievement of better breast contours with minimal scarring.

Special liposuction cannulas specifically designed for the treatment of gynecomastia (Fig. 11.3) have been successfully used for the treatment of more difficult or firmer breasts.[56,58–61] Cross-tunnel suctioning for larger breasts, ptotic breasts, and those with excess skin or well-defined inframammary folds makes SAL more effective. Such extensive cross-suctioning enables more consistent contraction of the skin and allows it to redrape with less waviness and irregularity. The inframammary crease can be obliterated by sharp dissection[62] or by suction cannulas.[61] In our practice we do not employ special sharp cannulas due to the potential risk of intra- and postoperative bleeding.

After infiltration, a suction cannula is inserted through the same access incision used for infiltration. The laterally placed incision in the inframammary fold allows better access for the liposuction to the whole breast laterally and medially. This contrasts with the axillary and transareolar incisions preferred by others, but provides less access and greater risk of accidental penetration of the chest wall. A 4.6 mm or 5.2 mm Mercedes cannula is used for the initial suction employing the palm down and pinch techniques. The refinement and final contouring is performed with a 3 mm or

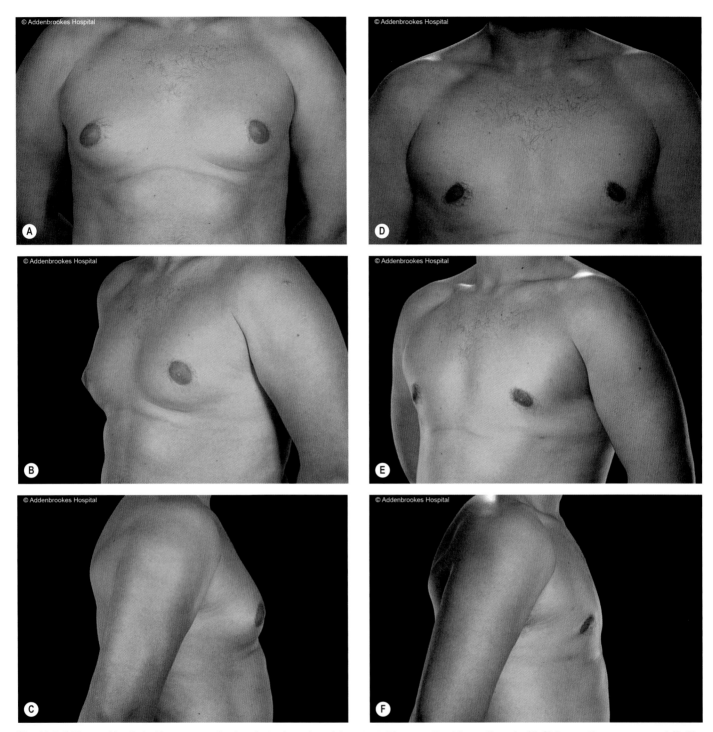

Fig. 11.2 A 25-year-old patient with gynaecomastia of moderate size and consistency treated by conventional liposuction only. **(A–C)** Preoperative appearance and **(D–F)** postoperative result 6 months later. *(From: Wong KY, Malata CM. Conventional versus ultrasound-assisted liposuction in gynaecomastia surgery: a 13-year review.* J Plast Reconstr Aesthet Surg. *2014;67:921–926.)*

3.7 mm Mercedes cannula. It is important to make a concentrated effort to suction the breast tissue and not just the subcutaneous tissue. During suction, contour changes are constantly assessed by direct observation, while the thickness of the breast is evaluated intermittently with the contralateral hand by palpation between the fingers and thumb. A close watch is also kept on the color (blood-staining) and volume of the aspirate. Once a satisfactory contour is obtained, the surrounding fat is feathered to avoid a noticeable saucer deformity, and any well-defined inframammary fold as determined preoperatively is deliberately disrupted in order to avoid the gynecoid (female) contour of the breast. This also enables the liposuction to extend well beyond the confines of the breast in order to facilitate postoperative redraping of the skin as popularized by Rosenberg.[55,58,61]

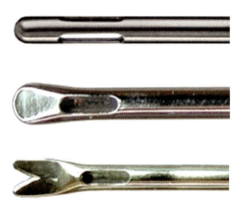

Fig. 11.3 Examples of different liposuction cannulas. (Top) Mercedes tip, (middle) spatula tip, and (bottom) V-shaped tip.

Conventional liposuction can be used in the traditional manner (as in our practice) and employ power assistance alone or in combination with open glandular excision.[63] We have a low threshold for conversion to open excision based on the contour, lump palpability, and pinch test. Therefore, if unsuccessful based on the contour, palpation, and pinch, a semicircular inferior periareolar incision should be made and the disc resected by open excision. This is easily accomplished within a few minutes because of the prior liposuction.

Ultrasound-assisted liposuction

Ultrasound-assisted liposuction (UAL) was developed by Zocchi in the 1980s based on selective destruction of adipose tissue while protecting other tissues from damage.[14] UAL is far more effective for firmer breasts than SAL (Fig. 11.4, UAL). By emulsifying breast fat, it is particularly useful for addressing dense, fibrous gynecomastia.[7,14,54,57,64] It has also been suggested that UAL results in less postoperative bruising, a smoother breast contour, better postoperative skin contraction, and less surgeon fatigue.[7,54,57,65–67] Furthermore, in our study of 219 consecutive patients over a 13-year period, compared to conventional liposuction, UAL had significantly lower rates of intraoperative conversion to open excision (25% vs. 39%) and postoperative revision (2% vs. 19%).[54] Patients treated with UAL were therefore 8.5 times less likely to undergo subsequent revision surgery and 1.5 times less likely to have intraoperative conversion to open excision. As a result, when available, UAL has become our preferred modality of treatment.

UAL employs either solid or hollow cannulas. After infiltration with the wetting solution (at a rate of 400 mL/min for the Mentor Contour Genesis or Mentor Lysonix 3000 machines; Mentor Medical Systems, Santa Barbara, California), a hollow UAL cannula with or without a skin-protective port is inserted through the same stab incisions as those used for conventional liposuction. In addition to the better mechanical leverage of the liposuction, the laterally placed incisions avoid trauma and thermal burns to the nipple areolar complex.[6,7,57] UAL is technically demanding and a number of precautions have to be undertaken to prevent morbidity (Box 11.3).[68–72] Routine safety measures to avoid thermal injuries[6,7,57] are taken including continuous saline irrigation through the sheath system (40 mL/h for the Mentor based machines listed above), use of a probe sheath, skin guard, wet towels around the entry site, and avoidance of "end hits". The cannula is continuously moved in fan-like long strokes, starting deep and working superficially. The strokes should go beyond the marked boundaries of the breast enlargement, and, as with SAL, a special effort is made to disrupt the inframammary fold where this is well formed. The well described UAL endpoints[73] are determined by loss of tissue resistance, aspirate volume, blood-tinged appearance of the aspirate, and planned treatment time. Final fat evacuation and contouring is performed using conventional liposuction (3.7 mm Mercedes cannulas) with the suction set at the machine's maximum (see Video 11.1 ⏵).[74]

Other minimally invasive techniques

An increasing number of minimally invasive techniques have also been described including endoscopically-assisted,[75,76] pull-through,[15,77–79] arthroscopic shavers,[8,15,80] and mammatome excision.[81,82] Their exact roles remain to be established. The most promising is the arthroscopic shaver which provides a less invasive alternative to open excision with no visible periareolar scar, and can be combined effectively with liposuction.[8] Additionally, it is readily available in most hospitals in the UK and USA. These minimally invasive techniques have been

---

BOX 11.3 Disadvantages of ultrasonic liposuction

- Limited availability and expensive equipment
- Increased operating time
- Labor intensive for the nurses
- Specific risks of:
  - Thermal injury
  - Skin necrosis
  - Demyelination of peripheral nerves
- Cavitation and potential DNA changes
- Meticulous precautions are needed including:
  - Skin guard
  - Ultrasonic liposuction probe sheath
  - ±Continuous fluid irrigation
  - Wet towel around the skin
  - Continuous movement technique of the probe
  - Avoidance of end hits

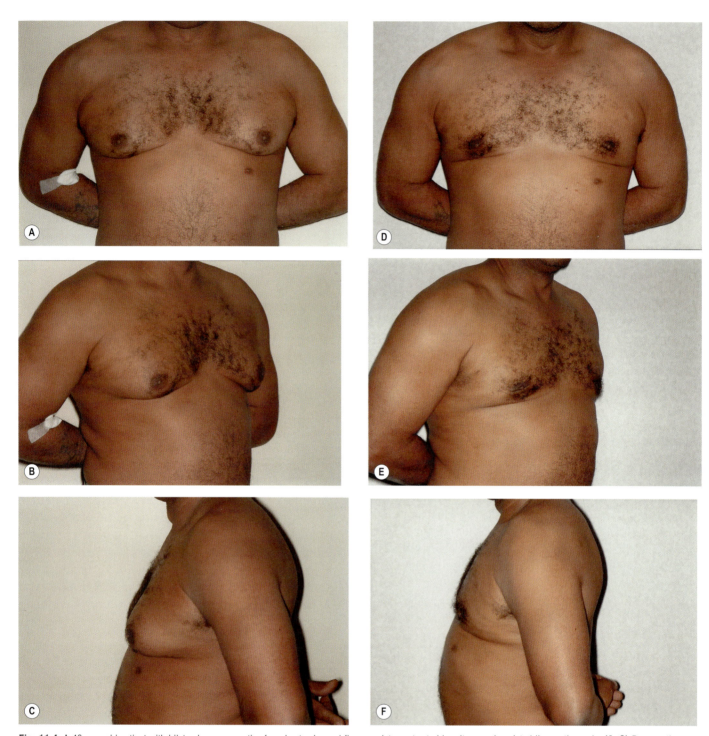

Fig. 11.4 A 46-year-old patient with bilateral gynecomastia of moderate size and firm consistency treated by ultrasound-assisted liposuction only. **(A–C)** Preoperative appearance and **(D–F)** postoperative result 5 months later.

advocated in an attempt to reduce unsightly scarring and the risk of nipple deformities. However, it remains to be seen whether they will be efficacious or widely adopted.

Open excision

Open excision via an inferior periareolar approach[11] is the traditional approach. Various other incisions have been described such as circumareolar, periareolar,

transareolar, and circumthelial.[11,83–94] Liposuction is frequently not effective for very glandular tissue, small discrete breast buds, and body builders as the latter have large amounts of glandular tissue with little fat.[95,96] Excisional techniques are effective for these groups of patients, although they are associated with a high complication rate with potential for adverse scars and contour abnormalities.[97,98] Open excision is currently used in combination with liposuction, as pioneered by

Teimourian and Perlman.[13] The liposuction serves a number of purposes such as pretunneling to facilitate resection, reducing bleeding and bruising, and partially breaking down the breast tissue. After liposuction the tissue can be resected via a number of access incisions.

We prefer the time-honored Webster's technique for open excision where breast tissue is excised via a semicircular incision along the inferior margin of the nipple areolar complex. To excise the excess tissue, Bostwick scissors are used to dissect inferiorly to the lower border of the breast before proceeding in a deep plane above the pectoralis major muscle to the superior border of the breast. At least a 1 cm disc of breast tissue is left under the areola to prevent a depression of the nipple areolar complex[6] (Figs. 11.5 & 11.6). Open excision

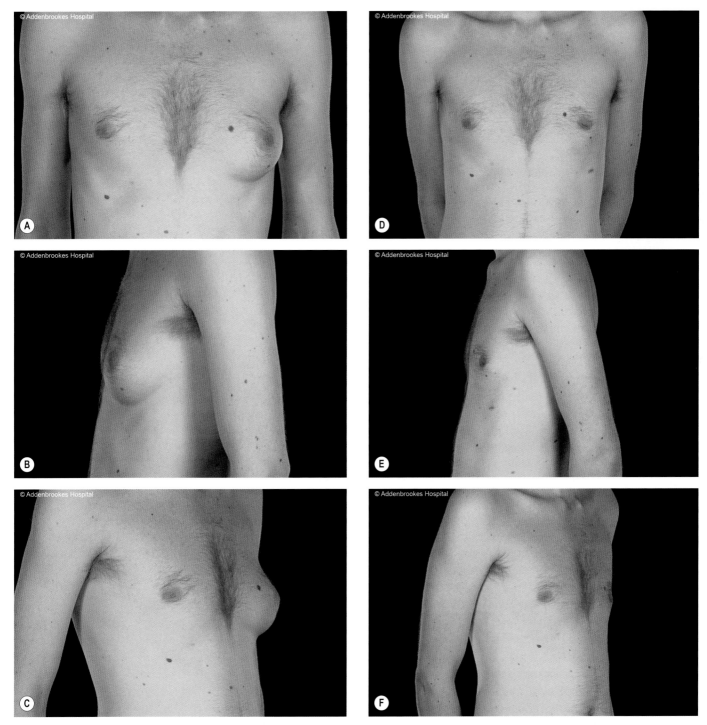

Fig. 11.5 A 20-year-old patient with left-sided gynecomastia of large size and moderate consistency, treated by conventional liposuction and open excision. **(A–C)** Preoperative appearance and **(D–F)** postoperative result 6 months later showing excellent symmetry.

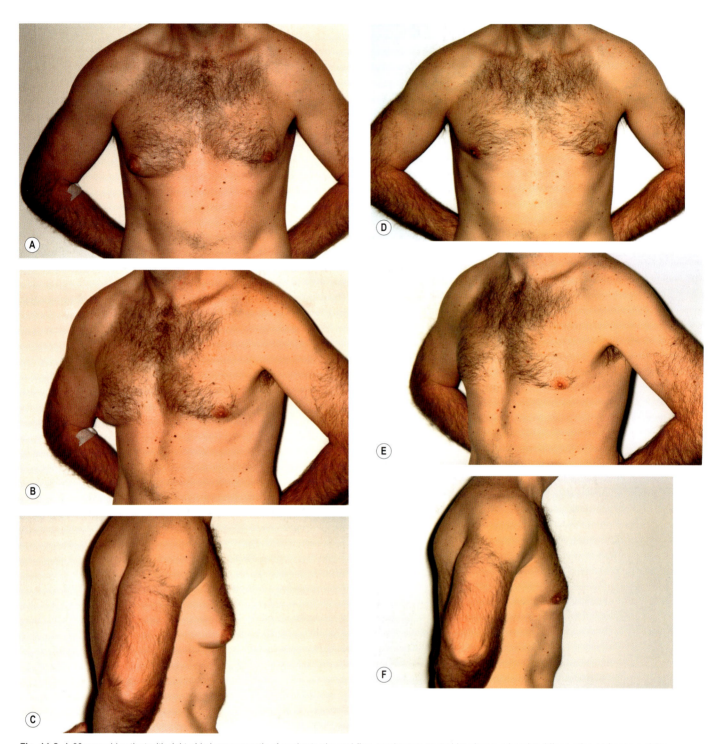

Fig. 11.6 A 30-year-old patient with right-sided gynecomastia of moderate size and firm consistency, treated by ultrasound-assisted liposuction and open excision. **(A–C)** Preoperative appearance and **(D–F)** postoperative result 6 months later showing excellent symmetry.

even when combined with liposuction sometimes does not fully correct large and ptotic breasts for which skin reduction is indicated. Some authors recommend eschewing skin resection leaving the skin to contract on its own over a 6–8 month period. We prefer to address the skin excess at the first operation if the patient is willing to accept the scars. This has practical benefits such as cost, a single operation, and reduced time away from work.

Skin reduction

There are a number of procedures used to reduce excess skin in gynecomastia. Although most of these techniques are similar to those used in females, it is important to reduce the resemblance to the female breast reduction pattern and (try as much as possible to) minimize the scars. Although skin reduction techniques can result in large scars as compared to liposuction and Webster's incision, they are well tolerated by patients with large breasts, significant ptosis, or poor skin quality.

In patients with obvious skin excess or very large breasts, skin reduction techniques should also be planned usually at the same time as the open excision of the breast tissue or as a second stage, a minimum of 4–6 months later. There is, however, no consensus on when and how to undertake skin resection. We base this decision on skin elasticity, presence of ptosis, skin excess, skin type, and the patient's willingness to accept a potential two-stage procedure. The surgeon's preference also plays a role in choosing the technique.

In patients in whom open excision is not mandated by the gynecomastia appearance and consistency, we always consent them for open excision in case the liposuction leaves significant residual stromal tissue. Whenever there is skin excess or ptosis, we prefer to address the skin excess at the original operation, especially in cases of poor or borderline skin elasticity. The choice of skin reduction technique (Box 11.4) also depends to a large extent on the surgeon's preference.

Concentric mastopexy pattern

The periareolar concentric mastopexy-type skin reduction is preferable to other skin reduction techniques principally because it avoids extra-areolar scars. We prefer to use the concentric periareolar technique[13,99] because of the less noticeable scarring (Figs. 11.7 & 11.8). There is still a risk of adverse scarring (widely stretched, hypertrophic, or keloid), particularly in dark skinned patients. In very large breasts this technique is

---

BOX 11.4 **Salient features of skin reduction surgery for gynecomastia**

- Indications:
  - Large gynecomastia (Simon's grade IIb or III)
  - Ptotic breasts
  - Poor skin quality
  - Post massive weight loss
- Options for skin reduction:
  - Concentric
  - Vertical scar (LeJour type)
  - Elliptical
  - T-scar (Wise pattern)
  - Lateral wedge
  - No vertical scar with nipple transposition (Lalonde type)

---

associated with excessive puckering of the periareolar skin, persistent discharge, and suture palpability. In patients with true ptosis, those aiming for complete resolution (flat breasts) or best possible cosmesis, skin reduction can be undertaken using the LeJour vertical mammaplasty skin pattern.

LeJour pattern

In patients with true ptosis or very large breasts, skin reduction and tissue resection can be undertaken using the LeJour vertical mammaplasty skin pattern. The skin and underlying breast tissue is resected in a vertical ellipse and then the pillars are approximated. However, the final vertical scar is very noticeable. This technique should be used as a last resort, especially in those who wish to avoid a T-scar (Figs. 11.9 & 11.10).

Other skin reduction techniques

Others resort to lateral wedge, elliptical, and inverted-T excisions (Fig. 11.11). All these scars are more noticeable even after 12–18 months. Patients with very large or ptotic breasts are suitable candidates for elliptical mastectomy and free nipple grafting or superior nipple transposition (Figs. 11.12 & 11.13). This also avoids the telltale features of female-type breast reduction scars. It should however be avoided in dark-colored skin because of nipple depigmentation. In an attempt to reduce unsightly scarring and risk of nipple deformities, less invasive excisional techniques have recently been advocated, but their role remains to be established. In patients with a high potential for keloid or hypertrophic scarring we frequently employ a Lalonde-type breast reduction no-vertical scar technique (Figs. 11.12 & 11.13). After de-epithelialization, liposuction is performed prior to open glandular excision and via the horizontal incision. After achieving hemostasis the nipple areolar complex is transposed superiorly and brought out through the predetermined "button-hole". The long inframammary incision is then closed over a suction drain.

Staged skin reduction

Skin reduction, with its resultant large visible scars, is sometimes resisted by patients, and thus another approach is to stage the surgery. Specifically, starting with liposuction followed by subsequent skin resection a minimum of 4–6 months later. This potentially reduces the incidence of skin resection and hence minimizes scarring. Occasionally patients planned for two-stage surgery accept the initial results and decline the second skin reduction procedure. The staged skin reduction is also likely to be smaller following some skin

Text continued on p. 191

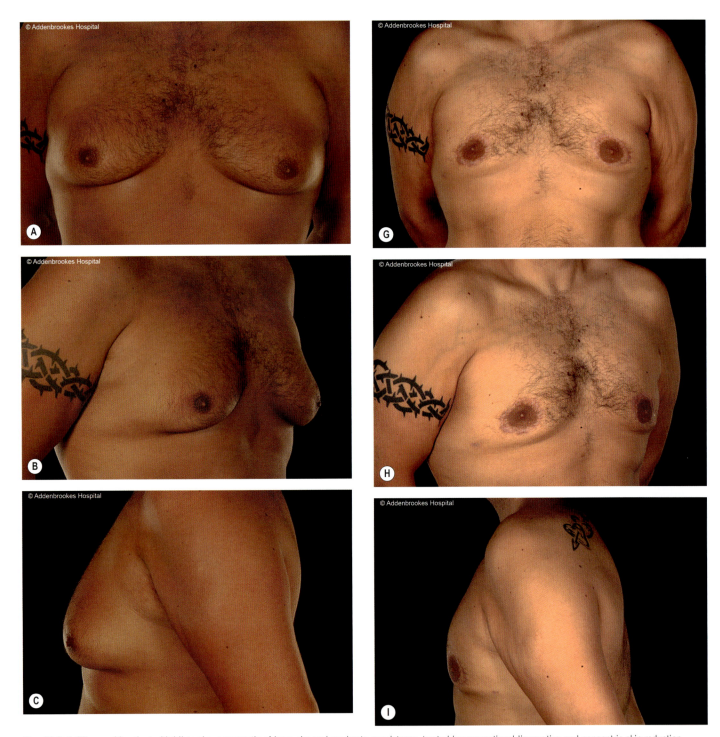

Fig. 11.7 A 30-year-old patient with bilateral gynecomastia of large size and moderate consistency, treated by conventional liposuction and concentric skin reduction. **(A–C)** Preoperative appearance, **(D–F)** markings, and **(G–I)** postoperative result 7 months later.

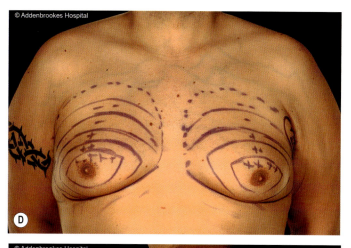

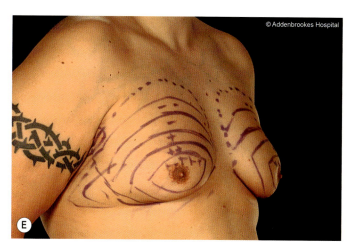

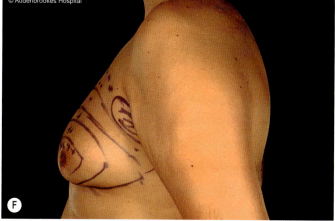

Fig. 11.7, cont'd

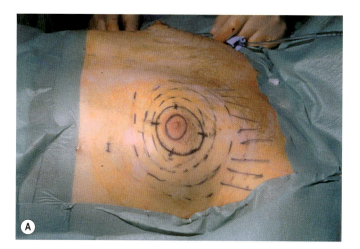

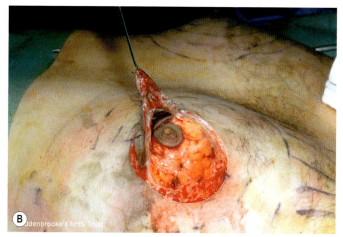

Fig. 11.8 Intraoperative images of conventional liposuction, glandular resection, and concentric skin excision. **(A,B)** The markings are similar to the Benelli periareolar mastopexy technique with the solid lines outlining the extent of skin resection. The doughnut is de-epithelialized.

Continued

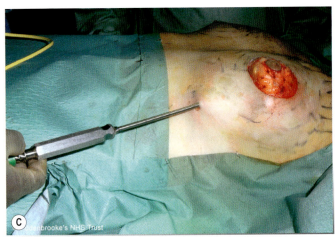

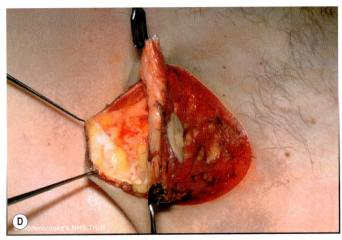

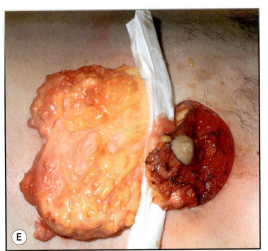

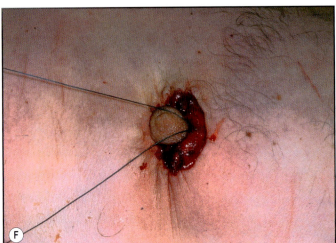

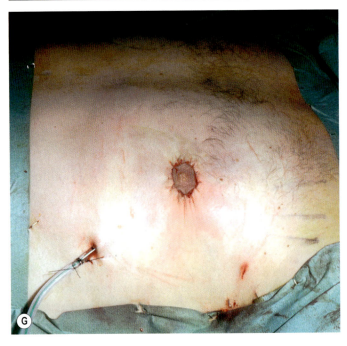

Fig. 11.8, cont'd (C,D) Conventional liposuction is subsequently performed, and the residual breast tissue then excised, leaving the nipple areolar complex vascularized on a superior pedicle. **(E–G)** Following tissue resection, a periareolar purse-string suture is placed with subsequent skin closure using 4/0 vicryl deep dermal and 4/0 monocryl subcuticular sutures. A suction drain is placed following extensive tissue resections.

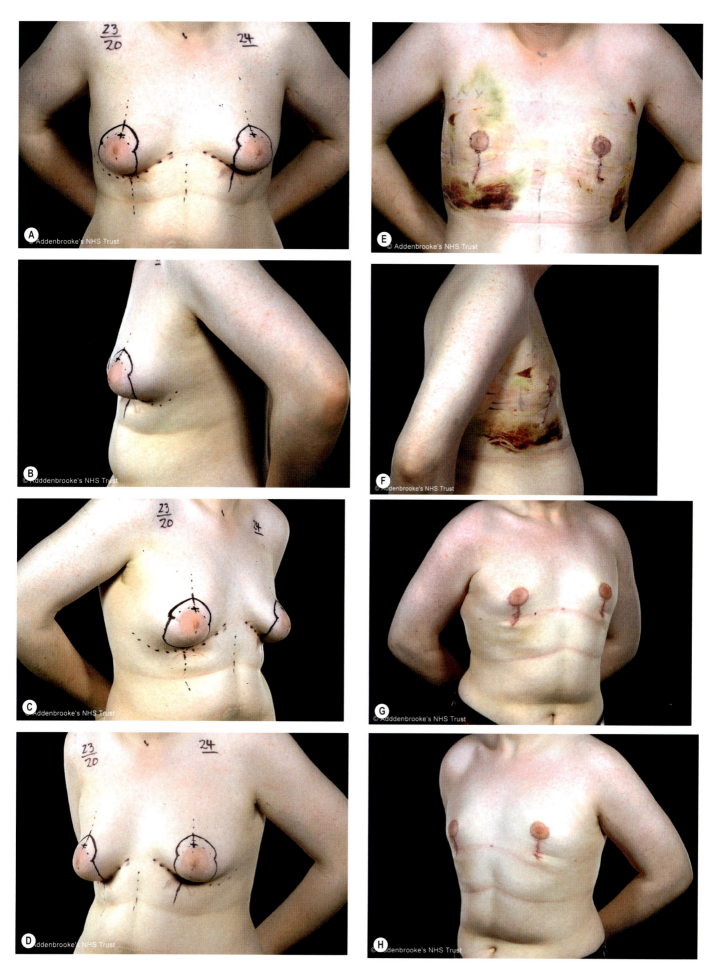

Fig. 11.9 A 17-year-old patient with bilateral gynecomastia of large size, firm consistency, and grade 1 ptosis treated by conventional liposuction, glandular resection, and LeJour skin pattern excision. **(A–D)** Preoperative appearance with markings and **(E,F)** postoperative results 1 week (top 2) and 2 months later **(G,H)**. Note the flat chest contour in the lateral and oblique views.

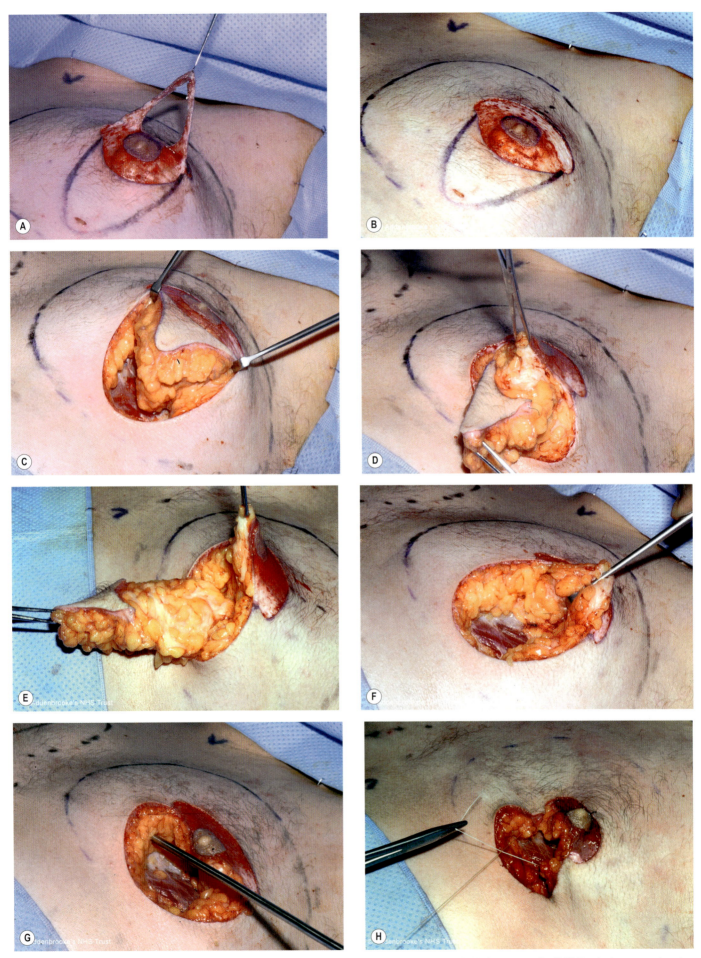

Fig. 11.10 Intraoperative images of conventional liposuction, glandular resection, and LeJour skin excision of left sided gynecomastia. **(A,B)** Standard area around areolar de-epithelialized. **(C,D)** Central glandular tissue with overlying skin resected. **(E,F)** Following resection, the nipple areolar complex is left on a thin pedicle to avoid excessive upper pole fullness. **(G,H)** The lateral pillars are clearly delineated and are approximated with 2/0 vicryl.

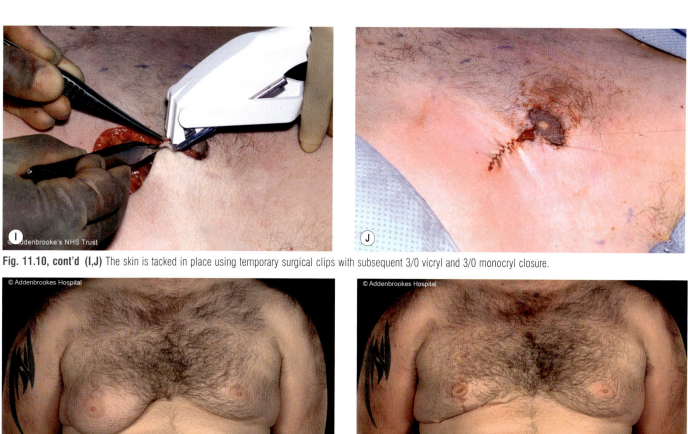

Fig. 11.10, cont'd (I,J) The skin is tacked in place using temporary surgical clips with subsequent 3/0 vicryl and 3/0 monocryl closure.

Fig. 11.11 A 45-year-old patient with right-sided gynecomastia of large size, firm consistency, skin excess, and pseudoptosis, treated with conventional liposuction, glandular resection, and Wise pattern skin excision. **(A–C)** Preoperative appearance and **(D–F)** postoperative result 5 months later. He had a suboptimal result with poor scars but good symmetry at 5 months.

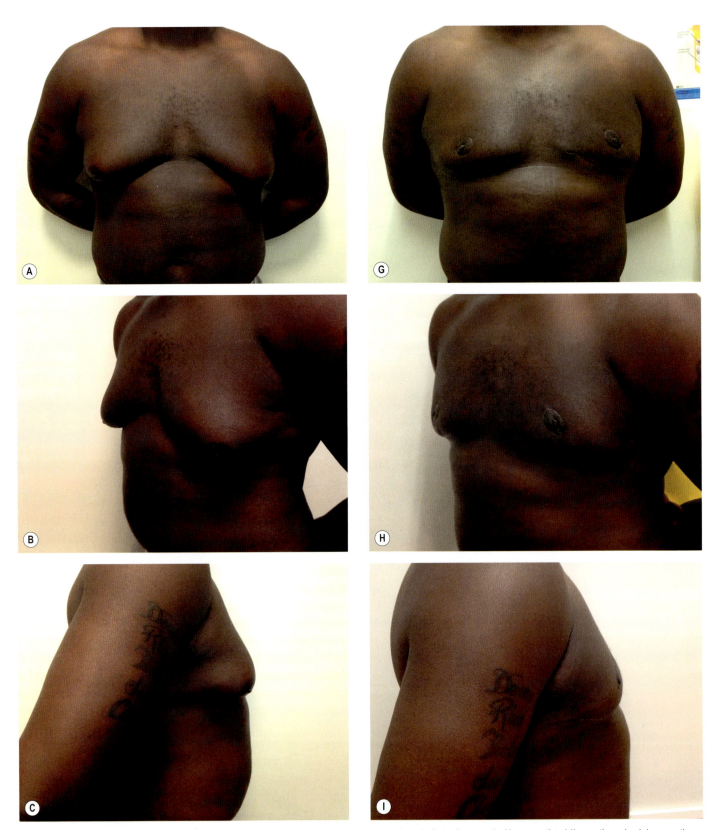

Fig. 11.12 A 37-year-old patient with bilateral gynecomastia of large size, firm consistency, and grade 2 ptosis, treated with conventional liposuction, glandular resection, and Lalonde-type skin excision with no vertical scar. **(A–C)** Preoperative appearance and **(D–F)** markings. The neoareola is 20 mm wide, and its lower border must be located at least 4 cm above the upper incision. **(G–I)** Postoperative result 4 months later. The horizontal scar is rather long, but the lack of a vertical scar avoids the telltale appearances of a female breast reduction.

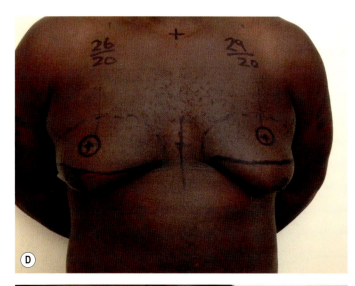

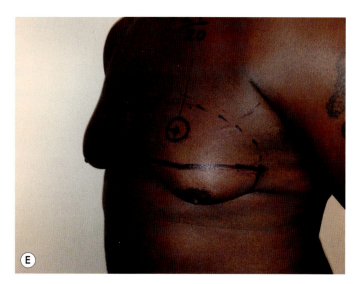

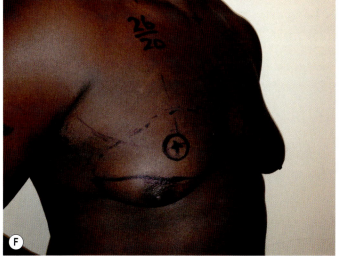

Fig. 11.12, cont'd

contraction. However, tight adherence to underlying tissues from internal scarring can sometimes be a problem. We reserve skin reduction and excisional techniques for severe gynecomastia with significant excess after attempted liposuction.

Algorithmic approach to gynecomastia surgery

From our experience we have proposed a unifying approach to gynecomastia surgery (Fig. 11.14) which seeks to maximize the strengths of the above different modalities while minimizing the drawbacks of each technique.[6] In our practice, the starting point for all cases is liposuction, even in those with firm subareolar discs. While the latter group may still need open excision, the initial liposuction facilitates the surgery[6,62] by pretunneling, reducing bleeding, and contouring the peripheries to prevent saucerization.

We always consent patients for the potential need for open excision. Webster's technique via an inferior peri-areolar incision is indicated for firm subareolar lumps and for residual glandular tissue following liposuction. It is also technically easier to undertake liposuction at the beginning of the operation rather than after excision. Liposuction should therefore be performed to the maximum extent to start with. Liposuction also stimulates skin contraction, particularly with the ultrasound-assisted modality. In our practice, conventional liposuction is only used when UAL is not available because the latter is more efficacious.[54] Although the superiority of UAL is not universally accepted, we have shown it to be a more effective modality in treating gynecomastia based on the objective parameters of intraoperative conversion to open excision and need for subsequent revisional surgery.[54]

Liposuction followed by open excision is very effective for most patients and has also been advocated for

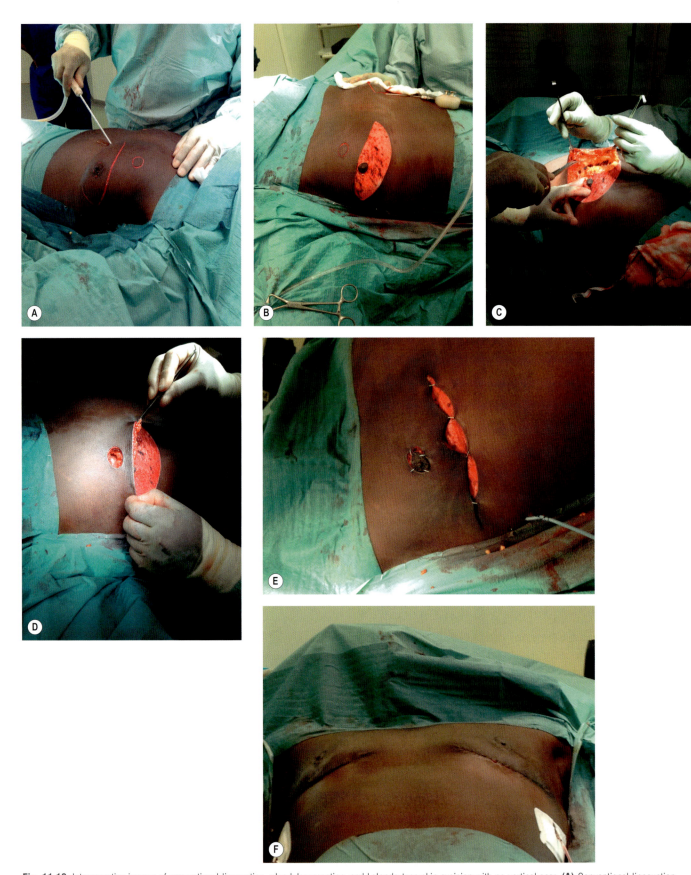

Fig. 11.13 Intraoperative images of conventional liposuction, glandular resection, and Lalonde-type skin excision with no vertical scar. **(A)** Conventional liposuction, **(B)** de-epithelialization of an ellipse extending from the inframammary folds to a horizontal line about 4 cm below the neoareola "button hole", **(C)** raising of skin flaps prior to glandular resection, **(D,E)** redraping of skin flaps and neoareola, **(F)** closure.

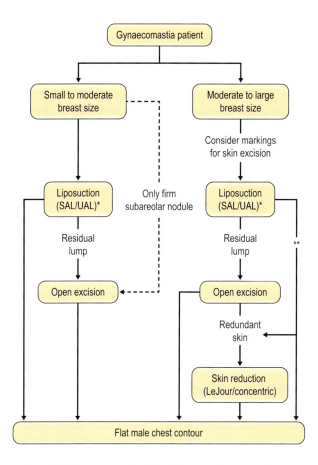

*If available UAL is preferred to SAL, as it is more efficacious and stimulates better skin contraction

**Excellent skin quality combined with the use of UAL may totally obviate the need for open excision and skin reduction

Fig. 11.14 Diagrammatic algorithm for a practical approach to the surgical treatment of gynecomastia. SAL, suction-assisted lipectomy; UAL, ultrasound-assisted liposuction. *(From: Fruhstorfer BH, Malata CM. A systematic approach to the surgical treatment of gynaecomastia. Br J Plast Surg. 2003;56:237–246.)*

marked gynecomastia with skin excess[95,99–102] as long as patients are made aware that they may need a second-stage procedure 6 months later to address any residual excess skin. Conventional liposuction is effective for soft to moderately firm breasts, especially those with a diffuse distribution. It is particularly unsuccessful in patients with firm discrete subareolar lumps.

When there is skin excess or ptosis, we prefer to address this at the original operation.[103] This is especially so in cases with poor or borderline skin elasticity. Such patients needing skin reduction also benefit from initial liposuction as it reduces the bulk; these patients are often obese and therefore need tapering at the breast–fat junction. The periareolar concentric mastopexy-type reduction results in pleats or skin folds that settle down satisfactorily after 2–3 months. However, the periareolar Benelli suture is sometimes palpable, and the knot needs

to be buried deep to the dermis. The scars may also stretch, and caution should be exercised in patients prone to hypertrophic or keloid scarring. The vertical component of the LeJour mammaplasty scar, like the lateral wedge excision, is noticeable but leads to dramatic improvement in contour. Surprisingly, it is quite well accepted by patients[6]. A lateral gathering and resection of the excess skin has been suggested by some, but it may lead to nipples being positioned too laterally. Skin reduction is an integral part of gynecomastia surgery.

Postoperative care

Drains are not routinely used, except for large resections or when skin reduction is performed, such as in post massive weight loss patients.[104] Following the procedure, a pressure dressing consisting of fluffed-up gauze or Reston foam (3M Health Care, Borken, Germany) is applied and held in place with Microfoam or Mefix tape. Patients are instructed to wear a gynecomastia pressure garment day and night for 4–6 weeks. Oral antibiotics are continued for a total of 5 days.

Outcomes, prognosis, and complications

Although many plastic surgeons can obtain excellent results using many treatment modalities, there is a plethora of techniques. Therefore, a logical and integrated approach along the above lines can lead to predictable results in the surgical management of gynecomastia. Our starting point for all cases of gynecomastia is liposuction, even in those cases with firm subareolar discs, because it facilitates subsequent open excision. It is also technically easier to undertake liposuction at the beginning of the operation rather than after excision. We only use conventional liposuction when ultrasonic liposuction is not available.

In patients in whom open excision is not mandated by the appearance and consistency we always consent them for open excision in case the liposuction leaves significant residual stromal tissue. Whenever there is skin excess and/or ptosis, we prefer to address the skin excess at the original operation especially in cases of poor or borderline skin elasticity. This is in order to avoid skin redundancy postoperatively. The choice of skin reduction technique depends to a large extent on the surgeon's preference. We favor the periareolar concentric mastopexy-type reduction.

The possible complications of gynecomastia surgery are shown in Box 11.5. Prior to the advent of liposuction,

- Bleeding and hematoma formation
- Seroma formation
- Infection
- Skin/nipple necrosis
- Contour deformity such as nipple inversion or depression
- Altered sensation of the nipples
- Skin redundancy
- Residual asymmetry
- Adverse scars (wide, hypertrophy, keloid, pigmentation)
- Overcorrection, undercorrection
- Occasional need for revision surgery: asymmetry, residual tissue, skin Xs, depressed nipples
- "Recurrence"

Table 11.3 Summary of gynecomastia surgery perioperative information for patients

Procedure time	90–120 min
Anesthetic time	General
Hospital stay	Day surgery, but occasionally 1 night stay
Time off work	1–2 weeks
No driving	1–2 weeks
Pressure garment	4–6 weeks
No sports	6–8 weeks

gynecomastia surgery was historically associated with a high rate of complication: notably hematoma formation, seromas, disfiguring scars, retraction of the nipple, and reduced nipple sensitivity.[97,98,105] Table 11.3 summarizes the perioperative advice we give to patients.

Secondary procedures

Gynecomastia patients are by and large a surgically challenging group of patients, not least because of their high expectations of surgery. In patients who have undergone surgical treatment it is sometimes necessary to perform revision surgery several months after the initial operation for a variety of reasons. These include inadequate correction, patient dissatisfaction[10], presence of painful residual lumps, asymmetries, and "recurrence" (often related to weight gain). Overcorrection is rare. Similar to other surgical conditions, the need for revision surgery is an objective indicator of the effectiveness of a particular treatment.

Conclusion

Today the surgeon is faced with a wide range of excisional and liposuction procedures for gynecomastia. We have presented an integrated approach to surgical management and highlighted the roles of the different treatment modalities. It is often difficult even for experienced surgeons to choose the most appropriate treatment. Sometimes combinations of these modalities are needed depending on the degree of gynecomastia.

In conclusion, surgical treatment of gynecomastia consists of three basic steps that may not all be necessary in a given patient: liposuction, open excision, and skin reduction. Liposuction should always be used in diffuse or large breast enlargements. It can be optional in the small breast with a firm, subareolar nodule, but facilitates the subsequent open excision. Our results with ultrasonic liposuction have led us to conclude that, when available, it is preferable to conventional liposuction because it is more efficacious and stimulates better skin contraction. Furthermore, there may also be less bruising. Following liposuction, the consistency of the breast is again assessed and open excision is performed if a residual lump is present. Skin excision is indicated if there is still noticeable skin excess. The choice between concentric, vertical scar (LeJour technique), and elliptical skin reduction depends largely on the amount of skin excess to be resected and also the surgeon's experience.

Although many plastic surgeons can obtain excellent results using many treatment modalities, today's surgeon who is faced with a plethora of techniques can achieve predictable results with high patient satisfaction by following a pragmatic approach along the lines that we have proposed.

6. Fruhstorfer BH, Malata CM. A systematic approach to the surgical treatment of gynaecomastia. *Br J Plast Surg.* 2003;56:237–246. *First comprehensive algorithmic approach to the surgical management of gynecomastia. It takes into account breast size, consistency, skin excess, and skin quality.*

8. Petty PM, Solomon M, Buchel EW, Tran NV. Gynecomastia: evolving paradigm of management and comparison of techniques. *Plast Reconstr Surg.* 2010;125:1301–1308. *An algorithmic approach to gynecomastia surgery, which establishes the role of minimally invasive*

arthroscopic excision of firm to moderately firm and large gynecomastia using remote incisions.

11. Webster JP. Mastectomy for gynecomastia through a semicircular intra-areolar incision. *Ann Surg.* 1946;124:557–575. *Original description of the time-honored Webster's technique of periareolar approach to open excision for gynecomastia.*

13. Teimourian B, Perlman R. Surgery for gynecomastia. *Aesthetic Plast Surg.* 1983;7:155–157. *First description of liposuction combined with open excision for gynecomastia treatment. This has become a widely accepted*

method because of the frequent difficulty of removing breast parenchyma by suction alone.

14. Zocchi M. Ultrasonic liposculpturing. *Aesthetic Plast Surg.* 1992;16:287–298. *Ultrasound-assisted liposuction was pioneered by Michele Zocchi in the 1980s as described in this paper.*

24. Braunstein GD. Gynecomastia. *N Engl J Med.* 1993;328:490–495. *Excellent overview of gynecomastia including prevalence, pathogenesis, and treatment.*

36. Simon BE, Hoffman S, Kahn S. Classification and surgical correction of gynecomastia. *Plast Reconstr Surg.* 1973;51:48–52. *Widely quoted practical clinical classification of gynecomastia taking into account the size of the breast and amount of redundant skin.*

54. Wong KY, Malata CM. Conventional versus ultrasound-assisted liposuction in gynaecomastia surgery: a 13-year review. *J Plast Reconstr Aesthet Surg.* 2014;67:921–926. *First paper to objectively compare suction-assisted and ultrasound-assisted liposuction in gynecomastia surgery.*

55. Rosenberg GJ. Gynecomastia: suction lipectomy as a contemporary solution. *Plast Reconstr Surg.* 1987;80:379–386. *Gary Rosenberg popularized the use of suction-assisted liposuction beyond the confines of the breast in order to facilitate contouring and postoperative redraping of the skin in gynecomastia surgery.*

57. Hodgson ELB, Fruhstorfer BH, Malata CM. Ultrasonic liposuction in the treatment of gynecomastia. *Plast Reconstr Surg.* 2005;116:646–653, discussion 654–655. *Evaluation of ultrasound-assisted liposuction for gynecomastia surgery.*

12

Breast implant-associated anaplastic large cell lymphoma (ALCL)

Mark W. Clemens II and Roberto N. Miranda

SYNOPSIS

- Breast implant-associated anaplastic large cell lymphoma (BIA-ALCL) is a distinct type of T-cell lymphoma involving the capsule or effusion surrounding a breast implant that can present in patients receiving either reconstructive or cosmetic breast implants.
- BIA-ALCL presents in two-thirds of cases as a delayed (>1 year) periprosthetic fluid collection, and as a capsular mass in one-third of cases. One in eight patients will present with lymphadenopathy.
- Optimal screening tools include ultrasound or positron emission tomography (PET)/computed tomography (CT) with directed fine-needle aspiration. Diagnosis should be made prior to surgical intervention.
- Tissue, implants, and fluid specimens from suspected cases should be sent to pathology for CD30 immunohistochemistry with a clinical history and to "rule out ALCL".
- Operative treatment of confirmed cases should include removal of bilateral implants, resection of the entire capsule, and complete excision of the disease including involved lymph nodes.
- The role of adjunctive treatments such as chemotherapy, chest wall radiation, anti-CD30 immunotherapy, and stem cell transplant for advanced disease is under investigation.

Introduction

BIA-ALCL is a rare T-cell lymphoma arising around breast implants placed either for reconstructive or cosmetic indications. Safety communications by the United States Food and Drug Administration (FDA) in 2011, 2016, and 2017 cautioning about BIA-ALCL and textured breast implants including clinical presentation, prognosis, and treatment options, and subsequently increased public and physician awareness.[1] This warning was based upon case reports dating back to a sentinel case described by Keech and Creech in 1997.[2] Since the FDA safety communication in 2011, a number of major government agencies around the world have developed BIA-ALCL patient and physician recommendations.

The National Comprehensive Cancer Network (NCCN) released standardized diagnosis and treatment guidelines for BIA-ALCL in 2016 which was subsequently adopted by the American Society of Plastic Surgeons (ASPS) and the American Society of Aesthetic Plastic Surgeons (ASAPS).[2a,3] The World Health Organization (WHO) has officially recognized BIA-ALCL as a subset of ALCL, and in 2014 its intergovernmental agency, the International Agency for Research on Cancer (IARC), designated BIA-ALCL a priority for further research to determine malignancy etiology and mechanism of pathogenesis.[4] In 2015, the US National Cancer Institute (NCI) posted specific surgical recommendations for the treatment of BIA-ALCL.[5] In 2015, the French National Cancer Institute (Agence Nationale de Sécurité du Médicament) released diagnosis and treatment recommendations for BIA-ALCL and mandated that all breast implants carry a warning that a clearly established link exists between breast implants and ALCL.[6] The past two decades have been marked by a transition from limited case reports of a novel periprosthetic T-cell lymphoma to our current understanding and recognition of BIA-ALCL.[7] Several evolving concepts have helped to define diagnostic tools, therapeutic strategies, and outcomes of BIA-ALCL and are the focus of this chapter.

Lymphoma background

Lymphoma is a cancer of the immune system developing from lymphocytes and is the most common malignancy of the blood.[8] Lymphoma broadly includes Hodgkin's lymphoma, non-Hodgkin's lymphoma (NHL), and a variety of lymphoproliferative disorders. In the USA, approximately 65 000 cases of NHL were diagnosed in

2010.[9] Stein and colleagues first described ALCL in 1985 as a novel type of NHL characterized by large anaplastic lymphoid cells that express the cell surface protein CD30.[10] Estimated incidence of T-cell NHL diagnoses in the USA in 2014 was 17 302.[11] This included 1982 cases of ALCL, 758 of which occurred in females.[12]

ALCL was added as a distinct entity to the Kiel classification in 1988 and to the Revised European-American Lymphoma (REAL) classification in 1994.[13] The WHO classification of lymphomas recognized the disease in 2001 and further delineated variants in their updated 2008 classification.[14,15] NHL prognosis is determined using the International Prognostic Index (IPI) based upon presence of recognized risk factors such as the Ann Arbor staging system, advanced age, elevated serum lactate dehydrogenase (LDH), poor performance status, and increased number of extranodal sites of disease.[16] Clinicopathologic subtypes of ALCL include a spectrum of diseases from the more aggressive systemic ALCL down to the indolent CD30 positive lymphoproliferative disorders of the skin that include a benign lymphomatoid papulosis and sometimes the indolent primary cutaneous ALCL (5-year OS (overall survival)>90–95%, lymph node metastases 5%).[17] Multiple sites of disease, frequent lymphadenopathy, and wide dissemination characterize systemic ALCL. Systemic ALCL is further classified by either the expression or absence of the anaplastic lymphoma kinase (ALK) tyrosine kinase receptor gene translocation. ALK is most commonly expressed as a result of the t(2;5) translocation involving the 2p23 and the 5q35 chromosomes that create an oncogenic fusion protein of the ALK gene and the nucleophosmin gene.[18] ALK+ ALCL accounts for approximately 50–80% of all ALCLs, occurs most commonly in males (male/female ratio: 6.5:1) under the age of 30 years, and has a 5-year OS by IPI point value of 0/1: 90%, 2: 68%, 3: 33%, 4/5: 23%.[5] In contrast, ALK– ALCL is an immunophenotypically and cytogenetically heterogeneous group and has a 5-year OS by IPI points value of 0/1: 74%, 2: 62%, 3: 31%, 4/5: 13%. Standard first-line chemotherapy is cyclophosphamide, hydroxy-daunorubicin, vincristine, and prednisone (CHOP), and refractory disease is treated with ifosfamide, carboplatin, etoposide (ICE), or etoposide, methylprednisone, cytarabine, cisplatin (ESHAP).[19] When treated with chemotherapy, ALK+ ALCL has a higher overall 5-year survival rate than systemic ALK– ALCL (58% vs. 34%, respectively).[20,21] As a percentage of all T-cell lymphomas, ALK+ ALCL is more common in North America than Europe or Asia (16.0% vs. 6.4% vs. 3.2%, respectively). Systemic ALK– ALCL is more common in Europe than North America or Asia (9.4% vs. 7.8% vs. 2.6%, respectively).[22]

BIA-ALCL: a new entity

BIA-ALCL is distinct from primary breast lymphoma (PBL), which is a disease of the breast parenchyma, representing 0.04–0.5% of breast cancers and 1–2% of all lymphomas.[23] PBL is predominantly a B-cell lymphoma (65–90%),[24,25] while BIA-ALCL is purely a T-cell lymphoma arising either in an effusion surrounding the implant or or in scar capsule surrounding a breast implant.[26,27] All confirmed reported cases of BIA-ALCL are ALK– and express the CD30 cell surface protein (Box 12.1, Figs. 12.1A,B & 12.2). Most cases are diagnosed during implant revision surgery performed for a late-onset (>1 year), persistent seroma and may be associated with symptoms of pain, breast lumps, swelling, or breast asymmetry. The number of BIA-ALCL cases reported in primary augmentation and reconstruction for breast cancer or prophylaxis are nearly equivalent; however, the number of women receiving augmentation implants outnumbers by double those women receiving reconstructive implants. BIA-ALCL most commonly follows an indolent course provided there is adequate surgical ablation of the implant and surrounding capsule without systemic therapy, but aggressive exceptions, disease progression, and death have been reported.[28] No risk factors have been clearly identified for ALCL though many have been theorized including the presence of a subclinical biofilm, response to particulate from textured implants, a consequence of capsular contracture or repeated capsular trauma (such as with closed capsulotomies), genetic predisposition, or an autoimmune etiology, but these observations have not been confirmed in formal epidemiological studies.[29] Recent studies have demonstrated a possible pathogenic mechanism of chronic T-cell stimulation with local antigenic drive, ultimately leading to the development of lymphoma.[30] Further research is required to identify modifiable risk factors, susceptible populations, and optimal screening and surveillance modalities.

BOX 12.1 Criteria for diagnosis of breast implant-associated anaplastic large cell lymphoma

1. A tumor with adequate pathologic specimen for analysis, involving an effusion either surrounding a breast implant or lining a breast implant capsule.

2. Neoplasm with large lymphoid cells with abundant cytoplasm and pleomorphic nuclei.

3. Tumor demonstrates uniform expression of CD30 by immunohistochemistry and a single clonally expanded T-cell population by flow cytometry.

4. Negative for anaplastic lymphoma kinase (ALK) protein or translocations involving the ALK gene at chromosome 2q23.

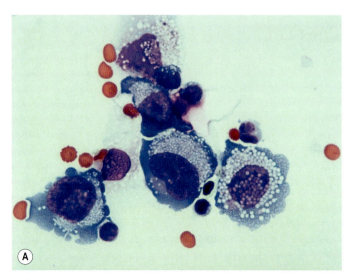

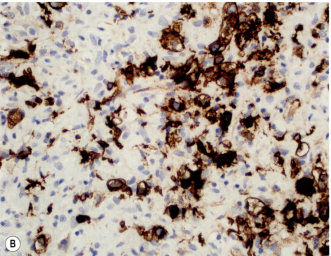

Fig. 12.1 (A) Wright Giemsa staining from a malignant effusion of breast implant-associated anaplastic large cell lymphoma (BIA-ALCL) demonstrating pleomorphic cells with horseshoe shaped nuclei, nuclear folding, and abundant vacuolated cytoplasm (1000× magnification). **(B)** Immunohistochemistry in tissue section demonstrates sheets of large cells positive for CD30 in a case of BIA-ALCL. *(From: Clemens MW, Miranda RN. Coming of age, breast implant-associated anaplastic large cell lymphoma after 18 years of investigation. Clin Plast Surg. 2015;42(4).)*

included nine patient deaths associated with the disease. de Jong and colleagues reported an individually matched case control study from the Netherlands nationwide pathology database.[60] The pathology database served a total population of approximately nine million women. The authors found a positive association for the development of ALCL in women with breast implants compared to those without an implant, with an odds ratio of 18.2 (95% confidence interval, 2.1–156.8). Based upon this data, the authors estimated an incidence of 0.1–0.3 per 100 000 BIA-ALCL cases for women with prostheses per year. A number of prior studies failed to show an association between breast augmentation and risk of lymphoma; however, these studies were limited by the number of patients enrolled or by the insufficient time period of follow-up.[61–63] These studies underscore the difficulty of determining the incidence and prevalence of a very rare and recently recognized clinical entity. The United States FDA Manufacturer and User Facility Device Experience (MAUDE) database has received 359 adverse event reports of ALCL in women with breast implants as of February 1, 2017.[59] However, the FDA deems this data as potentially duplicative, unverified, and unreliable. The ASPS/FDA collaboration PROFILE prospective registry reports 149 unique pathologically confirmed BIA-ALCL cases in the United States as of June 1, 2017. In a review of the top 40 global breast implant markets worldwide, 464 adverse event reports of BIA-ALCL were reported to government authorities.

An MD Anderson epidemiology study estimated a lifetime prevalence of BIA-ALCL of 1:30,000 by comparing pathologically confirmed cases in the United States (US) with US textured implant sales. This study presumed that BIA-ALCL occurs only in textured breast implants).[59b] This incidence was 67.6 times higher than that of primary ALCL of the breast in the general population. Mcguire and colleagues reported the results of

Epidemiology

Since 1997, approximately 99 patients have been reported either in case reports of BIA-ALCL or literature reviews (Fig. 12.3).[31–57] Reporting has benefitted from formal recognition and wider physician education, which has led to an exponential increase in published cases over the last few years. Reliable epidemiological data for the incidence and prevalence of BIA-ALCL has been difficult to determine for the estimated eleven million-plus women worldwide with breast implants.[58] The FDA database has received approximately 359 adverse event reports of ALCL in women with breast implants, which were reported to the Manufacturer and User Facility Device Experience (MAUDE) database as of February 2017. This

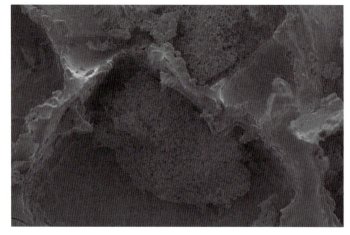

Fig. 12.2 Scanning electron micrograph (300× magnification) demonstrating aggregates of lymphoma cells clustered on the surface of a textured silicone implant.

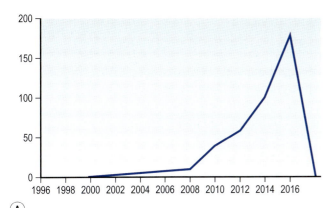

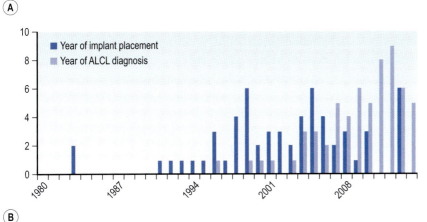

Fig. 12.3 (A) Timeline of published cases of breast implant-associated anaplastic large cell lymphoma (BIA-ALCL) as well as **(B)** year of implant placement and diagnosis of BIA-ALCL.

the US FDA mandated CA/CARE Trial of Biocell implants, which was the largest series ever reported for any type of textured implant, and included 17,656 women receiving 31,985 Biocell textured implants. Within that series, six cases of breast implant–associated ALCL cases occurred resulting in a risk of 1:2943 (95%CI:1350,8000).[59c] In 2016, the Australian Therapeutic Goods Administration released an update on BIA-ALCL estimating a disease risk of 1 in 1000 to 1 in 10,000 women with textured implants based on data from 60 national cases and reported manufacturer specific risks of Allergan Biocell (1:3705), Silimed polyurethane (1:3894), and Mentor Siltex (1:60631).[59d] This discrepancy in risk between Australia and US data may be due to geographic predisposition or physician reporting and requires further study.

Diagnosis and treatment

The diagnosis and treatment of BIA-ALCL follows standardized guidelines established by the National Comprehensive Cancer Network (NCCN). Diagnosis of BIA-ALCL can be difficult as it remains relatively rare at most medical centers. Two-thirds of BIA-ALCL patients will present as a malignant effusion associated with the fibrous capsule surrounding an implant occurring on average 9 years after implantation. Any seroma occurring greater than 1 year after implantation not readily explainable by infection or trauma should be considered suspicious for disease (Fig. 12.4).[48] One-third of patients present with a mass, which may indicate a more aggressive clinical course.[68] Adrada and colleagues reviewed 44 BIA-ALCL patients with imaging studies and reported on the sensitivity/specificity for detecting an effusion using ultrasound (84%/75%), computerized tomography (55%/83%), magnetic resonance imaging (82%/33%), and PET (38%/83%).[64] Additionally, the sensitivity/specificity to detect a BIA-ALCL mass was reported for ultrasound (46%/100%), computerized tomography (50%/100%), magnetic resonance imaging (82%/33%), and PET (64%/88%). The sensitivity of mammography was found to be inferior for BIA-ALCL effusion and mass. Ultrasound is utilized at our institution as a screening tool for suspected cases and in combination with PET for confirmed cases to determine extension and for surveillance of disease.

For suspected patients, any aspiration of periprosthetic fluid should be sent to pathology for cytologic evaluation and include a clinical history with the stated intent to "rule out BIA-ALCL". Pathologic evaluation may demonstrate BIA-ALCL as individual cells, cell clusters in aggregates, or as coherent sheets. Diagnosis by hematoxylin and eosin staining alone can be difficult; however, BIA-ALCL will demonstrate strong and uniform membranous expression of CD30 immunohistochemistry. Other T cell antigens are expressed variably

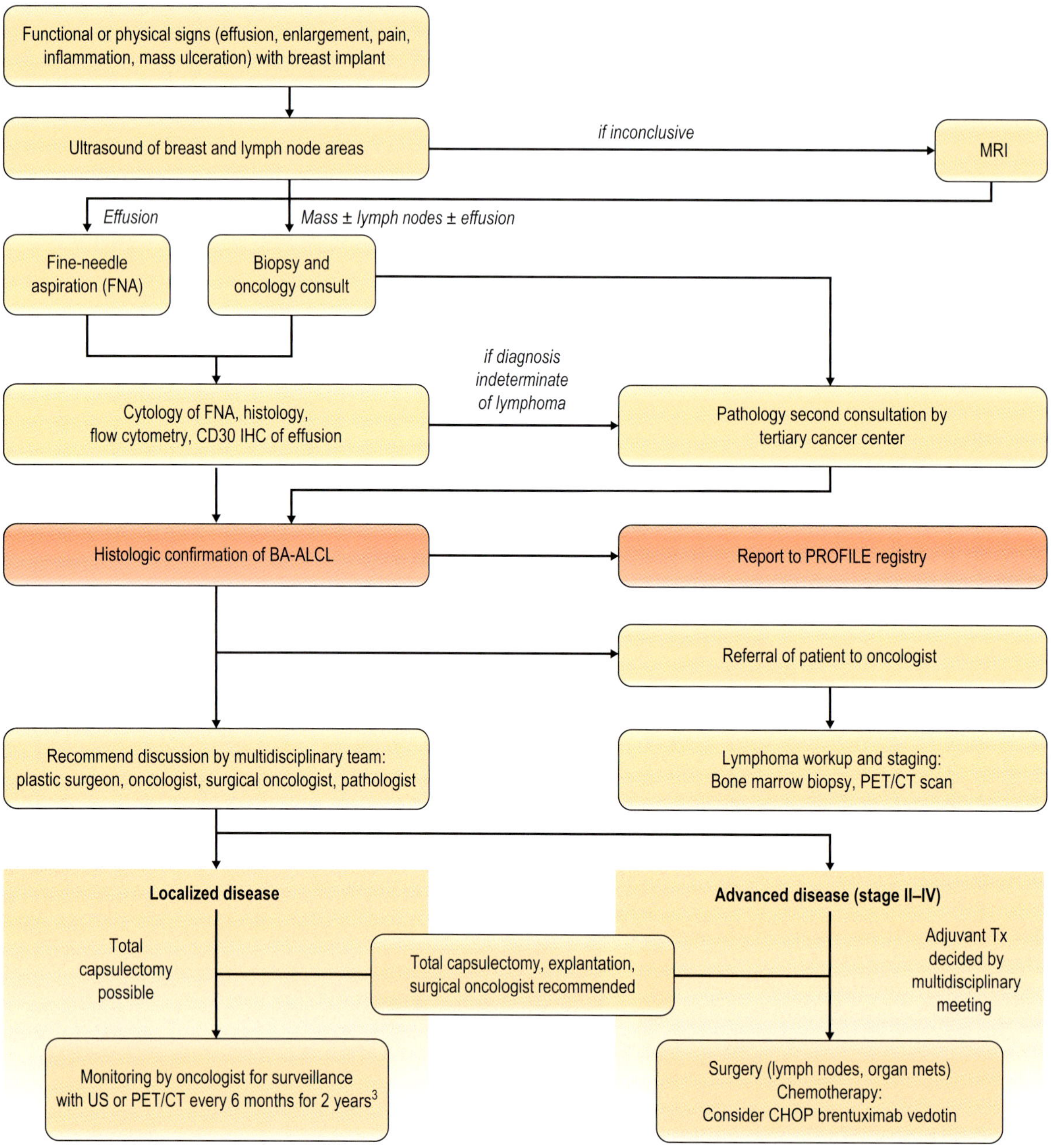

Fig. 12.4 Diagnosis and Management of BIA-ALCL follows standardized guidelines of the National Comprehensive Cancer Network (NCCN). Approach to a patient with a delayed seroma and treatment of BIA-ALCL are summarized above per NCCN guidelines. Abbreviations: CHOP: cyclophosphamide, hydroxydaunorubicin, vincristine, and prednisone; IHC: immunohistochemistry; PROFILE: Patient Registry and Outcomes For breast Implants and anaplastic large cell Lymphoma etiology and Epidemiology, www.thepsf.org/PROFILE (From: Clemens MW, Butler CE. ASPS/PSF efforts on BIA-ALCL. Plastic Surgery News. 2015;26(7).)

with the most common being CD4 (80–84%), CD43 (80–88%), CD3 (30–46%), CD45 (36%), and CD2 (30%).[65] Expression of CD5, CD7, CD8, or CD15 is rare. Ultrasound may help define the extent of a seroma and can be helpful in identifying any associated capsule masses. Clinical examination should include evaluation of regional lymph nodes. Volumes of an effusion can range from 20 to 1000 mL and is typically viscous. The surrounding capsule may be thickened and fibrous or may be deceptively normal in appearance, consistent with the under appreciation of this lymphoma. If a mass is present, it can protrude into the implant creating a mass

effect distortion on imaging, or the mass may protrude outward into the soft tissue.

Patients with biopsy proven BIA-ALCL must be referred to a lymphoma oncologist. Surgical treatment of BIA-ALCL requires complete tumor ablation, which includes removal of the implant, complete removal of any disease mass with negative margins, and total capsulectomy. Because an implant capsule may drain to multiple regional lymph node basins, there does not appear to be a role for sentinel lymph node biopsy in the treatment of BIA-ALCL. Fine-needle aspiration of enlarged lymph nodes can yield a false negative, and

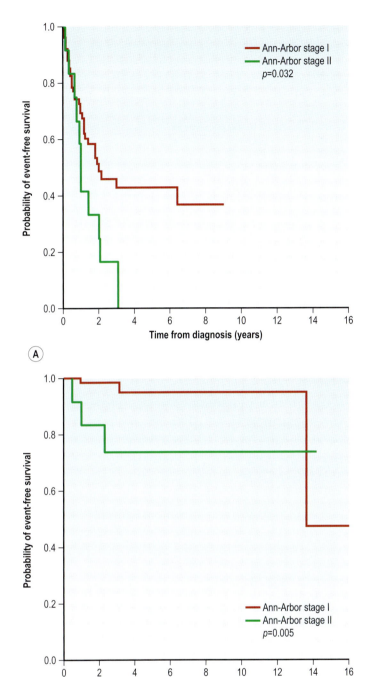

Fig. 12.5 Survival curves according to Ann Arbor stage. **(A)** Event-free survival, **(B)** overall survival. *(From: Clemens MW, Medeiros LJ, Butler CE, et al. Complete surgical excision is essential for patients with breast implant-associated anaplastic large cell lymphoma. J Surg Onc. 2016;34(2):160-168.)*

resection may be the definitive treatment in the majority of cases. Surgery should be performed with strict onco-logic technique including use of specimen orientation sutures, placement of surgical clips within the tumor bed, and use of new instruments if performing a contra-lateral explantation. At this time, the FDA does not recommend screening or prophylactic implant removal for asymptomatic patients or patients with familial susceptibility cancer. Although reimplantation is not recommended, several BIA-ALCL patients have received implant replacement with a smooth implant following definitive treatment, and these patients are being closely monitored for any disease sequelae.

Staging

Patients with BIA-ALCL or any type of lymphoma are traditionally staged by the 1971 Ann Arbor classifica-tion, which stages disease based upon progression as a "liquid tumor".[66] Under this classification, nearly all BIA-ALCL patients fall under one of two stages, either stage IE (84%) or stage IIE (16%) (Fig. 12.5A & B). Although most patients with BIA-ALCL have a relatively indolent clinical course, reports of deaths attributable to disease emphasize the importance of a timely diagnosis and adequate treatment with appropriate surveillance or else disease progression can occur with detrimental effect. Patients with BIA-ALCL who have died were described as having local or regional extension of their disease, and no patients with BIA-ALCL have developed widely disseminated disease. This pattern of progres-sion suggests that BIA-ALCL is a distinct entity, and displays progression more similar to solid tumors than to other non-Hodgkin lymphomas. This pattern of disease spread is also better suited to a clinical and pathologic staging system modeled after the American Joint Committee on Cancer (AJCC) TNM (tumor, lymph node, metastasis) system for staging solid tumors.[67]

A recent BIA-ALCL TNM staging system is more applicable than the Ann Arbor system for predicting prognosis and for evaluating treatment regimens in patients with BIA-ALCL (Figs. 12.6A,B & 12.7A,B; Table 12.1).[68]

Clinical characteristics and outcomes

The clinico-pathologic features of BIA-ALCL have been reported in several literature reviews. In 2014, Miranda *et al.* reviewed the long-term follow-up of 60 BIA-ALCL patients.[56] The mean age was 52 years old (range 28–87 years) with a median of 9 years (range 1–32 years) between implantation and lymphoma diagnosis. Patients presented with either a malignant effusion or

therefore excisional biopsies should be performed of any suspicious lymph nodes. The involvement of a surgical oncologist in the management of this lymphoma is strongly recommended with the aim of obtaining optimal surgical control. An incomplete resection or inadequate local surgical control may subject the patient to the need for adjunctive treatments such as chemo-therapy and radiation therapy, whereas complete

Table 12.1 Proposed TNM staging for breast implant-associated anaplastic large cell lymphoma

Tumor extent	T1	T2	T3	T4
T	Confined to effusion or a layer on luminal side of capsule	Early capsule infiltration	Cell aggregates or sheets infiltrating the capsule	Lymphoma infiltrates beyond the capsule
Lymph nodes	**N0**	**N1**	**N2**	
N	No lymph node involvement	One regional lymph node (+)	Multiple regional lymph nodes (+)	
Metastasis	**M0**	**M1**		
M	No distant spread	Spread to other organs/ distant sites		
Stages				
IA	T1N0M0			
IB	T2N0M0			
IC	T3N0M0			
IIA	T4N0M0			
IIB	T1-3N1M0			
III	T(4)N(1–2)M0			
IV	T(any)N(any)M1			

TNM, tumor, lymph node, metastasis.

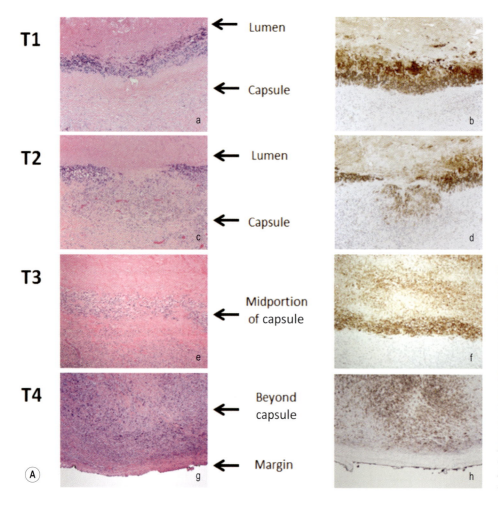

Fig. 12.6 Breast implant-associated anaplastic large cell lymphoma (BIA-ALCL) staging system: this TNM (tumor, lymph node, metastasis) staging system was modeled after the American Joint Committee on Cancer (AJCC) TNM system for solid tumors. T1: Lymphoma cells confined to the effusion or a layer on the luminal side of the capsule (Ia, Ib); T2: lymphoma cells superficially infiltrate the luminal side of the capsule (Ic); T3: clusters or sheets of lymphoma cells infiltrate into the thickness of the capsule (IIa); and T4: lymphoma cells infiltrate beyond the capsule (IIb), into the adjacent soft tissue or breast parenchyma (III, IV). *(From: Clemens MW, Medeiros LJ, Butler CE, et al. Complete surgical excision is essential for patients with breast implant-associated anaplastic large cell lymphoma. J Surg Onc. 2016;34(2):160-168.)*

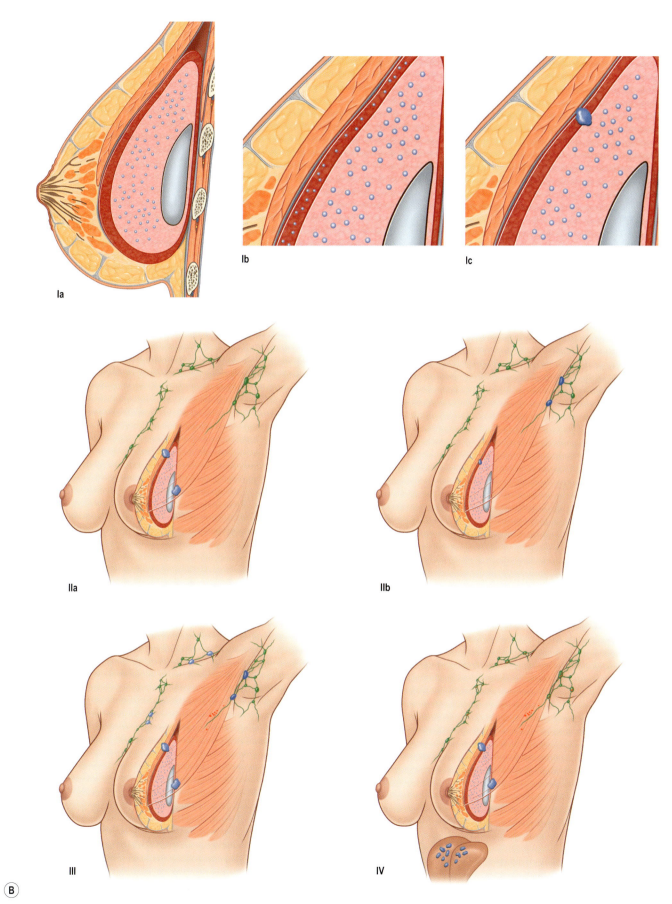

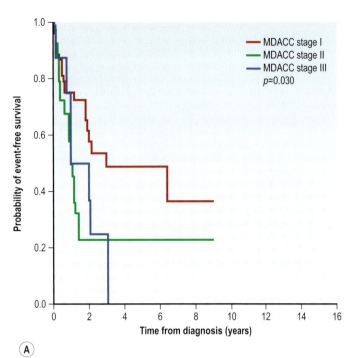

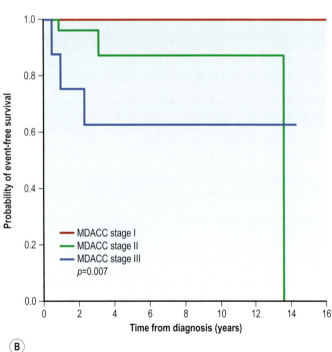

Fig. 12.7 Survival curves according to breast implant-associated anaplastic large cell lymphoma (BIA-ALCL) TNM (tumor, lymph node, metastasis) staging. **(A)** Event-free survival, **(B)** overall survival. MDACC, MD Anderson Cancer Center. *(From: Clemens MW, Medeiros LJ, Butler CE, et al. Complete surgical excision is essential for patients with breast implant-associated anaplastic large cell lymphoma. J Surg Onc. 2016;34(2):160-168.)*

seroma (70%) or a distinct mass (30%). The median OS was 12 years (median follow-up, 2 years; range 0–14 years). A total capsulectomy with implant removal was performed in 93% of patients. Overall survival and progression free survival (PFS) were similar between patients who received and did not receive chemotherapy (p=0.44 and p=0.28, respectively), suggesting that some patients may achieve optimal outcomes with

an adequate surgical approach. Radiation therapy has also been used for local control of disease, and further research is required to determine specific indications for adjunctive treatments. Patients with a breast mass had a worse OS and PFS (p=0.052 and p=0.03, respectively). At this time, it is unclear whether the association of mass and worse prognosis indicates a more aggressive variant, a more progressed disease, or perhaps a consequence of inadequate surgical ablation of tumor infiltration. Event free survival and overall survival by different treatment modalities are summarized in Fig. 12.8A & B.

Hart *et al.* performed a meta-analysis and identified 53 BIA-ALCL patients.[69] For patients with available clinical data, the authors noted rates of 17.3% extracapsular disease and 23.1% with the presence of a mass. Furthermore, 39.6% of patients were treated with surgery alone, 9.4% with surgery and radiation, 18.9% with surgery and chemotherapy, 30.2% with surgery, chemotherapy, and radiation, and 1.9% with chemotherapy alone. At a median follow-up of 15 months (3.6–90 months), disease recurrence was 28.3%, of which 73.3% were treated with salvage chemotherapy. BIA-ALCL was attributed to four patient deaths. Extracapsular disease extension was associated with increased risk for recurrence (p<0.0001) and patient death (p=0.0008). This study also found a statistically significant difference in 3- and 5-year survival rates between patients presenting with and without a mass (p=0.0308 and p=0.0308, respectively). While BIA-ALCL may follow a relatively indolent course in most patients, reports of disseminated cancer and deaths attributed to the disease emphasize the importance of timely diagnosis and adequate treatment with appropriate surveillance.

Brody and colleagues recently reported a summary of 79 published patients and 94 previously unreported cases.[70] The authors report that for all implants where surface characteristics were known, there was at least one textured device used within the patient's surgical history. The authors reconfirm that there are no known pure smooth implant cases and importantly note that BIA-ALCL has been reported in association with all major forms of implant texturing techniques from current implant manufacturers. Microbiology cultures were negative in all cases when taken, although formal biofilm evaluation was not performed. The authors noted that most patients had a slow disease progression and a good prognosis when adequately treated, but conceded occasional lymphadenopathy, metastases, and nine attributable deaths.

Setting research priorities

Further research into the development of primary cell lines and biologic models is important to fully elucidate

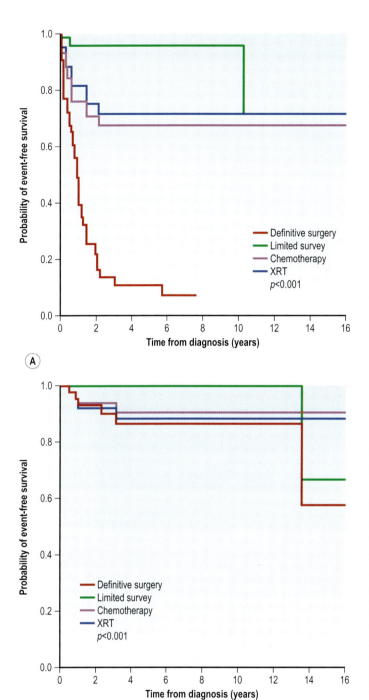

Fig. 12.8 Survival curves according to treatment approaches. **(A)** Event-free survival, **(B)** overall survival. XRT, x-radiation therapy. *(From: Clemens MW, Medeiros LJ, Butler CE, et al. Complete surgical excision is essential for patients with breast implant-associated anaplastic large cell lymphoma. J Surg Onc. 2016;34(2):160-168.)*

the exact etiology and pathogenesis of BIA-ALCL. Lechner and colleagues reported the establishment and characterization of a BIA-ALCL model cell line (TLBR-1) as well as heterotransplantation of the disease into immunocompromised mice. Establishment of cell lines from effusion or excisional biopsies will be important to completely characterize the disease and for the identification of potential molecular targets.

Future research is warranted to determine if certain patients have a predisposition to developing the disease and if any modifiable risk factors exist either with the patient or type of implant utilized. Kim and colleagues recently reported on an updated RAND corporation sponsored multidisciplinary consensus to evaluate current knowledge gaps in diagnosis, management, and surveillance of BIA-ALCL.[71] Panelists agreed that late seromas occurring >1 year after breast implantation should be evaluated via ultrasound, and, if a seroma is present, the fluid should be aspirated and sent to an experienced hematopathologist for culture, cytology, flow cytometry, and cell block. Surgical removal of the affected implant and capsule (as completely as possible) should take place, which is sufficient to eradicate capsule-confined BIA-ALCL; surveillance should consist of clinical follow-up at least every 6 months for at least 5 years and breast ultrasound yearly for at least 2 years; and BIA-ALCL is generally a biologically indolent disease with a good prognosis, unless it extends beyond the capsule and/or presents as a mass. (For patient management examples see Figs. 12.9A–F & 12.10A–C.) The panel disagreed as to whether chemotherapy and radiation therapy should be given to all patients with BIA-ALCL, or which patients may benefit, and recommended further investigation in larger studies with longer follow-up.

Advances in the treatment of T cell lymphomas gives promise for BIA-ALCL refractory to surgical therapy alone. Brentuximab vedotin is a novel anti-CD30 monoclonal antibody that has changed the management of systemic ALCL with a reported objective response rate of 86% and a complete remission rate of 59% in relapsed or refractory systemic ALCL.[72,73] Prospective trials of BIA-ALCL patients at major referral centers may help delineate chemotherapeutic sensitivity and efficacy of novel agents.

Medico-legal considerations

Following recommendations made by the FDA in 2011, implant manufacturers added a written warning, about the existence of BIA-ALCL, to breast implant package inserts within the USA and Canada. Breast implant informed consent examples, which include the risk of BIA-ALCL, were subsequently produced by the American Society of Plastic Surgeons (ASPS) and are available for download from www.plasticsurgery.org. With respect to BIA-ALCL, risk disclosure should have at least three basic objectives. The first objective is to make patients aware of the existence of this rare disease; the second is for patients to understand common presenting symptoms such as a breast mass or delayed-presentation seroma or effusion; and the third is to compel patients to take action and follow-up

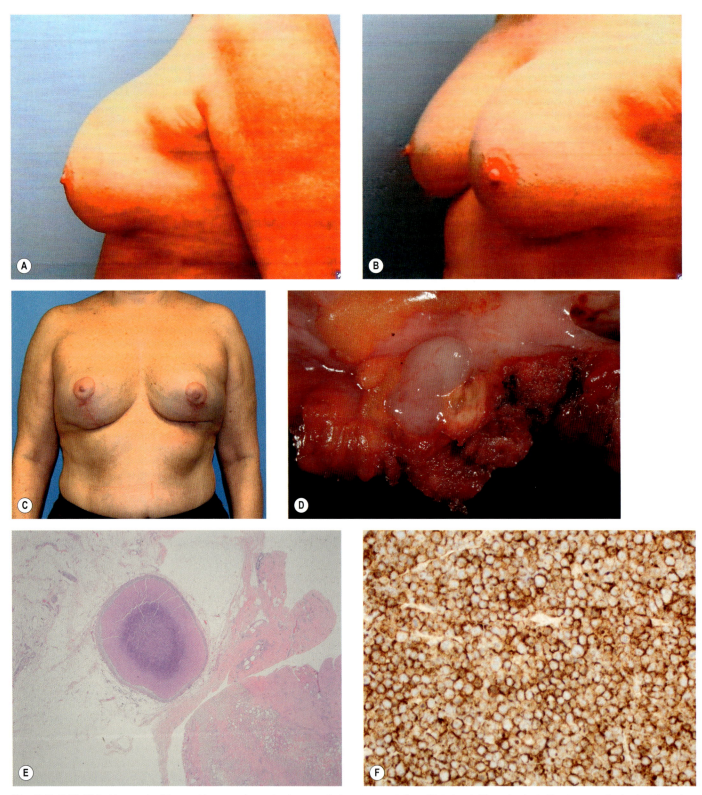

Fig. 12.9 (A,B) Clinical image of a 52-year-old woman who received a cosmetic breast augmentation with textured silicone implants. Twenty years after implantation, she developed swelling of the left breast of recent onset which was aspirated multiple times. The patient then received a partial capsulectomy, implant removal, and mastopexy. **(C)** Adequate tumor resection was questionable, and despite being asymptomatic, the patient underwent a completion capsulectomy with excision of the posterior capsular wall. **(D)** Postoperative pathology again demonstrated persistent breast implant-associated anaplastic large cell lymphoma (BIA-ALCL) disease of her chest wall and now with free margins. **(E)** Tissue section demonstrates a nodule with compact tumor cells. **(F)** Immunohistochemistry demonstrates most tumor cells that express CD30. Patient received no further adjunctive treatments and is currently 2 years disease free.

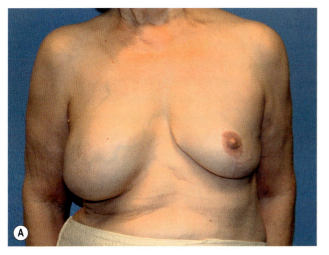

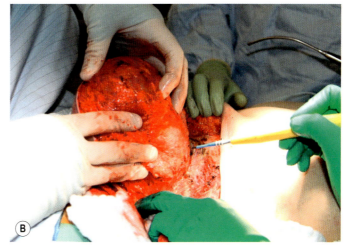

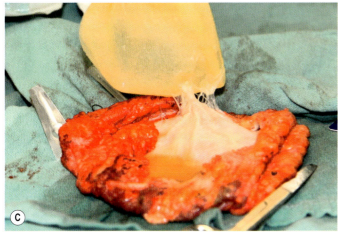

Fig. 12.10 (A) Clinical image of a 77-year-old woman who received a right mastectomy for breast cancer in 2003. Eleven years after implantation, she developed swelling of the right breast of recent onset. **(B,C)** Patient then received a total capsulectomy and implant removal. Patient is 2 years disease free and received PET-CT scans every 6 months for the first 2 years for surveillance. Patient declined further reconstruction.

with a physician should these symptoms occur. At an initial consultation, printed copies of a patient's signed consent as well as procedure specific informational pamphlets will enable patients to further digest surgical details at their leisure in their own homes, and engenders more effective recall. The legal threshold for inclusion of a specific risk in informed consent is unfortunately vague, and therefore the decision to include BIA-ALCL in informed consent should ideally be by self-obligation, not mandate. Despite the realities of a litigious society, it is important to remember that informed consent is a process, not an event, and there should be an ongoing conversation rather than just a form signing. Liability more frequently results from a lack of communication, and surgeons are most commonly judged not by their mistakes, but how they have managed them.

The future of insurance coverage of complications related to breast implants continues to evolve and is not guaranteed. An analogy has been raised with regards to screening for breast implant ruptures. When the US moratorium on silicone implants ended in 2006, the FDA recommended all women with silicone breast implants undergo MRI evaluation for implant failure at 3 years postimplantation. Because insurance policies do not cover this screening, the suggested study is not widely performed.[74] Fortunately, a similar trend has not been seen with regards to screening for BIA-ALCL. Whereas MRI screening is for a device failure, patients with delayed seromas are being screened for the presence of a malignant lesion of the breast. Therefore, physicians should not hesitate to perform pathologic review of an effusion with CD30 immunohistochemistry (which is not performed on routine specimen evaluation) if they have a reasonable clinical suspicion of a cancer. WHO is expected to address BIA-ALCL in their updated 2016 classification of lymphomas, and formal recognition will facilitate physician awareness, patient education, reporting, and management.

Reporting of cases

Many resources exist for oncologists and surgeons treating a BIA-ALCL patient. The Plastic Surgery Foundation paired the ASPS and the US FDA to form the PROFILE registry (Patient Registry and Outcomes For breast

Implants and anaplastic large cell Lymphoma etiology and Epidemiology). The purpose of PROFILE is to increase the scientific data on BIA-ALCL in women with breast implants as well as to support research to characterize BIA-ALCL and to elucidate the exact role of breast implants in the etiology of the disease. In addition to providing plastic surgeons, oncologists, and patients with the information they need about breast implants and treatment of BIA-ALCL, confirmed cases in the registry will be available for analytical epidemiological studies. Treating physicians are encouraged to report confirmed cases to the PROFILE website, which can be found at www.thepsf.org.

Conclusions

Timely diagnosis of BIA-ALCL will depend on the millions of women with breast implants having access to heightened surveillance, knowledgeable physicians, and appropriate testing and medical care. BIA-ALCL is a rare lymphoma associated with breast implants, although the exact etiology and pathogenesis remain unclear. Accurate diagnosis and complete surgical treatment is important for definitive treatment of patients. Further research is critical for prevention, diagnosis, and optimal treatment of BIA-ALCL.

🌐 Access the complete reference list online at **http://www.expertconsult.com**

28. Kim B, Roth C, Young VL, et al. Anaplastic large cell lymphoma and breast implants: results from a structured expert consultation process. *Plast Reconstr Surg.* 2011;128:629–639. *The authors conducted a structured expert consultation process to evaluate evidence for the association of breast implants with anaplastic large cell lymphoma (ALCL), and to determine the clinical significance and a potential biological model based on their interpretation of the published evidence. Panelists agreed that (1) there is a positive association between breast implants and ALCL development but possible under recognition of the true number of cases; (2) a recurrent, clinically evident delayed seroma after breast implantation should be aspirated and sent for CD30 immunohistochemistry analysis; (3) anaplastic lymphoma kinase-negative ALCL that develops around breast implants is a clinically indolent disease with a favorable prognosis that is distinct from systemic anaplastic lymphoma kinase-negative ALCL; (4) management should consist of removal of the involved implant and capsule, which is likely to prevent recurrence, and evaluation for other sites of disease; and (5) adjuvant radiation or chemotherapy should not be offered to women with capsule-confined disease. The authors' assessment yielded consistent results on a number of key issues regarding ALCL in women with breast implants, and was used as the basis for the Food and Drug Administration (FDA) safety communication in 2011.*

56. Miranda RN, Aladily TN, Prince HM, et al. Breast implant-associated anaplastic large-cell lymphoma: long-term follow-up of 60 patients. *J Clin Oncol.* 2014;32:114–120. *Miranda et al. reviewed the long-term follow-up of 60 breast implant-associated anaplastic large cell lymphoma (BIA-ALCL) patients. The mean age was 52-years-old (range 28–87 years) with a median of 9 years (range 1–32 years) between implantation and lymphoma diagnosis. Patients presented with either a malignant effusion or seroma (70%) or a distinct mass (30%). The median overall survival (OS) was 12 years (median follow-up 2 years; range 0–14 years). A total capsulectomy with implant removal was performed in 93% of patients. OS and progression-free survival (PFS) were similar between patients who received and did not receive chemotherapy (p=0.44 and p=0.28, respectively), suggesting that some patients may achieve optimal outcomes with an adequate surgical approach. Patients with a breast mass had a worse rate of OS and PFS (p=0.052 and p=0.03, respectively). The association of a mass may indicate either a worse prognosis of a more aggressive variant, more progressed disease, or perhaps a consequence of inadequate surgical ablation of tumor infiltration.*

60. de Jong D, Vasmel WL, de Boer JP, et al. Anaplastic large-cell lymphoma in women with breast implants. *JAMA.* 2008;300:2030–2035. *de Jong and colleagues reported an individually matched case control study from the Netherlands nationwide pathology database. The pathology database served a total population of approximately nine million women. The authors found a positive association for the development of ALCL in women with breast implants compared to those without implants, with an odds ratio of 18.2 (95% confidence interval, 2.1–156.8). Based upon this data, the authors estimated an incidence of 0.1–0.3 per 100 000 BIA-ALCL cases for women with prostheses per year. This study contradicted a number of prior studies that failed to show an association between breast augmentation and risk of lymphoma. In addition, those prior studies were woefully limited in power and length of follow-up.*

This study emphasized the difficulty in determining the incidence and prevalence of a very rare and recently recognized clinical entity.

68. Clemens MW, Medeiros LJ, Butler CE, et al. Complete surgical excision is essential for patients with breast implant-associated anaplastic large cell lymphoma. *J Clin Oncol.* 2015:160–168 *The authors evaluated the efficacy of different treatment modalities utilized for BIA-ALCL in order to determine an optimal treatment approach. A total of 128 patients were reviewed for pathologic findings, and clinical follow-up and malignant tissue specimens were centralized for 87 patients with BIA-ALCL. At a median follow-up of 45 months (range 3–217 months), the median OS after diagnosis of BIA-ALCL was 13 years, and the OS rate was 93% at 3 years and 89% at 5 years. Patients with lymphoma confined by the fibrous capsule surrounding the implant had better event-free survival (EFS) and OS than patients with lymphoma spread beyond the capsule (p=0.03). Patients who underwent a complete surgical excision that included total capsulectomy with breast implant removal had better OS (p=0.022) and EFS (p=0.014) when compared with patients who received partial capsulectomy, systemic chemotherapy, or radiation therapy. Based upon observed disease progression characteristics, a novel solid tumor TNM (tumor, lymph node, metastasis) staging system was proposed. The authors concluded that surgical management with complete surgical excision is essential to achieve optimal EFS in patients with BIA-ALCL.*

69. Hart A, Lechowicz MJ. Breast implant-associated anaplastic large cell lymphoma: treatment experience in 53 patients. *Aesthet Surg J.* 2014;34(6):884–894. *Hart et al. performed a meta-analysis and identified 53 BIA-ALCL patients. For patients with available clinical data, the authors noted rates of 17.3% with extracapsular disease and 23.1% with the presence of a mass. A total of 39.6% of patients were treated with surgery alone, 9.4% with surgery and radiation, 18.9% with surgery and chemotherapy, 30.2% with surgery, chemotherapy, and radiation, and 1.9% with chemotherapy alone. At a median follow-up of 15 months (3.6–90 months), disease recurrence was 28.3%, of which 73.3% were treated with salvage chemotherapy. BIA-ALCL was attributed to four patient deaths. Extracapsular disease extension was associated with increased risk for recurrence (p<0.0001) and patient death (p=0.0008). This study also found a statistically significant difference in 3- and 5-year survival rates between patients presenting with and without a mass (p=0.0308 and p=0.0308, respectively).*

70. Brody GS, Deapen D, Clive T, et al. Anaplastic large cell lymphoma (ALCL): occurring in women with breast implants analysis of 173 cases. *Plast Reconstr Surg.* 2015;135(3):695–705. *Brody and colleagues recently reported a summary of 79 published patients and 94 previously unreported cases. The authors report that for all implants where surface characteristics were known, there was at least one textured device used within the patient's surgical history. The authors reconfirm that there are no known pure smooth implant cases and importantly note that BIA-ALCL has been reported in association with all major forms of implant texturing techniques from current implant manufacturers. The authors noted most patients having slow disease progression and a good prognosis when adequately treated, but conceded occasional lymphadenopathy, metastases, and nine attributable deaths.*

13

Oncological considerations for breast reconstruction

Grant W. Carlson

SYNOPSIS

- In the US 35% of women treated for breast cancer with total mastectomy receive immediate or early breast reconstruction. The percentage is higher in young women and those treated in tertiary care medical centers.
- Immediate breast reconstruction (IBR) has several advantages: it can prevent some of the negative psychological and emotional sequelae seen with mastectomy; the aesthetic results of immediate reconstruction are superior to those seen after delayed reconstruction; and it also reduces hospital costs by reducing the number of procedures and length of hospitalization.
- IBR has the potential to impact the treatment of breast cancer. It could affect the delivery of adjuvant therapy and the detection and treatment of recurrent disease. Chemotherapy and radiation therapy could also impact the complication rates of reconstruction.

Introduction

Approximately 35% of women treated for breast cancer with total mastectomy receive immediate or early breast reconstruction. The percentage is higher in young women and those treated in tertiary care medical centers. IBR has several advantages: it can prevent some of the negative psychological and emotional sequelae seen with mastectomy; the aesthetic results of immediate reconstruction are usually superior to those seen after delayed reconstruction; and it also reduces hospital costs by reducing the number of procedures and length of hospitalization. Therefore, IBR has the potential to impact the treatment of breast cancer. It could affect the delivery of adjuvant therapy and the detection and treatment of recurrent disease. In addition, chemotherapy and radiation therapy could also impact the complication rates of reconstruction. The oncological considerations for breast reconstruction are outlined in this chapter.

Immediate breast reconstruction impact on survival

There are concerns that breast reconstruction may negatively impact breast cancer survival. Studies have shown that breast reconstruction does not interfere with the detection of local recurrences (LRs). Skin and nipple-sparing mastectomy are increasingly used to improve the results of breast reconstruction. Despite their relative surgical conservatism compared to traditional mastectomy, these techniques have not been associated with an increase in breast cancer recurrence. Complications after reconstruction have the potential to delay the administration of adjuvant therapy and potentially impact survival.

Agarwal et al. used the SEER cancer registry from 1998 to 2002 and assessed 52 249 patients to evaluate the breast cancer specific survival of patients treated with immediate or early delayed breast reconstruction after mastectomy.[1] Demographic covariates included age, race, marital status, income, education, and county metropolitan status; oncologic covariates included tumor stage, histologic grade, lymph node status, hormone receptor status, receipt of radiation, and unilateral or bilateral mastectomy. Breast reconstruction patients had significantly lower hazard of death (HR 0.73, p<0.0001) compared to those treated with total mastectomy alone when controlling for demographic and oncologic covariates.

Access to breast reconstruction is a surrogate marker for quality of breast cancer care, so these results are not surprising. Patients in cancer centers are more likely to be referred to plastic surgeons and undergo more aggressive treatment and surveillance in follow-up. There is also a selection bias that large multi-institutional cancer registries, like the SEER registry, cannot overcome. These registries do not collect data on patient comorbidities that impact the selection process of who receives breast reconstruction. Healthier people are more committed to their medical care and are more likely to undergo breast reconstruction and ultimately have a better survival.

The effects of the stress of surgery including anesthesia, blood loss, and opioid use may impact cancer progression. Reconstructive surgeries, especially using autologous tissue, are longer operations with greater blood loss and postoperative pain. Studies are needed that examine the impact of different reconstructive techniques on breast cancer survival.

Immediate breast reconstruction and local recurrence of breast cancer

Skin sparing and nipple sparing mastectomy

Skin sparing mastectomy (SSM) has markedly improved the aesthetic results of IBR (Fig. 13.1). Preservation of the native skin envelope and the inframammary fold reduces the amount of tissue necessary for reconstruction.[2] Breast symmetry can often be achieved without operating on the contralateral breast and the periareolar incisions are inconspicuous under clothes.

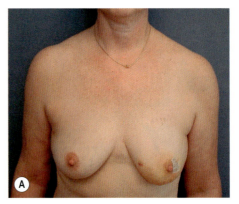
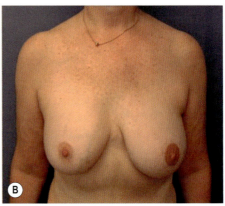

Fig. 13.1 Skin sparing mastectomy and immediate transverse rectus andominis musculocutaneous flap (TRAM) flap breast reconstruction.

There have been concerns that skin, nipple, and inframammary fold preservation reduces the effectiveness of total mastectomy. There is a large body of evidence that LRs after SSM are comparable to non-skin sparing mastectomy (Table 13.1).[3–5] Care must be taken, however, in patients with superficial cancers or diffuse ductal carcinoma in situ (DCIS) to assure adequate surgical margins.

Table 13.1 Published series of local recurrence of breast cancer after skin sparing and non-skin sparing mastectomy

Author	Follow-up (Months)	SSM (N)	LR in SSM (%)	Non-SSM (N)	LR in Non-SSM (N)
Newman et al.[85]	50	437	6.2	437	7.4
Carlson et al.[3]	41.3	187	4.8	84	9.5
Kroll et al.[4]	72	114	7.0	40	7
Simmons et al.[5]	15.6–32.4	77	3.9	154	3.2
Rivadeneira et al.[86]	49	71	5.6	127	3.9
Medina-Franco et al.[87]	73	176	4.5	-	-
Carlson et al.[10]	64.6	565	5.5	-	-
Slavin et al.[88]	44.8	51	3.9	-	-
Toth et al.[89]	51.5	50	0	-	-
Spiegel et al.[90]	117.6	221	4.5	-	-
Foster et al.[91]	49.2	25	4.0	-	-

LR, local recurrence; SSM, skin sparing mastectomy.

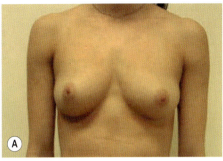
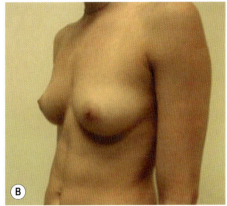
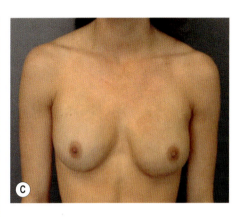
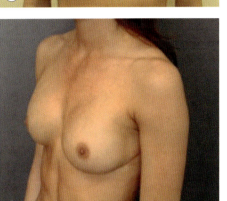

Fig. 13.2 Nipple sparing mastectomies and immediate implant reconstruction via inframammary fold incisions. **(A,B)** Preoperative appearance. **(C,D)** Postoperative appearance.

Nipple-sparing mastectomy (NSM) is growing in popularity because of its perceived aesthetic benefits (Fig. 13.2). Patient satisfaction with nipple areolar reconstruction following SSM can be disappointing.[6] Data regarding the oncological safety of NSM is hampered by small sample size, varying indications and surgical techniques, and short follow-up (Table 13.2). There are limited oncological and reconstructive indications for performing NSM. Large tumors and those located in the central breast have an increased incidence of nipple involvement. Larger, more ptotic breasts are not good candidates for the procedure. Nipple elevation cannot be achieved without preservation of a dermoglandular pedicle, which impacts the completeness of mastectomy. The ideal candidate for an NSM has small to moderate sized breasts with minimal ptosis.

Detection of local recurrence after breast reconstruction

The role of postreconstruction imaging after the treatment of breast cancer remains controversial. There is a paucity of data that addresses the issue, and there are no established guidelines.[7] The incidence of LR of breast cancer is related to tumor stage. Most LRs after total mastectomy are in the skin and subcutaneous tissue and are readily detected by physical examination.[8] A flap or implant could potentially delay the discovery of chest wall recurrences.

Systemic relapse is not inevitable following LR, especially after the treatment of DCIS.[9,10] This argues that early detection of LRs may have a potential survival impact. All forms of mastectomy leave residual breast tissue, and the differences are in terms of the microscopic breast tissue left behind in the skin and inframammary fold, which is largely preserved after SSM. Torresan *et al.* evaluated residual glandular tissue in the skin flaps that would have been preserved after SSM.[11] They found that 60% contained residual glandular tissue and it correlated with skin flap thickness.

Table 13.2 Published series of nipple areolar complex recurrence after therapeutic nipple sparing mastectomies

Author	Year	N	Median follow-up (months)	NAC recurrence
Petit et al.[92]	2005	579	41	0%
Sacchini et al.[93]	2006	68	24.6	0%
Paepke et al.[94]	2008	94	34	0%
Babiera et al.[95]	2010	53	15	0%
Kim et al.[96]	2010	152	60	1.3%
Jensen et al.[97]	2011	77	60.2	0%
Peled et al.[98] Lohsiriwat et al.[99]	2012	152	45	0%
Lohsiriwat et al.[99]	2012	861	50	1.3%
Sakurai et al.[100]	2013	788	78	3.7%
NAC, nipple areolar complex.				

The completeness of mastectomy is important in the treatment of DCIS because most cases of recurrence represent unexcised residual disease. Several authors have reported LR of DCIS treated by SSM and IBR.[9,12,13] They found that the majority of LRs were invasive carcinomas. This suggests that postreconstruction mammography can have a role in the early detection of recurrences prior to the development of invasive carcinoma.

Physical examination of implant reconstruction is relatively easy. There is minimal soft tissue covering the implant except along the inframammary fold and in the axillary tail. Deep chest wall recurrences are extremely unlikely because the implants are placed in the submuscular plane. Conventional mammographic evaluation has limited utility because the implants obscure soft tissue visualization. MRI, which has been used extensively to evaluate the integrity of silicone gel implants, may have a role in the selective surveillance after implant reconstruction.[14–17]

The sensitivity of physical examination of autologous reconstruction is lower than that seen with implant reconstruction. Deep chest wall recurrences often avoid detection until symptoms develop. Autologous reconstruction causes less impairment of mammographic tissue visualization.[18] Benign mammographic findings after transverse rectus abdominis myocutaneous (TRAM) flap reconstruction include fat necrosis, lipid cysts, calcifications, lymph nodes, and epidermal inclusion cysts (Fig. 13.3).[19] Breast cancer recurrences in

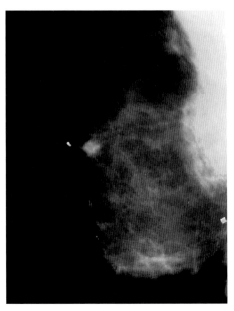

Fig. 13.4 Mammographic appearance of local recurrence after TRAM flap reconstruction.

autologous tissue reconstruction are mammographically similar to that of primary tumors (Fig. 13.4).[20,21] Proponents of surveillance mammography feel that screening breast cancer patients with autologous reconstructions can detect non-palpable recurrences before clinical examination.

Helvie *et al.* evaluated surveillance mammography in 113 patients after TRAM flap reconstruction.[22] Six patients underwent biopsy for suspicious mammographic findings, and two LRs were detected. Two patients in the study group went on to develop recurrences that were detected by physical examination. There was one false negative mammogram resulting in a sensitivity of 67% and specificity of 98% for surveillance mammography after TRAM flap reconstruction.

There is a paucity of data regarding the efficacy of MRI of the breast following autogenous breast reconstruction.[23,24] Breast MRI has been shown to clearly delineate autogenous flaps from residual mammary adipose tissue. The absence of contrast medium uptake during breast MRI precludes recurrent carcinoma to a high probability. Fat necrosis in a TRAM flap will show early postoperative contrast enhancement, but this resolves within 6–12 months. Rieber *et al.* evaluated MRI of the breast in the follow-up of 41 patients who had undergone autogenous tissue breast reconstruction.[25] MRI was able to distinguish flaps from surrounding residual breast tissue in all cases. It excluded disease recurrence in four patients with suspicious mammographic or sonographic findings, and returned false positive findings in three cases.

The potential indications for postreconstruction imaging include patients with close surgical margins

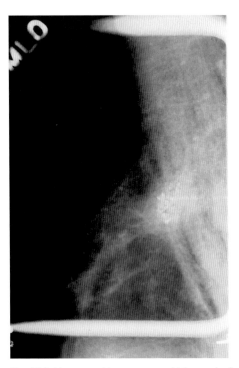

Fig. 13.3 Mammographic appearance of fat necrosis after TRAM flap reconstruction.

and patients with diffuse DCIS treated by SSM. Its routine use after autologous reconstruction after SSM for invasive carcinoma warrants further study. The low detection rate and specificity does not justify the routine use of MRI in the follow-up of patients postreconstruction. MRI is most useful in patients with abnormal findings on physical examination or mammography and ultrasound. It is also helpful to delineate the extent of local disease recurrence.

Treatment of local recurrence after breast reconstruction

Surgical options following LR after breast reconstruction depend on the location and number of metastatic deposits and previous treatment. Imaging of the reconstructed breast and body scans are necessary to delineate the extent of tumor involvement (see Fig. 13.4). Isolated LRs can be treated with removal of as much reconstructed tissue as necessary to achieve negative margins. Adjuvant chest wall radiation is usually administered (Fig. 13.5).

In cases of implant reconstruction, it may be necessary to remove a portion of the implant capsule necessitating implant removal in most cases. Howard *et al.* reviewed 16 cases of LR after TRAM flap reconstruction.[26] Eight recurrences occurred in the skin and were detected on physical examination. Eight recurrences occurred in the chest wall and were symptomatic, being detected on physical examination or diagnostic imaging. Twelve were felt amenable to surgical resection, and three required removal of the entire TRAM flap.

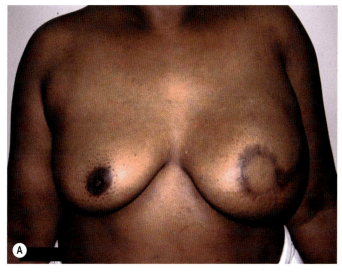

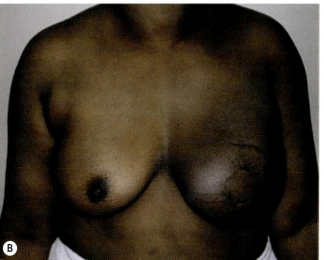

Fig. 13.5 (A) Preoperative and **(B)** postoperative appearance of local breast cancer recurrence in a left TRAM flap treated by wide local excision and radiation.

Immediate breast reconstruction and adjuvant therapy

Chemotherapy

There are concerns that IBR may delay the administration of adjuvant chemotherapy. A survey of 376 consultant breast surgeons in the UK and Ireland found that the majority (57%) preferred delayed reconstruction because of these concerns.[27] Breast reconstruction does have a high complication rate especially in patients that are obese, smoke tobacco, or have a history of chest wall irradiation. Alderman *et al.* performed a multi-institutional study of complication rates after tissue expander or TRAM flap reconstruction.[28] They reported a 52% complication rate, with major complications occurring in 30% of patients.

It seems logical that the high complication rate of IBR could potentially delay the administration of adjuvant therapy. Studies comparing onset of chemotherapy after IBR and control group treated with mastectomy alone have failed to show significant differences.[29–32] Alderman *et al.* examined the impact of breast reconstruction on the administration of adjuvant chemotherapy. Data from eight National Comprehensive Cancer Network institutions was used. They found that IBR did not result in the omission of adjuvant chemotherapy, but there was a modest but statistically significant delay in the time to administration.[32] The authors concluded that this short delay would not impact survival.

Wound complications after IBR must be treated aggressively to remove necrotic, potentially infected tissue. Patients with clean, open wounds can receive chemotherapy with minimal compromise in wound healing. These patients must be followed closely to detect early signs of infection.

Patients with locally advanced, stage III breast cancer are generally treated with chemotherapy followed by total mastectomy and adjuvant radiation. The 5-year survival rate is 50–80%, and patients with a poor response to chemotherapy have an especially bad prognosis. It may be preferable to delay reconstruction until after mastectomy and adjuvant radiation in these patients. This avoids the potential problems from radiation delivery and the adverse effects of postmastectomy radiation therapy (PMRT) on immediate reconstruction. These issues will be discussed in detail later in this chapter.

There is conflicting data regarding the impact of neoadjuvant chemotherapy on complications after IBR. Mehrara *et al.* found that neoadjuvant chemotherapy was an independent predictor of overall complications in free flap breast reconstruction.[33] Zweifel-Schlatter *et al.* compared 47 patients undergoing immediate free flap breast reconstruction after neoadjuvant chemotherapy with 52 patients who did not receive preoperative therapy, and found no delay in beginning adjuvant therapy.[34] The use of neoadjuvant chemotherapy did not impact wound complications or delay adjuvant radiation therapy.

Radiation

Rationale for postmastectomy radiotherapy

The goals of postmastectomy radiotherapy are to optimize locoregional control and improve survival. Studies have shown that extensive lymph node involvement, large tumor size ($\geq$5 cm), tumor lymphovascular invasion, and positive margins predispose to locoregional recurrence (LRR) after total mastectomy for breast cancer. Randomized trial and a meta-analysis have shown that PMRT can reduce this risk by approximately 67%.[35–37] Locoregional recurrences and systemic recurrence should not be considered as separate events. An improvement in locoregional control of breast cancer directly effects the development and spread of subclinical tumor deposits.

Two randomized trials have shown a survival benefit for postmastectomy radiotherapy in patients with 1–3 metastatic lymph nodes.[38,39] These studies were criticized because the high rate of regional failure in the non-irradiated group was felt to be the result of inadequate axillary surgery and the use of non-anthracycline based chemotherapy. A meta-analysis by the Early Breast Cancer Trialists' Collaborative Group has provided strong evidence supporting the use of postmastectomy radiotherapy.[40] The group studied the results of 22 trials of PMRT conducted between 1964 and 1986 and noted that 1133 women had axillary dissection and 1–3

positive lymph nodes. Radiotherapy reduced LRR (2p<0.00001), overall recurrence (RR 0.67, 2p=0.00009), and breast mortality (RR 0.78, 2p=0.01) in this group.

Improvements in breast screening, lymph node analysis, and better system therapy have resulted in lower absolute risks of recurrence than are seen in the older studies analyzed, which could lower the impact of PMRT. Many centers currently recommend PMRT for patients with early breast cancer. This policy has increased the complexity of planning breast reconstruction in patients who potentially have nodal involvement. In patients with stage III breast cancer, the best policy may be to perform delayed breast reconstruction. There are two concerns when administering PMRT after IBR: technical difficulties with radiation delivery and negative effects of radiation on the aesthetic outcome.

Impact of breast reconstruction on the administration of radiotherapy

The chest wall is the single most important target to receive radiation. The majority of LRR are seen in the chest wall only and not the LNs. The sites at greatest risk are the skin overlying the tumor bed and the mastectomy scar. There are technical problems related to irradiation of the reconstructed breast. Distortion of the chest wall anatomy means that radiotherapy portals need to be modified. The treatment is more difficult, particularly irradiating the internal mammary lymph nodes (IMLNs). This may require changing the depth of tangential fields resulting in an increased volume of irradiated lung or heart. The steeply sloping medial contour from inflated expanders may produce problems with field matching resulting in a less precise junction and underdosing of the area under the junction. This adversely affects electron dosimetry and increases the negative effects of PMRT as a result of the higher energy beam requirements and tangential irradiation of the skin surface.

Chen *et al.* performed a survey of radiation oncologists with regard to the treatment of breast cancer in women who have had breast reconstruction.[41] A total of 358 radiation oncologists responded, and 57% of them felt reconstruction challenged their ability to deliver effective breast radiation. With regard to patients with tissue expander reconstruction, 60% preferred treating moderately filled implants with 150–250 cc rather than completely deflated or fully inflated implants. The reason given was to minimize the dose to the heart and lungs.

The routine treatment of IMLNs is controversial. All of the randomized trials that showed a survival benefit of PMRT in node positive patients used IMLN irradiation.[35,36,40] The results of retrospective studies examining IMLN irradiation specifically are conflicting. It is the single greatest predictor of high heart and lung doses in patients with implant-based reconstruction whether unilateral or bilateral reconstruction is performed and is a risk factor for cardiac toxicity. Long-term results of randomized trials will hopefully answer this important question with regard to IMLN irradiation.

Motwani *et al.* examined the effect of immediate autologous breast reconstruction on the technical delivery of PMRT.[42] Two radiation oncologists reviewed radiotherapy plans in 110 patients. These were compared to matched controls that had mastectomy alone. A qualitative scoring system was used that evaluated chest wall coverage, treatment of the IMLN chain, minimization of lung exposure, and avoidance of the heart. They found that patients having immediate breast reconstruction had compromise of their radiation therapy plans compared to that of the control group. If coverage of the IMLNs was eliminated, the risk of compromise was significantly reduced. The authors suggested that in patients with locally advanced breast cancer, the option for delayed reconstruction should be considered.

Several studies from other centers that do not routinely treat IMLNs have shown excellent chest wall coverage, local control, and acceptable doses to the heart and lungs.[43-45] Interpretation of these studies is hampered by different radiation techniques being used for reconstruction patients compared to matched controls without reconstruction.

Immediate implant-based reconstruction in the setting of postmastectomy radiotherapy

There is increasing level III data indicating that radiation increases surgical morbidity after implant-based breast reconstruction.[46-49] Lam *et al.* reviewed 12 studies involving 1853 patients to examine the impact of PMRT on immediate two-stage implant reconstruction.[49] Postreconstruction radiotherapy of the tissue expander resulted in a significantly higher overall reconstructive failure compared to controls (29.3% vs. 5%, p<0.00001). Barry and Kell in a meta-analysis of 11 studies found that patients receiving PMRT after implant reconstruction had a significantly increased risk of complications (OR=4.2, 95% CI: 2.4–7.2) compared to those that did not receive radiation.[46] Autologous reconstruction was associated with less morbidity (OR=0.21, 95% CI: 0.1–0.4) in the setting of PMRT.

The impact of radiation therapy on implant breast reconstruction from the patients' perspective is less well documented. Albornoz *et al.* performed a multicenter study that evaluated patient reported outcomes for implant-based breast reconstruction with or without radiation using the Breast-Q.[50] The Breast-Q is a validated patient-reported outcome measure (PROM) designed to quantify a patient's experience in terms of postsurgical satisfaction and health-related quality-of-life (QOL) after breast surgery and reconstruction. It can provide patients and providers with important information to assist in decision-making with regard to breast reconstruction. The questionnaire was completed by 633 patients after implant reconstruction: 414 did not receive radiation, and 219 received radiation (preoperative radiotherapy 47, postoperative radiotherapy 172). Patients that received postoperative radiotherapy had a significant reduction in all domains (satisfaction with breasts, satisfaction with outcome, psychosocial well-being, sexual well-being, and physical well-being) in a univariate analysis. Patients that received radiation were younger and had higher rates of axillary dissection and chemotherapy. Multivariate analysis confirmed the negative impact of radiotherapy on the satisfaction with breasts domain (p=0.03) when adjusted for patient and treatment factors. The authors hypothesize that this may be a reflection of radiation side effects including capsular contracture and fibrosis. They conclude that the potential decrease in patient satisfaction after irradiation of implant reconstruction should be part of the informed decision-making process.

These results confirmed the findings of a similar study using the Breast-Q by Eriksson *et al.*[47] They also found that radiotherapy significantly impacted all questionnaire domains when administered in the setting of implant reconstruction. These authors also reported the impact of radiotherapy on reconstructive failure: no radiotherapy 6%, preoperative radiotherapy 25%, and postoperative radiotherapy 15% (p<0.001). Patients with reconstructive failure were not included in the questionnaire analysis. Eriksson noted that a large majority of women who were successfully reconstructed would choose breast reconstruction again regardless of whether they received radiation or not. They concluded that autologous reconstruction should be considered in the setting of radiotherapy, especially in previously irradiated patients. The reported high satisfaction rates showed that implant-based reconstruction is not contraindicated in the setting of radiotherapy.

There are many patients who do not desire or are not candidates for autologous reconstruction. It is incumbent upon the treating surgeon to provide the patient with accurate information so that she can make an informed decision with regard to implant reconstruction in the setting of radiation therapy.

Radiation impact on TRAM flap reconstruction

The body of evidence in the literature has shown that radiation therapy increases the risk of TRAM flap complications and negatively impacts the aesthetic outcomes. Early work showed that chest wall radiation increased the risk of complications after delayed pedicled TRAM flap reconstruction.[51] Overall, a history of chest wall irradiation resulted in a statistically significant increase in both fat necrosis and flap necrosis. Bipedicle TRAM flap reconstruction showed a reduced risk of these complications, arguing that improved blood supply can overcome some of the effects of radiation.

Williams et al. reviewed 19 cases of pedicled TRAM flap irradiation.[52] Complication rates were compared to delayed TRAM flaps performed after the administration of radiation and a control group of TRAM flap reconstruction alone. The overall flap complication rate is the same whether radiation was administered before or after reconstruction. Ten patients (52.6%) demonstrated postirradiation changes to the TRAM flap and 6 required surgical interventions (31.6%).

Carlson et al. performed a retrospective review of 199 patients undergoing 232 pedicled TRAM flap reconstructions to identify patients who received radiotherapy.[53] Patients were stratified into 5 groups by the use and timing of radiation as well as the timing of the reconstruction. Blinded reviewers assessed the overall aesthetic appearance. The incidence of flap complications was 34.2% in the immediate non-irradiated group, 10.7% in the delayed non-irradiated group, 44% in the post-TRAM radiation group, 60% in the immediate pre-TRAM radiation group, and 33% in the delayed pre-TRAM radiation group (p=0.010). Patients who had immediate TRAM flap reconstruction and did not receive radiation had a better global aesthetic outcome (p<0.001) than the other 4 groups. The aesthetic outcome was similar whether radiation was administered pre- or post-TRAM flap reconstruction.

Tran et al. compared immediate and delayed free TRAM flap reconstruction in patients receiving PMRT.[54] The study groups included 32 immediate and 70 delayed TRAM flaps. The incidence of early complications did not differ between the groups. However, the incidence of late complications (fat necrosis, volume loss, or flap contracture) was significantly higher in the immediate reconstruction group. Nine patients (28%) in the immediate group required an additional flap to correct distorted contours. The authors concluded that in patients who need PMRT, TRAM flap reconstruction should be delayed until radiation therapy is completed.

A paper by Rogers and Allen has demonstrated similar deleterious effects of radiation on deep inferior epigastric perforator (DIEP) flap reconstruction.[55] They examined 30 DIEP flaps that received PMRT compared to a control group of 30 non-irradiated DIEP flaps. They reported a 23.3% incidence of fat necrosis in the radiated group vs. 0% incidence in the control group. Radiation fibrosis was seen in 56.7% of cases with 5 (16.7%) requiring surgical revision.

Spear et al. reviewed 171 pedicled TRAM flaps in 150 patients to determine the effect of radiation therapy.[56] This was the first study that critically evaluated the cosmetic effects of radiation therapy on TRAM flap reconstruction. Radiation, whether administered before or after reconstruction, had a negative impact on the aesthetic appearance, symmetry, contracture, and hyperpigmentation of the flap reconstruction. This was based on the evaluation of postoperative photographs by blinded judges. There was a two-fold increase in the incidence of fat necrosis in the post-TRAM flap group compared to a control group. The authors recommended that TRAM flap reconstruction be postponed in patients who will receive postmastectomy radiotherapy.

Delayed-immediate breast reconstruction

MD Anderson Cancer Center advocates a two-stage approach to "delayed-immediate breast reconstruction" in patients who may potentially receive PMRT to avoid potential complications and interference with radiation delivery.[57] Stage I consists of performing a SSM with insertion of a subpectoral tissue expander that is filled to the appropriate volume in an attempt to preserve the skin envelope. After review of the permanent pathological analysis, if PMRT is not required, patients undergo IBR. In patients who require PMRT, the expander is deflated to provide a flat surface for radiotherapy. After its completion, the expander is re-inflated and the skin envelope expanded. This second staged is a form of delayed skin preserving reconstruction.

An animal study has shown that partial deflation of a tissue expander exacerbated the adverse effects of radiation, as evidenced by a reduction in epidermal thickness, an increase in seroma formation, and an increase in capsular thickness compared to a study group that received radiation to a fully inflated expander.[58] MD Anderson Cancer Center performed a 5-year review of 47 patients with stage III breast cancer who underwent delayed-immediate breast reconstruction.[59] The overall expander loss occurred in 15 patients (32%), including 9 (22%) during re-inflation after PMRT.

Timing of delayed reconstruction after PMRT

In performing autologous delayed breast reconstruction, the optimum delay to allow the acute effects of

PMRT to resolve appears to be 6–12 months. Baumann *et al.* reviewed their experience with delayed free TRAM flap reconstruction after PMRT to determine the impact of timing on surgery complications.[60] In total, 189 patients were identified and stratified into 2 groups: reconstruction performed less than 12 months from PMRT and reconstruction performed after 12 months. They found that complications were decreased in the longer delay group including total flap loss and re-operation. Momoh *et al.* reviewed their experience with 100 patients having delayed free flap reconstruction after PMRT and found no difference in complication rates whether the operation was performed early (within 6 months) or delayed (greater than 6 months after PMRT).[61]

Breast reconstruction after failed breast conservation

Breast conservation therapy (BCT) is the treatment of choice for most early stage breast cancers. Despite survival rates equivalent to total mastectomy, BCT is associated with a 0.5% per year risk of in breast recurrence over 20 years. The primary treatment after failed breast conservation is total mastectomy. Reconstruction in this setting is poorly understood and presents a unique set of challenges.

There is a rise in data indicating that the complication rates of implant-based IBR are increased in the setting of preoperative radiotherapy. Mastectomy skin flap necrosis, capsular contracture, and reconstructive failure have all been well documented.[47,62–64] Cordeiro *et al.* found the aesthetic grades to be lower in patients having immediate tissue expander reconstruction after failed breast conservation.[62] Hirsch *et al.* reviewed their experience with immediate tissue expander reconstruction after breast conservation.[63] They found a 29.6% (21/71) rate of explantation with the rates being similar during the first stage (tissue expander) and the second stage (permanent implant placement).

Good results can be achieved with implant-based reconstruction after failed breast conservation, but the patients must be counseled on the increased risk of complications (see Fig. 13.1). The literature provides no data on how time after breast conservation affects the results of immediate tissue expander reconstruction.

Contralateral prophylactic mastectomy

Women diagnosed with breast cancer increasingly elect to undergo a contralateral prophylactic mastectomy (CPM) at the time of breast cancer treatment. Data from a large national registry spanning most of the last decade document a more than doubling of the incidence of CPM.[65] The potential drivers of this trend are many, but in general they stem from a perception held by patients, the medical community, and the general public that there is a risk of subsequent primary breast cancer. Some risk factors are better understood than others. For instance, heritable genetic mutations substantially heighten the risk of a contralateral primary breast cancer, but indeterminate findings on MRI or certain histopathology have unknown implications.

Younger age has been widely demonstrated to increase the likelihood of electing for CPM.[66–72] Among women with early stage disease, younger women face a longer life expectancy and thus a longer window in which to develop a second primary breast cancer. On the other hand, younger women with very early presenting cancers may be more likely to harbor a predisposing genetic mutation, which clearly confers an increased risk of a subsequent cancer to the opposite breast and may motivate the pursuit of CPM. It is also known that younger women are more likely to pursue postmastectomy breast reconstruction in general.[2–4] Some have postulated that better symmetry and a superior aesthetic outcome can be achieved with bilateral breast reconstruction, which may make some women more accepting of a contralateral procedure.

Women of racial minorities are less likely to choose CPM, a trend that likely reflects cultural preferences and socioeconomic differences.[67,69–71,73] A family history of breast cancer was a strong predictor of prophylactic mastectomy.[66,69,72,74,75] Furthermore, a family history consisting of multiple first-degree relatives is among the indications for prophylactic mastectomy put forward by the Society of Surgical Oncology.[76]

The use of MRI in the diagnostic workup of a breast cancer increases the use of CPM by two- to three-fold.[69,74,77] Sorbero *et al.* propose two mechanisms for this association.[77] Firstly, women imaged by MRI are more likely choose mastectomy over breast conserving surgery, which introduces the option of CPM that a subset of women will take. Secondly, indeterminate findings in the contralateral breast, some of which will necessitate further breast biopsies, generate uncertainty and distress for the patient and perhaps even their surgeon, which then spurs a decision for CPM.

Occult breast cancer is discovered in approximately 5% of CPM specimens.[75,78] While these lesions may have been identified on surveillance imaging and effectively treated, most evidence points to an overall improvement in disease-free survival following CPM, at least among women at high risk, such as those with a strong family history or hormone receptor negative cancer.[77,79,80]

Nationwide data on breast reconstruction demonstrates an overall increase in IBR, as well as a significant increase in the use of breast implants.[81] The increasing proportion of women who undergo CPM is undoubtedly a substantial contributor to these trends. The benefits of prophylactic mastectomy must be weighed against the added morbidity of a second procedure, which in the vast majority of cases involves not only mastectomy but also reconstruction. Because the procedure is elective and the breast is healthy, patients and even clinicians may underestimate the potential risks. Crosby *et al.* examined immediate postmastectomy bilateral reconstruction for an index cancer combined with a CPM in 497 patients.[82] The findings showed that 154 patients developed a complication in the reconstruction, and 42 patients (27.3%) developed a complication in the prophylactic side. In implant reconstruction, they found a 22.5% complication rate in the index breast and a 19.2% risk of a complication in the prophylactic breast. The risk of having a complication in both breasts was 11.1%.

The considerable added morbidity of prophylactic mastectomy has been demonstrated in other series.[75,82–84] Miller *et al.* reviewed a single institution experience of 600 patients treated by total mastectomy (unilateral 391, CPM 209).[83] When adjusting for confounding variables (age, BMI, smoking, diabetes, reconstruction, and radiation), patients undergoing CPM were 1.5 times more likely to have any operative complication (p=0.029) and 2.7 times more likely to have a major complication (p=0.004) when compared with patients undergoing unilateral mastectomy.

The incidence of CPM has risen dramatically over recent years. Women who choose CPM are more often young, white, and have a family history of breast cancer. Failure of breast conservation and pursuit of postmastectomy breast reconstruction are other contributing factors. Reconstructive trends in this cohort, namely the prevalence of immediate implant-based reconstruction, are mirrored by national trends among *all* patients who undergo mastectomy. As the incidence of CPM continues to increase, the outcomes of this procedure must be critically assessed. The added morbidity appears to be substantial.

🌐 **Access the complete reference list online at** **http://www.expertconsult.com**

1. Agarwal J, Agarwal S, Pappas L, et al. A population-based study of breast cancer-specific survival following mastectomy and immediate or early-delayed breast reconstruction. *Breast J.* 2012;18(3):226–232. *Large population based study using the SEER database of over 52 000 breast cancer patients. Regression analysis showed that IBR had no impact on breast cancer survival.*

3. Carlson GW, Bostwick J 3rd, Styblo TM, et al. Skin-sparing mastectomy. Oncologic and reconstructive considerations. *Ann Surg.* 1997;225(5):570–575, discussion 575-578. *A large retrospective review comparing the outcomes of non-skin sparing and skin sparing mastectomies in the treatment of breast cancer.*

8. Langstein HN, Cheng MH, Singletary SE, et al. Breast cancer recurrence after immediate reconstruction: patterns and significance. *Plast Reconstr Surg.* 2003;111(2):712–720, discussion 721-722. *Review of 39 local recurrences after IBR. The majority of local recurrences occurred in the skin and subcutaneous tissue.*

32. Alderman AK, Collins ED, Schott A, et al. The impact of breast reconstruction on the delivery of chemotherapy. *Cancer.* 2010;116(7):1791–1800. *Multi-institutional study that found IBR did not lead to omission of chemotherapy but was associated with a modest delay in initiating treatment.*

40. EBCTCG, McGale P, Taylor C, et al. Effect of radiotherapy after mastectomy and axillary surgery on 10-year recurrence and 20-year breast cancer mortality: meta-analysis of individual patient data for 8135 women in 22 randomised trials. *Lancet.* 2014;383(9935):2127–2135. *Landmark meta-analysis that examines the impact of postmastectomy radiotherapy on breast cancer survival.*

47. Eriksson M, Anveden L, Celebioglu F, et al. Radiotherapy in implant-based immediate breast reconstruction: risk factors, surgical outcomes, and patient-reported outcome measures in a large Swedish multicenter cohort. *Breast Cancer Res Treat.* 2013;142(3):591–601. *Study that evaluates the impact of postmastectomy radiotherapy on surgical morbidity and patient reported outcomes after immediate implant-based reconstruction.*

62. Cordeiro PG, Snell L, Heerdt A, et al. Immediate tissue expander/implast breast reconstruction after salvage mastectomy for cancer recurrence following lumpectomy/irradiation. *Plast Reconstr Surg.* 2012;129(2):341–350. *This text highlights that implant-based reconstruction after failed breast conservation has poorer aesthetic outcomes for patients without a history of radiation.*

67. Cemal Y, Albornoz CR, Disa JJ, et al. A paradigm shift in U.S. breast reconstruction: part 2. The influence of changing mastectomy patterns on reconstructive rate and method. *Plast Reconstr Surg.* 2013;131(3):320e–326e. *Review of the National Inpatient Sample database showing the increase in implant-based breast reconstruction and the use of contralateral prophylactic mastectomy.*

98. Peled AW, Foster RD, Stover AC, et al. Outcomes after total skin-sparing mastectomy and immediate reconstruction in 657 breasts. *Ann Surg Oncol.* 2012;19:3402–3409. *Single institution experience with nipple sparing mastectomies that highlights changes in technique to reduce complication rates.*

14

Preoperative evaluation and planning for breast reconstruction following mastectomy

John Y.S. Kim and Nima Khavanin

SYNOPSIS

- The specific details of an individual patient's preoperative context can optimize shared decision-making and yield better reconstructive outcomes while concomitantly managing patient expectations.
- Preoperative evaluation for breast reconstruction generally includes understanding a patient's oncologic status, treatment plan, past medical and surgical history, medications, anatomy, and postoperative expectations.
- A patient's oncologic history will guide important decisions including eligibility for nipple-sparing mastectomy as well as the need for chemoradiation.
- Perioperative medication management plays an important role in decreasing the risk for adverse events, and decisions to continue or withhold specific medications should be made on a case-by-case basis.
- Risk calculators convert a patient's demographic information and comorbidities into an individualized measure of risk, facilitating patient education and shared decision-making.

Introduction

The surgical management of breast cancer requires a multidisciplinary approach that involves medical oncologists, radiologists, pathologists, breast/oncologic surgeons, and reconstructive surgeons. This integration is especially germane for breast reconstruction patients since there are diverse technique choices available, each with its attendant profile of risks and benefits. The specific details of an individual patient's preoperative context can optimize shared decision-making and yield better reconstructive outcomes while concomitantly managing expectations. Accordingly, in this chapter we will review current literature on how patient and disease factors, including pre-reconstruction radiation, chemotherapy, patient anatomy, medications, and comorbidities, play into medical, surgical, and cosmetic outcomes following breast reconstruction.

Patient history

A detailed patient history should focus on a patient's oncologic history and treatment plan, relevant medical and surgical history, and risk factors that may affect wound healing and/or reconstructive outcomes.

Oncologic status and treatment plan

A patient's stage is not only an important predictor of life expectancy but also the need for neoadjuvant or adjuvant chemoradiation. Details such as tumor size and location can affect a patient's candidacy for nipple-sparing mastectomy, and information on cancer type, e.g., inflammatory cancer, can affect the extent of skin resection and consequent need for soft-tissue coverage. The magnitude of the oncologic problem can also dictate a decision to potentially delay reconstruction if there is limited life expectancy or if the urgency of adjuvant treatment mandates a deferral of potentially complex reconstructive procedures.

Stage

As a prognostic factor, cancer stage is among the most important predictors of a patient's long-term cancer survival. Recent SEER (Surveillance, Epidemiology, and End Results) statistics demonstrate nearly 100% 5-year survival rates for Stage 0 or I, 93% for stage II, 72% for stage III, 22% for stage IV.[1] This data often plays an important role in a woman's decision between

Table 14.1 Factors in the evaluation for postmastectomy radiation[12-16]
Indications
• Locally advanced disease – T4 tumor • T3 tumor with evidence of node involvement upon pathology • Margins positive for invasive disease upon pathology • Tumor of any size with 4+ involved nodes
Possible indications
• T1–2 disease & 1–3 involved nodes • T3N0 • DCIS identified at the surgical margin • Node negative, triple negative breast cancer
DCIS, ductal carcinoma *in situ*.

breast-conserving therapy and mastectomy, as well as her decision on whether or not to pursue reconstruction. Recently, trends in mastectomy for early-stage breast cancer increased to 37.8% in 2011, with 36.4% of these patients electing to undergo reconstruction.[2] Although patients with early disease (stage I or carcinoma *in situ*) are more likely to undergo reconstruction,[3,4] some centers report no association between cancer stage and reconstruction rates,[5] and this relationship likely varies across institutions.

Cancer stage is also one of many variables, including tumor size, margins, nodal involvement, and tumor histology, that factors into the decision regarding postmastectomy radiation and systemic chemotherapy. Indications for postmastectomy radiotherapy are presented in Table 14.1. The possibility of adjuvant and neoadjuvant therapies can affect both the timing and even modality of reconstruction and should be reviewed with every patient.

Special case: inflammatory breast cancer

Inflammatory breast cancer is an aggressive form of cancer marked by the classic finding of peau d'orange and a relatively poor prognosis.[6] These cancers may require aggressive surgical resection in addition to chemotherapy and irradiation, and have a relatively high recurrence rate.[7,8] Reconstruction in this setting can be particularly challenging as the diffuse skin and lymphatic involvement can require extensive resection of the breast, chest wall, and skin, resulting in an extensive mastectomy defect. Furthermore, the need for radiotherapy increases the rate of poor patient outcomes. While some surgeons consider inflammatory breast cancer a relative contraindication to reconstruction, others note the utility of autogenous flaps in helping to provide durable, vascularized coverage over the chest wall in anticipation of postmastectomy radiation.[9,10]

Relatively little reconstructive data exists on this rare cohort.[10] In the largest study to date,[9] 59 women, all of whom received chemotherapy and radiation, underwent 52 delayed and 7 immediate autogenous reconstructions. Complications occurred in nearly 36% of patients, with one total flap loss.

Special case: nipple-sparing mastectomy

As its name suggests, nipple-sparing mastectomy (NSM) preserves the nipple and areola, in addition to the typical mastectomy skin flap, allowing for potentially improved cosmetic outcomes.[11] Generally, NSM is only indicated in carefully selected patients, particularly those undergoing mastectomy for prophylactic reasons or those with smaller, unifocal lesions a reasonable distance away from the nipple areolar complex.[12-14] Other variables favoring this potential approach include negative axillary node involvement, negative lymphovascular involvement, no extensive intraductal component, grade 1 or 2 tumor, HER2/neu negativity, and ER/PR positivity. Contraindications include inflammatory breast cancer, clinical involvement of the nipple areolar complex, nipple retraction, Paget's disease, bloody nipple discharge, and multicentricity (Table 14.2).[15,16]

Retrospective studies of nipple pathology in patients with nipple removal have demonstrated subclinical nipple involvement rates ranging from 0 to 58% depending on the tumor size and location, multicentricity, and lymph node positivity among other variables.[11] These data have led researchers to develop oncologic criteria for NSM including peripheral tumor location, size under 2–5 cm, and a tumor to nipple distance greater than 2 cm.[17] Using similar patient selection criteria, local

Table 14.2 Criteria for nipple-sparing mastectomy	
Indications[11-18]	**Contraindications**
• Tumor location >2 cm from the nipple • Negative axillary nodes • No lymphovascular involvement • No extensive intraductal component • Tumor grade 1 to 2 • HER2/neu negative • Tumor size <2–5 cm* • ER/PR positive*	• Inflammatory breast cancer • Clinical involvement of the nipple areolar complex • Nipple retraction • Paget's disease • Bloody nipple discharge • Multicentricity • HER2/neu positive • Tumor grade 3
Supporting factors	
• No prior breast surgery or radiation • Young, <45 years old • Non-smoker • No adjuvant radiation	
*Ongoing topics of research	

cancer recurrence rates of 1–12% have been noted at follow-ups of 13–66 months, respectively,[11] and some authors even advocate for further expanding these inclusion criteria.[18] A recent systematic review and meta-analysis found the pooled nipple areolar complex cancer recurrence rate to be 0.9%, compared to a 4.2% recurrence rate in the skin flap beyond the nipple areolar complex.[16]

In addition to the risk of cancer recurrence in the nipple, NSM creates an added reconstructive–aesthetic conundrum in that patients expect that the nipple will be preserved, which is not always the case. In fact, nipple necrosis rates with NSM range from 1 to 9.7% for partial necrosis, and 0 to 7.9% for total necrosis.[11] From a reconstructive standpoint, a number of variables, including active smoking, patient age, BMI, preoperative radiation, incision type, flap thickness, and breast size, have been identified as risk factors for nipple necrosis.[19–22] Full-thickness periareolar incisions for mastectomy access have been consistently demonstrated to increase the rate of nipple necrosis compared to alternatives, whereas an inferolateral inframammary fold incision is relatively well-tolerated.[20,23,24] Another study found that a C or larger bra cup size is associated with a 34% nipple necrosis rate (32% partial necrosis, 2% total necrosis) compared to a 6% nipple necrosis rate (all partial necrosis) with an A or B bra cup size ($p = 0.003$).[21] Although theoretically a concern, the degree of breast ptosis and the distance between the sternal notch and the nipple areolar complex has not been shown to impact complication rates following NSM.[22] Similarly, the use of a bio-prosthetic sling or concurrent axillary/nodal surgery is not associated with greater rates of nipple necrosis.[21]

Chemotherapy

Neoadjuvant chemotherapy is well established in breast cancer and can reduce the tumor burden in the breast and axilla, allowing for less extensive surgical operations.[25] As many of these agents are cytotoxic, they may theoretically increase a patient's risk for complications such as infection or wound healing issues.[26] However, multiple large cohort studies and meta-analyses have not demonstrated association between neoadjuvant chemotherapy and infection, skin necrosis, seroma, unplanned return to the operating room, or reconstructive failure.[27–29]

Adjuvant chemotherapy similarly plays a crucial role in improving disease recurrence and overall survival in breast cancer,[30,31] and has been extensively studied with regards to its association with reconstructive outcomes. Many chemotherapeutic agents have well-documented systemic side effects involving the heart, lungs, kidneys, and liver, among others that will vary depending on a

patient's particular regimen. The most recent regimens from the National Comprehensive Cancer Network guidelines are presented in Tables 14.3 and 14.4. Despite these systemic effects, the use of adjuvant chemotherapy after immediate breast reconstruction has been consistently demonstrated to be safe with regards to the risk of surgical complications, wound healing issues, and reconstructive failure.[32–34] Even in the setting of

Table 14.3 Neoadjuvant/adjuvant chemotherapy regimens for HER2-negative invasive breast cancer

Preferred regimens
• Dose-dense AC (doxorubicin/cyclophosphamide) followed by paclitaxel ever 2 weeks
• Dose-dense AC (doxorubicin/cyclophosphamide) followed by paclitaxel weekly
• TC (docetaxel and cyclophosphamide)

Other regimens
• Dose-dense AC (doxorubicin/cyclophosphamide)
• AC (doxorubicin/cyclophosphamide) every 3 weeks
• FAC/CAF (fluorouracil/doxorubicin/cyclophosphamide)
• FEC/CEF (cyclophosphamide/epirubicin/fluorouracil)
• CMF (cyclophosphamide/methotrexate/fluorouracil)
• AC (doxorubicin/cyclophosphamide) followed by docetaxel every 3 weeks
• AC (doxorubicin/cyclophosphamide) followed by weekly paclitaxel
• EC (epirubicin/cyclophosphamide)
• FEC/CEF (cyclophosphamide/epirubicin/fluorouracil) followed by docetaxel or weekly paclitaxel
• FAC (fluorouracil/doxorubicin/cyclophosphamide) followed by weekly paclitaxel
• TAC (docetaxel/doxorubicin/cyclophosphamide)

(Modified from the NCCN Guidelines version 2.2015 for Invasive Breast Cancer.)

Table 14.4 Neoadjuvant/adjuvant chemotherapy regimens for HER2-positive invasive breast cancer

Preferred regimens
• AC (doxorubicin/cyclophosphamide) followed by paclitaxel + trastuzumab ± pertuzumab
• TCH (docetaxel/carboplatin/trastuzumab) ± pertuzumab

Other regimens
• AC (doxorubicin/cyclophosphamide) followed by docetaxel + trastuzumab ± pertuzumab
• Docetaxel + cyclophosphamide + trastuzumab
• FEC (cyclophosphamide/epirubicin/fluorouracil) followed by docetaxel + trastuzumab + pertuzumab
• FEC (cyclophosphamide/epirubicin/fluorouracil) followed by paclitaxel + trastuzumab + pertuzumab
• Paclitaxel + trastuzumab
• Pertuzumab + trastuzumab + docetaxel followed by FEC (cyclophosphamide/epirubicin/fluorouracil)
• Pertuzumab + trastuzumab + paclitaxel followed by FEC (cyclophosphamide/epirubicin/fluorouracil)

(Modified from the NCCN Guidelines version 2.2015 for Invasive Breast Cancer.)

expander/implant-based breast reconstruction, adjuvant chemotherapy affected neither the timing of expander inflation nor surgical complication rates, including seroma, infection, or skin necrosis.[35]

Concomitantly, concerns that immediate breast reconstruction may delay the initiation of adjuvant chemotherapy have been largely refuted.[5,36–38] The largest study to date, including 3643 patients, concluded that while immediate reconstruction resulted in a modest but significant overall delay, it was unlikely to be clinically significant and did not lead to frank omission of chemotherapy.[39] Nonetheless, it is important to carefully coordinate the surgical plan with potential delays in mind. For example, patients with multiple risk factors for wound healing complications may benefit from modalities that offer the lowest risk of wound healing problems in order to facilitate transition to adjuvant therapy. Although the optimal timing of mastectomy, reconstruction, and adjuvant chemotherapy is an active topic of research, a significant survival benefit has been demonstrated with the initiation of chemotherapy even as late as 44 days[40] to 12 weeks[41] postoperatively.

Hormonal and biologic therapies

Targeted hormonal and biologic therapies have also emerged as important parts of the oncologic armamentarium in treating of breast cancer, with varying degrees of evidence on their impact on breast reconstruction outcomes. Estrogen has been understood to promote cutaneous wound healing via signaling through epidermal estrogen receptors.[42] Selective estrogen receptor modulators (SERMs) including tamoxifen and raloxifene have demonstrated similar accelerated cutaneous wound healing properties in an *in vivo* mouse model.[43] In an *in vitro* study of human fibroblasts, however, tamoxifen delayed cell proliferation, growth factor production, and consequently wound healing, but did improve scar formation.[44] A randomized controlled trial of tamoxifen in patients with a history of keloids

demonstrated a 40% absolute reduction in the risk of keloid development when compared to placebo.[45] With respect to safety, SERMs are largely considered low risk. However, tamoxifen has been associated with grade 2+ subcutaneous fibrosis when administered with concomitant radiotherapy,[46] as well as increased risk of venous thromboembolic disease, particularly in older women during their first 2 years after exposure.[47] The 5 year risk for venous thromboembolism in tamoxifen patients has been reported as 1.2%, compared to 0.5% within the control arm.[47]

Fewer studies to date have addressed the effects of relatively new biologic agents on surgical outcomes. The VEGF inhibitor bevacizumab has been associated with multiple wound complications, including dehiscence, ecchymosis, surgical site bleeding, and infections.[48] However, its evidence in breast reconstruction is currently limited. Golshan *et al.*[49] reviewed data on 13 patients with triple negative breast cancer undergoing mastectomy with immediate reconstruction, 5 of which received cisplatin alone (3 transverse rectus abdominis myocutaneous [TRAM] flaps and 2 expander/implant) and 8 cisplatin plus bevacizumab (2 TRAMs and 6 expander/implant). Of these, 4 patients (50% total, 66% of expander/implant reconstructions) in the bevacizumab plus cisplatin cohort experienced reconstructive failure after tissue expander placement with AlloDerm. To date, no studies have been published on the effects of HER2/neu pathway inhibitors, trastuzumab or lapatinib, on breast reconstruction outcomes.

Radiotherapy

For many patients with extensive nodal involvement, locally advanced breast cancers, or those undergoing breast conserving therapy, external beam radiation is a routine part of a multimodal treatment plan that has been shown to decrease loco-regional disease recurrence and even overall survival (Table 14.5).[50–52] Radiation exposure does, however, lead to fibrosis as well as

Table 14.5 Impact of postmastectomy radiotherapy on oncologic outcomes							
Citation	Follow-up time	No. of patients	Nodal status	Locoregional recurrence		Overall survival	
				PMRT	No PMRT	PMRT	No PMRT
Overgaard *et al.*, 1999	10 yr	135	N0	3%	17%	82%	70%
		1061	1–3N +	7%	30%	62%	54%
		51	≥4N +	14%	42%	32%	20%
Katz *et al.*, 2000	10 yr	132	N0	6%	23%	56%	55%
		794	1–3N +	6%	31%	55%	44%
		448	≥4N +	11%	46%	24%	17%
Truong *et al.*, 2005	20 yr	183	1–3N +	9%	20%	61%	53%
		112	≥4N +	17%	41%	30%	16%
PMRT, postmastectomy radiotherapy							

vascular and structural compromise of the skin and underlying tissues, putting patients at an increased risk of complications and poor aesthetic outcomes.[53] The best method for integrating breast reconstruction and radiation remains controversial and is an active area of ongoing research.

Preoperative radiation – prosthetic reconstruction

Patients with a history of radiation exposure generally present in one of two ways: immediate reconstruction after failed breast conserving therapy or delayed reconstruction following postmastectomy radiotherapy. One study of 76 patients comparing these two cohorts – in the setting of expander/implant reconstruction – did not identify any significant differences in outcomes between the two.[54]

When compared to those with no radiation exposure, patients undergoing prosthetic reconstruction in a previously irradiated field are at an increased risk for multiple complications including capsular contracture, wound dehiscence, implant extrusion, re-operation, and reconstructive failure.[55-60] Severe capsular contracture rates in the setting of prior radiotherapy can be as high as 20% at 10 years; compared to patients without any radiation exposure, the risk is increased 3.3- and 7.2-fold in one- and two-stage implant reconstruction, respectively.[56] Overall, this increased risk of complications manifests itself in relatively low rates of successful reconstruction, with reports as low as 60% in two-stage procedures.[54] In this cohort, nearly 56% of explantations or conversions to a flap occurred after tissue expander insertion, and 44% following expander/implant exchange. The most common underlying reasons included infection, pain or tightness, prosthesis exposure, or poor cosmesis.[54]

Despite conflicting early results within the literature, the deleterious effects of prior radiation are largely believed to decrease patient satisfaction and aesthetic outcomes in the setting of prosthetic reconstruction. A 2006 study of 315 expander/implant reconstruction found very good or excellent surgeon-reported aesthetic results in 55.1% of patients with prior irradiation, good results in 24.1%, fair in 17.2%, and poor in 3.4%, with no significant difference when compared to those whore never irradiated ($p = 0.225$).[61] More recently, however, multiple studies of patient collected data using the validated BREAST-Q (Reconstruction Module) have demonstrated a significantly negative effect on satisfaction with breast appearance as well as overall health-related quality of life.[62,63]

Preoperative radiation – autologous reconstruction

Because of concerns regarding the deleterious effect of radiation, many have historically favored autologous reconstruction in the setting of an irradiated field.[64] Nonetheless, these patients are generally still at an increased risk for complications, particularly fat necrosis, when compared to a cohort that is never irradiated.[65-68] A recent meta-analysis of reconstructive outcomes in this cohort demonstrated a 10% wound healing complication rates, 10% fat necrosis rates, 4% infection rate, 2% hematoma rate, and 4% seroma rate.[69] Of the 1011 total flap reconstructions performed on an irradiated field within the meta-analysis, the pooled flap loss rate was only 1% and partial flap necrosis rate 6%.[69] Overall, autologous reconstruction of previously irradiated chest is widely considered the safest and most reliable option and should be encouraged in patients willing to undergo a flap-based procedure.

Mantle radiation for lymphoma

Historically, the pattern of radiation for Hodgkin's lymphoma has covered lymph nodes in the neck, mediastinum, and axilla, and was referred to as "mantle radiation" because of its similarity to the distribution covered by a mantle.[70] Mantle radiation differs from postmastectomy radiation in that it focuses on the mediastinal lymph nodes; patients present with targeted area of irradiated tissue on the medial portion of the breast while the central and lateral portions generally remain healthy.[70] The overall dose of radiation is also typically less, ranging from 35–44 Gy compared to 60 Gy in whole-breast radiation.[70]

Only two case series of 23 total patients have been reported of breast reconstruction following mantle radiation.[70,71] Overall, eleven patients developed one or more complications, including 5 with mastectomy flap necrosis, 5 severe capsular contractures (1 grade IV, 4 grade III), 6 cellulitis, 4 seroma, 1 hematoma, and 1 chronic breast pain. Four patients undergoing initial expander/implant reconstruction required implant removal and salvage with an autologous tissue flap. Although these patients may not demonstrate significant radiation-induced changes to the skin,[70,71] physicians must remain cognizant of the increased risk in this unique cohort.

Postoperative radiation

The final determination regarding postmastectomy radiation is generally made only after a thorough evaluation of tumor and lymph node specimens by pathology. While there is some institutional and physician variation in treatment protocols, some current indications for postmastectomy radiotherapy generally include locally advanced tumors with positive nodes or positive surgical margins (see Table 14.1). In these treated patients, benefits include significant reductions in long-term loco-regional recurrence and overall survival rates (see Table 14.5). The optimal management of breast reconstruction in the setting of anticipated post-mastectomy radiation is somewhat controversial with some promulgating an immediate conversion to implant prior to radiation, and others advocating a delayed approach.[54,57,72,73] For those considering autologous reconstruction, there is also the variant known as the "delayed-immediate" approach wherein the expander is placed deliberately in advance of anticipated radiation to hold and preserve the native skin envelope and volume until after radiation when definitive autologous (or prosthetic) reconstruction can be performed.[74–76] A traditional alternative in this setting is to delay the reconstruction altogether until after radiation, in which case an autologous reconstruction will almost certainly be necessary.

Medications

A complete medication history should include all over-the-counter and herbal/alternative drugs, in addition to prescription medications. In this section we will review the evidence for some of the most common medications that a reconstructive surgeon may encounter.

In general, medications associated with withdrawal syndromes should be continued or tapered as needed in the perioperative period. Oral medications may be substituted for a transdermal, transmucosal, or intravenous form in order to compensate for impaired absorption secondary to decreased gastrointestinal function or decreased oral intake.

Aspirin/NSAIDs

Aspirin irreversibly inhibits platelet cyclooxygenase, increasing perioperative blood loss and the risk for hemorrhagic complications.[77,78] Despite potential benefits with regards to minimizing cardiovascular complications, the POISE-2 trial found that in patients undergoing non-cardiac surgery aspirin increases bleeding risk without any improvement in cardiovascular outcomes or overall mortality.[79] In breast reconstruction, the hematoma rate increases to 9.2% in patients on aspirin compared to 4.7% in the control group.[80] Although its plasma half-life is only 20 minutes, the irreversible effects of aspirin may take up to 10 days to resolve. In general, most patients taking aspirin monotherapy benefit from holding their doses for one to two weeks prior to surgery.[81]

Other nonsteroidal anti-inflammatory drugs (NSAIDs) exhibit reversible inhibition of cyclooxygenase isoforms resulting in a similar antiplatelet effect and increased risk for bleeding.[82] Selective COX-2 inhibitors, including

celecoxib, have minimal effects on platelet function, but appear to have deleterious cardiovascular effects instead.[83] In general, many surgeons similarly recommend discontinuing NSAIDs, including selective COX-2 inhibitors, one to two weeks prior to surgery, although in a healthy individual, ibuprofen's effect on platelet function appears to normalize within 24 hours.[84]

Oral contraceptives

Oral contraceptives are a widespread class of medication used to both prevent pregnancy and treat a number of gynecologic conditions. Their prevalence makes them a leading cause of thromboembolic events in young women, with baseline rates as high as 0.1% that only further increase in the setting of surgery and an active malignancy.[85,86] Most surgeons recommend discontinuing birth control pills 4–6 weeks prior to surgery so that estrogen/progestin levels may return to physiologic levels. It is important to remind patients that other methods of contraception should be used to prevent unwanted pregnancies through at least the first week after resuming the medication.

Glucocorticoids

Patients on corticosteroids must balance their benefit in treating the disease process against the risks of immunosuppression, increased protein catabolism, and poor wound healing.[87]

Generally, the human body produces 10–12 mg of cortisol daily. This number increases to approximately 25–50 mg/day with moderate stress, and 75–150 mg/day with major stress, returning to baseline within 24–48 hours of the inciting event.[87] With patients on chronic steroid therapy, decision-making surrounding the possibility of a suppressed hypothalamic–pituitary–adrenal axis is generally guided by the duration and dosing leading up to the operation.[88–90] Patients who have taken steroids for less than three weeks, or who are on chronic alternate-day therapy, are unlikely to have a suppressed axis and may continue their usual dose. Alternatively, patients taking greater than a dose equivalent of 20 mg of prednisone for three or more weeks will require greater doses perioperatively. Those on a dose equivalent to 5–20 mg of prednisone for greater than 3 weeks can either undergo testing or receive an empiric postoperative glucocorticoid burst.

Past surgical history

A focused surgical history in the breast reconstruction patients must include details of all prior surgical procedures, particularly those involving the breast, abdomen, or other potential donor sites.

Breast surgery

It has been estimated that over 2 million women in the United States have undergone augmentation mammaplasty, with another 300 000 procedures being performed each year.[91] When faced with breast reconstruction, this cohort has demonstrated a predilection for implant-based procedures, either alone or with a latissimus dorsi flap.[92–95] This preference is, at least in part, due to their willingness to receive implants as well as their relatively low BMIs, with less soft tissue available for flaps.[92,96]

Complication rates following reconstruction in this cohort do not appear to be affected by the location of the previous implants or the reconstructive procedure (i.e., direct to implant vs. expander/implant),[96] and are largely the same as complication rates for the general population.[97,98] Only one small study found a significant difference driven largely by capsular contracture, which the authors hypothesize may be a result of residual biofilm or capsule from the previous augmentation.[96] Nonetheless, patient satisfaction rates with their reconstruction have been noted to be greater in patients with a history of augmentation.[92]

Abdominal surgery

Abdominal scars of all types (e.g., subcostal, Pfannenstiel, midline laparotomy, etc.) may devascularize portions of an abdominal flap compromising its survival[99] and increasing donor site morbidity.[26,100,101] In order to counteract any potential flap unreliability, strategies to improve abdomen-based flap perfusion, including surgical delay, flap design modifications, and microvascular augmentation of flap perfusion may be indicated.[102–106] With careful planning, DIEP flaps have been successfully reported in patients with vertical or short-transverse scars from prior intra-abdominal surgery[99] as well as Pfannenstiel incisions.[107]

A history of abdominoplasty is particularly concerning as the perforators supplying the tissue flaps have been previously transected during the undermining and resection of the upper abdominal flap. Although a handful of small studies have noted the ingrowth of new perforators through the rectus abdominis, allowing for successful abdominal flap reconstruction,[99,108–110] prior abdominoplasty should be considered a relative contraindication to abdominally-based breast reconstruction.

Comorbidities

Knowledge of a patient's medical comorbidities facilitates patient-centered discussions regarding the optimal timing and modality of reconstruction. Combined with a nomogram[60] or individual risk calculator[111,112] these data allow surgeons to characterize a patient's individual risks for complications, facilitating patient education and perioperative decision-making. Below we discuss the effect of common comorbidities on patient outcomes.

Diabetes mellitus

Diabetes mellitus is itself an end result of a variety of metabolic processes, which can be largely classified into two distinct processes: type 1, insulin-dependent diabetes and type 2 diabetes. Regardless of the underlying process, diabetes has been traditionally associated with a number of systemic effects including peripheral artery disease, microvascular disease, neuropathy, and immune compromise.[113] Over 100 cytologic factors have been identified that may lead to increased wound healing complications in diabetes.[114] More recently, a number of studies are beginning to explore potential differences in the adverse effects of insulin-dependent, type 1 diabetes and type 2 diabetes – potentially as a surrogate for effects of both short and long-term glycemic control.[115]

One recent study using a nationwide patent registry found an increased risk of wound complications in diabetics on univariate analysis (4.6% vs. 9.8%, $p < 0.001$), that went away upon adjusting for potential confounding variables, including obesity, which is often associated with type 2 diabetes as a part of the larger "metabolic syndrome".[116] A handful of smaller studies have recapitulated this finding in smaller, single-center cohorts, demonstrating no increase in wound complications or reconstructive failure in diabetics.[117,118] The largest study on this topic to date, including nearly 30 000 patients, found a small but significant increased risk of overall complication, including wound complications, in diabetics undergoing autologous reconstruction; this effect was a greater in insulin-dependent, type 1 diabetics than in type 2 diabetics.[115]

It is important to note that these studies are all limited in that they are retrospective in nature and potentially influenced by selection bias. Also, a history of diabetes does not necessarily suggest poor glycemic control, particularly since the Surgical Care Improvement Project (SCIP) guidelines have recommended postoperative blood glucose ≤200 mg/dL on postoperative days one and two.[119] Although additional studies are indicated to better characterize the risks associated with diabetes mellitus following breast reconstruction, the effect of poor glycemic control on wound complications is generally well accepted.[113,114] Proper medical management of a patient's diabetes leading up to and following breast reconstruction should be emphasized.

Smoking

Smoking exerts a variety of well-understood negative effects on wound healing, microvascular blood flow, and oxygen delivery, increasing the risk for wound complications and their downstream sequelae following breast reconstruction.[60,120–126] Particularly following autogenous reconstruction, smoking can increase rates of flap necrosis and donor site complications, such that many surgeons suggest excluding smokers from candidacy for such procedures.[126–128]

Interestingly, the adverse effects of smoking may persist even after quitting. One study of 227 TRAMs demonstrated a step-wise decrease in postoperative complication rates between current smokers, ex-smokers (quit within the past 12 months), and non-smokers.[126] More recently, an analysis of nearly 12 000 patients demonstrated a 2.46-times increase in the odds of flap loss in former smokers when compared to never smokers, regardless of the particular reconstructive procedure.[111] Additional studies are required to clarify these still controversial findings[129] and better characterize the true effect of former smoking on patient outcomes.

All smokers seeking consultation for breast reconstruction should be strongly urged to quit at least 3–4 weeks prior to their operations in order to reduce the occurrence of complications.[130] For patients who are concerned of relapse, nicotine replacement therapy has been demonstrated to increase smoking cessation rates by 50–70% without any added risk of wound healing complications.[130–132]

Obesity

Breast reconstruction in obese patients is a challenging procedure as these patients are not only prone to increased complication rates compared to non-obese patients,[133–138] but their relatively large and ptotic breasts can be aesthetically difficult to reconstruct, particularly in the setting of a unilateral procedure. Obesity exerts its negative effects on surgical outcomes via two broad categories of mechanism. The first involves the direct effects of a patient's body habitus on the surgical procedure, and the second the comorbid conditions with which obesity is strongly associated. These include coronary artery disease, diabetes, obstructive sleep apnea, hypertension, hyperlipidemia, microvascular disease, abdominal wall hernias, and venous disease, among others.[139]

The use of tissue expander/implant reconstruction in this cohort remains a contentious issue. The increased risk of reconstructive failure and patient dissatisfaction with aesthetic results[140,141] has led some surgeons to advocate for the use of autologous breast reconstruction in obese patients.[142] Nonetheless, others argue that although elevated, both overall complication and reconstructive failure rates remain acceptable, and expander/implant reconstruction should be offered along with autologous procedures to all women who are interested, regardless of their BMI.[143,144]

One of the major cosmetic challenges in this cohort stems from difficulties in achieving large volumes and ptosis in reconstructed breasts, particularly in the setting of unilateral reconstruction. One study of 262 patients found that obese patients undergoing an expander/implant procedure had an odds ratio of 0.14 for aesthetic satisfaction when compared to normal weight individuals.[141] In these patients the use of acellular dermal matrix or other bioprosthetic slings may facilitate the accommodation of large expanders or implants, and allow for the recreation of a more natural-appearing inferior pole projection and ptosis similar to the pre-mastectomy state.[145–147]

In addition to providing ample tissue for the reconstruction of large, ptotic breasts, flap reconstruction provides the added benefit of excising excess soft tissue from potential donor sites including the abdomen, inner thigh, and buttocks. In this high-risk cohort, however, traditional TRAM flaps may decrease upper abdominal strength, particularly in bilateral reconstructions.[148] Muscle-sparing TRAMs and perforator flaps[149–151] present attractive alternatives with significantly less abdominal wall morbidity (<5% incidence of abdominal weakness) and excellent overall results (<2% flap failure) in the hands of an experienced surgeon.[152]

Connective tissue disease

Although no clear link has been demonstrated between connective tissue disease (CTD) and breast cancer, their relative commonality makes it likely for reconstructive surgeons to encounter this challenging cohort of patients.[153,154] Many CTD patients develop severe reactions to radiotherapy likely mediated by a TGF-β response to radiation and the reactivation of quiescent disease[155] that drives tissue fibrosis, often manifesting as a late tissue response.[156] Interestingly, this reaction is more common with radiotherapy for breast cancer than other malignancies and is most prevalent in patients with scleroderma and systemic lupus erythematosus.[157] Although this concern does not preclude breast conservation and whole breast radiotherapy, many women with CTD seek to avoid radiotherapy and opt for a mastectomy with or without reconstruction instead.[157]

In general, a combination of disruptions in the TGF-β pathway, autoantibodies against collagen or other structural molecules, vasculopathy or disorders of angiogenesis, and the effects of anti-inflammatory or immune-modulating drugs all increase the risks of wound dehiscence in CTD patients.[158] Additionally, in some patients secondary conditions including antiphospholipid syndrome may result in a hypercoagulable state and increased risk of venous thromboembolism.[159] Other complications of interest include persistent seroma, particularly at the donor site for autologous reconstructions, and even delayed hematoma formation, believed to be secondary to platelet abnormalities.[158] To date, only small case series have been published on breast reconstruction in this high-risk cohort, and the true risk for complications remains to be determined.

Respiratory disease

For patients with a history of underlying lung pathology, normal perioperative pulmonary physiology may prove to be enough of a burden to drive the development of postoperative pulmonary complications. Particularly after operations exceeding 2.5 hours,[160] postoperative diaphragmatic dysfunction, pain, and splinting drive a reduction in lung volumes that may persist for up to 1 week in these patients.[161]

A known history of COPD increases the risk of postoperative pulmonary complications by 2.7- to 6-fold.[162] One large study using data from the National Surgical Quality Improvement Program registry found that COPD is associated with an adjusted odds ratio of 1.71 for postoperative pneumonia, 1.54 for unplanned re-intubation, and 1.45 for failure to wean from the ventilator.[163] Despite this increased risk, there does not appear to be a single prohibitive level of pulmonary function below which surgery is absolutely contraindicated in this population.[164,165] Only a handful of studies have specifically explored the effect of COPD on breast reconstruction and found similar relationships with major complications and delays in reconstruction.[166] Nonetheless, the risks and benefits of surgery, and potentially multiple operations in the context of breast reconstruction, must be weighed carefully on an individual basis.

Unlike COPD, despite initial beliefs that patients with underlying asthma experienced greater rates of pulmonary complications, more recent studies have failed to demonstrate a link between well-controlled asthma and adverse outcomes. That said, optimal medical management of a patient's asthma should be emphasized before moving forward with an elective operation.[167]

Bleeding/clotting disorders

At either end of the spectrum, disorders of the body's natural response to endothelial damage and clot formation may predispose the breast reconstruction patient to a number of potentially serious complications. Thrombophilia is the manifestation of a wide range of hereditary or acquired conditions that places patients at a significantly increased risk of venous thromboembolism (VTE).[168] The increased risk of postoperative VTE has been reported to range between 5- and 20-fold in these patients,[169] and may be increased even further in relatively prolonged autologous procedures.[170]

Of particular interest to the breast reconstruction patient is the potentially increased risk for anastomotic thrombosis and flap loss in hypercoagulable patients undergoing microsurgical reconstruction. Only a handful of small studies and case reports have explored this topic to date.[171–174] The largest series includes 100 patients undergoing free tissue transfer, of which 11 tested positive for pathologic heterozygous factor V Leiden mutation.[171] Although this study failed to identify a significant correlation between the thrombophilic disorder and flap failure secondary to thrombotic occlusion, their analyses were significantly underpowered to detect a difference in such a rare complication. A number of other, recent studies have demonstrated flap failure rates close to 15% in hypercoagulable patients,[172,173,175] much greater than the 1–2% typically seen in contemporary series of free tissue transfers.[176]

Ultimately, the majority of patients safely undergo free flap breast reconstruction, and the odds are that many undiagnosed patients have, and will continue to do so, as well. Nonetheless, the strong likelihood of an increased risk is enough for some surgeons to recommend against free tissue transfer in these patients,[172,174] promoting the use of prosthetic or pedicled flap reconstruction. Still, others will cautiously offer free tissue transfer along with the administration of therapeutic anticoagulation with the understanding of an increased risk for flap loss.[173,177,178]

At the other end of the spectrum, the presence of a bleeding disorder puts patients at an increased risk of developing a potentially life-threatening bleed or hematoma. One study of over 16 000 breast reconstructions identified a history of bleeding disorders as a risk factor for both major medical and surgical complications, demonstrating the utility of this information in perioperative risk stratification and decision-making.[116] When a bleeding disorder is known or suspected, the most crucial step is accurate diagnosis and treatment in order to prevent a potentially life-threatening perioperative bleed.[179] Preoperative screening, however, is not currently indicated in patients with a negative history and physical examination.[180,181]

Physical examination

The specific details of the physical exam as relevant to each reconstructive procedure will be reviewed in its respective chapter. In general, the physical exam should include basic vital signs, including height, weight and BMI, in addition to a detailed examination of the breasts and potential donor sites for autologous reconstruction.

The breast examination should focus on a number of factors including the position of the inframammary fold and nipple, asymmetries, skin thickness and quality, scars, and an axillary exam. This information can help determine a patient's aesthetic goals, particularly in unilateral reconstructions, and clarify the role of potential symmetry procedures at the time of reconstruction. Additionally, measurements of the sternum to the nipple, nipple to the inframammary fold, and the base diameter of the breast are taken to facilitate implant selection. Other findings such as the overall size of the mass, clinically positive lymph nodes, nipple inversion or discharge, Paget's disease, or peau d'orange will affect a patient's candidacy for NSM and/or post-mastectomy reconstruction, and should be incorporated into the discussion of reconstructive modality.

For patients considering autologous breast reconstruction, a variety of donor sites including the abdomen, buttocks, thigh, and back should be examined closely with an eye towards adequate volume for reconstruction. Previous scars following abdominal or pelvic surgery are discussed earlier in this chapter and should be noted as a potential source of damage to the vasculature and incisional hernias.

Preoperative photographs

Pre- and postoperative photography is now the standard of care in breast reconstruction, facilitating documentation, collaboration, patient education, and research.

Reviewing photographs with a patient during the initial consultation shifts the conversation from a one-sided discussion – a surgeon talking *to* the patient – into a collaborative environment in which the surgeon talks *with* the patient about what they can expect,[182] although care must be taken to avoid the implication of a guaranteed result.[183] Postoperatively, photographs allow patients and surgeons alike to more objectively assess results *vis-à-vis* expected outcomes, guiding the need for additional surgeries and/or symmetry procedures. Moreover, systematically reviewing postoperative images over time can even allow surgeons to track and study the evolution of their practice, promoting quality improvement and evidence-based decision-making.

Images of the breast can vary significantly based on their framing as well as the patient's configuration, and a systematic approach is critical in obtaining high quality, standardized images. The borders should extend from above the suprasternal notch in the lower neck

superiorly to below the midcostal margins inferiorly. Arms may be positioned either at the side, on the hips, or behind the lower back, and common views include anteroposterior (AP), lateral, and oblique images. Although conditions may vary based on the setting and available equipment, DiBernardo *et al.*[184] recommend positioning the patient in front of a suitable background and using a 50 mm lens at a distance of 3 feet and with a reproduction ratio of 1:12 in order to obtain high quality and standardized photographs. A medium blue or 18% gray background has been suggested in order to provide the best skin tones without affecting exposure.

Markings

The preoperative markings vary from one procedure to the next and will be discussed in detail within each procedure's respective chapter. General landmarks on the breast are depicted in Fig. 14.1 and include the position of the inframammary fold, midline, and mastectomy incision, among others. Donor site markings may include the anatomic boundaries of the flap, incision sites, the anticipated course of the vascular pedicle, and potential Doppler marking.

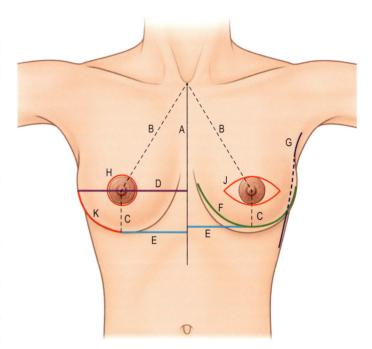

Fig. 14.1 Example of preoperative markings for breast reconstruction. Landmarks and measures of interest include (A) the midline, (B) sternal notch to nipple areolar complex, (C) nipple to inframammary fold (IMF) distance, (D) breast width, (E) projection of the IMF onto the midline and IMF offset, (F) the inframammary fold, and (G) the lateral border of the torso. The red lines represent potential mastectomy incisions: (H) circular and (J) elliptical periareolar incisions are common approaches to skin-sparing mastectomy with autologous and prosthetic reconstruction, respectively, whereas an inferolateral inframammary fold incision (K) is commonly used in nipple-sparing mastectomy.

Imaging

Perforator vessels vary significantly in size and distribution from one patient to the next, and even in the same patient from one hemi-abdomen to the other. Preoperative imaging of vascular anatomy has demonstrated good correlation with actual perforator locations and plays an important role in the work-up for a perforator-based flap reconstruction.[185-189] On average, vascular imaging decreases operative time by more than an hour in bilateral cases[189] and is associated with significantly fewer complications including partial flap loss, donor site morbidity,[189] and, in the abdomen, even increase the percentage of flaps successfully raised as DIEPs.[188] Cost–utility analyses favor the use of preoperative angiography in abdominal perforator flaps for breast reconstruction.[190]

Table 14.6 broadly outlines some of the available imaging techniques for perforator flaps. Considerations in perforator selection as well as details regarding specific imaging modalities are beyond the scope of this chapter and will be covered elsewhere.

Risk/benefit communication

Successful patient education facilitates informed decision-making and has been demonstrated to increase patient satisfaction as well as their overall postoperative quality of life.[191-194] Multiple comprehensive frameworks[191,195-198] exist to aid in this process. Most recently, the movement towards evidence-based decision-making has made quantitative risk assessment, particularly risk calculators, a popular new option.

Risk calculators

Effective communication of risk is contingent upon both the use of accurate, applicable data and patient

Table 14.6 Preoperative imaging modalities for perforator flaps	
Modality[185-190]	**Pros/Cons**
Doppler ultrasound	Fast, readily available at the beside, but unreliable compared to other modalities
MRA	Avoids radiation and use of IV contrast, but costly with generally poorer quality images than CTA
CTA	Fast with superior images, but at the cost of radiation exposure (effective dose of 5.6 mSv) and IV contrast
Angiography	Very accurate, but invasive and requires contrast. Largely replaced by CTA or MRA

CTA, computed tomography angiography; MRA, magnetic resonance angiography.

comprehension. Qualitative terms like "unlikely" or "rare" are vague and can be difficult to interpret,[198] whereas quantitative estimates eliminate any uncertainty, conveying a clear and consistent message. Even then, the challenge becomes providing accurate data that is relevant to the patient at hand. Population-derived measures of average risk often disguise the heterogeneity of breast reconstruction patients within a single number that either underestimate or overestimate most individuals' risk significantly.[112] Risk calculators have emerged across a variety of fields as a potential solution to this problem.[199,200] By tailoring a risk estimate to a patient's unique combination of comorbidities and demographic information, these calculators obviate the inaccurate extrapolation of average measures in an objective and reproducible manner.

This was the genesis for the Breast Reconstruction Risk Assessment (BRA) score.[112] The web-based BRA score calculator (Fig. 14.2) utilizes data from various multicenter patient registries including NSQIP, MROC, and TOPS to provide robust, validated models for a wide range of medical and surgical outcomes.[111,112,201] Acknowledging the inherent limitations of registry data, post-hoc modifications from systematic review of the literature help to enhance clinical relevance of the BRA score models.

Shared decision-making

Even to the well-informed patient, the decisions regarding the ultimate timing and modality of reconstruction are often very challenging to make.[195] A number of algorithms and guidelines exist to assist in shared decision-making between the surgeon and patient, facilitating these otherwise difficult decisions and increasing the acceptance of breast reconstruction altogether.[191,195,202,203]

While the specific relative indications and contraindications for varying procedures will be elucidated in subsequent, dedicated chapters, suffice it to say that from a global perspective autologous procedures allow for (1) a more natural reconstruction using the patient's own tissue; (2) a concomitant excision of soft tissue from donor sites including the abdomen; (3) potentially enhanced long-term patient satisfaction;[204] (4) relative resistance to radiation-induced complications *vis-à-vis* prosthetic reconstructions;[64] (5) a skin paddle where there is a functional or aesthetic need for enhancement or supplementation; and (6) obviated concerns for prosthetic malfunction or maintenance (Table 14.7). The downsides, however, include (1) longer operations with concomitantly longer hospital stays and postoperative recovery periods; (2) donor site morbidity including an additional surgical site and scar as well as functional and aesthetic concerns;[148,205,206] and (3) that these procedures are technically more challenging, often requiring additional training and specialized equipment (see Table 14.7).

Prosthetic-based reconstruction, in contrast, offers (1) shorter individual procedures and faster recovery; (2) reasonable control over breast volume and projection; (3) avoidance of a donor site with concomitant morbidities; (4) specialized training or surgical equipment – such as that needed for microsurgery – is generally unnecessary[207–212] (Table 14.8). Nonetheless, there are

sundry disadvantages, including additional surgery in the case of a two-stage expander implant process (conversely direct-to-implant procedures may be subject to limitations in volume and potentially higher rates of secondary revision) limited with regards to symmetry and implant size, and two-stage procedures necessarily require an additional operation, frequent office visits for expansion, and a prolonged period of time until definitive reconstruction is achieved. Furthermore, patients require long-term implant maintenance and are subject to potential implant-related complications, including capsular contracture, rippling and contour hollowing,

Breast Reconstruction Risk Assessment (BRA) Score

To calculate the estimated risk for postoperative complications in a patient who underwent mastectomy with immediate tissue expander or autologous reconstruction, complete the following worksheet.

Some models abstracted from participant use files of the Mastectomy Reconstruction Outcomes Consortium (MROC) database.
Some models abstracted from participant use files of the Tracking Operations and Outcomes for Plastic Surgeons (TOPS) database.
Some models abstracted from participant use files of the National Surgical Quality Improvement Program (NSQIP).

Height [62] ● in ○ m
Weight [145] ● lb ○ kg
Age [55]

	Yes	No
Do you have high blood pressure or are you taking medications for high blood pressure?	●	○
Have you been diagnosed with diabetes mellitus?	●	○
Have you experienced difficult, painful, or labored breathing? (only count if 30 days or fewer prior to procedure)	○	●
Have you undergone chemotherapy? (only count if 30 days or fewer prior to procedure)	○	●

American Society of Anesthesiologists (ASA) Physical Status Classification [2 ▼]
What is this?

Smoking status [Never ▼]

Are you having one or both breasts reconstructed? [Both ▼]

Have you had, or do you predict having, radiation therapy? [No ▼]

Bleeding risks:

	Yes	No
Vitamin K deficiency	○	●
Thrombocytopenia	○	●
Hemophilia	○	●
Other diagnosed clotting disorder	○	●
Coumadin, NSAIDs, or other anti-Coagulant NOT discontinued prior to surgery	○	●
Chronic aspirin therapy	○	●

Have you ever had a:

	Yes	No
Balloon angioplasty	○	●
Stent placement	○	●
Coronary artery bypass graft	○	●
Valve replacement/repair	○	●
Implantation of pacemaker/defibrillator	○	●
Other major cardiac surgery	○	●

Calculate Risk

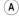

Fig. 14.2 User interface for the BRA Score web application. (**A**) Users may enter a series of data on patient demographics and medical comorbidities in order to obtain individualized risk estimated for postoperative complications. Estimates are generated from the NSQIP, MROC, and TOPS databases.[111,112,201] Web application is available at www.BRAscore.org.

Outcome	Reconstructive Modality				
	Tissue Expander	Pedicled Abdominal (TRAM) Flap	Latissimus Flap	Microvascular Reconstruction	Single-Stage Implant
Overall Complications	13.01%[1] – 13.86%[2]	29.69%[2] – 34.53%[1]	21.30%[2] – 41.78%[1]	22.48%[2] – 34.82%[1]	26.39%[1]
Overall Medical Complications[3]	1.37%	4.99%	1.88%	10.9%	
Overall Medical Complications[2]	13.86%	29.69%	21.30%	22.48%	
Surgical Site Infection[3]	3.53%	5.64%	2.61%	5.83%	
Seroma[2]	1.65%	2.87%	5.25%	2.48%	
Dehiscence[2]	3.99%	14.30%	5.45%	6.71%	
Flap Loss (Partial or Total)[2]	n/a	11.85%	3.40%	11.48%	
Explantation[2]	5.12%	n/a	n/a	n/a	[1] Abstracted from MROC data [2] Abstracted from TOPS data [3] Abstracted from NSQIP data
30-Day Reoperation[2]	5.20%	8.32%	3.84%	9.15%	

Fig. 14.2, cont'd (**B**) Risks are presented for overall complications, including medical and surgical complications, as well as 30-day hospital readmission. Surgical complications include surgical site infection, seroma, wound dehiscence, flap loss, or explantation. Complication rates are compared side by side for tissue expander based, pedicled TRAM, latissimus, and microvascular reconstructions.

Table 14.7 Benefits of autologous reconstruction[204–209]
Benefits
• Allows for a more natural feel and appearance of the reconstructed breast • No risk for implant related complications or long-term maintenance* • Improved reconstructive outcomes in the setting of prior radiotherapy • Offers skin paddle for functional or aesthetic enhancement or supplementation • Potential upside of excision of excess tissue from donor sites • Possibly improved long-term patient satisfaction • Generally a one-stage procedure • In the case of perforator flaps, potentially amenable to favorable reimbursement exceptions
Disadvantages
• Longer operative times • Longer postoperative hospitalization and recovery period • Potential complication of total flap loss • Donor site morbidity including reconstructive complications, functional disability, aesthetic deformity • Heightened problems with flap contracture and volume loss if subject to post-reconstruction radiotherapy • Can be technically more challenging, potentially requiring additional training and technology
*With the exception of a latissimus flap with prosthesis or other flap–implant combinations

Table 14.8 Prosthetic reconstruction[204–209]
Benefits
• Relative technical simplicity • Faster operation • Shorter hospitalization • More rapid postoperative recovery • Lack of donor site morbidity • Better potential control of breast size and projection • Ideal for women with minimal tissue at potential donor sites • Does not require specialized microsurgical training or technology
Disadvantages
• Less able to replicate natural, ptotic breast • Long-term implant maintenance and complications (i.e., need for MRI surveillance with silicone implants, possible implant rupture, capsular contracture, rippling and contour hollowing, malposition, rupture, palpability or visibility, exposure) • Less resistance to the deleterious effects of radiotherapy • Potentially decreased long-term patient satisfaction • Second surgery with expander/implant reconstruction • Frequent clinic visits for expansion of tissue expander

malposition, rupture, implant palpability or visibility, or frank exposure.[213,214]

The choice of immediate vs. delayed reconstruction has a similar profile of divergent advantages and disadvantages.[215] Immediate reconstruction may (1) minimize psychosocial effects associated with the mastectomy defect in the interim period; (2) combine reconstruction with the oncologic resection in a single operation; 3) potentially avoid the functional and aesthetic ramifications of scarring and loss of normal anatomy that occurs with delaying reconstruction. On the other hand, the delayed reconstruction can allow for demarcated tissue healing without further stressing mastectomy flaps and, in the setting of autologous reconstruction, can avoid subjecting the flap to the tissue-deforming sequelae of radiation.

Conclusion

Preoperative evaluation for breast reconstruction generally includes understanding a patient's oncologic status, treatment plan, past medical and surgical history, medications, anatomy, and postoperative expectations. Given the diverse array of reconstructive techniques available, such preoperative evaluation can also help generate risk–benefit profiles that can, in turn, guide shared decision-making between surgeon and patient. In this way, more thorough preoperative planning not only enhances patient understanding but may also yield superior, more *predictable* outcomes for breast reconstruction.

Access the complete reference list online at http://www.expertconsult.com

16. Mallon P, Feron JG, Couturaud B, et al. The role of nipple-sparing mastectomy in breast cancer: a comprehensive review of the literature. *Plast Reconstr Surg.* 2013;131:969–984. *Mallon and colleagues provided a thorough review of the literature examining the safety of nipple-sparing mastectomy and the factors influencing occult nipple malignancy in breast cancer patients. Many of the tumor characteristics they found to influence occult malignancy, including tumor–nipple distance less than 2 cm, grade, presence of nodal metasteses, lymphovascular invasion, HER-2 positivity, ER/PR negativity, tumor size, location, and multicentricity, are widely used in clinical decision-making regarding nipple-sparing techniques.*

26. Mehrara BJ, Santoro TD, Arcilla E, et al. Complications after microvascular breast reconstruction: experience with 1195 flaps. *Plast Reconstr Surg.* 2006;118:1100–1109, discussion 1110-1111. *The authors examined nearly 1200 cases of microvascular breast reconstruction, benchmarking the incidence of both major and minor complications as well as elucidating many of the risk factors associated with adverse events. The low major complication rate, and 0.5% total flap loss rate in particular, highlights the safety of microvascular techniques for breast reconstruction in highly-trained hands.*

39. Alderman AK, Collins ED, Schott A, et al. The impact of breast reconstruction on the delivery of chemotherapy. *Cancer.* 2010;116:1791–1800. *Concerns regarding the potential for an undue delay in the initiation of systemic chemotherapy in immediate breast reconstructions remained a significant barrier for surgeons and patients alike prior to this 2010 article by Alderman and colleagues. This multicenter study of over 3600 patients provided strong evidence that immediate breast reconstruction does not lead to omission of chemotherapy and that the modest delay in the initiation of treatment is unlikely to be of any clinical significance.*

64. Kronowitz SJ, Robb GL. Radiation therapy and breast reconstruction: a critical review of the literature. *Plast Reconstr Surg.* 2009;124:395–408. *This critical review of the literature provides thoughtful discussion on the optimal timing and technique of breast reconstruction in patients who may require postmastectomy radiation therapy. The article weights the risks and benefits of both delayed and immediate prosthetic reconstruction and autologous reconstrion, as well the alternative "delayed-immediate" technique in light of the most up-to-date evidence at the time of its publication, and provides a great foundation for continued study of this important topic.*

76. Kronowitz SJ, Hunt KK, Kuerer HM, et al. Delayed-immediate breast reconstruction. *Plast Reconstr Surg.* 2004;113:1617–1628. *In this 2004 study, the authors describe their two-stage, "delayed-immediate" approach to breast reconstruction. In an attempt to capitalize on the benefits of an immediate reconstruction while minimizing the deleterious effects of postmastectomy radiation therapy on the final*

outcomes, the authors advocate for the immediate insertion of a tissue expander at the time of mastectomy with definitive delayed reconstruction following the completion of radiation therapy. The authors also present the cases for 16 breasts treated in this manner and conclude that "delayed-immediate" breast reconstruction can achieve the aesthetic outcomes of immediate reconstruction while avoiding the aesthetic and radiation-delivery concerns of immediate reconstruction.

79. Devereaux PJ, Mrkobrada M, Sessler DI, et al. Aspirin in patients undergoing noncardiac surgery. *N Engl J Med.* 2014;370:1494–1503. *Perioperative medication management is an important part of ensuring patient safety and minimizing adverse events. This randomized control trial of aspirin use in non-cardiac surgery found that in all patients, even those already taking aspirin routinely, the initiation or continuation of aspirin therapy perioperatively did not significantly affect the rate of death of non-fatal myocardial infarction at 30 days. Aspirin use was, however, associated with a greater risk of major bleeding (4.6% in aspirin group vs 3.8% in placebo; HR = 1.23; P = 0.04).*

112. Kim JY, Khavanin N, Jordan SW, et al. Individualized risk of surgical-site infection: an application of the breast reconstruction risk assessment score. *Plast Reconstr Surg.* 2014;134:351e–362e. *Individualized risk calculators take the concept of preoperative risk assessment one step beyond the traditional cohort study by individualizing estimates given a patient's unique combination of demographic and clinical characteristics. The Breast Reconstruction Risk Assessment score (BRAscore) risk calculator is the first individual risk calculator available to plastic surgeons, leveraging data from a variety of sources to provide relevant and accurate estimates for a number of complications across the various breast reconstruction modalities. This article by Kim and colleagues details the development and internal validation of the first iteration of one of these models, focusing on a patient's risk for postoperative surgical site infection.*

118. Miller RB, Reece G, Kroll SS, et al. Microvascular breast reconstruction in the diabetic patient. *Plast Reconstr Surg.* 2007;119:38–45, discussion 46–48. *Diabetes mellitus is a very common and potentially significant risk factor in a number of surgical procedures because of its tendency to affect endothelial and red blood cell function, platelet function, and blood viscosity, among other effects. Miller and colleagues' retrospective review of nearly 900 free TRAM flaps aimed to more clearly define the effects of this condition on microvascular breast reconstruction. Their finding that flap complications did not differ significantly between diabetic (type 1 or 2) and non-diabetic patients is reassuring that this common condition is not a contraindication (relative or absolute) to microvascular breast reconstruction.*

122. Padubidri AN, Yetman R, Browne E, et al. Complications of postmastectomy breast reconstructions in smokers, ex-smokers, and nonsmokers. *Plast Reconstr Surg.* 2001;107:342–349, discussion

350–351. *Not unlike diabetes and hypertension, smoking is another common risk factor in patients presenting for an evaluation for breast reconstruction. The poor effects of smoking on wound healing and surgical results in general are well defined; however, this study by Padubidri et al. comprehensively quantifies its effects on the breast reconstruction cohort, highlighting its negative influence on total complication rates, mastectomy flap necrosis, and fat necrosis. Interestingly, however many of these risks returned to rates similar to those of non-smokers in ex-smokers who had quit at least 3 weeks prior to surgery, suggesting an important role for smoking cessation in improving patient safety and outcomes.*

204. Hu ES, Pusic AL, Waljee JF, et al. Patient-reported aesthetic satisfaction with breast reconstruction during the long-term survivorship period. *Plast Reconstr Surg.* 2009;124:1–8. *With improving long-term survivorship within the breast cancer community, patient reported outcomes, particularly regarding satisfaction with their breasts following reconstruction, are becoming ever more important in clinical decision-making on the modality of breast reconstruction. With fairly well understood differences in the aging process of expander/ implant and autogenous reconstructions, the authors set out to evaluate patient satisfaction, not only in the immediate postoperative period but long-term as well, with these TRAM and expander/implant breast reconstruction. While no difference was found in the short-term aesthetic satisfaction between the cohorts, in the long term satisfaction with expander/implants seemed to decrease, resulting in a significant difference when compared to their TRAM counterparts.*

15

One- and two-stage prosthetic reconstruction in nipple-sparing mastectomy

Amy S. Colwell

 Access video and video lecture content for this chapter online at expertconsult.com

SYNOPSIS

- Nipple-sparing mastectomy is increasingly performed for treatment or prevention of breast cancer.
- Key points of the history and physical exam determine if the patient is a candidate for nipple preservation.
- Reconstructive goals include rebuilding the breast with nipple centralization.
- Outcomes data show excellent results in cosmesis and complication rates.

Introduction

Nipple-sparing mastectomy (NSM) and immediate reconstruction are chosen when there is no oncologic involvement of the nipple by cancer and when it is in an acceptable anatomic location. Decision-making centers on incision location, one- vs. two-stage reconstruction, round or shaped implants, and utilization of acellular dermal matrix (ADM) or mesh. Technical pearls maximize results and minimize complications.

Reconstructive outcomes following NSM show low rates of complications and high rates of nipple retention.

 Access the Historical Perspective section online at
http://www.expertconsult.com

Basic science

The breast is a glandular structure composed of ductal and lobular units. The lactiferous ducts converge and empty into the nipple (Fig. 15.1). Breast cancer most commonly arises within the breast ducts. Treatment involves surgery to remove gross pathology with a clear margin, and this can be supplemented with chemotherapy and/or radiation for control of local, regional, or metastatic disease. A mastectomy proceeds in an anatomic plane between the breast tissue and subcutaneous fat to the sternum, clavicle, latissimus dorsi, and inframammary fold (IMF).

A subcutaneous mastectomy was a preferred technique years ago to remove the majority of breast tissue yet leave a small amount behind to ensure nipple and skin survival. These patients had an overall higher risk of breast cancer recurrence, and the technique was largely abandoned. Anatomical studies then showed lactiferous ducts empty into a central core of nipple surrounded by a subdermal plexus of blood vessels. Therefore, it was possible to remove the ductal tissue from the nipple core while preserving blood supply. Since then, NSM is gaining traction as a preferred method for breast cancer treatment or prevention. Absolute contraindications to NSM include involvement of the nipple, locally advanced cancer with skin involvement, inflammatory cancer, or bloody discharge from the nipple.[3] For each breast, the nipple ductal tissue is sent as a separate specimen for pathological evaluation. If this margin is positive for cancer, nipple removal is warranted.

The anatomical considerations in breast reconstruction center on pocket control, restoration of desirable breast contour, and nipple centralization. Mastectomy boundaries extend laterally beyond the desired breast border; thus, this border must be redefined. Furthermore, if the IMF is violated, then restoration is necessary

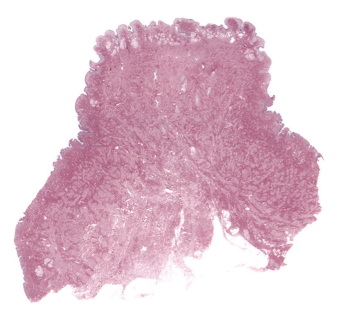

Fig. 15.1 The lactiferous ducts converge into the central nipple as shown on this low power view of a nipple in cross-section (stained with H&E). These ducts can be removed with a nipple-sparing mastectomy leaving the outer skin and subdermal plexus of blood vessels intact.

for proper implant placement. The aesthetic goals of many patients include more medial and superior fullness than is present in the native breast. Nipple preservation imposes challenges in achieving medial fullness while centralizing the nipple. Incision placement,

volume, and implant style are selected in order to optimize these results.

Diagnosis/patient presentation

Patient history

The patient typically has breast cancer or high risk for developing cancer. If the patient has genetic predisposition, the mastectomies are bilateral (Fig. 15.2). Patients with unilateral breast cancer may choose unilateral or bilateral mastectomy. The breast oncology surgeon decides relative safety and feasibility of nipple preservation, while the plastic surgeon determines if preservation would be beneficial to the aesthetic outcome. It is relevant to know if the patient received neoadjuvant chemotherapy or if they will receive postoperative chemotherapy; it is critical to know if the patient had prior radiotherapy. Planning for postoperative radiotherapy most often occurs when the final pathology is reported after the mastectomy, but on occasion this is known preoperatively.

The overall health status of the patient determines candidacy for immediate reconstruction. Poor prognostic factors include congestive heart failure, stroke, cardiac stent, requirement for home oxygen, and transplant recipients. Select high-risk patients may receive

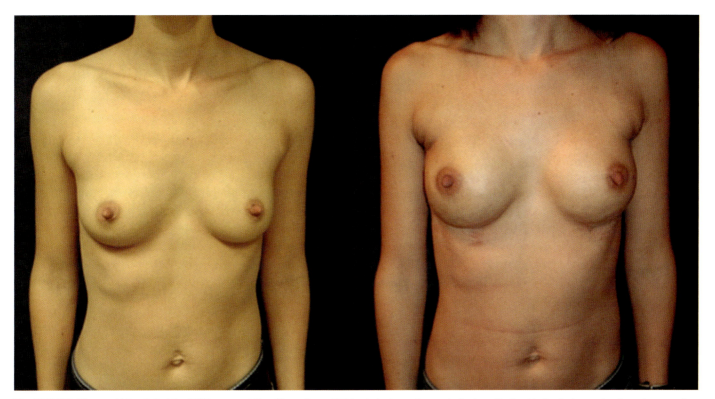

Fig. 15.2 This 33-year-old female had the *BRCA* gene mutation. She underwent bilateral nipple-sparing mastectomies with direct-to-implant reconstruction using smooth round moderate–plus profile 250 cc silicone gel implants.

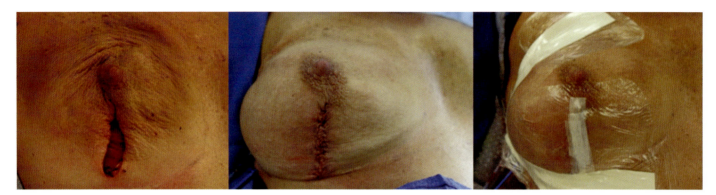

Fig. 15.3 For significant grade 2 or grade 3 ptosis, an inferior vertical incision is the safest approach to lift the nipple while keeping it centered. This patient is shown following tissue expander reconstruction. (Right) Microfoam tape is placed laterally for expander support and nipple positioning.

delayed reconstruction. With diabetes, perioperative sugar control is important. If possible, immunosuppressants and anticoagulants should be discontinued perioperatively if medically safe. Mental health conditions are optimized through a psychiatrist or therapist as conditions may worsen with postoperative recovery or complications. Smoking is strongly discouraged and may require transition to delayed reconstruction. Patients in healthcare or with MRSA exposure should have a nasal swab sent for culture.

The patient's reconstructive goals are considered. Overall goals for size, preference for number of surgeries, and the desired amount of uplift factor into decision-making.

Physical exam

The patient's height and weight are noted. A general inspection for skin quality, symmetry, and scars on the breast and abdomen are performed. The breast notch-to-nipple, nipple-to-fold, and breast base diameter are measured. The vertical position of one IMF is compared to the opposite breast. An overall estimate of volume is obtained.

Assessment

The history and physical help decide if implant or autologous reconstruction is the procedure of choice. With implant reconstruction, silicone is recommended over saline due to the more natural look and feel. Further discussion ensues to decide on nipple preservation, incisions, one- or two-stage reconstruction, ADM or mesh, and round or anatomic/shaped implants.

Patient selection

Nipple preservation

Surgical oncology determines if the patient is a candidate for nipple preservation based on tumor location

and characteristics. Plastic surgical considerations focus on the degree of ptosis and desired uplift of the breast. All patients with grade 1 ptosis and the vast majority of patients with grade 2 ptosis are considered surgical candidates for NSM. A 1 or 2 cm uplift of the nipple is expected as a skin response to mastectomy alone. If the patient desires a larger amount of uplift, or if there is grade 3 ptosis, a skin-sparing or areolar-sparing approach is typically preferred, although an inferior vertical approach to NSM can also be considered (Fig. 15.3). For prophylactic mastectomies in patients with grade 3 ptosis, a vertical mastopexy preserving circumareolar dermal blood supply can be performed before NSM to lift the nipple position; however, timing may not be optimal for cancer patients. Circumvertical mastopexy at the time of NSM has a higher potential risk for ischemic complications.

Incisions on the breast, prior radiotherapy, or post-mastectomy radiotherapy are not absolute contraindications to NSM.[4,5] Patients with prior lumpectomy, breast augmentation, mastopexy, or reduction can have successful NSM with immediate reconstruction.[6] Previous breast surgery should be considered in planning the mastectomy incision. Although prior radiotherapy is a general risk factor for implant-based reconstruction, NSM and immediate reconstruction can be performed in properly selected patients with minimal skin damage. If the patient will need post-mastectomy radiation, NSM can be considered. Radiation will often induce a tightening of the skin around an implant with an overall superior shift of the reconstruction superiorly. However, the nipple moves with the reconstruction. Nipple reconstructions following breast radiation of implants have limited success and may lead to cellulitis or implant exposure. Therefore, in select patients nipple preservation with mastectomy may offer the best chance for a safe, effective outcome (Fig. 15.4).

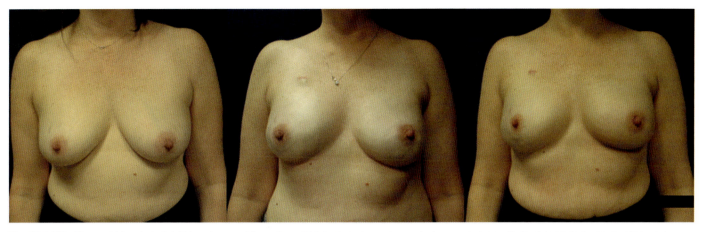

Fig. 15.4 This 43-year-old female had right breast cancer. She underwent bilateral nipple-sparing mastectomy procedures with direct-to-implant reconstruction using 470 cc moderate height, full-projection anatomic implants. (Right) She is shown 6 months after radiation to the left breast.

Incisions

The best incision is one that gives good access for both the mastectomy and reconstruction while minimizing the scar burden if possible[5] (Fig. 15.5). The inferolateral IMF incision is an excellent option to meet these goals for many patients.[7] The incision starts at approximately the 6 o'clock position under the breast and extends to approximately the 3 or 9 o'clock position lateral on the breast. This incision provides good access for sampling of axillary lymph nodes and avoids some inframammary perforators located more medially. A periareolar incision is often preferred by breast oncologists; however, this incision removes 50% of the blood supply to the nipple and is associated with a higher incidence of nipple necrosis in some series.[5] A lateral radial incision is a good option if there is concern about

viability of the skin and nipple from prior breast surgery or from an inexperienced breast surgeon. A radial incision takes away the least amount of blood supply from the nipple and can be extended medially to remove the nipple if necrosis ensues. An inferior radial incision provides the most uplift to the breast and the best centralization of the nipple in cases where ptosis exists. Although an ellipse of skin can be removed with the inferior incision, it is typically not necessary and can lead to a constricted inferior pole. If a patient has prior breast surgery, these scars can be used and extended if necessary for the mastectomy and reconstruction. If the scars are medial or superior to the nipple, these are typically ignored whereas a lateral or inferior scar is often utilized. An inferior periareolar scar from a prior breast augmentation can be utilized, or it can be ignored and a lateral radial incision or IMF incision used instead, which is the author's preference. Radiated lumpectomy scars should be avoided as these are associated with a higher risk of complications and wound healing problems.[6]

One- or two-stage reconstruction

Decision-making in one- or two-stage reconstruction centers on patient goals for size, minimizing number of surgeries, and quality of the mastectomy skin envelope.[8] In general, if the patient wants to be significantly larger in size, this is more safely accomplished in two stages (Fig. 15.6). In select cases with skin redundancy and an excellent skin envelope, it is possible to increase the size of the breast in one stage. Interestingly, if a patient wants to be significantly smaller and retain the nipple, this is also often better accomplished in two stages to allow skin shrinkage and a mastopexy at the time of tissue expander exchange. Breast and/or nipple asymmetry and ptosis can often be improved in one stage; however, two-stage surgery allows a second opportunity for

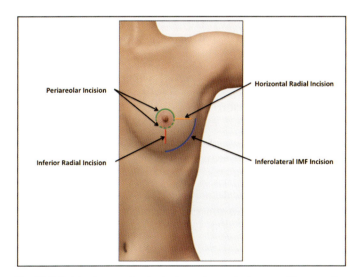

Fig. 15.5 Incisional approaches to nipple-sparing mastectomy combine ease of access and overall cosmesis. IMF, inframammory fold. *(Reproduced with permission from Colwell AS, Tessler O, Lin A, et al. Breast reconstruction following nipple-sparing mastectomy: predictors of complications, reconstruction outcomes, and 5-year trends.* Plast Reconstr Surg. *2014;133(3):496–506, Fig. 1.)*

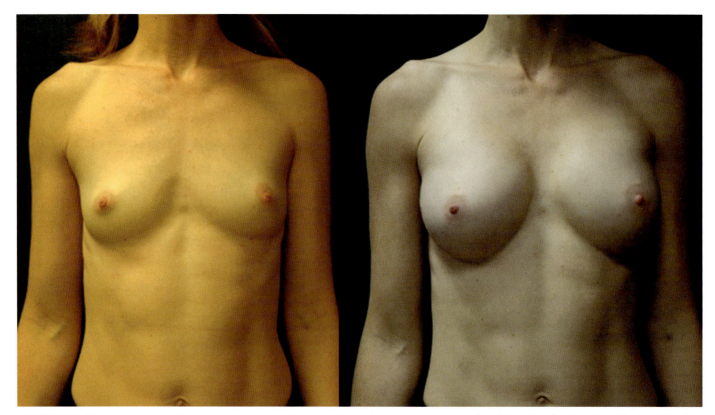

Fig. 15.6 This 36-year-old female had the breast cancer gene mutation. She underwent tissue expander reconstruction with acellular dermal matrix and is shown following her exchange to 495 cc full height, extra-full projection anatomic implants.

nipple and implant adjustment to optimize results. The quality of the mastectomy skin envelope is influenced by quality and thickness of the patient's skin, and technical ability of the breast oncology surgeon to remove all breast tissue in its natural plane atraumatically while preserving the subcutaneous fat and subdermal blood supply. The quality can also be damaged by the reconstructive surgeon if sharp retractors and extensive traction are used during the reconstruction, or if too much pressure is placed on the skin from a large implant or too much fill in the expander. Two-stage reconstruction is more common than one-stage; however, it is becoming increasingly common for patients to request one-stage reconstruction. A breast cancer diagnosis or positive *BRCA* gene test often comes at an inconvenient time with family life and jobs more important considerations. Although a one-stage reconstruction does not always offer the same opportunities for finesse and fat grafting commonly employed with two-stage reconstruction, it does get the patient back to her life more quickly.

Round or anatomic/shaped implants

Silicone implants are preferred over saline for breast reconstruction, as the cohesive gel more closely resembles breast tissue in look and feel. Smooth round silicone implants are the most common type of implant used in

the United States. Although the anatomic (shaped) textured silicone implants have been available for years worldwide, only recently were they approved in the United States. The advantages of round implants include more upper pole fullness, mobility, and softer feel compared to anatomic implants. The advantages of shaped implants include less visible rippling, more natural shape for a unilateral reconstruction, and more improvement in ptosis (Fig. 15.7). Theoretically, the texturing of the shaped implants may help mitigate the contractive forces of radiation.

Acellular dermal matrix or mesh

Breast reconstruction was initially performed in the subcutaneous plane over the muscle; however, capsular contracture often ensued. Placement of the implant or expander under the muscle improved capsular contracture, but it was hard to achieve a natural appearance with ptosis. Partial muscle coverage offered the advantage of submuscular placement and inferior pole release to create a more normal-appearing breast. Creative suture methods were employed to help prevent pectoralis muscle retraction and tissue expander migration. The development of ADM offered a more predictable means of tissue expander or implant placement and lower pole support. Human ADM is the most common material used in the United States and is popular for its

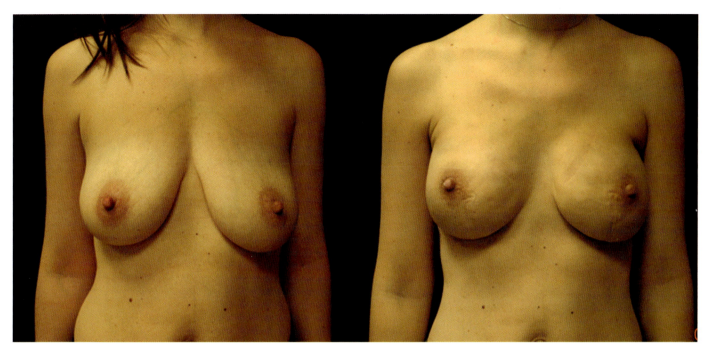

Fig. 15.7 This 34-year-old female had right breast ductal carcinoma in situ and a *BRCA* mutation. She was turned down for a nipple-sparing procedure at another facility. She underwent direct-to-implant reconstruction with an inferolateral inframammory fold incision and shaped full height, full projection 475 cc anatomic implants.

pliability, strength, integration into the tissues, and potential role in the mitigation of capsular contracture. A number of different products are currently available including porcine and bovine dermal matrix as well as synthetic silk, titanium, and vicryl mesh.[8] The choice of material may be guided by the needs for reconstruction. The material should be strong enough to help support the reconstruction initially and predictably for as long as the body needs the support. It should not induce enough inflammation to promote capsular contracture, nor should it have risk for extrusion. In the setting of infection, it should not be a permanent nidus for bacteria. If the breast skin is thin, a material is selected to integrate into the body's tissue and provide an extra layer of support and coverage.

Treatment/surgical technique

Preoperative planning

Important preoperative markings include the IMF on both sides and desired lateral border of the breast (Fig. 15.8). An incision is planned with the surgical oncologist. A paravertebral block can be performed to provide analgesia in the first 24–36 hours following the surgery and decrease overall narcotic requirement. Preoperative intravenous antibiotics are administered 30 minutes before start of the procedure, most commonly a first generation cephalosporin. This can be combined with gram-negative coverage if the patient is high risk. Some hospital policies advise preoperative Hibiclens®

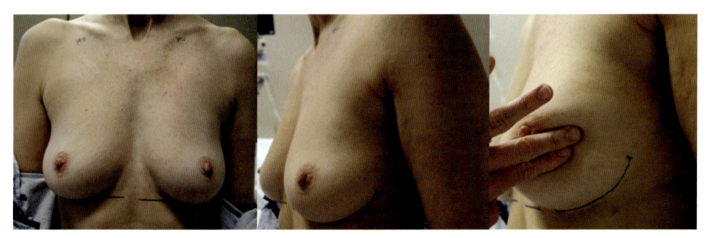

Fig. 15.8 Important preoperative markings include the inframammary fold and its relation to the opposite breast and fold. The ideal lateral border of the breast is marked and serves as the lateral extension for the inferolateral inframammary fold incision.

scrubs three days before surgery. The skin is prepped with chlorhexidine or DuraPrep™. After the mastectomy, the skin is reprepped with an antiseptic solution and new drapes are placed over pre-existing drapes placed at the surgical start. The arm position is angled downward to approximately 75 degrees with the operating room table. Paralysis is administered to make subpectoral dissection easier and facilitate implant placement. The mastectomy specimens are weighed on each side. It is helpful to double-glove for this procedure for sterility.

Technique for one- or two-stage breast reconstruction with partial pectoralis muscle release and acellular dermal matrix or mesh

The technique for one- or two-stage breast reconstruction follows a similar progression of events. Reconstruction is most commonly performed immediately with the mastectomy and with partial pectoralis muscle coverage and ADM or mesh. Total muscle coverage can be used in two-stage reconstruction and for small breasts in one-stage reconstruction following principles similar to those used in skin-sparing mastectomy.

Initial inspection

The skin is first inspected for color, thickness, and traumatic injury. If the skin and/or nipple has pink, red, blue, or gray discoloration, it suggests ischemic injury and may not be suitable for one-stage reconstruction. If there is severe damage, delayed reconstruction is considered. If the undersurface of the flap has exposed dermis, it is less conducive to one-stage reconstruction. The ideal skin envelope has a normal skin color and marbling of fat on the undersurface of the skin flaps (Fig. 15.9). The extent of dissection is then assessed. If the inframammary fold has been violated it will need to be re-established with sutures and/or ADM. The lateral extent of the dissection is the latissimus dorsi muscle. The lateral pocket border must be medialized with ADM, a serratus muscle flap, and/or suturing of the lateral skin envelope to the chest wall. If the medial extent of the dissection is medial to the sternal attachment of the pectoralis muscle, this may require fat grafting in the future.

Pectoralis muscle elevation (Video 15.1 ⊙)

The pectoralis muscle is placed on stretch and the fine subpectoral areolar tissue is divided with electrocautery to create a subpectoral pocket (Fig. 15.10). This is most easily performed with a short lighted retractor with serrated edges. This retractor is not used on the skin flaps. If subpectoral vessels are visualized, care is taken to grasp the vessel with a forceps in two places and use electrocautery before dividing. Dissection proceeds

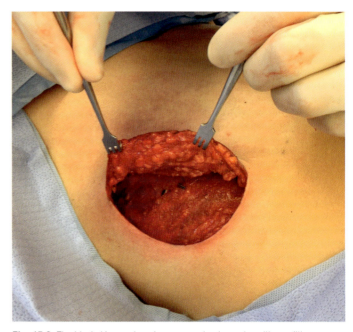

Fig. 15.9 The ideal skin envelope has a normal color and capillary refill on exam and a mottling of fat on the undersurface of the skin envelope.

from lateral to medial until the pectoralis insertion to the sternum is encountered. The inferior pectoralis muscle is then divided while on stretch using electrocautery. If the inframammary fold is intact, the muscle is released approximately 1 cm superior to the insertion to avoid lowering the fold. If the fold is not intact, the muscle can be released at its insertion. The inferior release is performed to approximately the 4 o'clock or 8 o'clock position on the chest wall. If the muscle is not released to this extent, the implant is often lateralized. It is sometimes necessary to extend the release to the 3 or 9 o'clock position. However, with extended release of muscle,

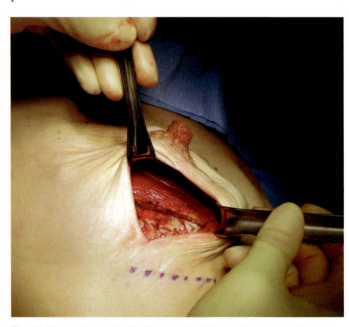

Fig. 15.10 A subpectoral pocket is created and the muscle is released from its inferior border to approximately the 4 or 8 o'clock position on the chest wall.

there is more muscle retraction. This leads to less muscle coverage, a greater proportion of subcutaneous/ADM coverage, and requires a larger piece of ADM to span the inferior pole. It is not necessary to limit superior subpectoral dissection as the natural inclination of the implant with gravity is inferior. The lateral attachment of the pectoralis muscle to the pectoralis minor is also released to allow redraping around the implant and to prevent indentation at the attachment, which often lies medial to the lateral border of the implant.

Determine pocket dimensions

Once the pectoralis muscle is released, ADM is used to define the lateral border of the implant. To determine where to sew the ADM laterally, consideration is given to the breast base diameter measured preoperatively, the volume of the breast/desired new volume of breast, and expander or implant base diameter options. The pocket is typically created about 1 cm narrower than the anticipated implant or expander diameter to account for the stretch inherent in human ADM. If using a more rigid type of ADM or mesh, the pocket diameter may more closely approximate the diameter of the expander/ implant. Once the diameter is determined, a ruler is used to measure from the medial subpectoral border to the position on the serratus muscle laterally (Fig. 15.11). For bilateral procedures, the same distance is measured on both sides.

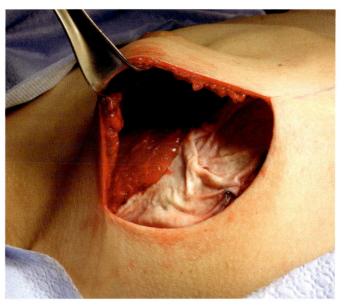

Fig. 15.12 The acellular dermal matrix (ADM) acts as the inferior and lateral extension of the pectoralis muscle to form a complete pocket around the implant or expander. The ADM is typically sewn to the chest wall using buried braided non-absorbable sutures, though it is possible to use absorbable sutures and sew to an intact inframammary fold.

Acellular dermal matrix (Video 15.2 ⊙)

ADM is used as an extension of the pectoralis muscle for complete implant coverage (Fig. 15.12). Although partial muscle release with two-stage reconstruction can be performed without ADM, it is less predictable. The addition of ADM or mesh allows precise positioning of the implant or expander, which is important for reconstruction of NSM. With skin-sparing mastectomy, expander malposition can often be corrected at the second stage with capsulotomy and capsulorrhaphy. However, with NSM, attaining symmetrical results relies in large part on the initial reconstruction for both one- and two-stage surgery.

A rectangular or contour ADM is chosen for reconstruction. The contour ADM is easy to use and adapts well to most breast base diameters, whereas most rectangular ADM will need to be trimmed. The size of ADM is chosen to fit the breast base width and anticipated volume. In general, a smaller piece is needed for tissue expander reconstruction compared to one-stage reconstruction.

Suturing the ADM can begin superiorly to the pectoralis muscle or inferiorly to the chest wall/inframammary fold according to surgeon preference. The diameter of the inferior suture line will be longer than the diameter of the superior suture line; thus, it is expected to have some bunching or pleating of the superior suture line. With human ADM, these pleats are not palpable or visible. However, if a stiffer material is used, it is

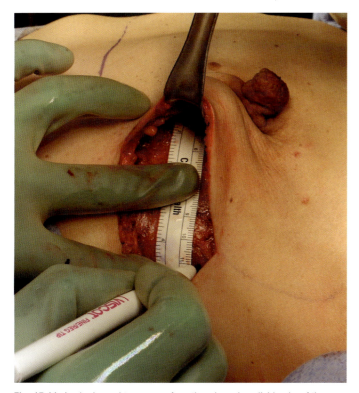

Fig. 15.11 A ruler is used to measure from the released medial border of the pectoralis muscle to the desired extent on the lateral chest wall.

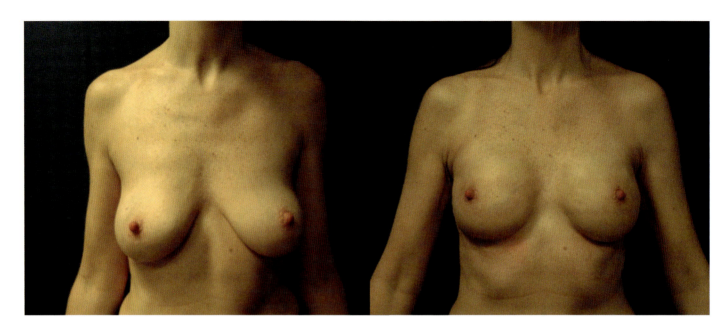

Fig. 15.13 This 47-year-old female had right ductal carcinoma in situ and underwent bilateral nipple-sparing mastectomy procedures. She had immediate direct-to-implant reconstruction using smooth round moderate classic 320 cc implants. Sewing the acellular dermal matrix to the chest wall allows raising the inframammary fold with redraping of the skin envelope.

sometimes necessary to excise these pleats and suture the material closed. The author finds it easiest to sew the ADM to the chest wall first to create the desired pocket dimensions. If the IMF is intact, the ADM can be sewn to the IMF directly. However, it is expected that round silicone implants will drop 1–2 cm using this technique and that textured anatomic implants will also drop but to a lesser degree. For less anticipated drop, ADM is sewn directly to chest wall at the level of the fold (Fig. 15.13). If the IMF is not intact, suturing ADM to chest wall is important to prevent bottoming out. Suturing begins medially with the ADM sewn to the released pectoralis muscle medial border with a buried simple stitch. The second stitch is sewn from the ADM to the inframammary fold to avoid medial restriction of the implant with a chest wall stitch. Care is taken to leave redundancy horizontally between stitches medially in anticipation of space needed for an implant or partially filled tissue expander. Suturing progresses laterally. If needed, the ADM can be trimmed if it is too wide for the pocket. Horizontal mattress sutures are preferred laterally from ADM to chest wall with the knots on the chest wall side. The author prefers a non-absorbable braided stitch (0 Ethibond) for the chest wall stitches, but Vicryl or PDS can be used. If the ADM does not reach the lateral/superior junction of the pectoralis muscle, a figure-of-eight suture can be placed from the lateral border of the pectoralis muscle to the chest wall in anatomic alignment with the newly created lateral border of the breast. If the surgeon anticipates the ADM is going to be too narrow for the pocket, suturing can start laterally to control the lateral and then inferior borders of the

implant and potentially leave a small space medially uncovered. These small areas are rarely visible clinically. One or two absorbable figure-of-eight or horizontal mattress sutures are then placed from the ADM to the pectoralis muscle medial and lateral. These help assess the pocket with sizer placement and furthermore help hold the implant in the pocket with initial insertion.

Variation: If desired, the serratus muscle can be elevated to provide the lateral border to the implant pocket. In this case, the serratus is dissected laterally to the desired width of the implant pocket. The ADM is then sewn to the serratus flap laterally. The advantage of this approach is that a smaller piece of ADM is needed for the inferior pole. In addition, the muscle flap sometimes spans the inferolateral IMF incision, which can be helpful in cases of incisional breakdown or radiotherapy.

Check pocket dimensions/size (Video 15.3 ⊙)

Once the pocket has been created, a sizer is placed to check pocket dimensions and to determine the volume of implant or fill the skin will allow. Although silicone sizers are optimal, saline sizers are widely used as they are inexpensive and convenient. The saline sizers can be filled with air or saline. The sizer is placed into the pocket and tacking stitches are placed to hold the sizer in place (Fig. 15.14). Increasing pinkness or redness with addition of volume to the sizer is indicative of ischemia (Fig. 15.15). The patient is sat upright to 90 degrees on the operating room table and symmetry is assessed. The final implant is chosen based on the acceptable volume and breast base diameter. A moderate classic or

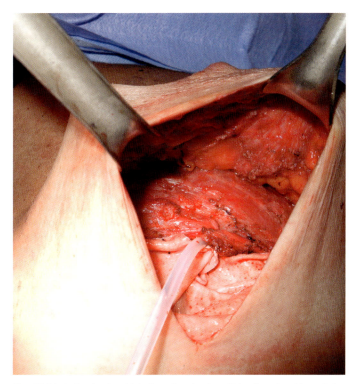

Fig. 15.14 A sizer is placed into the subpectoral–acellular dermal matrix pocket and sewn in place. The skin envelope is stapled shut, and the sizer is inflated to assess the pocket and determine implant size or expander fill.

moderate plus profile implant most commonly fits the volume and diameter goals for small to medium-size breasts while centralizing the nipple for one-stage reconstruction. A higher profile implant with a more narrow base width may lead to nipple lateralization or a medial pocket divot in smaller breasts; however, for larger breasts (>500 cc) the higher profile implant is used more frequently. A tissue expander is chosen based

upon breast base diameter and size goals. A tabbed expander can help maintain position but is more expensive than expanders without tabs. A higher profile implant is often chosen in two-stage reconstruction since the final volume is larger than the original breast volume with the same breast base width.

Preparation for implant or tissue expander

The pocket is assessed for hemostasis and irrigated with a triple antibiotic solution composed of 1 gram cefazolin, 50 mg gentamycin, and 50000 units of bacitracin per liter. Two 15 bard drains are tunneled 1–2 cm away from the pocket. If the skin exit site is above the IMF, the scars are hidden with most bathing suits. One drain is placed inside the ADM pocket along the inframammary fold, and the other is placed into the axilla and over the pectoralis muscle. Drains serve to remove fluid and also to oppose the skin to the ADM for vascularization and integration and prevent dead space. The skin is washed with an antibiotic-soaked sponge, and the surgeon's gloves are changed. The anesthesiologist ensures the patient has complete muscle relaxation.

Implant or tissue expander placement

Two retractors are placed inside the pectoralis–ADM pocket. The implant or tissue expander is inserted and expander filled to desired size using a closed system. Proper orientation is obtained. The ADM is sutured to the pectoralis with figure-of-eight or horizontal mattress absorbable braided sutures (2-0 Vicryl) (Fig. 15.16). Although it may be tempting to use permanent stitches here, the knots can often be palpated and serve as a concern for cancer. Excess ADM in the vertical dimension is trimmed whereas sutures may be tied more loosely or spanned if the vertical height is short.

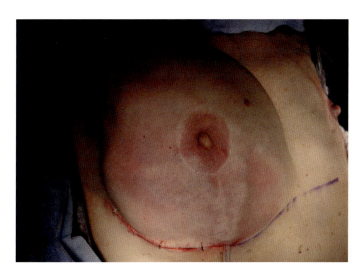

Fig. 15.15 If the sizer is inflated and the skin appears deep pink/red or blue/gray, this indicates relative ischemia at that volume. In this patient who had a prior inferior pedicle breast reduction followed by nipple-sparing mastectomies, the deep pink discoloration indicated that direct-to-implant reconstruction would not be possible. Instead, a tissue expander was placed with minimal volume fill, and she recovered uneventfully with no nipple or skin necrosis.

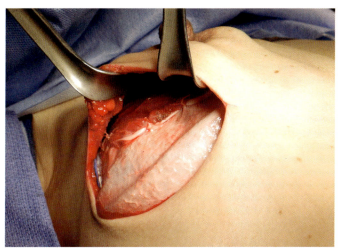

Fig. 15.16 Once the implant or expander is placed, braided absorbable sutures are used to close the muscle–acellular dermal matrix pocket.

Closure

The skin edges are trimmed or de-epithelialized 2–3 mm and closed in layers with absorbable sutures. Incisions are dressed with a surgical glue (Dermabond) and/or Steri-Strips. Microfoam tape is often used for implant stabilization and nipple positioning. Biopatches are placed around the drains. Tegaderm is then placed over the incisions and drain sites (Fig. 15.17).

Postoperative care

The patient stays in the hospital for 1 or 2 nights. On the first postoperative day, a loose-fitting surgical bra or ace wrap is placed for mild compression. Constricting garments are avoided to prevent additional ischemic injury to the skin. Showering is permitted if Tegaderm covers the incisions. Drain removal is performed when output is less than 30 cc per day, and oral antibiotics are maintained until the drains are out. Most commonly, one drain per breast is removed one week after surgery and the other is removed two weeks after surgery. Drains are not kept in place longer than 4 weeks. The skin often appears bruised and lumpy immediate after surgery, and a scab may form on the nipple (Fig. 15.18). These changes often worsen the first week following surgery but improve thereafter. The nipple may appear dusky with purple discoloration, but it has a remarkable ability to recover from ischemia. Nipple removal for necrosis is often best delayed 3–4 weeks following surgery to determine how much is viable. An antibiotic ointment is used on the nipple during the recovery

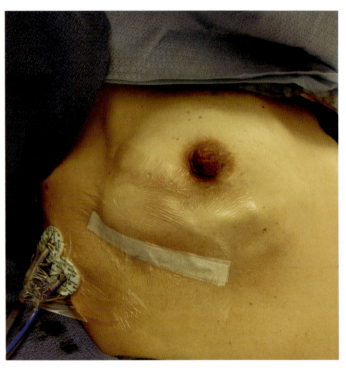

Fig. 15.17 The skin edges are trimmed and closed in two layers using absorbable stitches. The incision is dressed with surgical glue and/or Steri-Strips. The drain exit sites are covered with Biopatches. Tegaderm is used to cover the drain exit sites and incisions, which allows the patient to shower after discharge from the hospital.

phase. Walking is encouraged immediately after surgery, and patients may return to light activity and exercise in 6 weeks. However, more vigorous exercise and immersion in a pool or ocean are best delayed for 3 months. Tissue expander fills start 3 weeks after surgery and can occur weekly thereafter. The second surgery for tissue

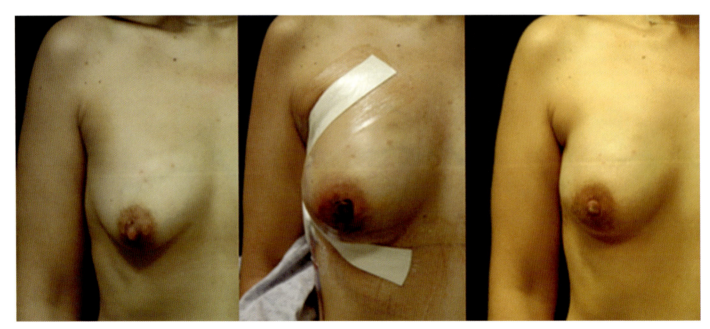

Fig. 15.18 It is common to see a scab on the nipple following nipple-sparing mastectomy (NSM) and immediate reconstruction. This is treated with a topical antimicrobial agent and typically falls off in a few weeks with no clinical sequelae. This patient is shown after NSM and direct-to-implant reconstruction one week after surgery (middle) and four weeks after surgery (right).

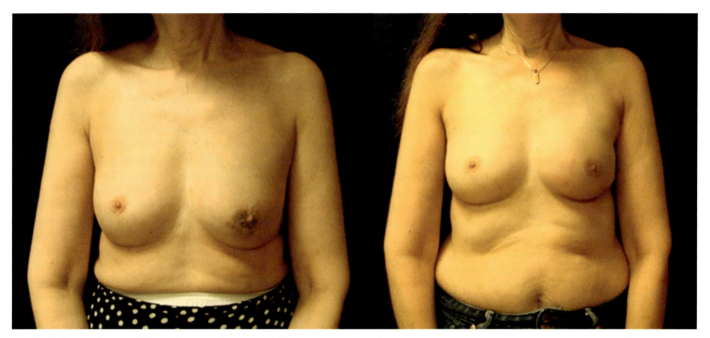

Fig. 15.19 Direct-to-implant (DTI) is performed most commonly in bilateral reconstructions; however, it can be performed in unilateral reconstructions. DTI offers good symmetry with small breasts such as in this 59-year-old female with left breast cancer that had immediate reconstruction with a smooth round moderate classic 325 cc implant.

expander exchange to implant typically occurs three months after the initial surgery. Once the reconstruction is complete, patients are followed every 1–2 years for implant checks.

Outcomes, prognosis, and complications

Outcomes following NSM and immediate reconstruction are largely successful in experienced hands with a high rate of nipple retention[5,9] (Figs. 15.19–15.20). In 500 consecutive one- and two-stage reconstructions after NSM, the overall complication rate was low and over 90% of nipples were retained.[5] Complications included hematoma, seroma, skin necrosis, and nipple necrosis. The risk of infection was 3.3%, which is comparable to some of the lowest reported rates of infection in implant-based reconstruction, and suggests nipple preservation does not increase overall risk of infection. There were

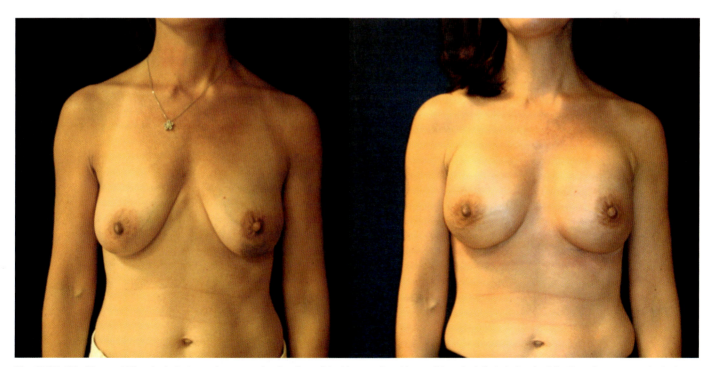

Fig. 15.20 This 45-year-old female desired one-stage reconstruction if possible. However, her skin was thin and relatively ischemic at the time of surgery, so she had tissue expanders placed with exchange to smooth round 500 cc silicone gel implants and fat transfer to the upper poles three months later.

no recurrences of cancer in the nipple, and the explant rate was less than 2%. Risk factors for complications included radiotherapy, smoking, and a periareolar incision.

Secondary procedures

Tissue expander exchange to implant

The tissue expander is filled to goal size. Position changes, mastopexy, and/or fat grafting can be performed at the second-stage surgery. The prior scar is typically used to access the expander, which is punctured and removed. A capsulotomy is routinely performed medial and superior to allow the implant to fill these areas. Capsulotomy is avoided inferior and lateral if possible with the partial muscle release technique due to unpredictable final implant position; however, in select cases it is required and ADM reinforcement of new position can be considered. Capsulorrhaphy is performed to medialize the pocket or raise the inframammary fold position. Most women who have two-stage reconstruction after NSM choose a size larger than their native breast. Therefore, a high profile implant diameter is often suitable for both nipple centralization and maximal projection. Fat grafting is performed to fill in divots and help minimize postoperative implant visibility. A mastopexy can be performed to help lift and centralize nipple position; however, there is a limit to the amount of lift and centralization that can be performed while keeping the blood supply intact. The nipple may be removed at the second stage if it is in an unacceptable position.

Nipple removal (with or without reconstruction)

If the pathology on the nipple specimen is positive for cancer, nipple removal with a margin of areolar tissue is warranted. This can be performed 3 weeks to several months following the initial surgery depending upon adjuvant treatment and can be performed with tissue expander exchange. Nipple reconstruction is offered three months after nipple removal.

Revision

Revisional surgery in one- or two-stage breast reconstruction is performed for implant malposition or size change, fat grafting, mastopexy, or capsular contracture. In our experience, the rate of revisions following reconstruction for skin-sparing or NSM was similar between one- and two-stage reconstruction with an overall rate of about 20% at 5 years.[10] Nipple position can be shifted with crescent mastopexy, a crescent with lateral extension, circumvertical or partial circumvertical mastopexy, or by changing the implant position (Fig. 15.21). A free nipple graft can be performed if there is enough laxity in the skin to allow skin closure and adequate soft tissue to support the graft.

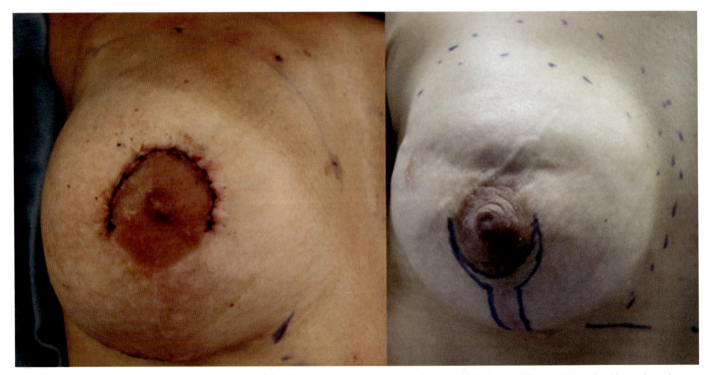

Fig. 15.21 With tissue expander exchange to implant or in revisional surgery, a mastopexy can be performed to shift nipple position and tighten the skin envelope. A crescent mastopexy and preoperative markings for a partial circumvertical mastopexy are shown.

References

1. Uroskie TW, Colen LB. History of breast reconstruction. *Semin Plast Surg*. 2004;18:65–69. *This paper offers a historical perspective on breast reconstruction and allows the reader to learn from prior trials and tribulations of the past.*

2. Colwell AS, Damjanovic B, Zahedi B, et al. Retrospective review of 331 consecutive immediate single-stage implant reconstructions with acellular dermal matrix: indications, complications, trends, and costs. *Plast Reconstr Surg*. 2011;128:1170–1178. *This paper was one of the first comparative outcomes studies on direct-to-implant breast reconstruction with ADM compared to traditional two-stage tissue expander-implant reconstruction without ADM. In this series, single-stage reconstruction had similar complication rates and costs compared to two-stage reconstruction.*

3. Coopey SB, Tang R, Lei L, et al. Increasing eligibility for nipple-sparing mastectomy. *Ann Surg Oncol*. 2013;20:3218–3222. *In this paper, the authors offer new guidance on who is a candidate for nipple-sparing mastectomy. They suggest that if the nipple is not involved by cancer grossly or radiologically that the patient may be considered for the nipple-sparing approach.*

4. Reish RG, Lin A, Phillips NA, et al. Breast reconstruction outcomes after nipple-sparing mastectomy and radiation therapy. *Plast Reconstr Surg*. 2015;135:959–966. *The authors perform an outcomes study on breast reconstruction after NSM and radiotherapy. They find that in patients with preoperative or postoperative radiotherapy, the complication rate is slightly higher, but most patients have successful reconstructions with implant and nipple retention.*

5. Colwell AS, Tessler O, Lin AM, et al. Breast reconstruction following nipple-sparing mastectomy: predictors of complications, reconstruction outcomes, and 5-year trends. *Plast Reconstr Surg*. 2014;133:496–506. *This paper presents 500 consecutive nipple-sparing mastectomy procedures with immediate reconstruction. The authors find a low overall complication rate in one- and two-stage implant reconstruction and outline risk factors for complications and reconstructive failures.*

6. Frederick MJ, Lin AM, Neuman R, et al. Nipple-sparing mastectomy in patients with previous breast surgery: comparative analysis of 775 immediate breast reconstructions. *Plast Reconstr Surg*. 2015;135:954e–962e. *The authors present a consecutive series of 775 implant-based reconstructions where 187 reconstructions had prior breast surgery. They find that NSM was successful in patients with prior scars from lumpectomy, breast augmentation, or breast reduction without an increased risk of nipple loss or reconstructive failure.*

7. Colwell AS, Gadd M, Smith BL, Austen WG Jr. An inferolateral approach to nipple-sparing mastectomy: optimizing mastectomy and reconstruction. *Ann Plast Surg*. 2010;65:140–143. *In this paper, the authors describe an inferolateral inframammary fold incision for nipple-sparing mastectomy that offers excellent access for both mastectomy and reconstruction.*

8. Scheflan M, Colwell AS. Tissue reinforcement in implant-based breast reconstruction. *Plast Reconstr Surg Glob Open*. 2014;2:e192. *This paper reviews patient selection and technique in implant-based reconstruction with acellular dermal matrix or mesh to optimize breast reconstruction.*

9. Spear SL, Willey SC, Feldman ED, et al. Nipple-sparing mastectomy for prophylactic and therapeutic indications. *Plast Reconstr Surg*. 2011;128:1005–1014. *In this paper, the authors provide early experience and guidance for patient selection in nipple-sparing mastectomy.*

10. Colwell AS, Clarke-Pearson E, Lin A, et al. Revision rates in implant-based breast reconstruction: how does direct-to-implant measure up? *Plast Reconstr Surg*. 2016;137:1690–1699. *The authors follow a cohort of direct-to-implant and tissue expander-implant reconstructions for an average of 5 years. They find a similar rate of complications and revisions in the two cohorts of patients.*

16

Skin-sparing mastectomy: Planned two-stage and direct-to-implant breast reconstruction

Mitchell H. Brown, Brett Beber, and Ron B. Somogyi

 Access video content for this chapter online at expertconsult.com

SYNOPSIS

- Alloplastic breast reconstruction is the most common approach used today for postmastectomy breast reconstruction.
- Traditional breast implant reconstruction is performed as a planned two-stage procedure with the use of a tissue expander followed by exchange to a breast implant.
- Changing demographics of the mastectomy patient, improved devices and support matrices, as well as refinements in mastectomy techniques have allowed for expanded indications of direct-to-implant breast reconstruction.
- Enhanced collaboration between oncologic surgeons and plastic surgeons is necessary in order to maximize outcomes in immediate breast reconstruction.
- Increasing awareness of the indications for skin and nipple preservation together with improved devices, internal scaffolds, and judicious use of fat transfer allow for results that may approximate the appearance and feel of a natural non-operated breast.

 Access the Historical Perspective section, including Fig. 16.1, online at

http://www.expertconsult.com

Introduction

Alloplastic reconstruction is the most common type of postmastectomy breast reconstruction worldwide. The increasing frequency of this form of reconstruction can be explained by several factors, including changing demographics of the mastectomy patient, improvements in devices and technologies used in reconstruction, and an increased appreciation for the morbidity associated with autologous reconstruction.

Traditional alloplastic breast reconstruction begins with the insertion of a tissue expander followed by a period of serial expansions. The expander is exchanged for a permanent prosthesis in a second procedure, which is often performed in conjunction with balancing surgery or other adjunctive procedures. This planned two-stage approach is predictable, allows for reconstruction of variable breast sizes, provides a period for review of pathology, and minimizes early tension on the skin envelope. Unfortunately, it necessitates a minimum of two surgeries as well as repeated visits for expansion of the device.

Direct-to-implant breast reconstruction, often referred to incorrectly as a single-stage procedure, attempts to create the final breast mound at the time of mastectomy. In carefully selected patients, this approach offers the benefit of fewer surgeries, a more rapid return to normal life, and avoidance of the period of expansion. Challenges include limitations on breast size, the potential for early skin or nipple necrosis, a higher priority for excellence in one procedure, and the risk of postoperative radiation of the permanent breast prosthesis.

This chapter will present the current thoughts on indications, contraindications, patient selection, and surgical technique in both the planned two-stage as well as the direct-to-implant postmastectomy breast reconstruction.

Patient presentation

The ideal alloplastic reconstruction should provide a close degree of symmetry with a soft and natural-feeling breast. It should be predictable and require the fewest number of surgeries possible, with minimal morbidity and minimal time to full recovery. Surgeons and patients would clearly prefer a single-stage approach to breast reconstruction, but not at the expense of inferior outcomes or unnecessary risks. The traditional and most common approach is a planned two-stage procedure involving the insertion of a tissue expander followed by a period of expansion and then exchange to a permanent prosthesis. In some circumstances, consideration can be made for avoidance of the period of expansion with insertion of the final prosthesis at the time of the mastectomy. Initially, this was called a single-stage alloplastic reconstruction; however, the term "direct-to-implant" reconstruction is more accurate. The advantages and disadvantages of direct-to-implant versus planned two-stage reconstruction are summarized in Fig. 16.2.

Patient selection for direct-to-implant reconstruction is critical. Patients must be good candidates based upon the shape and size of their breasts, nipple position on the breast mound, indication for mastectomy, likelihood of adjuvant therapy, size expectations, and risk factors for vascular compromise to the skin or nipple. The ideal candidate is a healthy non-smoker with an A–B cup breast who desires a similar or slightly larger size, minimal ptosis, prophylactic or early stage disease, and low likelihood for postoperative adjuvant therapy. Direct-to-implant patients must also have realistic expectations.

Direct-to-implant breast reconstruction

The combination of skin-sparing or nipple-sparing mastectomy with immediate reconstruction has allowed for excellent results in implant-based reconstruction.

The advantages of implant-based reconstruction have always been the relative straightforward nature of the procedure as well as the avoidance of distant donor site morbidity. The disadvantages, however, have been the need for tissue expansion with the inconvenience of repeated office visits and the inherent risks and discomfort of the expansions as well as the need for a second surgery for exchange of the expander. With the recent increase in high risk and gene positive patients, there is an additional population that is highly motivated to decrease their cancer risk through prophylactic mastectomy while maximizing their aesthetic outcomes and minimizing the number of procedures and postoperative recovery time. There have also been significant psychological benefits demonstrated with earlier completion of reconstruction,[2] and cost savings described with the use of a direct-to-implant approach.[3–6] A direct-to-implant approach for immediate reconstruction would be ideal for many of these reasons. This approach, however, is limited by the difficulty in providing adequate stable soft-tissue coverage for an implant in a fresh mastectomy pocket. Placement of an implant in a partial subcutaneous plane can cause significant stress to the lower pole mastectomy flaps leading to soft-tissue necrosis in the short term and significant thinning in the long term. Total submuscular coverage, while possible, limits the size of an implant that can be placed and does not allow for a natural fill of the lower pole. In both these cases, the lateral and inframammary folds are disrupted and poor definition is seen postoperatively. The recent addition of various soft-tissue support matrices to cover the implant in the lower pole has significantly improved our ability to perform safe and aesthetically pleasing direct-to-implant reconstruction. Nevertheless, given the increased constraints regarding patient selection and the increased material costs, direct-to-implant reconstruction is still used in a limited fashion and ultimately makes up only 10–15% of all reconstructed breasts.[2]

The concept of a direct-to-implant reconstruction can satisfy all our reconstructive goals and represents an attractive alternative to more established reconstructive techniques. Ultimately, the success of direct-to-implant reconstruction will depend on four key factors: (1) careful patient selection; (2) accurate device and material selection; (3) planning and execution of a mastectomy that leaves behind healthy, viable skin flaps; and (4) the timely and effective management of complications.

Patient selection

The ideal patient for a direct-to-implant reconstruction is a healthy woman with small to moderate sized breasts who desires to stay about the same breast size or slightly larger. Women with larger size and ptotic breasts may be candidates for skin reduction mastectomy with direct-to-implant reconstruction; however, the ability to preserve the nipple will be limited by the degree of ptosis and overall breast size.

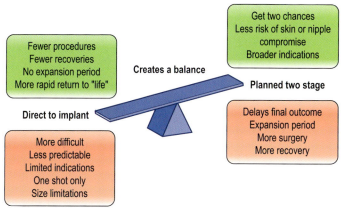

Fig. 16.2 Advantages and disadvantages of direct-to-implant versus planned two-stage breast reconstruction.

The main concerns with direct-to-implant reconstruction are skin flap viability and stable soft-tissue coverage. The consultation and surgical planning must adequately assess all factors related to these two issues. These factors include tumor location and biology, the ablative plan, the size and shape of the breast, access incision, as well as patient comorbidities. Of course, the aesthetic goals of the patient, including their willingness or desire to have contralateral balancing procedures, must also be considered.

There are few absolute contraindications to direct-to-implant breast reconstruction. Patients with poor skin quality or medical comorbidities that affect vascularity to mastectomy skin flaps are not good candidates. Obese patients and those with large, ptotic breasts that require significant adjustments to the skin envelope are difficult to reconstruct in a direct-to-implant approach. Patients with a history of breast radiation and those likely to require postmastectomy radiation have traditionally been offered autologous reconstruction or a two-stage implant-based reconstruction. Boundaries for implant-based reconstruction in these patients are being extended and several recent studies have shown good aesthetic results with acceptable complication profiles through the use of direct-to-implant reconstruction using acellular dermal matrix.[7,8]

Several recent studies have looked at predictors of failure in direct-to-implant reconstruction. Factors associated with less favorable aesthetic outcomes and higher rates of complications include active smoking, periareolar incisions, increasing body mass index, increasing breast cup size, preoperative irradiation, and prolonged operative time.[4,9–11]

Table 16.1 Types of soft-tissue support matrices used in breast reconstruction
Biologic
Human dermis
Autoderm
Human acellular dermal matrix
AlloDerm
Allomax
FlexHD
Dermacell
DermaMatrix
Porcine acellular dermal matrix
Strattice
Bovine acellular dermal matrix
Veritas
Surgimend
Silk
Seri Surgical Scaffold
Synthetic
Absorbable
Vicryl mesh
Non-absorbable
Prolene mesh
Marlex mesh

Internal support matrices can be classified as biologic or synthetic. Current options are summarized in Table 16.1.

There are three ways in which the body can respond to an internal tissue matrix. Material that is not recognized as self will stimulate the natural immune defenses of the body. Less complex materials such as absorbable mesh will undergo **resorption**.

If a material is more complex and unable to be resorbed, the body will respond through a process of **encapsulation**. On the other hand, if the body recognizes a material as self, then it will respond through a process of **revascularization** and cell repopulation. This is the outcome that we expect to see with the use of biologic devices. Acellular dermal matrix (ADM) is a tissue prepared from human, bovine, or porcine tissue from which cellular components that promote rejection have been removed. The resulting structurally intact tissue matrix provides the biologic scaffold necessary for normal tissue in-growth and cellular repopulation.

There are several reasons why the use of ADM has not been universally accepted. First, these materials are expensive and therefore not available at all institutions. Their cost can even offset the potential economic benefit of performing breast reconstruction in a single stage. In addition, there are several published reports of increased complications with the used of ADM including higher rates of infection, seroma, mastectomy flap necrosis, and explantation.[4,13–20]

Implant and material selection

The two primary requirements for direct-to-implant reconstruction are a breast implant as well as a support matrix to hold the implant in place under the pectoral muscle. There are multiple reasons for using an internal support matrix. These include:

1. Support the implant under the pectoral muscle
2. Maintain position of the pectoral muscle
3. Define the inframammary fold and lateral mammary fold
4. Eliminate the need to elevate serratus or rectus muscle/fascia
5. Minimize tension on the skin of the lower pole
6. Add soft-tissue cover to the lower pole and over the implant

A further benefit that has been attributed to some acellular dermal matrices is the potential to resist capsular contracture.[10,12] Although debate continues as to whether or not a protective effect truly exists, if it does, this would have particular benefit in patients who have either been radiated or are expected to undergo post-reconstruction radiation.

Vicryl mesh is widely available, relatively inexpensive, resistant to bacteria biofilm formation, and easy to use. It demonstrates little inflammatory response, is non-allergenic, and has a low complication profile in many surgical settings. Recent reports using Vicryl mesh instead of ADM in the lower pole during immediate direct-to-implant breast reconstruction have shown similar complication profiles with equally pleasing results and significant cost savings over both two-stage reconstruction or direct-to-implant reconstruction with ADM.[20–22] Longer term studies that assess soft-tissue changes in the lower pole as well as the incidence of capsular contracture will be important in assessing the efficacy of absorbable mesh. Also, these materials do not provide additional soft-tissue coverage and may not protect the implant if skin necrosis or wound dehiscence leads to a small area of exposure.

Characteristics of the ideal internal support matrix are summarized in Table 16.2.

Implant selection

The choice of a round or shaped implant is based on multiple factors and is highly dependent on surgeon and patient preference. Factors to consider in implant selection include desired breast shape, quality of overlying soft tissues, requirement for a form-stable gel, and ability to control the dimensions of the implant pocket. Of course, in unilateral reconstruction, this choice is heavily influenced by what shape will best match the opposite breast. Regardless of the device used, it is important to follow accepted principles of dimensional planning with attention paid to the base width of the breast, the breast footprint on the chest wall, and the anatomy of the underlying chest wall. With the pocket created, the implant selected must provide a hand-in-glove fit to limit seroma formation, undesirable implant movement, or rotation. A stable implant and soft-tissue

---

Table 16.2 **Characteristics of ideal internal soft-tissue support matrix in breast reconstruction**

Safe
Biologically inert
Body responds through revascularization
Low cost
Readily accessible
Long shelf life
Ease of storage
Sterile
Ready to use
Range of size and shape options
Consistency of thickness
Low risk of disease transmission

---

relationship will ultimately decrease the number of revisionary procedures.

Size selection begins during the initial consultation. Chest wall dimensions must be accurately measured specifically focusing on breast width, height, and projection. This allows the surgeon to estimate the existing breast volume. Additionally, a three-dimensional volumetric computer program, such as the VECTRA 3D may be helpful with implant selection. Intraoperatively, mastectomy weights together with the use of sterilizable implant sizers and clinical judgment are used to select the final implant. A small overcorrection from the mastectomy weight is suggested in order to accommodate for the laxity created in the skin envelope as a result of the mastectomy.[23]

Immediate direct-to-implant reconstruction – surgical technique

Effective collaboration between the oncologic and the reconstructive surgeon is paramount to a successful patient outcome. This includes a discussion regarding the type of mastectomy, importance of gentle tissue handling, preservation of the **inframammary fold** (IMF) as well as the serratus fascia, and minimizing unnecessary lateral dissection of the breast pocket. Preoperative selection of the incision should be discussed to ensure access to the entire breast gland for excision while minimizing tension placed on flaps during retraction. A longer, strategically placed incision that minimizes the need for flap retraction is preferred to a shorter, well-hidden scar that causes the breast surgeon to struggle while performing the mastectomy.

The most common incision for a skin-sparing mastectomy (with nipple removal) is a mid-breast incision. The length of the incision is determined by the size of the breast and the need to reduce excess skin (Fig. 16.3). When a nipple-sparing mastectomy is indicated, an inframammary approach is preferred as this will minimize visualization of the scar (Fig. 16.4).

There is benefit for the plastic surgeon to assist the oncologic surgeon during the mastectomy. Not only does this provide an opportunity for improved collaboration, it also allows an opportunity to educate regarding the importance of gentle tissue handling, minimal skin flap retraction, uniform mastectomy flaps, and preservation of deep fascia. Once the mastectomy is performed, the skin flaps are carefully assessed for viability as described below. Any doubt as to skin flap viability would necessitate conversion to expander-based reconstruction or to a delayed procedure. The pectoralis muscle is elevated beginning at its inferomedial attachment on the sternum and divided from its inferior rib attachments working

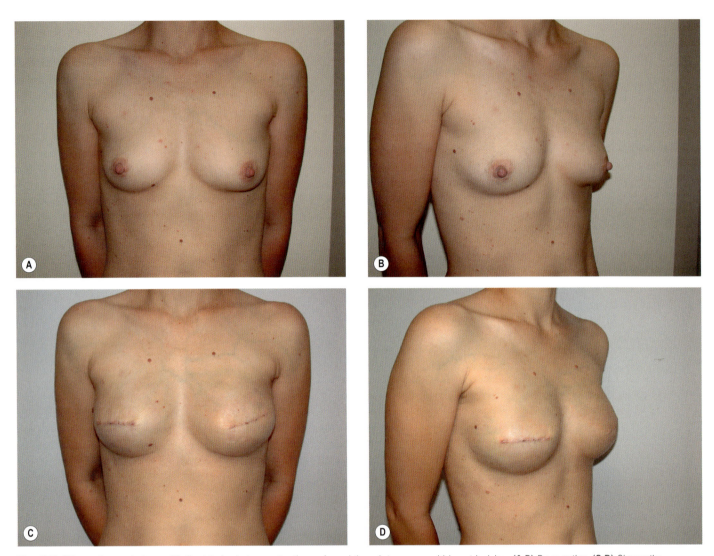

Fig. 16.3 Skin-sparing mastectomy with direct-to-implant reconstruction performed through transverse mid-breast incision. **(A,B)** Preoperative. **(C,D)** Six months postoperative.

laterally to the lateral mammary fold (LMF). At this point, the elevation includes part of the serratus fascia and ultimately results in a rectangular flap of pectoralis/serratus fascia that maintains a well-defined medial and lateral breast pocket. Pocket dissection is determined by the implant selection. When using shaped implants, it is important to make the pocket an appropriate size to fit the implant. A "hand-in-glove fit" is necessary to avoid implant rotation and malposition. Dissection is similar with the use of textured round devices; however, when a smooth surface implant is selected, the pocket is made slightly larger to allow for postoperative displacement exercises. This will help to minimize the risk of capsular contracture.

The internal support matrix can be inserted in two ways. When using an IMF incision, the matrix is first sutured to the free edge of the muscle and final closure is carried out along the IMF. If a mid-breast incision is used, it is easier to first place the matrix along the IMF and then close over the top of the implant to the free edge of the muscle. It is helpful to transpose the IMF and LMF from the skin markings onto the chest wall using methylene blue in order to ensure accurate fold placement. Following initial placement of the support matrix, sizers are inserted and the patient is placed in a sitting position. Breasts are inspected for symmetry, and the appropriate implant is selected. The patient is returned to a supine position, and the pockets are irrigated with antibiotic solution. A drain is placed along the inframammary crease in the subcutaneous plane and brought out through a separate incision in the anterior axillary line. Many surgeons place a second drain within the submuscular/ADM pocket. The authors have found that it is rare for fluid to collect deep to the muscle, and therefore they typically use a single drain. Several support matrices used today are fenestrated or

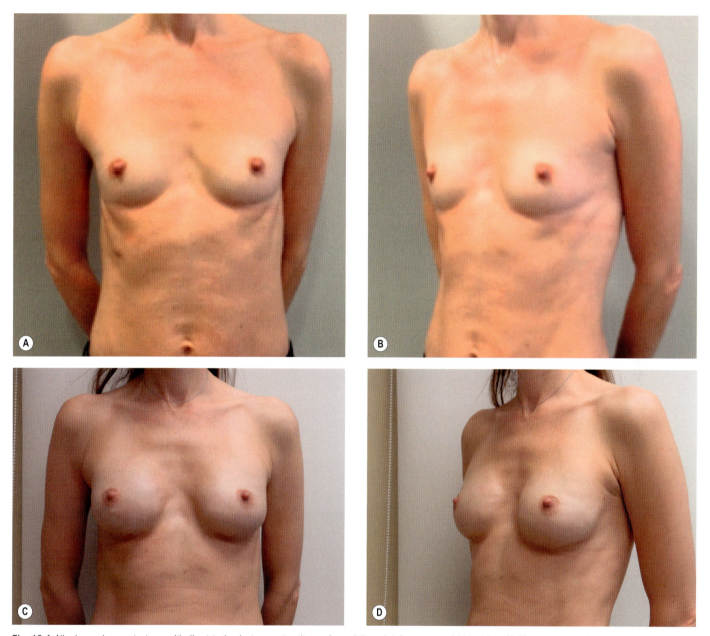

Fig. 16.4 Nipple-sparing mastectomy with direct-to-implant reconstruction performed through inframammary fold incision. **(A,B)** Preoperative. **(C,D)** One year postoperative.

perforated, which makes the need for a second drain less important (Fig. 16.5).

The implant is inserted using a minimal touch technique, and final closure of the pocket is performed. It is important to avoid excessive superior migration of the muscle, and therefore the muscle should be advanced inferiorly until the desired upper pole contour is achieved. The matrix is then trimmed as necessary to create a tight and supportive pocket. When a mid-breast incision is used, the muscle should be advanced inferiorly enough to place the muscle deep to the incision. This will be helpful in the event of any wound dehiscence or breakdown. Final closure is carried out in two layers, and a light protective dressing is applied.

Special consideration should be given to the patient that desires a significant decrease in their breast size at the time of mastectomy. In this case, the decision to forego preservation of the nipple in light of decreased complications should be considered. Direct-to-implant reconstruction is an excellent option in conjunction with skin-reducing mastectomies. In these cases, both Wise pattern and vertical skin patterns can be used and excess de-epithelialized skin can be used to provide additional implant coverage to the lower pole. When using a Wise pattern skin reduction, it is critical to preserve the medial perforators at the time of the mastectomy as the medial flap is most at risk for skin necrosis (Figs. 16.6 & 16.7).

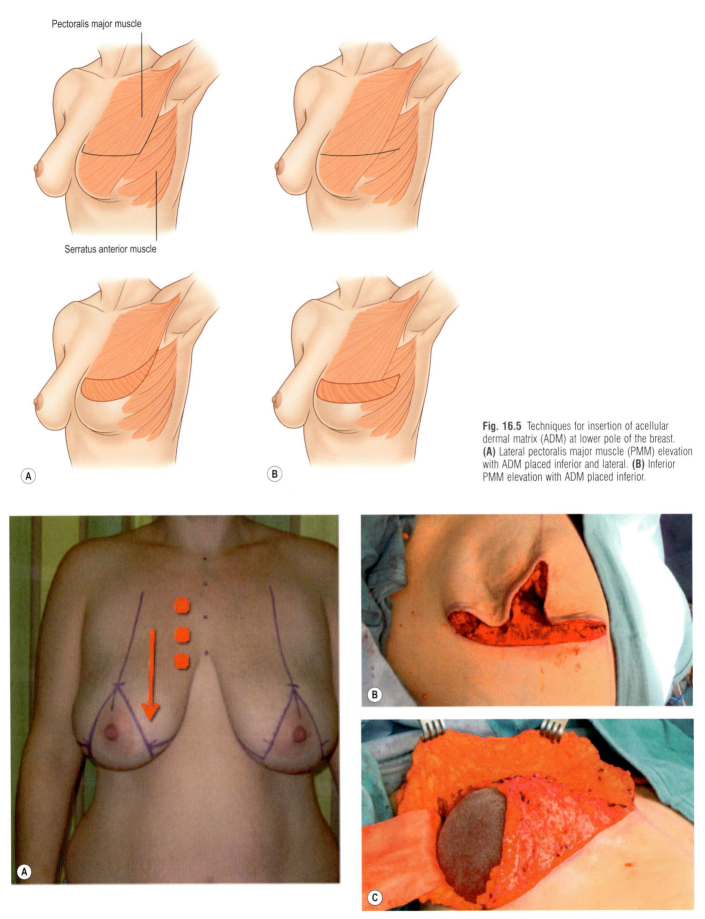

Pectoralis major muscle

Serratus anterior muscle

(A)

(B)

Fig. 16.5 Techniques for insertion of acellular dermal matrix (ADM) at lower pole of the breast. **(A)** Lateral pectoralis major muscle (PMM) elevation with ADM placed inferior and lateral. **(B)** Inferior PMM elevation with ADM placed inferior.

(A)

(B)

(C)

Fig. 16.6 Skin reduction mastectomy with inverted T pattern. **(A)** Skin markings. Note location of medial perforators. **(B)** Mastectomy completed. **(C)** Implant placed under pectoralis major muscle and dermal flap. Acellular dermal matrix to be sutured laterally.

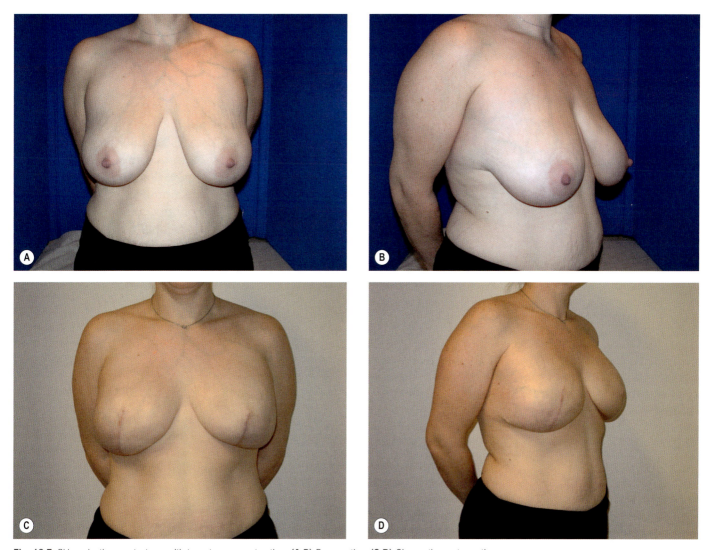

Fig. 16.7 Skin reduction mastectomy with two-stage reconstruction. **(A,B)** Preoperative. **(C,D)** Six months postoperative.

Assessment of skin flap viability

The success of breast reconstruction is dependent on avoidance of complications. Mastectomy skin flap necrosis, which occurs at a rate of 10–15%, can have significant consequences including major morbidity, delays in further oncologic treatment, implant loss or revision procedures, as well as poor aesthetic outcomes.[24]

Ischemic injury to the breast skin may occur during the mastectomy if the skin flaps are made too thin or if there is excessive traction on the skin flaps. Ischemic injury can also occur during reconstruction as placement of an implant can put direct stress on the skin flaps, thereby limiting perfusion. Traditional methods for assessing the likelihood of mastectomy skin flap necrosis rely almost exclusively on clinician judgment that includes intraoperative skin color, dermal edge bleeding, capillary refill time, and skin temperature. More recently, the incorporation of objective measures,

including laser-assisted ICG angiography have significantly decreased rates of skin flap necrosis.[25] Although promising, the use of these technologies must be determined based on institutional rates of tissue compromise versus cost of the technology itself.

Under any circumstance, if there is doubt as to the intraoperative viability of the skin flaps, the procedure should be converted to an expander-based reconstruction or a delayed procedure. When an expander is used, it can be inflated to gently fill the skin envelope, but without unnecessary tension on the overlying mastectomy skin flaps. This approach also provides the opportunity for postoperative expander deflation in the event of continuing tissue compromise.

Postoperative care

Postoperatively, patients are placed into supportive surgical bras. A tight compressive bra or wrap is avoided as it may compromise blood flow to the breast skin. Patients are maintained on oral antibiotics until the drains are removed. Gentle arm range-of-motion exercises are encouraged immediately. Activity is limited for 4–6 weeks after surgery. When smooth surface devices are used, displacement massage is started two weeks after surgery or as tolerated by the patient.

Complications

Significantly lower complication rates are currently being reported as compared to those published in earlier studies owing to better materials, increased surgeon experience, and better coordination between breast surgeons and plastic surgeons.[6,26] Major complications have been reported with an overall incidence as low as 6%, and individual complications including implant loss, skin necrosis requiring re-operation, infection, hematoma, seroma, and capsular contracture as low as 2% each.[10,23] Minor complications such as suture exposure, delayed healing, and epidermolysis are rare and usually self resolving with conservative and supportive care.

The largest multi-institutional report comparing early complications of direct-to-implant reconstruction with two-stage reconstruction found a higher rate of overall complications (6.8% compared with 5.4%) and prosthesis failure (1.4%, compared with 0.8%) in direct-to-implant reconstruction. No significant difference was found with regard to infection, re-operation, or major medical complications. Overall, low rates of early complications were found in both groups.[2] It is important to remember that complication rates will be highly dependent on the type of mastectomy performed as well as the selection of mastectomy incision.[27]

In direct-to-implant reconstruction, postoperative complications must be managed aggressively and in a timely fashion. Seromas and hematomas must be drained immediately to prevent excess tension on the overlying skin flaps and to minimize long-term implant malposition. Skin flap necrosis must be followed closely and if not healing quickly should be excised and closed primarily to avoid the possibility of implant exposure. Skin edge necrosis (2–5 mm) can often be managed with debridement and closure under local anesthesia. If the area of necrosis is larger, the implant may need to be downsized, replaced with an expander, or removed altogether.

Refinements and secondary procedures

When first described, the insertion of a permanent prosthesis at the time of mastectomy was erroneously referred to as a "single-stage reconstruction". Today, we understand that secondary revisions and refinements are necessary in 10–30% of patients, depending on patient selection and surgeon experience.[4,10,27] Common indications include adjustment of implant size, refinement of the inframammary or lateral mammary folds, or managing soft-tissue contour irregularities. Lipofilling has become a common adjunct to improve contours and camouflage the periphery of the implant. It is our practice to discuss secondary lipofilling with all of our patients. As techniques improve to monitor skin flap viability, primary lipofilling of both the pectoral muscle as well as the subdermal component of the mastectomy flap will be considered more frequently. This may assist in decreasing the need for secondary minor revisions.

Planned two-stage breast reconstruction

Patient selection

Regardless of timing of the reconstruction, patients undergoing planned two-stage implant-based reconstruction should ideally be healthy non-smokers who have good quality expandable chest wall skin and soft tissues. Patients seeking larger breast sizes may be reconstructed with implants; however, the surgeon should assess whether the native soft tissues are of sufficient quality to support the weight of larger implants. Where this concern exists, consideration is made for autologous reconstructive options. Patients who are undergoing unilateral reconstruction to match a moderately ptotic breast may also achieve a better result with autologous options.

Contraindications to planned two-stage alloplastic reconstruction include a lack of available expandable skin or a lack of underlying bony support to withstand the forces of the overlying expansion. Patients with existing chronic postmastectomy chest wall pain may also be poor candidates. Although an accepted risk factor, pre- or post-reconstruction radiation is not an absolute contraindication to expansion. In the delayed setting, we have found two-stage implant reconstruction to provide acceptable results in the radiated patient provided the chest wall tissues are soft and compliant and the patient desires a smaller breast size. Increasingly we have incorporated pre-treatment of the mastectomy flaps with fat grafting to improve the quality, thickness, and compliance of the mastectomy flaps.[28,29]

Immediate two-stage implant reconstruction in patients requiring postoperative radiotherapy has also been well established.[8,30–33] Various protocols exist, some advocating rapid expansion and expander to implant exchange prior to radiation versus exchanging the expander for the implant post-radiotherapy. The authors' preference in this scenario is to rapidly expand and exchange prior to radiation when possible. In situations where postoperative radiation therapy is anticipated, the use of ADM as a lower pole support may assist in minimizing the risk of capsular contracture. Fig. 16.8 shows the interface between normal capsule and ADM at the time of expander exchange. The lack of formation of a capsule in the area of the ADM decreases the ability of the capsule to tighten in a circumferential manner, making clinical contracture less likely.

Differences in approach for delayed and immediate two-stage alloplastic reconstruction

Important differences exist in the approach to the delayed versus the immediate two-stage breast reconstruction. In the delayed setting, the quality, compliance, and vascularity of soft tissues is already known. This results in less uncertainty regarding the possibility of mastectomy flap necrosis, wound dehiscence, and expander exposure. As these effectively represent delayed skin flaps, they may be more tolerant of the tension created by the initial fill of the expander.

In addition, in the delayed setting, the position and extent of the expander pocket dissection is controlled by the plastic surgeon, not determined by the existing mastectomy pocket. This confers a greater degree of control over the expander position, eliminating the need for muscle flaps or internal support matrices to control the lateral position of the expander. Finally, the pectoralis major is adhered to the overlying mastectomy flaps, therefore inferior pectoralis attachments to the ribs can be divided as in the case of a primary augmentation, facilitating anterior projection during the expansion process without the risk of over-retraction of the free muscle edge superiorly.

By contrast, in the setting of immediate reconstruction, the vascularity of the mastectomy flaps are less predictable, therefore less skin tension on wound closure is recommended. In addition, the anterior surface of the pectoralis major is completely detached from the overlying skin envelope. As a result the muscle must be controlled by either maintaining lower pole attachments to the rectus fascia, or by using internal support matrices to function as a pectoral extender down to the IMF. Finally, the lateral border of the mastectomy pocket often extends well beyond the desired lateral border of the tissue expander, necessitating the use of either serratus anterior flaps or an internal support matrix to control the lateral position of the expander.

Immediate two-stage reconstruction – surgical technique

The insertion of a tissue expander in breast reconstruction can be looked at as a "dress rehearsal" for the final outcome. The process of planning in reverse requires the surgeon to estimate the size and shape of the final implant and then select an expander to produce a pocket that is acceptable for the final device. This is especially critical when planning to use a shaped implant. Under-expansion is the key to success. The footprint of the expander should be narrower and shorter than the final implant. The authors prefer to use aggressively textured shaped tissue expanders with integrated ports due to their ability to provide preferential expansion of the lower pole of the breast. Suture tabs may help to decrease expander rotation and malposition. The base width of the expander is determined by the desired final width of the reconstructed breast, which may differ from the width of the original breast. Expander height and projection is then determined based on the patient's goals and on the proportions of the contralateral breast in the case of unilateral reconstruction.

Markings are made with the patient in the sitting position, and a team approach is used with both the oncologic and plastic surgeon present for the markings. Anatomic landmarks are then marked including the chest midline, breast meridians, medial and superior breast borders, and LMFs and IMFs. The choice of incision is based on a variety of factors including the preoperative size and shape of the breast, the desired postoperative breast size and position, and the location of pre-existing scars. Ultimately, skin incisions are performed in order to allow the surgeon to carry out a safe oncologic mastectomy with acceptable margins around the tumor.

There are several incision options for a skin-sparing mastectomy in conjunction with immediate expander

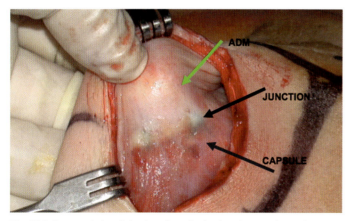

Fig. 16.8 Incorporated acellular dermal matrix showing absence of capsule formation over matrix surface. ADM, acellular dermal matrix.

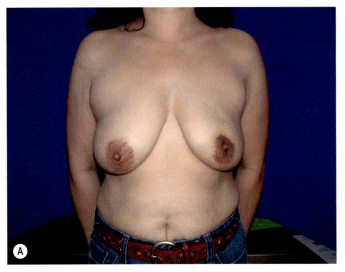

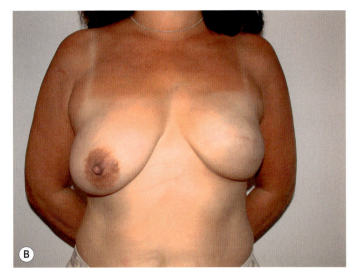

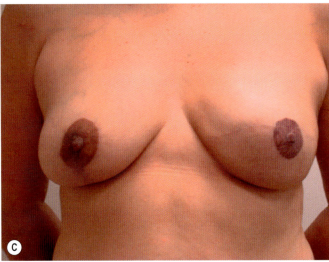

Fig. 16.9 (A) Preoperative view of large breasts with vertical skin excess. **(B)** Postoperative view following left mastectomy and reconstruction using a horizontal mastectomy incision. **(C)** Final view of same patient following left nipple areolar reconstruction and right breast balancing reduction.

insertion. In large breasts with vertical skin excess, a traditional transverse ellipse provides the opportunity to decrease the size of the skin envelope with minimal risk for skin flap compromise (Fig. 16.9). In cases where the breast should be lifted and narrowed, the ellipse can be oriented in a more oblique fashion (Fig. 16.10).

Nipple-sparing mastectomies with immediate reconstruction are becoming increasingly common due to the large number of prophylactic mastectomies performed at our center. In smaller breasts, mastectomies are generally performed through inframammary or lateral mammary incisions. Occasionally, periareolar incisions with or without a lateral extension are used for moderate sized breasts. When significant breast ptosis exists, skin reduction with nipple sacrifice is usually indicated. Mastectomies are designed using either a vertical or inverted "T" incision (Fig. 16.11). The inverted "T" skin-reducing mastectomy can be designed with an inferiorly based dermal flap to provide better lower pole soft-tissue coverage in case of delayed healing at the "T" junction.[34,35]

Patients are positioned on the operating table in the supine position with arms abducted at 90° and supported on arm boards. All patients receive perioperative antibiotic prophylaxis. Several staples or sutures are placed along the IMF in case the inked markings are lost during the mastectomy procedure.

Following completion of the mastectomy, skin flap viability is assessed clinically. Any questionable tissue is conservatively removed, and the decision as to whether to proceed with immediate reconstruction is made. Precise hemostasis is achieved with electrocautery. No blunt dissection is performed. In cases where the expander is to be placed in a total submusculofascial pocket, the pectoral muscle is elevated on its lateral border and dissected down to the rectus fascia. The rectus fascia is elevated to a point just inferior to the IMF. The serratus muscle is lifted laterally, and then the serratus is closed over the expander to the lateral edge of the pectoral muscle (Fig. 16.12). Transverse division of the rectus fascia below the level

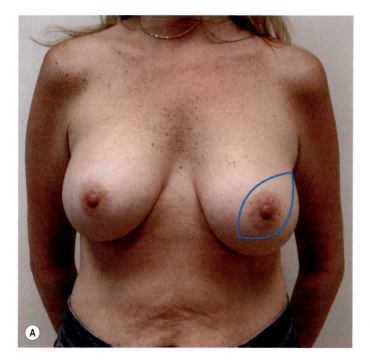

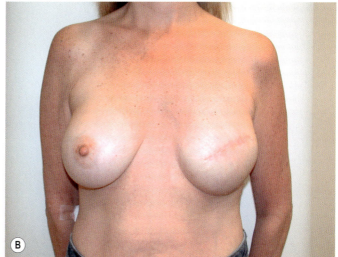

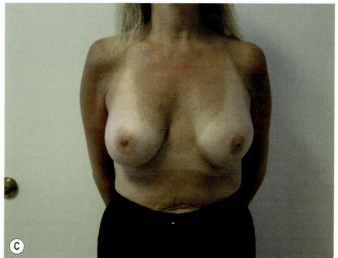

Fig. 16.10 (A) Preoperative view of breast showing vertical and horizontal skin excess with planned left oblique mastectomy incision indicated. **(B)** Postoperative view of same patient following left mastectomy and reconstruction using an oblique mastectomy incision. **(C)** Final result following nipple areolar reconstruction.

of the mastectomy pocket can then be performed to facilitate anterior projection during the expansion process.

Today, many surgeons choose to minimize muscle dissection by lifting the pectoral muscle with a lateral serratus extension and covering the lower pole of the expander with an internal support matrix. In this case, the pectoral muscle is lifted along the IMF maintaining the lateral attachments to the serratus muscle (Fig. 16.13). This approach allows for improved definition of the IMF and the LMF as well as accelerating early lower pole expansion. The pocket is then irrigated with antibiotic solution and the skin re-prepped. Using a minimal touch technique the expander is prepared by bathing it in antibiotic solution, removing the air, and positioning it in the pocket. A drain is placed in the subcutaneous pocket. Meticulous closure is performed with two layers of absorbable suture. The expander is then partially inflated with saline, avoiding unnecessary tension on the incision (see Video 16.1 ▶).

Patients are kept on postoperative oral antibiotics until the drain is removed. This is performed when the output falls below 30 cc per 24 hours for two consecutive days. Dressings are kept dry and intact for 5 days, at which point they are removed. Heavy lifting and strenuous activity is restricted for 6 weeks. Expander inflation begins approximately 2 weeks postoperatively and can be performed weekly as tolerated by the patient. Injection volumes per expansion can vary between 25 and 150 cc (average of 60 cc per inflation) and are based on patient comfort and avoidance of signs of skin blanching or over-tightening. Expansions are continued until patients are satisfied with breast volume and before tissues show signs of thinning or become overly tight. Overexpansion of the breast tissue is not recommended due to consequent thinning of the soft tissues, increased risk of exposure, and over-dissection and loss of control of the breast pocket. Depending on the skin quality, second-stage exchange is performed 1–3 months following completion of expansion.

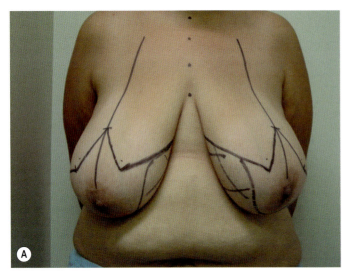

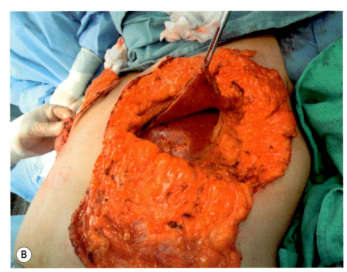

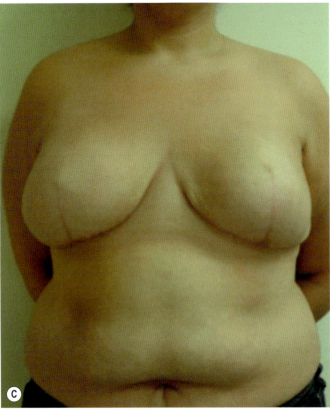

Fig. 16.11 (A) Preoperative view showing significant bilateral breast ptosis and planned inverted "T" pattern mastectomy with inferiorly based dermal flap. **(B)** Intraoperative view showing elevated pectoralis major muscle and undersurface of inferiorly based dermal flap reflected caudally. **(C)** Postoperative view of same patient prior to nipple areolar reconstruction.

Delayed two-stage reconstruction – surgical technique

In the delayed setting, the size of the expander is chosen preoperatively using the same dimensional approach described above. The base width of the expander is determined by direct measurement of the width of the chest wall. In unilateral reconstructions, the presence of a wide contralateral breast may necessitate the use of a wider tissue expander than the chest wall width measurement would suggest in order to achieve optimum symmetry. The height of the expander is then chosen based on the desired footprint of the final reconstructed breast. We prefer to avoid full height expanders to avoid unnecessary stretching of the upper pole tissues. As well, overexpansion of the upper pole of the breast beyond the desired final footprint may lead to loss of control of the pocket and the potential for superior implant malposition or rotation of shaped devices.

The patients are marked in the sitting position. Particular attention is paid to the position of the IMF, as this can often be blunted or obliterated as a result of the

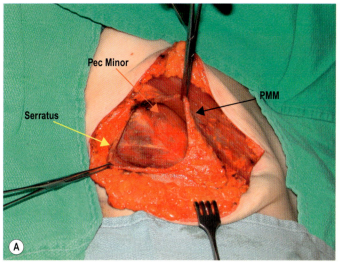

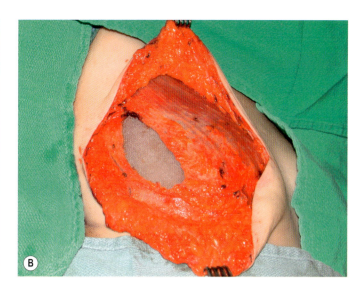

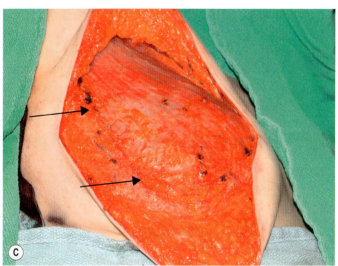

Fig. 16.12 (A) Intraoperative view of submuscular pocket dissection showing elevated pectoralis major (PMM) and serratus anterior muscles, and unelevated pectoralis minor muscle. **(B)** Tissue expander positioned in submuscular pocket. **(C)** Intraoperative view showing suture line (arrows) following closure of lateral border of PMM to anterior border of serratus anterior over the tissue expander.

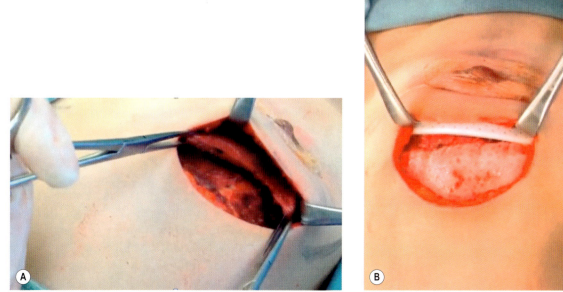

Fig. 16.13 (A) Intraoperative view of submuscular pocket dissection from an inferior approach with division of inferior pectoralis major fibers while maintaining attachments between pectoralis major and serratus anterior muscles. **(B)** Inset of acellular dermal matrix for inferior pole support and tissue expander coverage.

previous mastectomy. If absent, the IMF is marked according to the contralateral breast in unilateral cases, and according to the patient's bra position if available in bilateral cases. Patients are positioned and prepped as described above.

Typically the existing mastectomy scar is used for access. If the mastectomy flaps are robust with a healthy amount of subcutaneous fat, the authors prefer to open the incision laterally and approach the subpectoral pocket from the lateral border of the pectoral muscle. If, however, the mastectomy flaps are thin laterally, the authors will open the scar centrally, judiciously elevate skin flaps a few centimeters superiorly and inferiorly, and split the pectoral major muscle parallel to its fibers to enter the subpectoral pocket. All dissection is performed using electrocautery with preemptive hemostasis. No blunt dissection is used. The pocket is dissected exactly to the marked borders and the muscle is divided inferiorly as with a dual plane breast augmentation dissection. This facilitates greater projection of the lower pole during the expansion process. As the pectoralis major is in continuity with the overlying skin, windowshading of the muscle superiorly does not occur. After completion of the pocket dissection, expander preparation, insertion, and intraoperative inflation proceeds as described for immediate reconstruction (see Video 16.2 ⦿). Drains are not routinely used. Dressings are kept dry and intact for 5 days at which point they are removed and the patients are allowed to shower. Heavy lifting and strenuous activity is restricted for 4 weeks.

Expander to implant exchange – surgical technique

The second stage provides an opportunity to refine the breast shape and maximize symmetry between the two breasts. Today, many tools exist to assist the surgeon, including various implant styles, ADM, and selective lipofilling. Maxwell describes this as the bioengineered breast.[36] Implant selection is based on the patient's tissue characteristics, goals, and the final volume of the tissue expander. To account for the volume of the expander shell/port construct, as well as the greater compressibility of implants compared to expanders, the authors tend to insert implants which are 10–20% larger than the final expander volume. Silicone implants are almost exclusively used except in rare circumstances when the patient expresses a preference for saline. Debate exists regarding the ability of patients and plastic surgeons to reliably detect the visual differences between shaped and round implants. However, in the reconstructive population, the absence of breast tissue limits the ability of the

soft tissues to camouflage the shape of the underlying implant. When patients desire more upper pole fullness, either as an aesthetic preference or to better balance a contralateral breast, a round implant is chosen. When less fullness and a more gradual slope is desired in the upper pole of the breast, a textured, shaped, form-stable device is recommended.

In most cases, a portion of the existing scar is reopened for access. However, in cases where the anterior skin is very thin, when postoperative radiation to the expander has occurred, or when excision of the existing scar would significantly reduce the skin envelope, a new incision in the IMF is made. A circumferential capsulotomy is performed in the majority of cases, but this decision is based on the expander position. Selective capsulectomy is reserved for cases where the anterior capsule restricts breast expansion or to promote adherence of a textured surface device. Special attention is made to the position of the IMF. If the fold has become blunted from the expansion process, permanent sutures are passed through the superficial fascia at the level of the IMF via the capsulotomy incision, and then sutured to the chest wall fascia to create a more defined crease. In cases where the IMF has been completely obliterated by the expansion process, then a similar technique is used, but in this case the superficial fascia is grasped more inferiorly and elevated up to the planned IMF in order to try and recreate ptosis at the level of the fold (Fig. 16.14). Similar techniques are used to adjust the lateral mammary fold as indicated. Sizers are used to confirm the adequacy of pocket shape and size in both the sitting and supine positions prior to implant insertion.

Following all pocket modifications, the implants are prepared and inserted. Drains are occasionally used depending on the degree of capsule manipulation. Following skin closure, the soft tissues are inspected and lipofilling can be considered for areas of implant visibility or contour irregularity. Care must be taken to avoid injection within the implant pocket. If the tissues are too thin to allow for immediate lipofilling, then this can be performed in a delayed fashion. Representative cases are shown in Figs. 16.15 and 16.16.

Complications

Complications in two-stage alloplastic breast reconstruction are related to either the device or the soft tissues. Device complications include contracture, rupture, malposition, rotation, visibility, rippling, or late problems related to double capsule or seroma. Tissue complications include infection, thinning or stretching, necrosis, delayed healing, and dysesthesias of the breast.

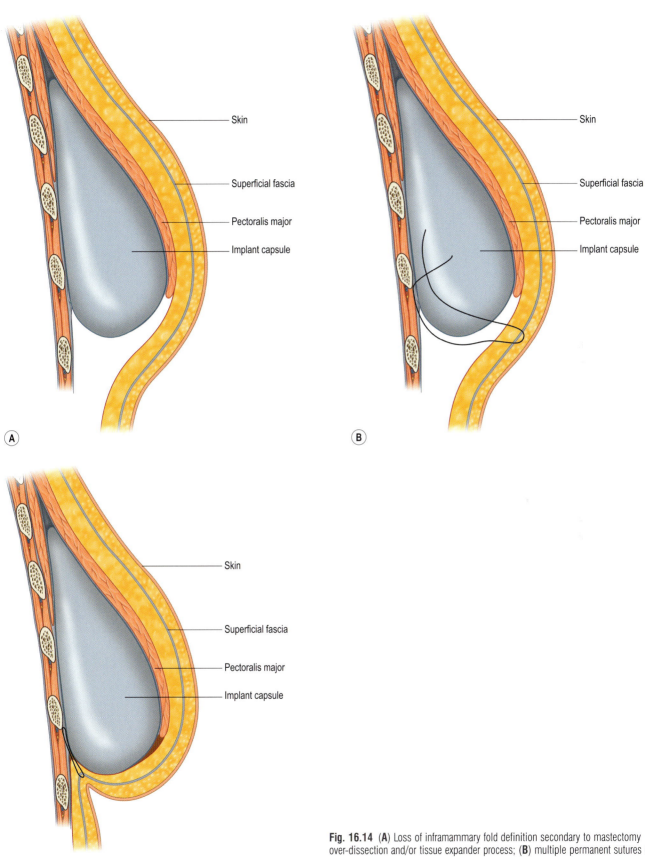

Fig. 16.14 **(A)** Loss of inframammary fold definition secondary to mastectomy over-dissection and/or tissue expander process; **(B)** multiple permanent sutures can be placed between the superficial fascial layer anteriorly and the chest wall posteriorly to re-define the inframammary fold; **(C)** placement of the anterior suture more inferiorly can recruit anterior skin to reproduce ptosis as necessary.

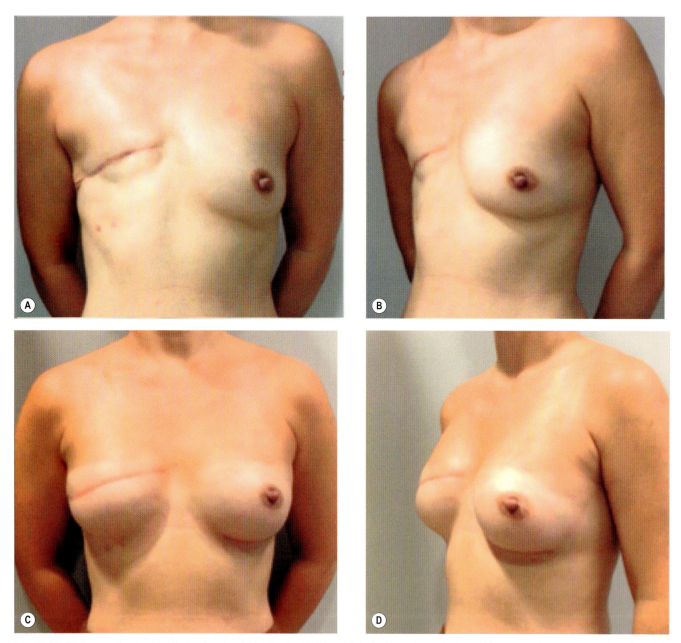

Fig. 16.15 (A) Preoperative view of patient undergoing right delayed and left immediate nipple-sparing mastectomy with two-stage breast reconstruction using 133MV12 tissue expanders. **(B)** Preoperative oblique view of same patient. **(C)** Postoperative view following bilateral exchange procedure with insertion of MX410 form-stable silicone implant and lipofilling to right breast. **(D)** Postoperative oblique view of same patient.

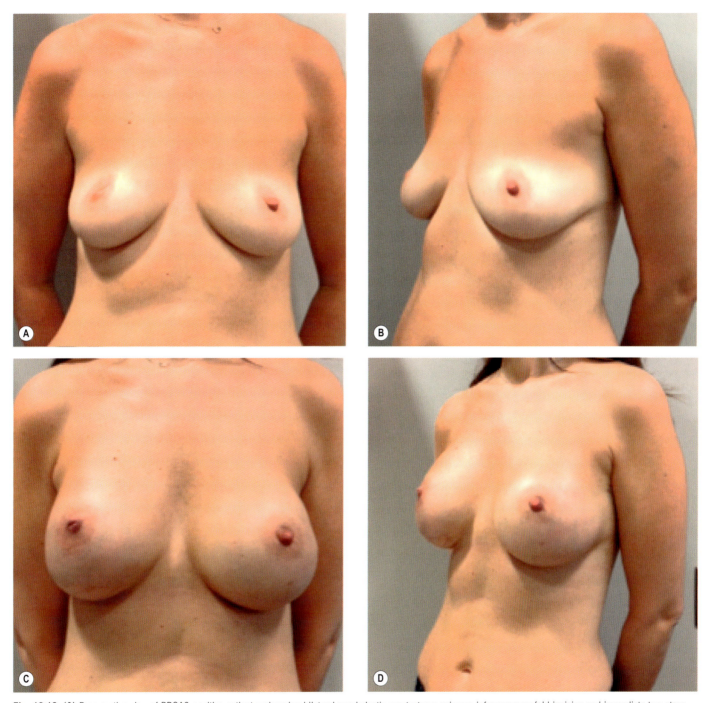

Fig. 16.16 (A) Preoperative view of BRCA2-positive patient undergoing bilateral prophylactic mastectomy using an inframammary fold incision and immediate two-stage breast reconstruction using 133MV500 tissue expanders. **(B)** Oblique view of same patient. **(C,D)** Postoperative view of final result following exchange procedure with insertion of round silicone 540 cc full projection implants and upper pole lipofilling.

Asymmetry or concerns with the aesthetic appearance are other concerns that are often raised by patients. Careful patient selection, dimensional planning, thinking in reverse, precise surgical technique, and a defined postoperative process will help to keep complications to a minimum.

Bonus image for this chapter can be found online at
http://www.expertconsult.com

Fig. 16.1 Bilateral nipple-sparing mastectomy through inframammary fold incision. Direct-to-implant reconstruction with shaped cohesive gel implants and acellular dermal matrix. **(A,B)** Preoperative. **(C,D)** One year postoperative.

Access the complete reference list online at **http://www.expertconsult.com**

2. Davila AA, Mioton LM, Chow G, et al. Immediate two-stage tissue expander breast reconstruction compared with one-stage permanent implant breast reconstruction: a multi-institutional comparison of short-term complications. *J Plast Surg Hand Surg*. 2013;47:344–349. *One of the largest multi-institutional reviews comparing complications in immediate one-stage versus two-stage alloplastic breast reconstruction. Series included over 10 000 patients and showed increased complication rates among those undergoing immediate implant placement.*

4. Gdalevitch P, Ho A, Genoway K, et al. Direct-to-implant single-stage immediate breast reconstruction with acellular dermal matrix: predictors of failure. *Plast Reconstr Surg*. 2014;133:738e–747e. *Retrospective cohort study to identify predictors of failure in single-stage immediate alloplastic breast reconstruction. Results shold help guide readers in patient selection for one-stage reconstruction and avoid those at high risk of early revision surgery.*

6. Colwell AS, Damjanovic B, Zahedi B, et al. Retrospective review of 331 consecutive immediate single-stage implant reconstructions with acellular dermal matrix. *Plast Reconstr Surg*. 2011;128:1170–1178. *This retrospective review of 331 consecutive single-stage implant reconstructions with ADM provides insight into the learning curve associated with incorporating single-stage implant reconstruction into a practice, as well as data on surgical complications, and a cost comparison between single and two-stage alloplastic reconstruction.*

11. Wink JD, Fischer JP, Nelson JA, et al. Direct-to-implant breast reconstruction: an analysis of 1612 cases from the ACS-NSQIP surgical outcomes database. *J Plast Surg Hand Surg*. 2014;48:375–381. *Retrospective review of direct-to-implant outcomes from the ACS-NSQIP database highlighting the importance of patient selection and providing population level data identifying groups of patients at higher risk of complications, including obese patients and smokers.*

15. Hoppe IC, Yueh JH, Wei CH, et al. Complications following expander/implant breast reconstruction utilizing acellular dermal matrix: a systematic review and meta-analysis. *Eplasty*. 2011;11:e40. *Meta-analysis of available studies evaluating the complications rates of ADM-assisted expander/implant breast reconstruction compared to traditional expander/implant breast reconstruction without ADM. The final analysis included 8 studies representing 977 ADM-assisted expanders and 3840 expanders without ADM. Data indicates a two-fold increase in infections when ADM was used and a three-fold increase in seroma formation when ADM was used. The use of ADM facilitated higher intraoperative expander filling in the ADM group.*

21. Ganz OM, Tobalem M, Perneger T, et al. Risks and benefits of using an absorbable mesh in one-stage immediate breast reconstruction. *Plast Reconstr Surg*. 2015;135:498e–507e. *Retrospective review of immediate one-stage implant reconstruction with total submuscular pocket compared to partial submuscular pocket with vicryl mesh. The authors conclude the use of vicryl mesh allows for larger implant volumes, better pocket control, and decreased need for contralateral balancing mastopexy. The authors advocate the use of vicryl mesh as a lower cost alternative to the use of biologic scaffolds or traditional two-stage reconstruction with expanders.*

23. Salzberg CA. Focus on technique: one-stage implant-based breast reconstruction. *Plast Reconstr Surg*. 2012;130:95S–103S. *Seminal article describing the technique of ADM-assisted one-stage immediate breast reconstruction, including indications, preoperative planning, implant selection, and detailed description of surgical staps and execution. Includes online videos of the technique.*

28. Sarfati I, Ihrai T, Kaufman G, et al. Adipose-tissue grafting to the post-mastectomy irradiated chest wall: preparing the ground for implant reconstruction. *J Plast Reconstr Aesthet Surg*. 2011;64:1161–1166. *One of the first publications demonstrating the benefits of autologous fat transfer to the irradiate mastectomy bed prior to performing implant-based breast reconstruction in patients who refused or were not candidates for autologous reconstruction. The authors describe their grafting technique, complications, and ratings of cosmetic outcomes.*

31. Cordeiro PG, Albornoz CR, McCormick B, et al. The impact of postmastectomy radiotherapy on two-stage implant breast reconstruction: an analysis of long-term surgical outcomes, aesthetic results, and satisfaction over 13 years. *Plast Reconstr Surg*. 2014;134:588–595. *The authors present the largest prospective long-term outcomes evaluation of women undergoing immediate two-stage alloplastic breast reconstruction with postmastectomy radiation compared to those not having radiation. The authors report that despite higher rates of implant loss, converting to flap reconstruction, and capsular contracture in the irradiated group, 90% of those who received radiation had good to excellent cosmesis and patient satisfaction.*

32. Nava MB, Pennati AE, Lozza L, et al. Outcome of different timings of radiotherapy in implant-based breast reconstructions. *Plast Reconstr Surg*. 2011;128:353–359. *Comparison of outcomes between delivery of radiation during tissue expansion versus radiating the final implant following expander to implant exchange. The authors report a six-fold increase in failure of the reconstruction when radiation was administered during the expansion phase.*

17

Secondary procedures following prosthetic breast surgery

G. Patrick Maxwell and Allen Gabriel

SYNOPSIS

- Breast augmentation is the most common aesthetic procedure performed in the US.
- Revisionary breast surgeries are complex, challenging, and unpredictable.
- The four main drivers for revisionary surgery are capsular contracture, implant malposition, ptosis, and implant visibility or palpability.
- Revisionary surgery techniques are introduced that utilize a site change operation with the use of acellular dermal matrix (ADM).
- Detailed recommendations are provided so that the reader can utilize advanced techniques to treat any secondary breast complication related to implants.

 Access the Historical Perspective section online at **http://www.expertconsult.com**

Introduction

It is estimated that over 300 000 primary breast augmentations were performed in the US in 2014, and therefore there are now over 3 million women with augmented breasts in this country.[1-3] Based on current data, between 15% and 30% of these women will have a re-operation within 5 years of their initial procedure.[1-3] Unfortunately, this rate climbs to 35% in patients with prior history of revisionary breast augmentation.[4] As procedures become more complex in nature and number, new techniques and solutions are required of surgeons who perform these challenging operations in order to improve long-term patient outcomes.

Capsular contracture has historically been the most common complication of aesthetic and reconstructive breast surgery and remains the primary reason for most revisionary surgeries.[2,3,5,6] While increasing data suggests capsular contracture can be minimized in primary augmentation by adhering to specific technical factors, such as precise, atraumatic, and bloodless pocket dissection; appropriate antibiotic irrigation of the breast pocket; and minimizing any points of contamination during the procedure,[4,7] treatment of an established capsule remains even more challenging than the application of these techniques alone.

With the enforcement of the United States Food and Drug Administration (FDA) restrictions on silicone gel implants in the early 1990s, many plastic surgeons in the US began to use saline implants.[1] Prior to the 1992 "moratorium", the majority of silicone gel implants were placed in the subglandular position, whereas saline implants (due to their palpability) were placed in the subpectoral position in an effort to conceal the untoward contour irregularities of these implants.[8] Many of these implants were of larger volumes, thus many patients experienced thinning of the breast parenchyma and the overlying soft tissues. This was independent of whether the implants were located in subglandular or subpectoral positions. The thinned parenchymal tissues in turn led to long-term complications that instigated some key drivers of revisionary breast surgery.

The four primary reasons (or "drivers") for aesthetic revisionary surgery in the premarket approval (PMA) studies were[9] (1) capsular contracture, (2) implant malposition, (3) ptosis, and (4) implant visibility or palpability. Frequently, these indications were not singularly distinct but were combined, with two or more being present in a given patient.

Basic science and disease process

Acellular dermal materials, biologically derived from allograft and xenograft, when placed in the human body, are thought to serve as a regenerative scaffold, promoting the organization of the healing process. These materials have become popular in aesthetic and reconstructive breast surgery where they are can serve as a tissue extension or tissue replacement ("soft-tissue patch") following cancer extirpation of the breast (so-called "sling technique").[23,24,28]

The authors' work with ADMs began in revisionary aesthetic breast surgery, attempting to prevent capsular contracture, rather than as a tissue replacement in breast reconstruction. Having previously employed "host-compatible" implant surfaces,[29] the authors utilized a similar concept in the clinical approach to breast revision: a dermal regenerative interface engaging the surface geometric contour of a breast implant.

Understanding the changes that occur in the breast tissue is part of management of the problem at hand. Following breast surgery many factors play a role in the changes that are observed in the breast form and at times are considered as late complications of breast augmentation. Patients lose or gain weight, which contributes directly to the breast shape. In addition, some patients may undergo surgical or non-surgical menopause, which has deleterious effects on the well-being of the skin and causes thinning of the breast skin, with decreased elasticity and increased ptosis. There are other physiological factors that play an important role in the pathophysiology of the changing breast forms. Patients present with any of the following complaints: capsular contracture, implant malposition, ptosis, and implant visibility or palpability. Interestingly, patients with capsular contracture do not realize the primary reason for the deformity of their breast and present to the office for other complaints as stated above.

Capsular contracture has plagued plastic surgery for many years as the most common complication of aesthetic and reconstructive breast surgery.[2,5] The majority of revisionary procedures are performed due to capsular contracture.[2,6] Many etiologies have been proposed for this process, and it is clear that prevention in primary cases is of utmost importance and is principally related to specific technical maneuvers that include precise, atraumatic, bloodless dissection; appropriate triple antibiotic breast pocket irrigation; and minimizing any points of contamination during the procedure.[4,7] Treatment of an established capsule can be more challenging and a variety of techniques have been described. It is important to understand the pathophysiological process and the disease at the cellular level in order to successfully manage capsular contracture. In this case, it is perspicuous at the cellular level that capsular contracture is most likely caused by any process that will produce increased inflammation, leading to formation of deleterious cytokines within the periprosthetic pocket. Consequently, in addition to all of the techniques for treating and preventing capsular contracture described by many of our colleagues,[4,5,8,30–36] the authors believe that the addition of ADM is another modality in fighting the evolution of the capsule. ADM can counteract the inflammatory process, adding additional availability of tissue ingrowth and controlling the interface of the pocket.

Acellular dermal matrix

The use of ADMs has been popularized in both breast and abdominal wall reconstructions and has been reported in a range of clinical settings.[14–24] In reconstructive cases, it has been used to replace tissue, extend existing tissue, or act as a supplement. In aesthetic cases it has been used to correct implant rippling and malposition as well as for symmastia.[26,27,37]

Immediate breast reconstruction using tissue expanders or implants has become one of the most commonly performed surgical techniques. As such, visible rippling and contour deformities have become a more frequently encountered problem because of thin tissues.[28] The recent use of allogenic tissue supplements avoids the problems of autologous tissue coverage and provides camouflage, thus decreasing rippling and increasing soft-tissue support.[28]

The rising demand for acellular dermal matrices has spurred tremendous growth in the number of available ADMs. Published research with regard to the use and efficacy of acellular dermal matrices in immediate breast reconstruction is growing but has not kept pace with the market explosion. The many features and indications of all ADMs can confound the decision-making process for surgeons who want to incorporate ADMs in their treatment armamentarium.

Acellular dermal matrices can be categorized under either xenograft or allograft in origin. All are produced with a similar objective of removing cellular and antigenic components that can cause rejection and infection. The lack of immunogenic epitopes enables the evasion of rejection, absorption, and extrusion.[15,16,24] Production processes allow basement membrane and cellular matrix to remain intact. This scaffold is left in place to allow ingrowth of the host's fibroblasts and capillaries, which are eventually incorporated as its own. Much of this scaffold matrix consists of intact collagen fibers and bundles to support tissue ingrowth, proteins, intact elastin, hyaluronic acid, fibronectin, fibrillar collagen, collagen VI, vascular channels, and proteoglycans – all of which allow the body to mount its own tissue regeneration process.[15,16,23,24]

All ADMs are FDA cleared for homologous use only. Although features and processing may vary between ADMs, the success of the product will ultimately depend on its ability to meet the desired characteristics of a model ADM for revisionary breast surgery. A list of ADMs that are available on the market for a variety of applications are included in Table 17.1.

Published literature

AlloDerm is clearly in the forefront with regard to published literature concerning ADMs for immediate breast reconstruction. A PubMed search using specific brand names and breast reconstruction reveals that the majority of publications involve AlloDerm. Ten of these papers relate directly to adjunctive ADM treatment of immediate breast reconstruction using AlloDerm,[15,16,23,24,28,38–40] DermaMatrix,[41] and Neoform.[42] All of these papers are recent publications, the oldest dating back to 2005,[15] and are non-controlled, retrospective case series. PubMed searches were also performed for all other human and xenograft ADMs – FlexHD, AlloMax, SurgiMend, Enduragen, Synovis, Permacol, and Strattice – with breast reconstruction and revealed no listings. It is likely that studies are underway and not yet completed.

As new products are introduced to the marketplace, it is always crucial to understand the science behind each technology. The device industry should be evaluated as critically as the pharmaceuticals, with regard to the science and mechanism of action.

When evaluating ADMs critically, it is important that we understand the differences in how the body responds to the various materials. Not all soft-tissue materials elicit the same biologic response. There are three unique processes that can take place with any tissue material that is placed into the body, whether it is a biologic or synthetic material. All products placed into the body elicit an inflammatory response with involvement of multiple cytoprotective and cytotoxic cytokines. The continuum of this reaction is controlled by the intrinsic mechanism unique to each scaffold.

Regeneration

With this process, the product is accepted by the body and the intact tissue matrix integrates and becomes part of the host through rapid revascularization and cellular repopulation. This is the process that is most beneficial and important to obtain good outcomes in breast surgery and perhaps the reason why we see less periprosthetic capsular contracture.

Resorption

This is the process where the human body attacks the replaced tissue and breaks it down by completely eliminating it, while depositing scar tissue in its place. This is commonly seen with absorbable mesh products.

Encapsulation

During this process, the product is encapsulated through an inflammatory response. The body is unable to break down the product due to its synthetic nature. Therefore, the product is encapsulated and walled-off from the host. This process is not unique to synthetic products but also applies to any foreign body (e.g., pacemakers and implants) that is placed into the host.

The goal of regenerating tissue is to recapitulate in adult wounded tissue the intrinsic regenerative processes that are involved in normal adult tissue maintenance.[43] Scar tissue does not have the native structure, function, and physiology of the original normal tissue. When a wound exceeds a critical deficit, it requires a scaffold to organize tissue replacement. Depending on the type of scaffold that is in place, different processes, as described earlier, will respond. At this point the intrinsic factors of the ADM will be important in aiding each specific regenerative or reparative process. While regenerative healing is characterized by the restoration of the structure, function, and physiology of damaged or absent tissue, reparative healing is characterized by wound closure through scar formation.[43] All biologic scaffolds are not the same because of differences in the methods used to process them – materials that encapsulate and scar do not offer the benefits of regenerative healing but lead to suboptimal results.

Diagnosis and patient presentation

ADM is utilized as an adjunct to the sound surgical principles necessary to diagnose and treat the

Table 17.1 Comparison of different commercially available acellular dermal matrices

Product name	Manufacturer	Origin	Method of preservation	Year introduced	Time to hydrate	Shelf life	Refrigeration required
AlloDerm	LifeCell	Human dermis	Lyophilized; patented freeze-drying process prevents damaging ice crystals from forming	1994	10–40 min, depending on thickness, with warmed saline solution in two-step bath with light agitation	2 years	No
DermaMatrix	Processed by Musculoskeletal Transplant Foundation (MTF) for Synthes CMF	Human dermis	Aseptic processing method; lyophilized	2005	3 min	3 years	No
FlexHD	Processed by Musculoskeletal Transplant Foundation (MTF) for Ethicon	Human dermis	Aseptic processing method; packaged in an ethanol solution	2007	None	18 months	No
SurgiMend	TEI Biosciences	Fetal bovine dermal collagen	Terminally sterilized with ethylene oxide	2007	60 s with room temperature saline	3 years	No
Strattice	LifeCell	Porcine dermal collagen	Terminally sterilized via low dose e-beam; retains critical biochemical components; significantly reduces the key component believed to play a major role in the xenogeneic rejection response	2008	Minimum of 2 min in sterile saline	2 years	No
Veritas	Synovis Surgical Innovations	Bovine pericardium collagen	Terminally sterilized; sodium hydroxide treatment for purification and microbiological security	2008	None	2 years	No
Surgisis	Cook Biotech	Porcine small intestinal submucosal	Sterilized with ethylene oxide	2004	3–10 min	1 year	No
AlloMax	Manufactured by Regeneration Technologies/ Tutogen Medical, Inc. for Bard Davol	Human dermis	Terminally sterilized	2007	Hydrates rapidly	5 years	No
MatriStem	ACell/Medline	Porcine bladder	Unavailable	2009	None	2 years	No

underlying cause(s) necessitating the revisionary aesthetic breast surgery. Clinical data shows the four main indications (drivers) for revisionary surgery: capsular contracture, implant malposition, ptosis, and implant visibility or palpability.[25-27] Each patient must be individually evaluated with regard to concerns, goals, knowledge of previous surgical and implant specifics, and careful evaluation of her breasts – dimensions, quality/quantity of overlying soft tissue, and scarring (critical in planning surgery and maintaining necessary vascularity to manipulated tissues).

Despite the apparent complexity of a given clinical presentation, there are five underlying basic components that may be the cause, or contribute to the cause, of the problem: the skin, soft tissue, capsule, implant, and chest wall. These underlying components must be carefully and systematically analyzed from outside in, or inside out, until all layers involved are evaluated.

Patient selection

The main drivers for revisionary surgery, as mentioned earlier, should always be kept in mind as the five components (see above) are evaluated. We have learned from revisionary and reconstructive breast experiences that one or more of these components and layers may need to be addressed in addition to the use of ADM. Such surgical manipulations may include skin envelope reduction, fat injection, lamellar separation, capsulectomy, capsulotomy, and site change of the replacement implant. In order to help plan for the surgery some general principles can be followed.

For patients whose original implants were subglandular, a pocket change to a subpectoral plane and lower pole coverage with ADM is generally performed. For those patients whose original implants were subpectoral, a neopectoral pocket with the addition of ADM is generally performed. For patients with adequate breast tissue, a subfascial pocket may be utilized with ADM coverage or support as indicated. As always, appropriate candidate selection is important for achieving a successful outcome, and high-risk patients (e.g., smokers and those with a BMI higher than 35) should be discouraged from elective surgery. The core principles for aesthetic breast revisions are summarized in Table 17.2.

Treatment and surgical technique

The use of ADM can be categorized into four distinct indications based upon the underlying clinical presentation: (1) coverage of implant lower pole (usually for revision mastopexy), (2) implant stabilizer (usually for malposition correction), (3) tissue thickener (usually

Table 17.2 The process of aesthetic breast revision core principles

Patient–physician education	
Patient evaluation	**Preoperative planning**
1. Listen to patient (concerns, dislikes, symptoms)	1. Dimensional and tissue evaluation (asymmetry)
2. Obtain accurate history	2. Implant evaluation
3. Interactive assessment	3. Periprosthetic pocket evaluation
4. Define problem	4. Define operative strategy
5. Craft solution(s)	5. Implant selection
6. Educate/expectations	6. Pocket selection
	7. Soft tissue management
	8. Adjunctive techniques
Surgical technique	**Postoperative management**
1. Access: incision location/length	1. Comprehensive patient experience
2. Implant removal/evaluation	2. Commitment to surgical excellence
3. Pocket alteration (location/size/capsule/technique)	3. Short-term postop care (movement, drains, dressings, sutures)
4. Implant selection (intraoperative info) (sizers?, upright evaluation)	4. Long-term postop care
5. Implant handling/irrigation/positioning	5. Management of revisions
6. Soft tissue alterations (tailor tac)	
7. Additional maneuvers (ADM, drains)	

ADM, acellular dermal matrix.
(Adapted from Adams WP, Jr. Process of breast augmentation. *Plast Reconstr Surg.* 2008;122(6):1892–1900.)

superomedially or inferiorly), and (4) treatment of capsular contracture (which may be technically similar to lower pole cover or superior-medial thickening) (Fig. 17.1).

Coverage of lower pole

This important concept and technique, which is our most frequently utilized ADM placement, is employed when performing soft-tissue and skin envelope alterations in revisionary surgery (revision mastopexy with augmentation). As many patients with previously placed implants develop laxity, sag, or tissue thinning over time, mastopexy or revision mastopexy over the replacement implant is required to achieve the aesthetic breast form. If the existing implant is subglandular, a subpectoral (subpectoral-fascial) pocket is created (after capsule treatment), the new implant inserted in the newly created subpectoral pocket, and the lower portion of the implant covered with ADM. This allows a circumvertical or "inverted T" mastopexy to be safely performed without underlying muscle, as the ADM separates the skin closure from the implant. If the existing implant is already subpectoral, a neopectoral

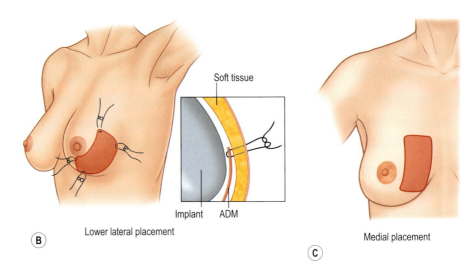

Center placement

(A)

Lower lateral placement

Soft tissue

Implant   ADM

(B)

Medial placement

(C)

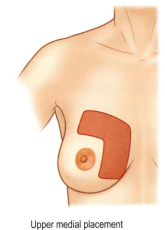

Upper medial placement

(D)

Fig. 17.1 The use of acellular dermal matrix (ADM) can be categorized into four distinct indications based upon the underlying clinical presentation: **(A)** center placement; **(B)** lower lateral placement; **(C)** medial placement; and **(D)** upper medial placement.

site change is carried out, and the ADM utilized similarly. If there has been a previous implant in both the subglandular and subpectoral pockets, "lamellar" separation (dissecting the pectoralis muscle from its superficial and deep scarred attachments) may be necessary (Fig. 17.2). ADM is considered to be the outer layer of the underling implant (to which it is intimately engaged by proximity of placement) and may also require suture stabilization. Thus the ADM may be tacked to the inferior border of the pectoralis major above and to Scarpa's fascia or deep fascia below (at the level of the inframammary fold [IMF]). Parachute pullout sutures may alternatively be used to redrape the ADM. When there is lamellar scarring requiring lamellar separation, the remaining pectoralis muscle may be "window shaded" up in the pocket, requiring lower muscle inferior pull following its release. This lower pole coverage situation is best achieved by suturing of the ADM along the entire length of the lower pectoral border, draping it over the implant inferiorly, and securing it (under more taughtness) at or near the IMF. This application is similar to

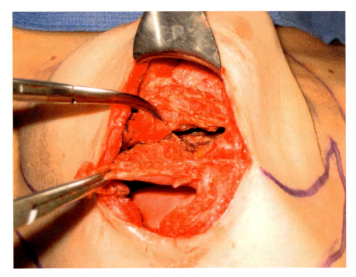

Fig. 17.2 "Lamellar" separation (dissecting the pectoralis muscle from its superficial and deep scarred attachments).

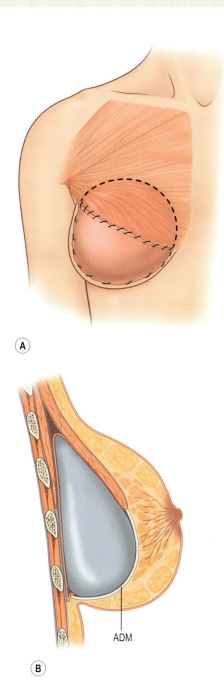

(A)

(B)

ADM

Fig. 17.3 When there is lamellar scarring requiring lamellar separation, the remaining pectoralis muscle may be "window shaded" up in the pocket, requiring lower muscle inferior pull following its release. This lower pole coverage situation is best achieved by suturing of the acellular dermal matrix (ADM) along the entire length of the lower pectoral border, draping it over the implant inferiorly, and securing it (under more taughtness) at or near the IMF. This application is similar to the "reconstructive model", as a "pectoral muscle extension".

the "reconstructive model", as a "pectoral muscle extension" (Fig. 17.3). In all instances, adequate environment, cover, and stability over the non-muscle covered portion of the implant (lower pole) by the ADM allows the skin envelope to be safely lifted and tightened (mastopexy), assuming adequate respect for the vascularity to the redraped tissue, as well as compliance with all sound surgical principles (Figs. 17.4–17.6).

With regard to the biomechanical properties of the desired ADM, rapid revascularization is required to provide conformability of the ADM and to redrape over the surface of the implant (with intimate engagement of surface contours). If the patient had capsular contracture, a more elastic material may be desired. If the patient had more laxity or stretch deformity, less elastic material might be preferable.

Implant stabilizer

ADM allows for the surgeon to gain enhanced control in maintaining the implant position in a newly created "neo" pocket or for re-enforcement after capsulorrhaphy in various forms of implant malposition correction. Inferior malposition (double bubble), medial malposition (symmastia), or lateral malposition are generally treated by capsulorrhaphy or site change (the author's preference and recommendation). In a certain percentage of patients, the tissue is strong enough to support this correction with a new pocket and appropriate suturing alone. A number of these patients, however, will have thin tissue, previous scarring, or problematic bony contour slopes, such that re-enforcement of the site change (i.e., neopectoral pocket of appropriate dimensions in the correct location with old pocket obliteration) with ADM is highly advised to re-enforce or buttress the corrected implant position (Figs. 17.6–17.8). These materials are sutured in the appropriate position with proper purchase to achieve support. The biomechanical properties of the ADM for this indication are strength and taughtness to maintain implant stabilization.

Tissue thickener

This concept is an extension of second stage breast reconstruction where expander to implant conversion is facilitated by a superomedial placement of an extra-thick ADM, to enhance soft tissue cover of the implant and give a better visual and palpable confluence of chest to breast form.[44] In aesthetic revisions this is also most frequently applied to the upper pole (or superomedial area) to thicken tissue, minimize visibility of traction rippling, camouflage implant edges, and enhance cleavage. An extra thick allograft material is generally utilized and appropriately trimmed. It is draped over the implant (with intimate engagement on its deep surface) and in contact with the existing capsule or new/neopocket on its superficial surface. Parachute 2-0 Prolene sutures with Keith needles are utilized in the ADM corners and interspersed on the medial side to facilitate placement and redraping. The suture ends are tied externally, under no tension, and covered with a Tegaderm for 7–10

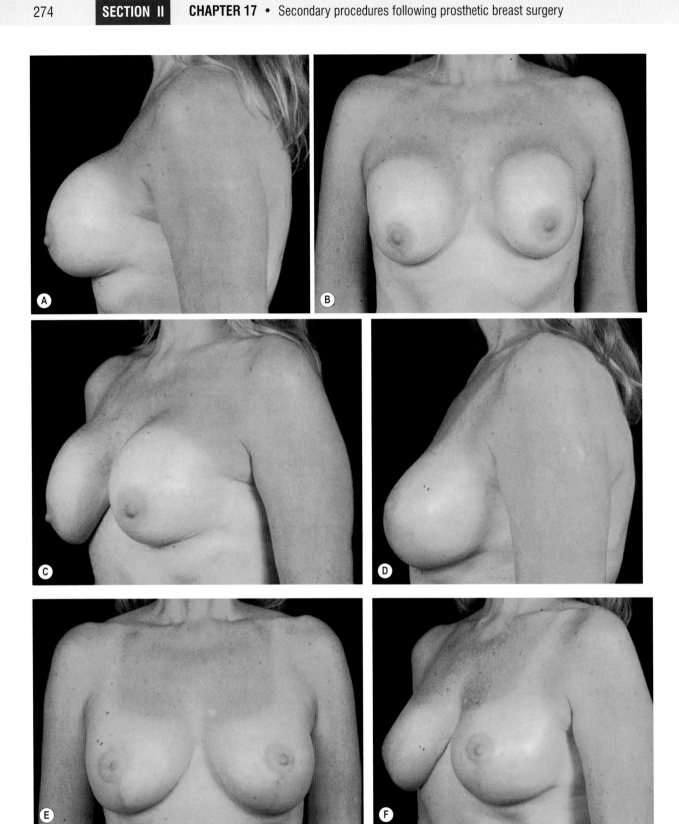

Fig. 17.4 (**A–C**) Preoperative views of a 37-year-old woman after breast augmentation. (**D–F**) Thirty-two months after revision augmentation mastopexy (inverted T), which included the development of a neopectoral pocket, lower pole coverage with acellular dermal matrix and replacement of implants with form stable, highly cohesive gel anatomic implants.

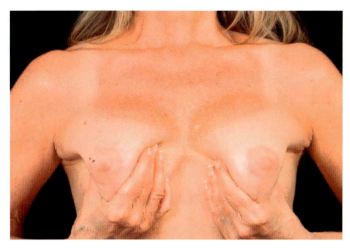

Fig. 17.5 Patient as seen in Fig. 17.4 demonstrating the softness of the implants 32 months following the treatment of her capsular contracture and ptosis.

The ADM should be conformed to, and in intimate contact with, the outer surface of the implant (like a hand in a glove). The appropriate pocket is created whether it is neopectoral, subpectoral, or subfascial.[8,11] Three to five half-mattress stabilizing "parachute" sutures are placed between the skin and the ADM to stabilize the tissue and place it in the desired location. Sizes selected are normally in the 6–8×10–16 cm range (depending on size of implant), rectangle or "contour" shapes, and trimmed as needed. Seroma formation should be prevented in all breast revisions in order to increase revascularization and cellular repopulation of the ADM, so drains are always recommended.

days. This same application is occasionally used laterally or inferolaterally for implant visibility or palpability, and inferiorly to "thicken" a very thin cutaneous cover (Figs. 17.7 & 17.8). The key to success is proper pocket alteration with incorporation of the extra thick ADM providing bulk, and including revascularization and cellular repopulation.

Treatment of capsular contracture

Even though the presenting problem may be capsular contracture, additional deformities may be identified following detailed analysis from the skin envelope to the chest wall, as noted above. This can include thinned tissue over an encapsulated implant, malposition of the encapsulated implant, or stretched deformity, snoopy, or ptosis over an encapsulated implant. If the encapsulation is in the subglandular position, a total capsulectomy with site change to the subpectoral position is usually performed. If the encapsulation is in the subpectoral position, a neopectoral pocket with partial anterior capsule excision and residual capsule obliteration, or total (perhaps partial) capsulectomy is performed. In these cases the ADM is again selected for rapid revascularization, conformability to the implant, and performance. The technique is most frequently similar to the "lower pole cover" concept, but may be closer to a "medial thickener", or "malposition reinforcer" dependent upon the presenting problem (Figs. 17.9 & 17.10). There is an increasing body of documentation that the coupling of the ADM to the implant will further reduce the incidence of capsular contracture.[13,25] If capsular contracture is the only clinical diagnosis, then we recommend a placement of the ADM at the lower or middle poles.

The surgical techniques used are based on the preoperative findings and the indications as described above.

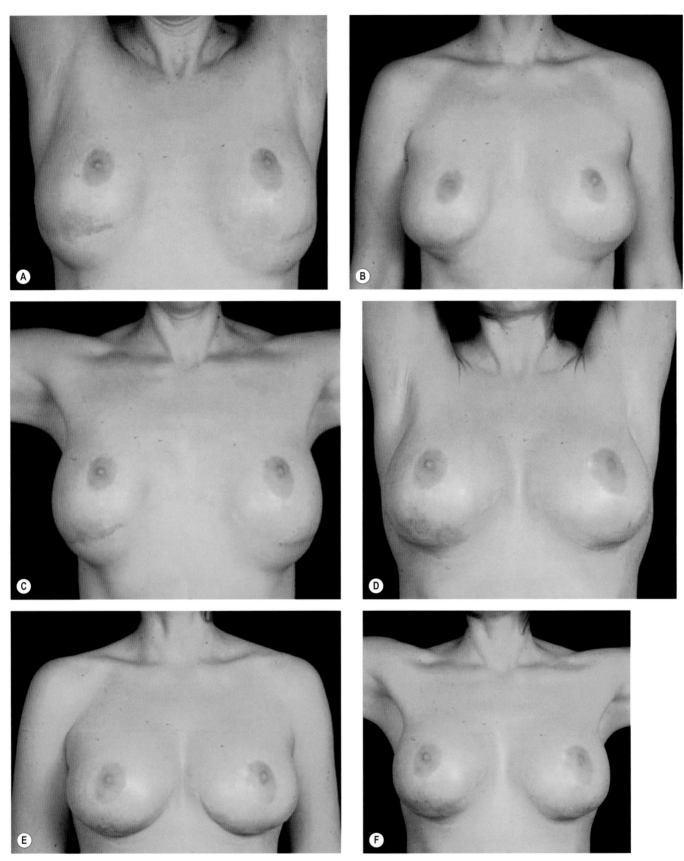

Fig. 17.6 (A–C) Preoperative views of a 49-year-old woman after augmentation mastopexy. **(D–F)** Thirty months after revision augmentation mastopexy (inverted T) that included the development of a neopectoral pocket, lower pole coverage and reinforcement of inferior and lateral walls with acellular dermal matrix (ADM), and replacement of implants form stable, highly cohesive gel anatomic implants. Successful correction of inferior and lateral malposition was achieved.

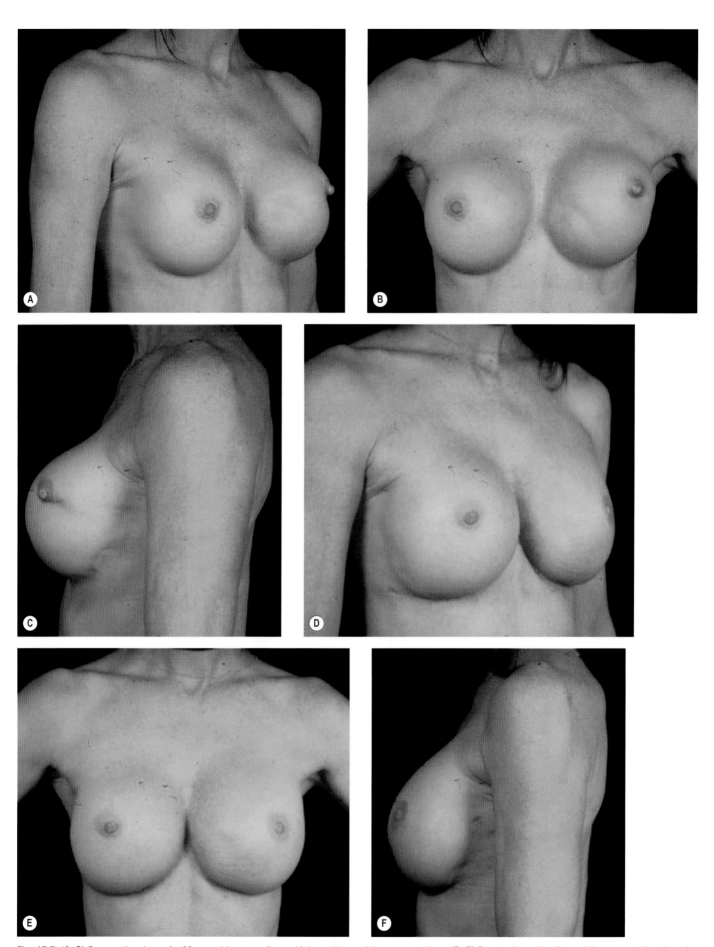

Fig. 17.7 **(A–C)** Preoperative views of a 38-year-old woman after multiple previous revision augmentations. **(D–F)** Twenty-six months after revision augmentation through IMF incision, which included the development of neopectoral pocket, lamellar separation, lower pole coverage with acellular dermal matrix, and replacement of implants with textured gel implants.

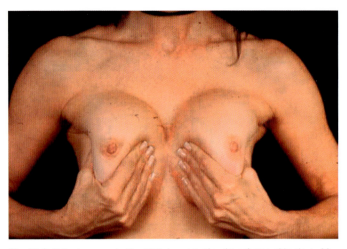

Fig. 17.8 Patient as seen in Fig. 17.7 demonstrating the softness of implants 26 months following the treatment of her implant malposition, lamellar scarring, and tissue thinning.

Outcomes, prognosis, and complications

Breast augmentation is the most common aesthetic procedure performed in the US and perhaps in the world.[45] It is in the nature of plastic surgeons to strive for perfection and continue to improve surgical techniques to achieve the best aesthetic form. Despite advances in implant technology and surgical techniques, undesired outcomes are encountered leading to revisionary surgeries. In preparing for a revisionary breast augmentation, one must understand patients' goals and expectations and evaluate the probability of their accomplishment, as well as the risk/benefit ratio. When a decision is made to move forward, the goal should be to plan and execute the most precise and efficient surgical correction. To achieve this goal, one must understand the problem(s) and variables involved and then look for new solutions.

In the past our options were limited to working with only the native tissues available to us for these procedures. With the advent of ADM, the indications and the

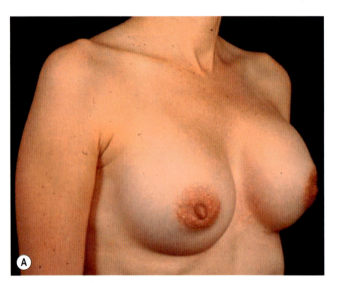

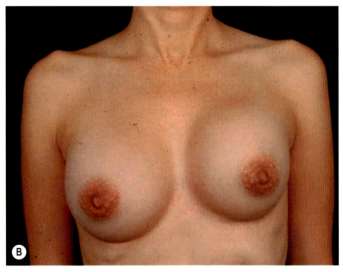

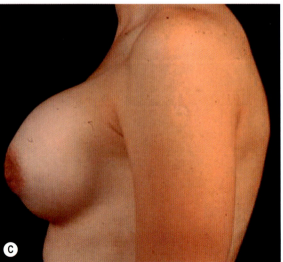

Fig. 17.9 (A–C) Preoperative views of a 45-year-old woman after multiple previous attempts at correction of capsular contracture.

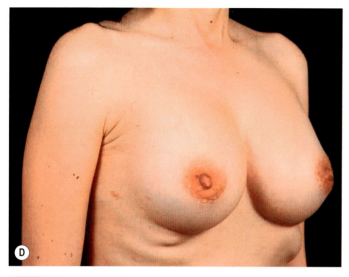

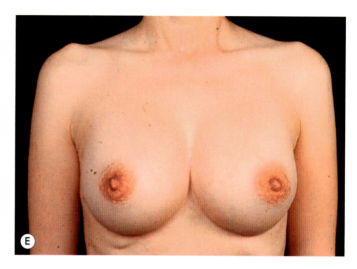

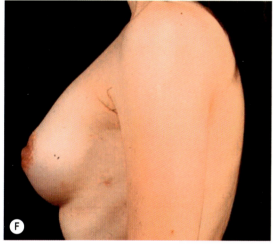

Fig. 17.9, cont'd (D–F) Twenty-two months after revision augmentation through IMF incision, which included the development of neopectoral pocket, lower pole coverage with acellular dermal matrix, and replacement of implants with higher profile, lower-volume textured gel implants.

spectrum of correcting secondary deformities has improved.

The use of acellular dermal products has been popularized in both breast and abdominal wall reconstructions.[14–24] In reconstruction cases, ADMs have been used to replace tissue, extend existing tissue, or act as a supplement. In aesthetic revisions, the ADM essentially becomes an outer conforming, regenerative layer around the implant. They have been used to correct implant rippling and displacement, ptosis, and capsular contracture.[26,27,37] ADMs are used as an alternative to other autologous tissue methods of coverage and provide camouflage, thus decreasing rippling and increasing soft-tissue padding.[28] In addition to all the indications described previously, we have also used ADMs as a mode of treatment for capsular contracture.[25] Breast capsular contracture is similar to lamellar scarring in the eyelids. At the cellular level, capsular contracture is most likely caused by any process that produces increased inflammation, which in turn leads to the formation of deleterious cytokines within the periprosthetic pocket. Consequently, in addition to the

many techniques described for treating and preventing capsular contracture,[4,5,8,30–36] we believe that the addition of ADM is another modality in fighting the evolution of the capsule. An ADM can counteract the inflammatory process, adding more tissue ingrowth

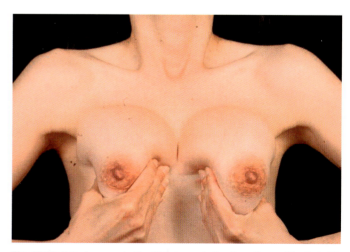

Fig. 17.10 Patient as seen in Fig. 17.9 demonstrating the softness of implants 22 months following the treatment of her capsular contracture.

availability and controlling the interface of the pocket by providing a regenerative layer between device and native tissue.

The rising demand for the use of ADM, coupled with good outcomes in breast reconstructions, has spurred tremendous interest in its use for aesthetic breast surgery patients. In the past, revisionary surgeries were generally performed with a total capsulectomy, removal of the implant from the subglandular plane, and placement of a new implant in the subpectoral position.[5,8,10] This is a fairly simple procedure, involving a change in implant placement from over the muscle to under the muscle. More recently, it has become necessary to perform revisionary surgery on volume-depleted or severely scarred breasts. In correcting these deformities as described in the indication section, in addition to the site change operation, ADMs can provide additional coverage where the repair is performed.

The recent published series of 197 consecutive patients who underwent revisionary breast augmentation/mastopexies with acellular dermal matrices was one of the largest series to date to address the use of ADM in revisionary aesthetic breast surgery.[46] Reasons for revision included capsular contracture (61.8%), implant malposition (31.2%), rippling (4.8%), ptosis (4.8%), implant exposure (1.6%), and breast wound (0.5%). The mean follow-up period was 3.1±1.1 years (range: 0.1–6.1 years). The complication rate was 4.8% including Baker grade III/IV capsular contracture (1.6%), infection (1.6%), implant malposition (0.5%), hematoma (0.5%), and seroma (0.5%). Ninety-eight percent of revisions were successful with no recurrence of the presenting complaint.

A challenge that plastic surgeons continue to face in aesthetic revisionary surgery is the cost of these products and their affordability by the patient. On the other hand, the biggest possible cost of performing a revisionary surgical procedure (to patient and surgeon alike) is the need to perform another surgical revision due to failure of the planned procedure. No doubt the coming years will be exciting as we further define the issues, advance the science, and increase our understanding via evidence-based medicine, for the benefit of our patient population.

🌐 Access the complete reference list online at **http://www.expertconsult.com**

2. Spear SL, Murphy DK, Slicton A, Walker PS. Inamed silicone breast implant core study results at 6 years. *Plast Reconstr Surg.* 2007;120(7 suppl 1):8S–16S, discussion 7S–8S. *The authors provide an update on the postapproval study for Allergan Corporation. The study demonstrates the safety and effectiveness of Natrelle (formerly Inamed) silicone-filled breast implants over 6 years, including a low rupture and high satisfaction rate.*

3. Cunningham B, McCue J. Safety and effectiveness of Mentor's MemoryGel implants at 6 years. *Aesthetic Plast Surg.* 2009;33(3):440–444. *The authors provide an update on the postapproval study for Mentor Corporation. The study shows that Mentor MemoryGel Silicone Breast Implants represent a safe and effective choice for women seeking breast augmentation or breast reconstruction following mastectomy.*

4. Adams WP Jr, Rios JL, Smith SJ. Enhancing patient outcomes in aesthetic and reconstructive breast surgery using triple antibiotic breast irrigation: six-year prospective clinical study. *Plast Reconstr Surg.* 2006;117(1):30–36. *The authors show the clinical importance for the use of triple antibiotic breast irrigation. This study shows the lower incidence of capsular contracture, compared with other published reports, and its clinical efficacy supports previously published in vitro studies. Application of triple antibiotic irrigation is recommended for all aesthetic and reconstructive breast procedures and is cost effective.*

8. Maxwell GP, Gabriel A. The neopectoral pocket in revisionary breast surgery. *Aesthet Surg J.* 2008;28(4):463–467. *The authors describe in detail (and with multiple illustrations) the operative technique for the creation of the neopectoral pocket.*

13. Maxwell GP, Gabriel A. Use of the acellular dermal matrix in revisionary aesthetic breast surgery. *Aesthet Surg J.* 2009;29(6):485–493. *The authors show the largest acellular dermal matrix (ADM) based revisionary surgeries, including both revisionary augmentation and revision of augmentation mastopexy. This series shows that the ADM can be used both safely and effectively in revisionary cases, resulting in decreased rates of capsular contracture and implant cushioning/stabilization.*

14. Bindingnavele V, Gaon M, Ota KS, et al. Use of acellular cadaveric dermis and tissue expansion in postmastectomy breast reconstruction. *J Plast Reconstr Aesthet Surg.* 2007;60(11):1214–1218.

23. Salzberg CA. Nonexpansive immediate breast reconstruction using human acellular tissue matrix graft (AlloDerm). *Ann Plast Surg.* 2006;57(1):1–5.

24. Spear SL, Parikh PM, Reisin E, Menon NG. Acellular dermis-assisted breast reconstruction. *Aesthetic Plast Surg.* 2008;32(3):418–425.

26. Duncan DI. Correction of implant rippling using allograft dermis. *Aesthet Surg J.* 2001;21(1):81–84.

43. Harper JR, McQuillan DJ. A novel regenerative tissue matrix (RTM) technology for connective tissue reconstruction. *Wounds.* 2007;2007(6):20–24.

18

The pedicled TRAM flap

Julian J. Pribaz and Simon G. Talbot

SYNOPSIS

- The pedicled transverse rectus abdominis myocutaneous (TRAM) flap is a consistent, predictable, and expeditious method of autologous breast reconstruction.
- The pedicled TRAM flap was introduced by Dr. Carl Hartrampf[1,2] in the 1980s and remains one of the most commonly used autologous methods of breast reconstruction today.
- The rectus abdominis muscle is a Mathes and Nahai type III muscle,[3] and the pedicled TRAM flap relies on the superior epigastric vessels and its terminal branches.
- The key contraindication to a pedicled TRAM flap is injury or absence of the vascular pedicle (for example, after open cholecystectomy).
- Many variations on this flap (for example, double pedicled flaps, supercharged flaps, and delay procedures) make this flap versatile and reliable.

Access the Historical Perspective section online at
http://www.expertconsult.com

Introduction

The goal of all breast reconstruction is to create a natural and aesthetically pleasing breast that is stable, long-lasting, with good symmetry to the opposite side. This can be most consistently and predictably achieved by using autologous tissue to perform the reconstruction. Of course, this entails more complex surgery, additional scars, and a longer recovery time than implant-based reconstruction, but in the long run these are often worthy trade-offs. Autologous breast reconstruction can be achieved with pedicled or free flaps, and these flaps can be used for many purposes other than breast reconstruction. However, the focus of this chapter will be on the use of the pedicled TRAM flap in breast reconstruction.

The pedicled TRAM flap remains a commonly used method of autologous breast reconstruction in the United States.

Careful patient selection is very important. The patient must be healthy enough to undergo an approximately 3-hour operation, have suitable anatomy, minimal comorbidities, and be aware of the 6–8 weeks needed for recovery.

Basic science/anatomy

The TRAM flap consists of a transverse island of abdominal skin and fat that is supplied by periumbilical perforators that are the terminal branches of the superior epigastric vascular pedicle. This arises from the internal thoracic artery and veins (also known as the internal mammary artery and veins). The superior epigastric artery and its venae comitantes course along the deep aspect of the rectus muscles and send perforators from posteriorly through the muscle just medial to the linea semilunaris and in the periumbilical area and connect with the terminal branches of the larger, deep inferior epigastric vessels, upon which free TRAM flaps and DIEP flaps are based (also used in breast reconstruction and described in other chapters). Multiple minor pedicles comprising the intercostal arteries and venae comitantes, supplied by the thoracic aorta and vena cava, contribute to the muscle perfusion, and may be preserved superiorly in the dissection. The rectus abdominis muscle is a Mathes and Nahai type III muscle.[3]

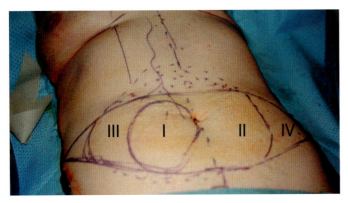

Fig. 18.1 Vascular zones (I, II, III, IV) of right sided transverse rectus abdominis myocutaneous flap.

Motor and sensory innervation to the flap are from the seventh through twelfth intercostal nerves; however, these are cut during flap dissection.

The TRAM flap is a very large flap, and an attempt has been made to quantify the vascularity of different parts of this flap. The skin island has been subdivided into four perfusion zones, with the number previously thought to reflect the degree of vascularity to the overlying skin and fat. Zone 1 overlies the rectus muscle, zone 2 overlies the contralateral muscle, zone 3 is lateral to the ipsilateral muscle, and zone 4 is lateral to the contralateral rectus muscle (Fig. 18.1).[8,9]

The best perfused area of the flap is in zone 1, directly over the perforators. Initially, it was thought that zone 2 over the contralateral muscle was next best perfused, but it has been shown that zone 3, lateral to zone 1 on the ipsilateral side, has better perfusion. The least perfused part is zone 4 on the contralateral lateral aspect.[10]

It is best to only use the best-perfused part of the flap for reconstruction to avoid fat necrosis: zone 1 and the adjacent parts of zone 3 and 2, depending on the volume of tissue required.

Ipsilateral versus contralateral TRAM

Although either can lead to a successful reconstruction, an ipsilateral flap is preferred, as this transfers zone 3 superiorly, which is better perfused than zone 2, which would be transferred superiorly if a contralateral flap is used. Use of an ipsilateral flap also helps to maintain the inframammary fold, a xiphoid hollow, and confers a potentially lower rate of fat necrosis.[11] However, prior abdominal scars may necessitate the use of a contralateral flap (Fig. 18.2).

Surface markings (Figs. 18.3 & 18.4)

The following markings are made preoperatively in a standing position for reference and to aid the mastectomy surgeon(s):

1. midline of chest and abdomen (including sternal notch reference point)
2. periareolar incision(s) with lateral extension
3. bilateral inframammary folds
4. limits of the breast mounds.

The flap design and markings are made intraoperatively after assessment of the mastectomy defect and skin island requirements:

1. costal margins as a guide where to stop upper flap elevation
2. abdominal flap incisions
   a. upper line approximately 2 cm above umbilicus to capture periumbilical perforators
   b. lower line assessed at where the upper abdominal flap will reach after the TRAM tissue is relocated and the patient is flexed
3. periumbilical incision for preservation of the umbilicus during dissection
4. expected location of the skin paddle(s) of abdominal skin when relocated to the chest to allow de-epithelialization of the flap(s) while remaining taut on the abdomen.

Diagnosis/patient presentation

The TRAM flap may be used for breast reconstruction stemming from almost any cause. Typically this is required after mastectomy for breast cancer. However, a multitude of other indications exist: partial mastectomy reconstruction, chest wall reconstruction, sternal reconstruction, congenital asymmetry reconstruction, etc.

The pedicled TRAM flap is a relatively large and very reliable flap that transfers the redundant soft tissue present in the mid and lower abdominal region to reconstruct a breast that has a very natural feel and shape and without the need for a prosthesis.

Breast reconstruction with a pedicled TRAM flap is expeditious and reliable with few complications at the recipient and donor sites if done properly.[12] The procedure can be performed either at the time of mastectomy (which is generally simpler) or secondarily in patients who prefer to have a delayed reconstruction (or patients who will need to have postoperative radiation as the effects of radiation to the flap itself are variable and unpredictable and may result in a suboptimal result). The authors typically wait at least 3–6 months after the completion of radiation and may leave a tissue expander as a "place-holder" while undergoing radiation to maintain breast contour and to make it possible to keep significantly more native breast skin. When this is undertaken, the pectoralis is typically elevated for insertion of a tissue expander, and replaced and re-suspended at the time of TRAM flap to prevent an animation deformity over the flap.

The main cited disadvantage of this procedure over alternative reconstructive options is that part of the rectus abdominus muscle is harvested with the flap, possibly resulting in abdominal wall weakness and a potentially increased incidence of an abdominal wall hernia. This will be discussed later in the chapter. Another cited disadvantage is that the pedicled TRAM flap has a less robust blood supply than the free TRAM flap or the DIEP flap, with a consequent increased incidence of fat necrosis. However, as described later in this chapter, if only the best-perfused parts of the flap are utilized, this has not been borne out to be a major problem in the authors' experience.

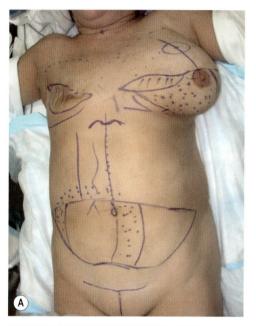

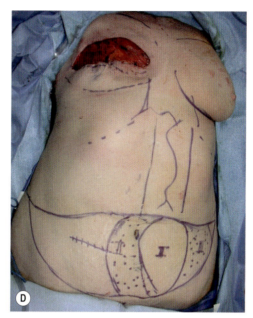

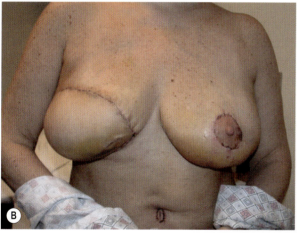

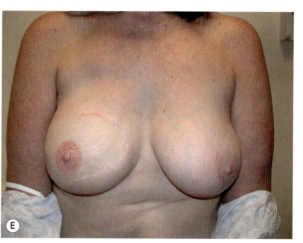

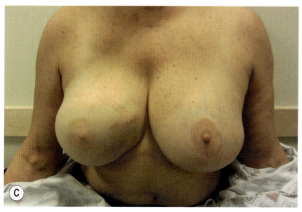

Fig. 18.2 Typical intra- and postoperative results of delayed ipsilateral and contralateral reconstructions. **(A–C)** Ipsilateral pedicled transverse rectus abdominis myocutaneous (TRAM) flap reconstruction. **(D,E)** Contralateral pedicled TRAM flap reconstruction.

Continued

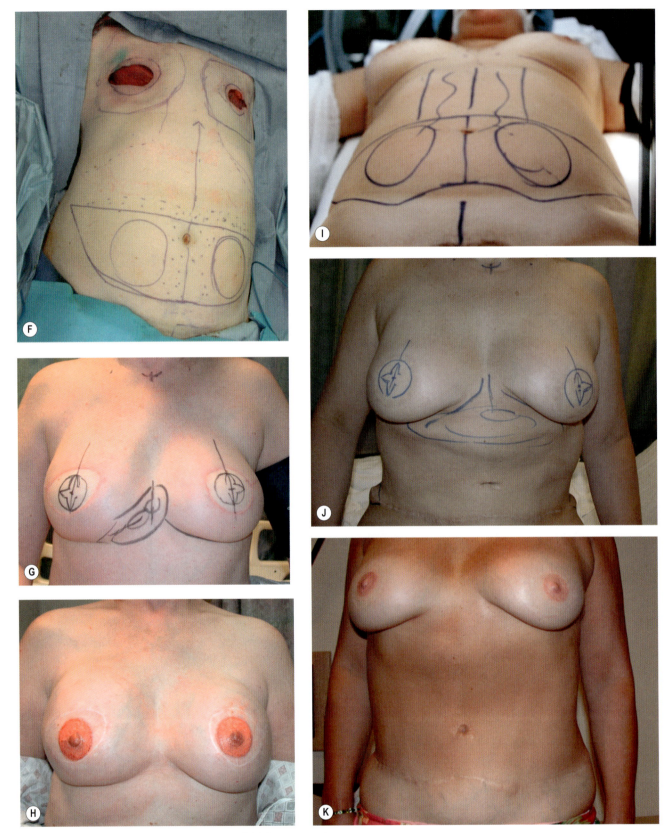

Fig. 18.2, cont'd (F–L) Bilateral immediate pedicled TRAM flap reconstructions.

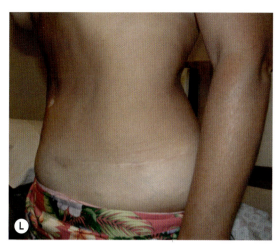

Fig. 18.2, cont'd

Patient selection

The primary goals of breast reconstruction include construction of a natural-appearing breast with contralateral symmetry, safely, with stability over time. An acceptable (or even improved) donor site is important.

Patient selection and operative planning should take into account the size and shape of the breast, plans for contralateral surgery (in unilateral cases), cancer stage and need for radiation, appearance of the abdomen, prior abdominal operations, general health of the patient, as well as lifestyle, goals, and expectations. These help in the decision-making between implant versus autologous techniques and the variety of autologous techniques available.

Most women are eligible for this method of breast reconstruction. However, patients with serious medical problems, psychiatric disorders, morbid obesity, and patients who continue to smoke heavily are not good candidates for this form of reconstruction.

Patients may not be candidates if they have insufficient abdominal tissue to create an adequate mound. However, thin patients typically also have relatively small breasts requiring less tissue for reconstruction, so this is only a relative contraindication.

The pedicled TRAM is contraindicated in patients with an extensively scarred abdomen. It is also contraindicated in patients with severe chronic back pain and patients with significant fibromyalgia symptoms.

An increasing number of patients who have had prior implant-based reconstruction are being referred for conversion to autologous reconstruction, and the pedicled TRAM flap is an excellent option.

Younger women still in their childbearing years, unfortunately, are also commonly referred for reconstruction after mastectomy, and they are concerned about the effects of the abdominal surgery on a successful vaginal delivery. Successful pregnancies (including twins) with vaginal deliveries have been reported after TRAM flap surgery.

Treatment/surgical technique

The steps involved are demonstrated for both a unilateral (see Fig. 18.3) and bilateral (see Fig. 18.4) breast reconstruction.

The umbilicus is first incised and dissected down to the abdominal wall. Although optional, we prefer to de-epithelialize the parts of the TRAM flap(s) that will later be buried under the mastectomy skin flap(s), leaving sufficient intact skin to allow for adjustment at the time of inset. It is easier to de-epithelialize while the flaps remain taut on the abdomen, but it is fine to do this later.

The skin island is then incised (beveling superiorly towards the deep fascia to capture as many perforators as possible) and dissected down to the abdominal wall. The abdominal wall is then dissected superiorly to the epigastric area and connected with the mastectomy site in the midline, leaving as much of the medial aspect of the inframammary fold intact as possible. Preserve the intercostal perforators to this upper abdominal skin flap by not extending the dissection above the costal margins laterally. Ensure an adequate width tunnel exists through which to pass the pedicle(s) into the breast pocket(s) – approximately large enough to pass a fist through. This tunnel should not be excessive, as it can distort the inframammary fold.

The lateral aspect of the TRAM flap is elevated off the underlying muscles to the lateral aspect of the anterior rectus sheath, where the lateral row of periumbilical perforators are seen. Medially, the flap is also elevated off the linea alba for approximately 1–2 cm. Any perforators visualized are preserved.

The fascia is then incised down to the muscle. Superiorly, a 2.5 cm strip of fascia is maintained along the length of the muscle in the central aspect of the muscle. This protects any vessels immediately beneath and also facilitates a more expeditious flap harvest.

The muscle is then separated from the fascia medially and laterally. Laterally, the multiple intercostal neurovascular pedicles are cauterized and divided. The muscle is divided at approximately the level of the arcuate line, and the inferior epigastric vessels are also ligated and divided. The flap is now developed as a superiorly based flap and dissected superiorly until the superior pedicle is visualized near the xiphoid process.

The flap is now ready to be introduced into the mastectomy pocket. To help with orienting the flap, it is marked with an arrow pointing laterally towards zone

Text continued on p. 290

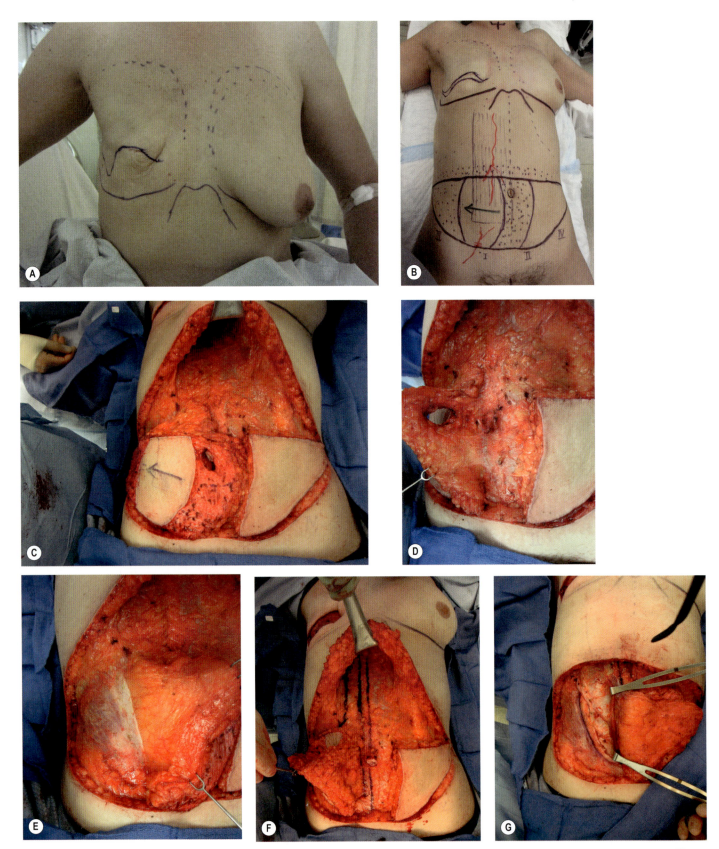

Fig. 18.3 Technique of unilateral ipsilateral transverse rectus abdominis myocutaneous flap reconstruction. **(A)** Preoperative markings. **(B)** Intraoperative markings. **(C)** Flap de-epithelialization and tunnel creation. **(D)** Medial flap elevation. **(E)** Lateral flap elevation. **(F)** Markings for anterior rectus sheath incisions. **(G)** Rectus muscle elevation. Note that these are of two patients (A,C,E and G are one patient; B,D, and F the other).

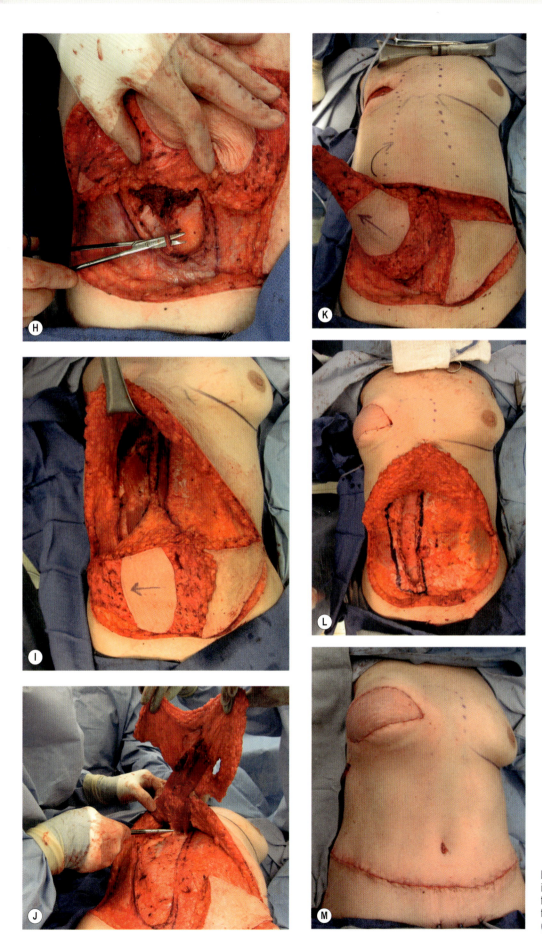

Fig. 18.3, cont'd **(H)** Division of deep inferior epigastric vessels. **(I)** Elevated flap. **(J)** Mobilization of the flap. **(K)** The flap is turned with zone 3 superiorly. **(L)** Flap insetting. **(M)** On-table result.

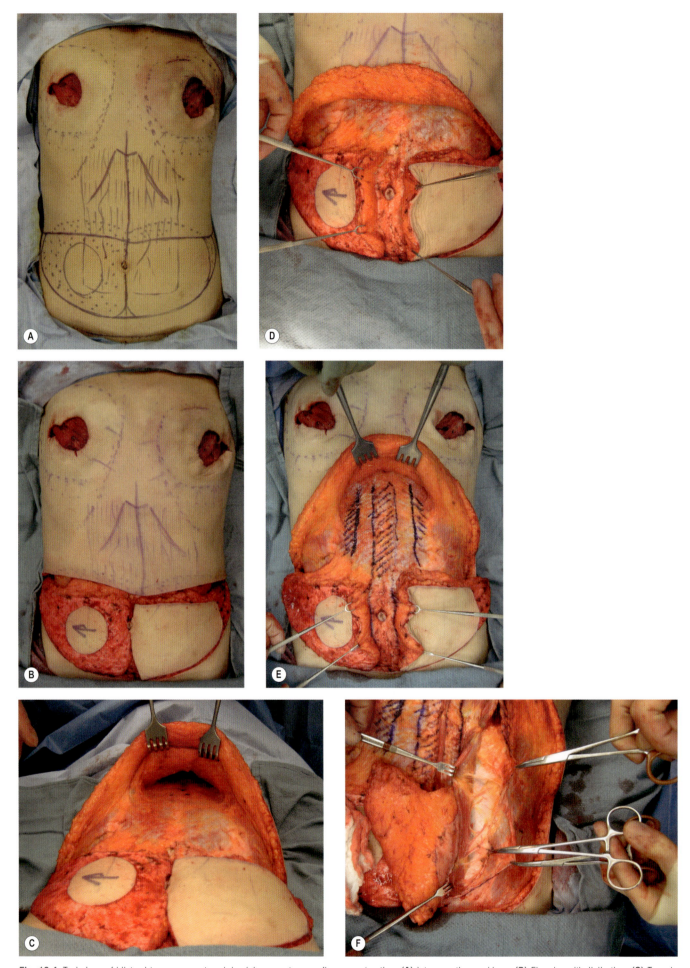

Fig. 18.4 Technique of bilateral transverse rectus abdominis myocutaneous flap reconstruction. **(A)** Intraoperative markings. **(B)** Flap de-epithelialization. **(C)** Tunnel creation. **(D)** Medial and lateral flap elevation. **(E)** Markings for anterior rectus sheath incisions. **(F)** Rectus muscle elevation.

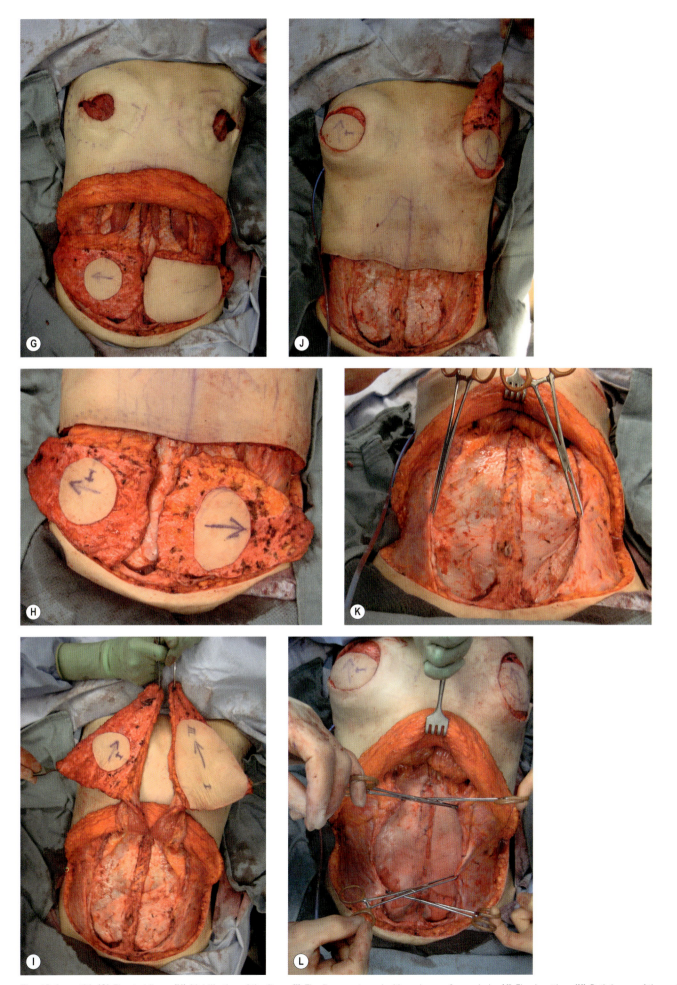

Fig. 18.4, cont'd **(G)** Elevated flaps. **(H)** Mobilization of the flaps. **(I)** The flaps are turned with each zone 3 superiorly. **(J)** Flap insetting. **(K)** Both leaves of the rectus sheath are included in the closure. **(L)** Mesh closure of the abdomen.

Continued

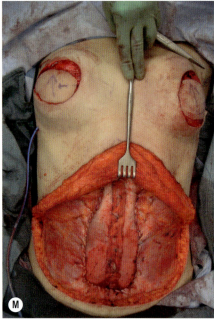

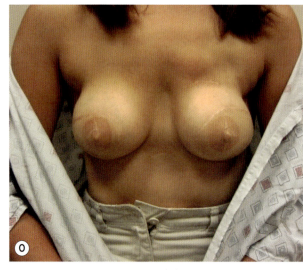

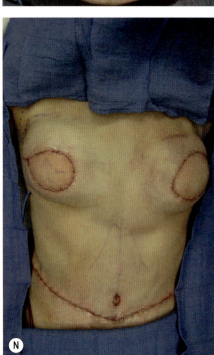

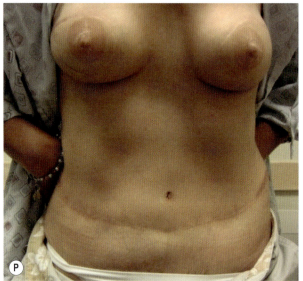

Fig. 18.4, cont'd (M) Completed mesh inset. **(N)** On-table result. **(O)** Final result after nipple creation and tattooing. **(P)** Final results of abdominal donor site.

3, and the flap is introduced into the breast cavity bringing zone 3 superiorly.

Preparation of mastectomy site and flap inset depends on the immediate or delayed nature of the reconstruction. In immediate breast reconstruction after mastectomy, not uncommonly the mastectomy pocket may have been resected beyond the aesthetic margins of the breast by the oncologic surgeon, and it is important to re-define the inframammary fold and the lateral aspect of the pocket. This is performed with multiple quilting sutures. A Blake suction drain is then inserted into the breast pocket along the inframammary fold and exits laterally and inferior to the fold. An additional drain into the axilla may be used, especially if an axillary node

dissection has been performed. In delayed reconstructions, the mastectomy defect must be recreated. It is often necessary to remove scarred skin from radiation.

The quality of the mastectomy skin flaps is also assessed, and if these appear ischemic, these are cut back to where healthy dermal bleeding is evident. The pedicled TRAM flap is now brought up from the abdomen and tunneled underneath the upper abdominal skin into the epigastric region and then introduced into the mastectomy pocket, bringing zone 3 superiorly. Twisting is not a problem if zone 3 is grasped and simply brought superiorly into the pocket. The flap will automatically orient itself into a satisfactory configuration. Ensure that the flap remains viable and non-congested despite being moved to the breast pocket. Additional widening of the tunnel or dissection to avoid tension or kinking of the pedicle may be required.

As mentioned, the ipsilateral flap is preferred, and in doing this transfer, for a right breast reconstruction, the flap rotates in a clockwise direction. On the left side, bringing zone 3 superiorly means that the flap rotates in an anti-clockwise direction. The final inset can then be performed. The use of an ipsilateral flap has the added benefit of producing less of a bulge in the epigastric area than a contralateral flap – although in both instances there is atrophy of the denervated muscle and the bulge diminishes with time.

Repair of TRAM donor site must be done with care to avoid the dreaded complication of hernias and bulges. All cases are best repaired with an inlay of a polypropylene mesh, which is fitted into the defect created by the muscle harvest, which is larger than the fascial defect. The mesh stretches in one direction only, and this stretch should be directed in a superior–inferior orientation to prevent bulging. The mesh is sutured with buried sutures to the linea alba in the midline and laterally to the conjoint fascia of the external and internal oblique within the anterior rectus sheath. A running polypropylene suture is then inserted advancing the fascia over the mesh, burying at least 50% of the mesh. This gives a very sound repair and has greatly reduced the incidence of bulging or hernia.

Finally, in order to close the skin, the patient is flexed at the hips. Quilting sutures are placed in the midline above the umbilicus between the linea alba and abdominal flap. In cases of bilateral TRAM flaps, the umbilicus is brought through a hole in the spanning mesh. Next, a vertical ellipse is excised in the abdominal skin overlying the umbilicus, together with some thinning of fat, and the umbilicus is brought to the surface.

The abdominal incisions are closed with interrupted and running 2-0 braided absorbable and 3-0 monofilament absorbable sutures and a running 5-0 chromic gut is used around the umbilicus. Typically three drains are inserted into the abdominal donor site.

Bilateral mastectomies are becoming increasingly common, and it is possible to safely perform bilateral TRAM flap reconstructions in these patients. This can only be done concurrently, as if only doing a single TRAM, the contralateral tissue is discarded and cannot be used subsequently. Each breast is reconstructed with the ipsilateral TRAM flap, which is dissected in the same manner as described above. In repairing the abdominal wall, a larger single piece of mesh is used to span the gap left by the bilateral muscle harvest. The mesh is sutured to the linea alba centrally and on each side to the fascia as described above, and again a running polypropylene suture on each lateral leaf of the rectus

fascia is advanced medially to cover a good part of the mesh. A hole is cut in the mesh over the umbilicus to allow it to be inset into its new location on the skin. Our experience has been very favorable with excellent outcomes and with minimal complications.

Modifications of TRAM flap reconstructions

Double pedicled TRAM flaps for single mastectomy reconstruction

In some cases where there is very large and/or ptotic opposite breast and the patient does not wish to have a reduction procedure, it may be necessary to utilize two flaps to achieve the necessary volume. In these cases, the ipsilateral flap is completely de-epithelialized and turned up first and the contralateral flap contains the skin island and it is stacked on top of the ipsilateral flap (Fig. 18.5).

Folded TRAM flap

Patients with a very large mastectomy or chest wall defect require a larger flap to adequately cover the defect that cannot be achieved with a single pedicle TRAM flap. Folding the flap expands the area that can be covered, and folding also produces a conical breast shape that enhances the reconstruction (Fig. 18.6).

Prior abdominal surgery

Prior abdominal surgery may necessitate modifications of the TRAM. For example, in cases where an open cholecystectomy has been performed and there is an existing scar, it is presumed that the rectus muscle and its blood supply has been transected, so the contralateral flap will be used to reconstruct the right mastectomy defect. Care must also be taken to avoid excessive undermining of the abdominal flap on the right to maintain vascularity of the abdominal skin which has lost the superior pedicle and associated perforators.

TRAM flap delay

In patients who potentially may have compromised vascularity and diminished perfusion of this flap, such as in the morbidly obese, smokers, or diabetic patients, a delay procedure can be performed whereby the inferior pedicle is exposed and ligated. In addition, the superficial epigastric vessels are also divided. This should be done two weeks or more prior to elevation of the flap (Fig. 18.7).

Modifications in flap design in obese patients or smokers

As an alternative to flap delay, the TRAM flap can be designed at a higher mid-abdominal level to capture more perforators from the superior epigastric vessels,

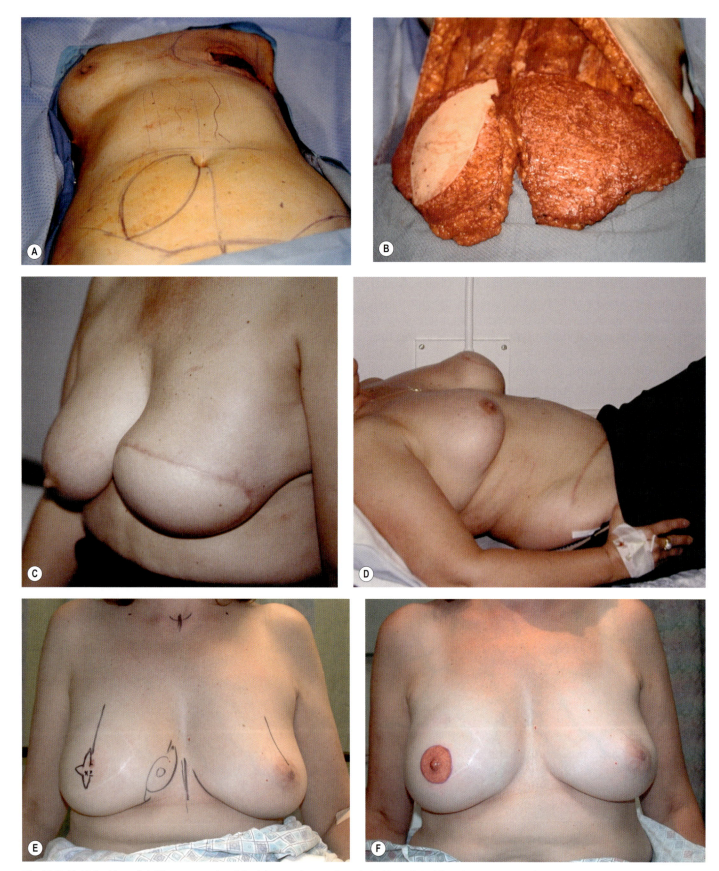

Fig. 18.5 (A–F) Double-pedicled transverse rectus abdominis myocutaneous flaps stacked for unilateral large breast reconstruction.

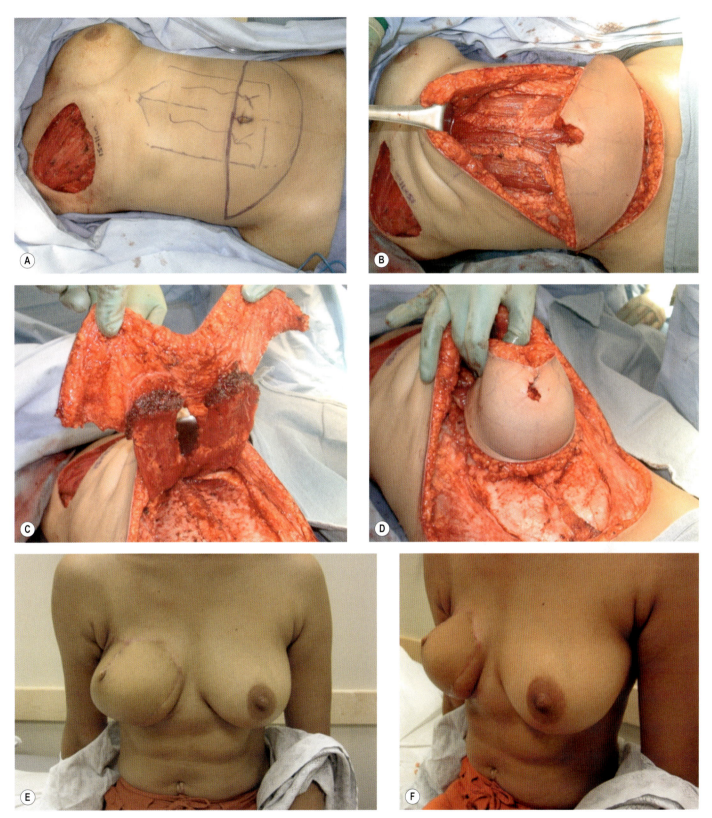

Fig. 18.6 (A–F) Folded bilateral pedicled transverse rectus abdominis myocutaneous flap to give volume and projection.

Continued

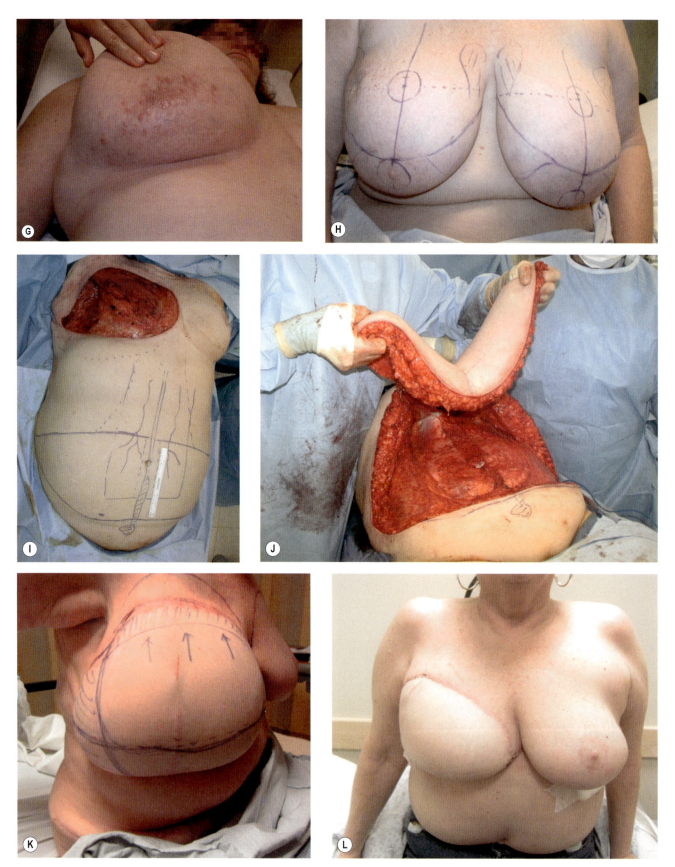

Fig. 18.6, cont'd   (G–M) In this patient a no-vertical-scar breast reduction was performed after breast lumpectomy and radiation following breast cancer. Post-operatively, angiosarcoma was diagnosed and a folded bilateral pedicled TRAM flap was performed with revisions shown here.

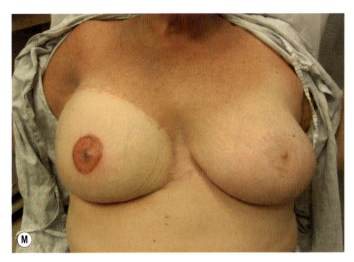

Fig. 18.6, cont'd

making the transfer safer, but the downside is that this results in a higher abdominal scar and a less aesthetic torso contour. This is only a relative disadvantage in very obese patients.

Secondary procedures

Secondary procedures, which include nipple and areolar reconstruction, revisions, and contralateral symmetry procedures, are performed once there has been adequate time for healing and settling of the initial reconstruction (Fig. 18.8). This is typically delayed for 4–6 months or until any adjunctive cancer related therapy is completed. Fat grafting has become a routine procedure especially to augment the deficient infraclavicular area and upper pole of the breast.

Hints and tips

1. Preoperatively, carefully select patients who will benefit from this procedure and who understand both the benefits and risks involved.
2. Address the opposite breast, as the goal is to obtain a symmetrical reconstruction. This may involve a breast reduction that can be safely done at the same time. The benefit is that less tissue is transferred with the TRAM flap, thus reducing the risks of fat necrosis. If the contralateral breast needs only a mastopexy, this is typically done secondarily.
3. Carefully assess the mastectomy site in the patients undergoing an immediate reconstruction. Firstly, the vascularity of the mastectomy flaps is assessed, and any compromised flaps are excised and adjustments made with a larger TRAM skin island. Also, the mastectomy pocket generally needs to be adjusted due to wide resection at the site of the inframammary fold and laterally.
4. In patients undergoing delayed reconstruction, the mastectomy scar is excised and the skin flaps are elevated off the pectoralis major muscle to recreate the mastectomy pocket. The skin below the mastectomy scar is usually excised down to the inframammary fold, as it is

generally too tight to accommodate the flap. Consequently, a TRAM flap with a larger skin island is required in delayed reconstruction.
5. Raise the pedicled TRAM flap as described above, and make a central subcutaneous tunnel that connects with the mastectomy site and which minimally encroaches into the inframammary fold of the side being reconstructed. Generally the tunnel is big enough to allow a hand to traverse, and thus the pedicled flap can be introduced into the cavity with minimal trauma. For safe passage through the tunnel, the TRAM flap should be pushed rather than pulled.
6. Zone 3 of the TRAM is brought superiorly and can be affixed with an absorbable suture.
7. It is helpful to make the TRAM flap slightly bigger than the opposite side, to allow for muscle atrophy. If it is still too large at the time of nipple-areolar reconstruction, it can be very simply liposuctioned to obtain symmetry.
8. A final assessment is made of the mastectomy flap vascularity, any tissue with dubious vascularity is excised, and the final de-epithelialization of the flap is performed and the inset completed. SPY technology (Novadaq, FL) may be helpful to evaluate compromised skin, if available.
9. The suturing of a thicker mastectomy flap to the edge of a de-epithelialized TRAM flap may lead to an uneven repair with an overriding of the mastectomy flap and relative depression of the TRAM flap. To avoid this, the use of a suturing technique that starts deep and takes a vertical mattress bite of the de-epithelialized side of the flap and a horizontal mattress of the surrounding mastectomy flap, results in a more even repair and better result.
10. Great care needs to be taken in repairing the abdominal wall using mesh as described above. The mesh is inlaid into the defect created by muscle harvest and attached to the conjoint tendon laterally and linea alba medially. The rectus fascia is then advanced with a running polypropylene suture, thereby covering up a significant part of the mesh and providing a strong repair. The mesh is used even if it is felt that the fascial defect can be closed primarily, as this provides a stronger repair, a reduced likelihood of hernia, and minimal displacement of the umbilicus. Care should be taken to ensure that the polypropylene mesh is inset with the direction of stretch in a vertical orientation and that the repair is not "too tight", as this can cause considerable discomfort postoperatively.
11. Drains are inserted at both the mastectomy site (usually one drain) and at the abdominal donor site (usually three drains—one on each lower abdomen and a central drain the helps drain the epigastric area).
12. The use of long-lasting local anesthesia agents delivered by an On-Q pump (I-Flow Corporation, CA) can help with postoperative pain.
13. Overall satisfaction: in the authors' unit, patients undergoing pedicled TRAM flap surgery (both unilateral and bilateral) tend to relate minimal interference with daily activities and report a satisfaction score of 8.3 out of 10, with most stating that they would have the surgery again.[13,14] Others, including Moscona et al.,[15] report that a total of 75% of women were satisfied with the operation, 73% declared high satisfaction, and only 12% were dissatisfied with the results. Also, Veiga et al.[16] similarly found a generic increase in health-related quality of life after TRAM breast reconstruction.

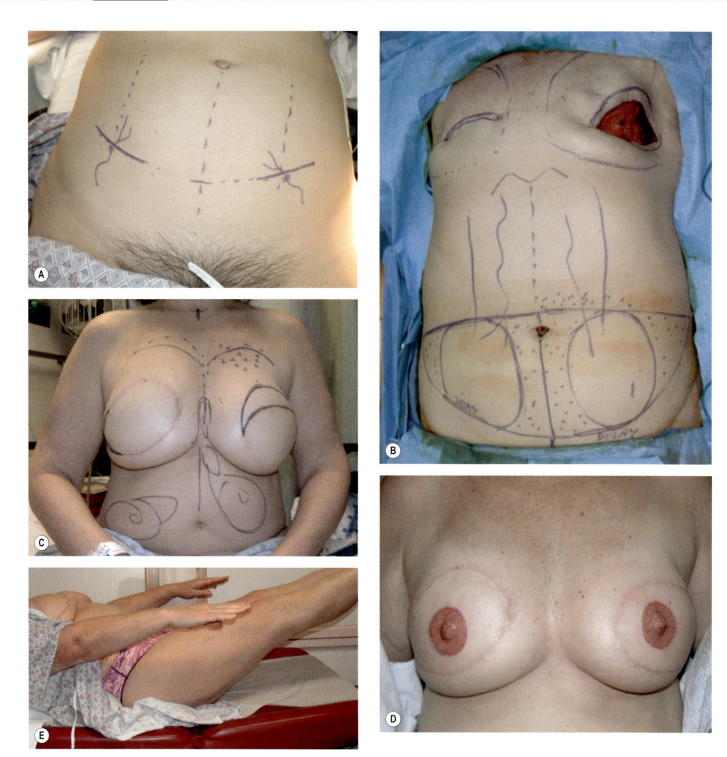

Fig. 18.7 (A) TRAM delay performed at time of first unilateral mastectomy (due to high probability for postoperative radiation). **(B,C,D)** Later contralateral mastectomy and bilateral delayed pedicled TRAM flaps were performed including revisions and nipple-areolar reconstruction. **(E)** Straight-leg raising is shown at 6 months postoperative.

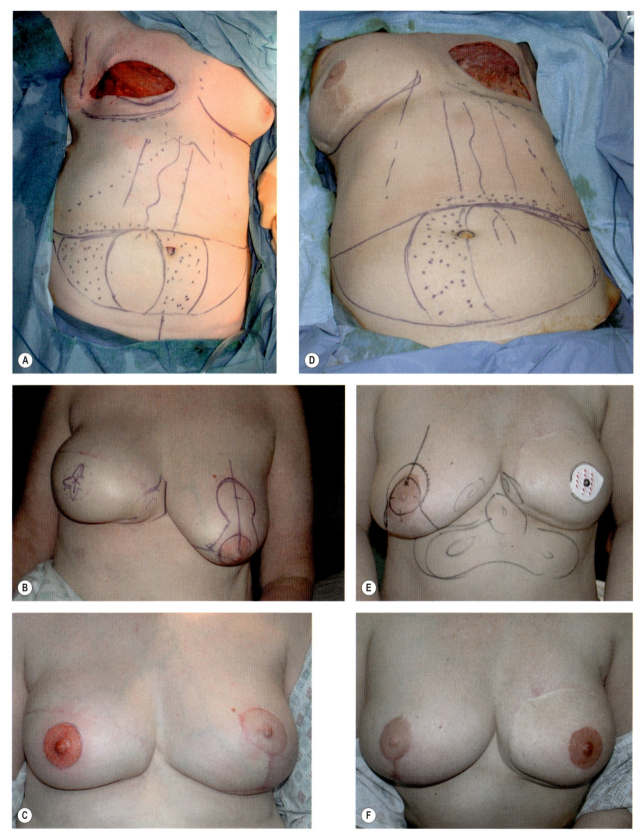

Fig. 18.8 Revision procedures. **(A–C)** Ipsilateral pedicled TRAM flap followed by nipple areolar reconstruction and contralateral mastopexy for symmetry. **(D–F)** Ipsilateral pedicled TRAM flap in a patient with a prior breast reduction (later revised at the time of nipple-areolar reconstruction).

Continued

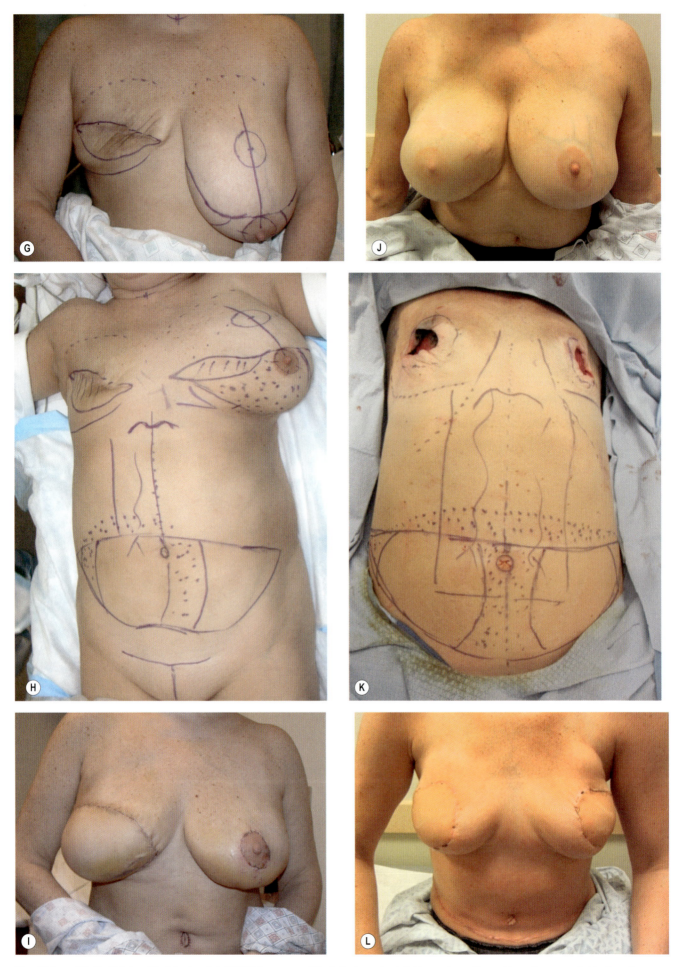

Fig. 18.8, cont'd (G–J) Delayed ipsilateral pedicled TRAM flap – more difficult due to contracted skin envelope with need to excise scar and skin above the inframammary fold; contralateral breast reduction at time of initial operation for symmetry. **(K–O)** Bilateral pedicled TRAM flaps with nipple-areolar reconstruction and fat grafting at 13 months; long-term appearance at 2.5 years postoperatively.

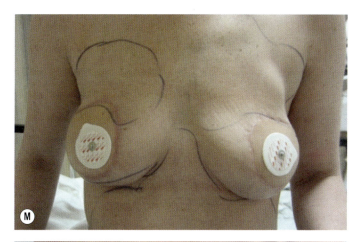

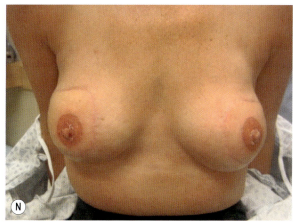

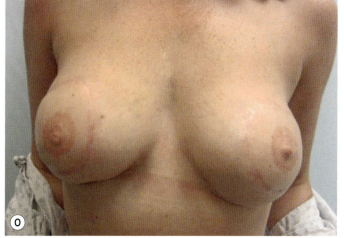

Fig. 18.8, cont'd

Postoperative care

After a pedicled TRAM flap procedure, patients are cared for on a regular floor. Typically, they remain in hospital for 3–5 days. They are treated with appropriate pain medication, which may include a PCA pump with transition to oral pain medications in 2–3 days. Additionally, the use of local anesthetic infusion products, such as the On-Q, can provide excellent postoperative pain control.

Patients receive DVT prophylaxis (compression boots during surgery and until fully ambulatory as well as subcutaneous heparin), and they are mobilized on the first postoperative day. They also remain on antibiotics whilst the drains are still in place, and they are instructed on drain output management in preparation for their discharge.

They are typically seen as outpatients one week later, at which time some (or all) of the drains are removed, if meeting criteria. The patients are reminded of the core strengthening exercises that were discussed and initiated at the initial consultation – namely to tighten their abdominal obliques and transversus muscles by "pulling in" their umbilicus. This improves their posture, exercises their core muscles, and hastens their recovery. These exercises can be safely and painlessly performed in the early postoperative period.

Outcomes, prognosis, complications

Complications may occur at either the recipient site or the donor site.

Recipient site

The most common complication in breast reconstruction is native chest flap necrosis. This can be minimized by initial debridement of compromised tissue. SPY technology can help determine viability of native skin.

Marginal fat necrosis may also occur. This usually involves only small areas that can be removed at the time of nipple-areolar reconstruction. Minor flap loss can also occur if a large flap extending into the distal parts of zone 2, 3 and 4 is used, but complete flap loss is extremely rare, and the authors have never seen this. There may be transient venous hypertension, which can be remedied with the insertion of a small angiocath into a distended peripheral vein or deep inferior epigastric venous pedicle and intermittent decompression of the venous hypertension is performed by withdrawing 1–2 cc of blood. This is not common, and the venous hypertension quickly equilibrates in the subsequent few hours. The angiocath can be safely removed the next morning.

The inframammary fold may also need to be revised. There may be an epigastric bulge medially from the muscle pedicle, most of which usually atrophies, and any residual fullness may be treated with liposuction of the overlying flap. The remaining inframammary fold may have been overdissected at the initial mastectomy and may need a formal repair and reconstruction.

At the time of nipple-areolar reconstruction, minor revisions to correct any asymmetries are usually required. There may be small areas of hardness due to fat necrosis that may need to be excised.[17] Structural fat grafting to upper infraclavicular areas or any other depressed areas are becoming routine to maximize aesthetic outcomes.

Procedures to the contralateral breast (reduction, mastopexy, etc.) may be required to obtain symmetry.

Donor site

Abdominal incision problems, when they occur, are usually minor wound issues that either heal secondarily or need minor revisions, such as with dog-ears. The drains are left in place until the output per 24 hours is less than 25 cc per drain. Premature drain removal can result in seroma formation.

Patients should be warned that full recovery will take several months, but typically patients are able to resume all activities of daily living that they were doing preoperatively.

Hernias are rare in the authors' experience, due to attention to detail with the repair.

Mesh infection is also extremely rare. Obese patients may experience some bulging despite mesh repair.[14,18,19]

Some patients complain of a sensation of tightness. This is typically transient and resolves in time. Care should be taken not to over-tighten the mesh repair initially.

General factors

Other factors that may contribute to an increased complication rate at both the recipient and donor sites include operating on patients who are obese, smokers, patients with multiple medical problems, psychosocial disorders, and the elderly. Surgeon inexperience can be a factor. Interestingly, complication rates do not appear to be elevated in bilateral versus unilateral TRAM flap reconstructions.[20–28]

Secondary procedures

The authors typically wait 3 months before further procedures to allow time for healing and reduced inflammation. Timeframes may be adjusted if radiation or chemotherapy is required until approximately 6 months post-radiation or until blood counts have returned to normal after chemotherapy.

Secondary procedures may include nipple-areolar reconstruction, resection of fat necrosis, structural fat grafting around the breast to improve contour deformities, and abdominal scar revisions. Nipple-areolar tattooing is then performed approximately 3 months following their creation.

🌐 Access the complete reference list online at   **http://www.expertconsult.com**

1. Hartrampf CR, Scheflan M, Black PW. Breast reconstruction with a transverse abdominal island flap. *Plast Reconstr Surg.* 1982;69: 216–225. *This paper details the early development of the TRAM flap by Dr. Hartrampf and colleagues and provides an excellent historical perspective.*

2. Scheflan M, Hartrampf CR, Black PW. Breast reconstruction with a transverse abdominal island flap. *Plast Reconstr Surg.* 1982;69:908–909. *This letter to the editor details some initial concerns with the TRAM flap and the article referenced in 1.*

3. Mathes SJ, Nahai F. *Reconstructive Surgery: Principles, Anatomy & Technique.* New York, St. Louis: Churchill Livingstone; Quality Medical Pub.; 1997. *Mathes and Nahai gives an clear and comprehensive description of the TRAM flap anatomy and classification.*

4. Millard DR Jr. Breast reconstruction after a radical mastectomy. *Plast Reconstr Surg.* 1976;58:283–291. *This paper is the first description of the use of lower abdominal tissue for reconstruction of a radical mastectomy defect.*

5. Holmstrom H. The free abdominoplasty flap and its use in breast reconstruction. An experimental study and clinical case report. *Scand J Plast Reconstr Surg.* 1979;13:423–427. *This paper details the first use of a "free abdominoplasty flap", later the free TRAM flap.*

6. Robbins TH. Post-mastectomy breast reconstruction using a rectus abdominis musculocutaneous island flap. *Br J Plast Surg.*

1981;34:286–290. *Prior to the pedicled TRAM, Robbins reported the pedicled vertical rectus abdominis flap – a further step towards the TRAM.*

7. Robbins TH. Breast reconstruction using a rectus abdominis musculocutaneous flap: 5 yr follow-up. *Aust N Z J Surg.* 1985;55:65–67. *The paper is a long-term follow-up of reference 6, showing the results of the pedicled VRAM flap.*

8. Scheflan M, Dinner MI. The transverse abdominal island flap: part I. Indications, contraindications, results, and complications. *Ann Plast Surg.* 1983;10:24–35. *These papers (references 8 and 9) show the early work of Scheflan and colleagues in reporting their experiences with the pedicled TRAM early in its development.*

9. Scheflan M, Dinner MI. The transverse abdominal island flap: Part II. Surgical technique. *Ann Plast Surg.* 1983;10:120–129. *These papers (references 8 and 9) show the early work of Scheflan and colleagues in reporting their experiences with the pedicled TRAM early in its development.*

16. Veiga DF, Sabino Neto M, Ferreira LM, et al. Quality of life outcomes after pedicled TRAM flap delayed breast reconstruction. *Br J Plast Surg.* 2004;57:252–257. *Any surgeon performing breast reconstruction should be familiar with the data regarding patient quality of life and satisfaction. This paper provides a broad overview of pedicled TRAM flap outcomes.*

19

Latissimus dorsi flap breast reconstruction

Michael S. Gart, John Y. S. Kim, and Neil A. Fine

Access video content for this chapter online at expertconsult.com

SYNOPSIS

- Latissimus dorsi flaps continue to play a significant role in primary and secondary reconstruction of total and partial mastectomy defects.
- Relative to other forms of autologous breast reconstruction, the latissimus flap is reliable, technically simpler, and associated with fewer and more modest short-term complications.
- The latissimus flap is an important salvage option following failed prosthetic or abdominal-based reconstruction.
- Surgical variations exist – including the extended and minimally-invasive latissimus flap – that allow the amount of autologous tissue to be tailored to the clinical situation.
- Complications at the flap donor site are generally minimal and limited mostly to seroma formation.
- The technical ease, favorable complication profile, and short operative/recovery times will ensure continued use of the latissimus flap in breast reconstruction.

 Access the Historical Perspective section online at
http://www.expertconsult.com

Introduction

The National Cancer Institute estimates nearly 232 000 women will be diagnosed with breast cancer in 2015, representing 14% of all new cancer diagnoses in the United States.[1] As the indications for external beam radiation therapy (XRT) and breast-conserving therapy (BCT) continue to expand, more women will require total or partial autologous tissue breast reconstruction. The latissimus dorsi flap is a powerful tool that can be applied to diverse oncologic defects of the breast, including partial mastectomy defects, autologous reconstruction of modified radical mastectomy defects, expander/

implant coverage prior to radiation therapy, and augmenting prosthetic reconstruction to improve symmetry. It is also important in treating radiation-induced complications and as a salvage flap for patients who have failed previous forms of reconstruction.

A critical advantage of the latissimus flap is that it does not require microsurgical techniques and can thereby afford patients faster recovery. Coupled with this relative technical ease is the modest frequency and magnitude of short-term complications.[2] Moreover, the latissimus flap is relatively resistant to the higher complications seen in obese patients undergoing prosthetic and abdominal-based reconstruction.[3,4]

Anatomy

The name "latissimus dorsi" is derived from the Latin *latus* (broad) and *dorsum* (back), literally translating to "the broadest [muscle] of the back". The latissimus is the most superficial and largest of the posterior trunk muscles, measuring approximately 25×35 cm (Fig. 19.1). It originates from the lower thoracic spine, the posterior iliac crest, and the thoracolumbar fascia, where it forms the roof of the superior lumbar triangle. The muscle fibers then converge toward the axilla, joining the teres minor to form the posterior axillary fold before inserting into the intertubercular groove of the humerus. The superior extent of the muscle overlies the tip of the scapula, and superomedially, the inferior trapezius muscle overlaps the latissimus (Figs. 19.2 & 19.3).

The latissimus myocutaneous flap is a Mathes and Nahai type V, with one dominant pedicle – the thoracodorsal artery – and a secondary segmental blood

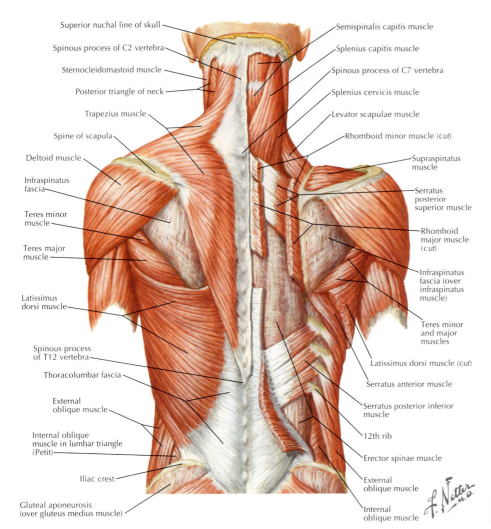

Superior nuchal line of skull

Spinous process of C2 vertebra

Sternocleidomastoid muscle

Posterior triangle of neck

Trapezius muscle

Spine of scapula

Deltoid muscle

Infraspinatus fascia

Teres minor muscle

Teres major muscle

Latissimus dorsi muscle

Spinous process of T12 vertebra

Thoracolumbar fascia

External oblique muscle

Internal oblique muscle in lumbar triangle (Petit)

Iliac crest

Gluteal aponeurosis (over gluteus medius muscle)

Semispinalis capitis muscle

Splenius capitis muscle

Spinous process of C7 vertebra

Splenius cervicis muscle

Levator scapulae muscle

Rhomboid minor muscle (cut)

Supraspinatus muscle

Serratus posterior superior muscle

Rhomboid major muscle (cut)

Infraspinatus fascia (over infraspinatus muscle)

Teres minor and major muscles

Latissimus dorsi muscle (cut)

Serratus anterior muscle

Serratus posterior inferior muscle

12th rib

Erector spinae muscle

External oblique muscle

Internal oblique muscle

Fig. 19.1 Superficial muscles of the back. (© Elsevier Inc. All Rights Reserved.)

supply, perforators from the posterior intercostal (lateral) and lumbar arteries (medial).[20] The axillary artery gives rise to the subscapular artery, which divides into two branches, the circumflex scapular artery and the thoracodorsal artery (Fig. 19.4). The thoracodorsal artery gives off a branch to the serratus anterior just before it enters the muscle, approximately 10 cm inferior to the tendinous insertion into the humerus. Within the substance of the muscle, the thoracodorsal artery bifurcates into transverse and lateral branches that demonstrate extensive intramuscular collateralization.[21–23] This intramuscular arborization forms the anatomic basis for the split latissimus flap.

The thoracodorsal nerve and vein accompany the thoracodorsal artery and together comprise the neurovascular bundle. Identifying the nerve positively identifies the thoracodorsal bundle, thus distinguishing it from other vessels in the area. The innervation to the latissimus muscle arises from the C6–C8 ventral roots via the thoracodorsal nerve, which has been shown to innervate several independent muscle groups,[24] pro-

viding additional rationale for the use of a split latissimus flap for maintenance of muscle function.

Patient presentation

The preoperative visit should include a discussion with the patient about her overall health, functional status, possible donor sites for breast reconstruction, and desires for reconstruction (pure autologous, pure prosthetic, or mixed). The pros and cons of immediate and delayed reconstruction should also be addressed to enable the patient to make the most informed decision possible.

The preoperative work-up generally consists of physical examination only. Provocative maneuvers – for example, having the patient place her hand on the examiner's shoulder and pull downwards – will allow assessment of the muscle bulk as well as the borders of the latissimus muscle. In some patients, this evaluation may be limited by body habitus. In the preoperative holding area, the anticipated skin paddle requirement

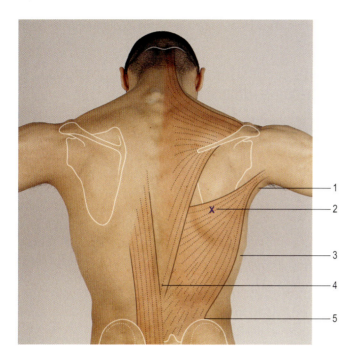

1. Axilla
2. Tip of scapula
3. Anterior margin of latissimus is palpable
4. Midline of back
5. Iliac crest

Fig. 19.2 Surface anatomy of the latissimus dorsi muscle. *(From Wei FC. Flaps and Reconstructive Surgery. Edinburgh: Saunders; 2009.)*

is marked and its location determined based on the anticipated breast skin defect. This allows evaluation of the quality and elasticity of the back skin and any final adjustments based on the location of soft-tissue deposits on the back to be made. This saves time in the operating room and can also allow surgeons to perform unilateral

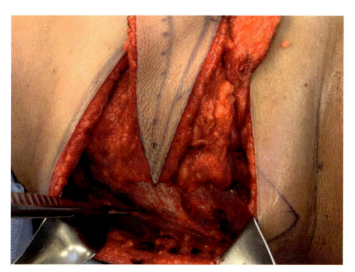

Fig. 19.3 Intraoperative view showing location of the inferior trapezius fibers (forceps) following release of the latissimus myocutaneous flap. The fibers should be identified and protected during flap dissection to avoid iatrogenic injury.

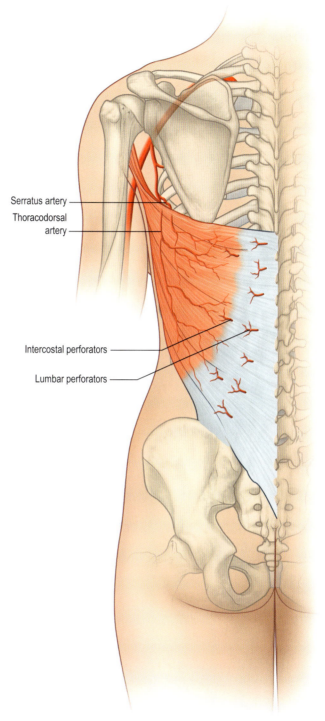

Serratus artery

Thoracodorsal artery

Intercostal perforators

Lumbar perforators

Fig. 19.4 Blood supply to the latissimus dorsi muscle.

latissimus flaps in the lateral decubitus position, shortening operative times.[25]

Due to the excellent reliability of this flap and the lack of variable vascular anatomy, preoperative vascular imaging studies are not considered necessary. In patients who have undergone previous axillary dissection, a weak or non-functional latissimus muscle may herald prior damage to the neurovascular pedicle. In these cases, preservation of the serratus branch may still allow for safe flap transposition.[26]

Patient selection

Ideal candidates for latissimus dorsi breast reconstruction include women who desire implant-based reconstruction but have previously undergone XRT as a component of their cancer therapy (women with local recurrence after previous BCT, women with existing expanders or implants after XRT, or women seeking delayed reconstruction after XRT who are not candidates for abdominally based flaps); women who desire fully autologous breast reconstruction but are not candidates for abdominal-based reconstruction; and women with failed prosthetic breast reconstruction. The latissimus flap can also be used to improve aesthetic outcomes following partial mastectomy. The use in women who have not yet undergone XRT should be avoided so as not to produce a tight, contracted soft-tissue envelope from the XRT, thus eliminating the latissimus as a salvage option. This is not a factor in most lumpectomy reconstructions as implants are not typically employed for this purpose and the soft tissue-only latissimus flap will blend with the irradiated breast to avoid severe contracture.

Mastectomy defects

Primary reconstruction of the mastectomy defect

The ideal candidate for a latissimus myocutaneous flap breast reconstruction is one who will undergo a skin-sparing mastectomy with immediate reconstruction using a supplemental prosthesis. The back skin can be used to replace the resected nipple areolar skin, while the muscle can provide durable coverage for the prosthesis. This will predictably lead to a more natural reconstruction than an implant alone, due to the replacement of a portion of the soft tissues removed with native soft tissue.

The extended latissimus flap can be used in primary or secondary reconstruction for complete autologous reconstruction in women with small to medium sized breasts,[27] and is possible in larger breasts if there is sufficient adipose tissue at the donor site.[28–30] The downside to this flap is the increased incidence in donor site seroma, particularly in obese patients, who often require larger flaps.[31] Lastly, for patients who may require significant skin excision to remove their breast cancer – for example, inflammatory breast cancer patients – the latissimus muscle can carry a large skin paddle, up to 30×40 cm.[32]

Primary reconstruction following previous breast-conserving therapy

The increasing use of BCT in early-stage breast cancers[33] has led to the rise of an important patient population, those who have failed BCT and present for reconstruction following previous XRT. Despite advances in radiation protocols, the rates of recurrence following BCT remain up to 11% at 10 years and up to 22% at 18 years.[34,35] The treatment of choice for local recurrence following BCT is salvage mastectomy. Most would agree that implants alone in the setting of previous radiation therapy will lead to a less favorable result, and autologous tissue is preferred to bring non-irradiated tissue into the reconstruction.[36] While some studies have reported poor aesthetic outcomes with latissimus flaps due to the addition of an implant[37,38] and others have reported better outcomes with TRAM flaps,[39,40] the latissimus flap remains relevant in patients who are not candidates for abdominal-based breast reconstruction. Some authors prefer to use these flaps primarily when prosthetic reconstruction is desired in the post-radiation mastectomy setting, citing high complication rates with prostheses alone,[34] while others use these flaps as a lifeboat if complications are seen following prosthetic reconstruction.[41] A review by Spear and colleagues showed that 40% of patients who had implant-based reconstruction in the setting of previous XRT ultimately required a latissimus flap to treat radiation-induced complications.[42] There have also been anecdotal reports of direct-to-implant reconstruction using the latissimus flap in prophylactic mastectomy and patients considered very low risk to require adjuvant XRT.[43,44]

Secondary reconstruction of the mastectomy defect

Delayed reconstruction allows the final pathologic status of the tumor and regional lymph nodes to be known and allows the patient to complete any adjuvant chemotherapy and/or radiation therapy prior to definitive reconstruction. Similarly, any mastectomy skin flap necrosis will have healed, and the amount of skin required for breast reconstruction can be determined with precision. The downside to delayed reconstruction is the formation of scar tissue and breast envelope skin contracture, which make dissection and flap inset more technically demanding. Perhaps the most significant current role of the latissimus dorsi flap is in secondary breast reconstruction – typically after radiation-induced problems with the primary reconstructive method.

At the authors' institution, they largely practice delayed-immediate breast reconstruction,[45] which minimizes the number of patients who present for secondary reconstruction following mastectomy alone. Placement of a tissue expander at the time of mastectomy preserves the skin envelope and limits scar contracture. For patients who have not undergone delayed-immediate reconstruction, the authors prefer to use abdominal-based reconstruction, but utilize the latissimus flap for patients who are not candidates for abdominal-based reconstruction. When a latissimus flap is used for secondary reconstruction, the possible need for supplemental breast prosthesis to optimize aesthetics is routinely discussed.

The latissimus dorsi flap also plays an important role in salvage reconstruction of the breast after previous failed reconstruction. Patients who have been radiated prior to or following prosthetic breast reconstruction are at increased risk for implant infection and exposure, both of which have successfully been treated with the latissimus.[41] Moreover, in patients with partial failure of abdominal-based flaps who require additional autologous tissue, the latissimus flap is an obvious choice.[46] Fortunately, the rates of free tissue transfer success are high; however, for patients with complete flap loss, the use of a latissimus flap with breast prosthesis can often provide a cosmetically acceptable result.

Lumpectomy defects

Increasingly, women are choosing to undergo breast-conserving therapy when possible, with one study showing a 2:1 preference for lumpectomy over mastectomy in women with early-stage breast cancer.[33] The plastic surgery literature is replete with articles detailing the deleterious effects of radiation therapy on the breast, including contracture, delayed wound healing, and skin hyperpigmentation. The latissimus flap plays an important role in both primary and secondary reconstruction of these defects.

Primary reconstruction of the lumpectomy defect

When a lumpectomy defect is of sufficient size to preclude the use of local, parenchymal-based techniques, the addition of a latissimus dorsi flap can improve aesthetic outcomes despite larger lumpectomy resections. For patients undergoing BCT, a muscle-only latissimus dorsi flap or a myocutaneous flap with a small skin paddle can be used to reconstruct the volume

deficiency, potentially preventing some of the sequelae of radiation therapy.

Secondary reconstruction of the lumpectomy defect

Lumpectomy defects may not be fully appreciated in the early postoperative setting, while the cavity remains filled with hematoma or seroma fluid. These defects, particularly when large (>10–20% of the breast volume), become more pronounced with time and radiation therapy. In these patients, a muscle-only latissimus flap can be used to restore lost breast volume, or a myocutaneous flap with a small skin paddle may be used to remove the constricted, radiated tissues.

Other specific indications

Patients who are not candidates for abdominal-based reconstruction

Patients who require autologous tissue as a component of their breast reconstruction may not be candidates for abdominal-based flaps. This includes women who lack sufficient abdominal skin and adipose tissue, either naturally or from previous surgery (abdominoplasty or abdominal-based breast reconstruction) and women who prefer to avoid the abdominal donor site due to its attendant morbidity. In these women, the latissimus flap is a clear choice.[47] In women who are active smokers, are morbidly obese, or have other medical comorbidities that would preclude the use of a pedicled or free abdominal-based flap, the latissimus may be a safer option and result in fewer complications while still providing a high degree of patient satisfaction.[2,48]

Limited availability of microsurgery

Those of us who work in academic medical centers may take for granted the availability of microsurgeons, microsurgical instruments, and appropriate postoperative care units with equipment and personnel to monitor a free tissue transfer. In a recent review of nationwide trends in breast reconstruction, 81.5% of all reconstructions were pedicled TRAM (48.8%) or latissimus (32.7%) flaps, with free flaps representing less than one in five reconstructions.[2] When microsurgical techniques are not available or feasible, the latissimus flap is an excellent autologous option.

Contraindications

The primary contraindication to latissimus dorsi flap breast reconstruction is a previous posterolateral thoracotomy, in which the latissimus muscle has been divided, making it unsuitable for use. Many thoracic surgeons will use a muscle-sparing approach that may leave this option open even with previous thoracotomy. The operative note and physical exam can clarify if the latissimus muscle has been spared. Some have suggested that an atrophic muscle may not provide adequate coverage or may herald damage to the neurovascular pedicle during a previous axillary dissection and consider this a relative contraindication. However, Fisher and colleagues demonstrated that even in patients with previous axillary dissection in which the thoracodorsal pedicle has been divided, reverse flow through the serratus branch can provide adequate blood supply for flap transposition.[26]

The other contraindication is a suspected or known need for postoperative XRT along with the need for a prosthetic device. If the latissimus flap will be used with a prosthetic device, XRT may cause significant and unpredictable contracture and having used it, it is not available for salvage.[42] The frequency with which the latissimus flap is used to improve or salvage prosthetic reconstructions that have been radiated makes this contraindication self-evident.

Surgical technique (see Video 19.1 ▶)

Marking

Patients are marked in the preoperative holding area in the standing position. When possible, immediate reconstructions should be marked in conjunction with the breast surgeon to appreciate the skin paddle requirements and identify important landmarks to be preserved during the mastectomy, including the inframammary fold. When reconstruction with a latissimus flap is planned, the nipple areolar complex can be excised in a circle rather than the standard ellipse to maximize the final aesthetic outcome of the reconstruction.[19]

At the donor site, important landmarks are the tip of the scapula, corresponding to the superior extent of the latissimus dorsi muscle, the posterior iliac crest, and the dorsal midline (see Fig. 19.2). As these are marked in the standing position, they must be rechecked once the patient is positioned on the operating table as landmarks may change (see Video 19.2 ▶).

Skin paddle design

Both the lateral and transverse branches of the thoracodorsal artery give off numerous perforating vessels to the overlying skin, making harvest of a skin paddle safe within the confines of the muscle borders; however, the most robust of these perforators arise from the lateral

branch. Therefore, the most reliable skin territory overlying the muscle is vertically oriented over the lateral aspect of the muscle, corresponding to the course of the lateral branch of the thoracodorsal artery.[21–23]

A number of skin paddle designs for the latissimus myocutaneous flap have been described, each with its own set of advantages and disadvantages. Which pattern is best for a patient depends on a number of factors, including surgeon and patient preference, anticipation of final scar location, the distribution of any excess soft-tissue deposits on the back, and, most importantly, the skin paddle requirements (see Video 19.3 ▶).

The mid-back transverse scar (Fig. 19.5) provides excellent exposure of the latissimus muscle, particularly near its humeral insertion, which facilitates its division and dissection around the pedicle; however, the final scar may be visible with a low-cut top. When possible, the authors prefer to have patients bring a bra from home to note the location of the strap and make efforts to place the final scar in this location. Moreover, this skin paddle has a tendency to be vertically oriented after transposition, which may make inset challenging, depending on the location of the breast skin defect. However, it is possible to safely elevate the corners of the flap to assist with skin paddle orientation at inset.

The low transverse or low oblique incision (Fig. 19.6) results in a final scar that is very well concealed with most clothing and can take advantage of any soft-tissue redundancy, increasing potential flap volume and providing the patient with contour improvement. This skin

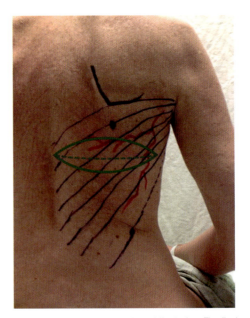

Fig. 19.5 High transverse skin paddle design. The final scar location (dashed line) is often well concealed beneath a bra strap, but will be visible in low-back tops. This incision pattern allows excellent access to the cephalad component of the muscle at the expense of more difficult dissection caudally.

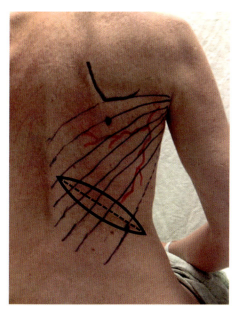

Fig. 19.6 Low transverse skin paddle design. The final scar location (dashed line) is well concealed in most clothing and often falls into a natural skin crease. This incision pattern can take advantage of any excess soft-tissue deposits, improving lower back contour. With this incision pattern, visualization of the cephalad portion of the muscle is limited, often requiring an axillary counter-incision.

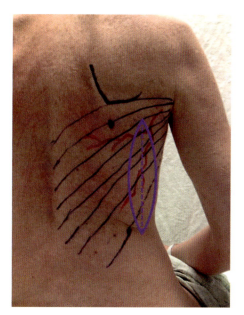

Fig. 19.8 Vertical skin paddle design. The final scar location (dashed line) may be concealed in clothing; however, it travels perpendicular to relaxed skin tension lines and is often noticeable. This incision pattern provides excellent exposure to the entire latissimus muscle, but is less preferred by patients.

paddle is ideal for skin defects located at or near the inframammary fold and provides nearly complete muscular coverage of an associated expander or implant. However, this design provides suboptimal exposure of the latissimus muscle, particularly near the axilla. A small axillary counter incision greatly facilitates this dissection and is well tolerated by patients (Fig. 19.7).

The vertical skin paddle (Fig. 19.8) provides excellent exposure of the latissimus muscle, but the final scar is oriented perpendicular to the relaxed skin tension lines. The oblique skin paddle (Fig. 19.9) has similar issues with the final scar and may not make efficient use of the

underlying muscle for implant coverage. These incision patterns are also less preferred by patients.[49]

In a recently published study, Bailey and colleagues surveyed 250 women to determine their preferences for incision placement and reasoning behind their preference.[49] The low, transverse incision was the most preferred (54% of respondents), followed by the

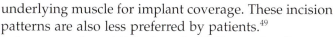

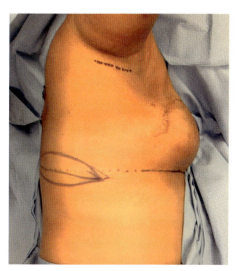

Fig. 19.7 Low transverse skin paddle design and marking for axillary counter incision.

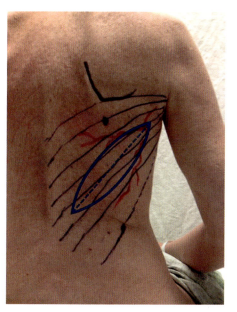

Fig. 19.9 Oblique skin paddle design. The final scar location (dashed line) is concealed in most clothing; however, depending on the location of the breast skin defect, this pattern may require adjustments to maximize muscle coverage of the expander. This incision pattern, like the vertical skin paddle, provides excellent exposure to the entire latissimus muscle, but is less preferred by patients.

mid-transverse skin paddle (22%); the vertical (3%) and oblique (9%) were the least preferred options. The most common reasons behind these preferences were the ability to conceal the scar in a low-back top and aesthetic contour improvement at the donor site. In this study, younger women were more concerned with concealing the scar, whereas older women were more concerned with contour improvement. These preferences for incision placement were not influenced by age, body mass index, body image, or preferred clothing.

Unilateral reconstruction

A unilateral latissimus flap is elevated with the patient under general anesthesia, in the lateral decubitus position. An IV bag wrapped in a thin towel makes a convenient axillary roll. In the case of immediate reconstruction, hemostasis is achieved in the mastectomy site and the incision temporarily closed with staples and covered with a sterile, adhesive dressing (Tegaderm or Ioban) before repositioning. The ipsilateral arm is prepped into the field and an extra, sterile mayo stand – or simply pillows stacked on the arm board – can be used to support the arm during flap harvest (Fig. 19.10). If using a mayo stand, it is important to make sure the edge is adequately padded to avoid excessive pressure on the arm. It is critical to confirm the landmarks, particularly the scapular tip, after patient positioning, as changes in arm movements can alter these markings and the location of the latissimus muscle relative to the skin paddle design on the back.

After confirming its location, the skin paddle is incised and dissection carried out through the superficial (Scarpa's) fascia, being careful to bevel away from the edges of the skin paddle to maintain flap volume and perfusion to the overlying skin. In the case of a purely autologous reconstruction or a patient who requires a large volume of tissue in addition to a prosthesis, all of the sub-Scarpa's fat is maintained with the muscle, and elevation proceeds directly beneath this layer (Fig. 19.11). This technique is also helpful in avoiding donor site contour defects, by maintaining

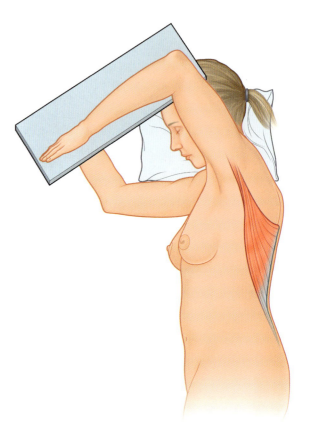

Fig. 19.10 The patient is positioned in the lateral decubitus position with the ipsilateral arm on a mayo stand. This allows access to the entire muscle and its insertion.

a constant thickness of the cutaneous flaps of the back.

The lateral border of the latissimus flap is identified first and then separated from the underlying serratus anterior muscle. This plane of dissection proceeds toward the caudal extent of the latissimus muscle, which is then divided, taking care not to violate the paraspinous or external oblique fascia. Doing so can make dissection more difficult and potentially risk lumbar herniation.[50]

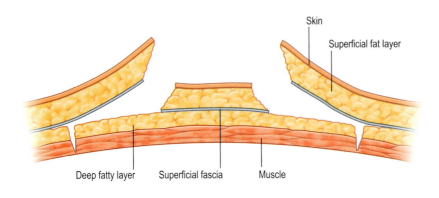

Skin

Superficial fat layer

Deep fatty layer   Superficial fascia   Muscle

Fig. 19.11 In purely autologous reconstructions, all of the fat beneath the Scarpa's fascia is maintained on the muscle surface to provide additional flap volume. Care is taken not to undercut the skin paddle.

Dissection then proceeds cephalad to the skin paddle, in a plane superficial to the latissimus muscle towards the axilla until the tendinous portion of the humeral insertion can be visualized. Depending on the location of the skin island, this dissection may require the use of a counter-incision placed near the axilla (see Fig. 19.7). This dissection can proceed rapidly, as the pedicle is located beneath the muscle, and there are no structures at risk in this plane. It is important to clearly define the latissimus muscle from the teres minor muscle, which converges toward the same insertion point and can be very closely associated with the latissimus.

The latissimus is then progressively freed from its midline attachments in a caudal to cephalad direction. During this part of the dissection, several large perforating vessels, representing the secondary segmental blood supply, will be encountered. Prospective hemostasis with bipolar electrocautery or clips will greatly facilitate dissection and prevent postoperative hematoma formation.

During the cephalad dissection beneath the latissimus muscle, the surgeon must be very careful to avoid iatrogenic injury to the serratus muscle, which can be easily incorporated by mistake if the dissection proceeds in an incorrect plane. The large perforating lumbar vessels will signal the inferior border of the serratus muscle. Superomedially, the fibers of the trapezius muscle that overlap and are superficial to the latissimus are identified and protected (see Fig. 19.3). Once the superior border of the muscle is reached, dissection continues in a medial to lateral direction, taking care to separate the latissimus from the teres minor muscle. Once all borders of the muscle are freed, the dissection proceeds beneath the latissimus muscle towards its neurovascular pedicle until the desired axis of rotation is achieved. We do not routinely skeletonize the pedicle to the latissimus, and prefer simply to visualize its pulsation beneath its protective fat pad to avoid iatrogenic injury.

Once the entire muscle is freed on its superficial and deep surfaces, the tendinous insertion is divided, taking care not to injure the insertion of the teres minor muscle or the underlying neurovascular pedicle (see Video 19.4 ▶). The authors prefer to disinsert the muscle completely and do not routinely divide the thoracodorsal nerve (Fig. 19.12). We find that leaving the tissue surrounding the pedicle avoids the concern of putting undue tension on the neurovascular pedicle and limits potential twisting of the pedicle. Patients do not complain of animation deformity from an intact nerve due to the complete division of the insertion into the humerus, as there is no "pulling" sensation without an origin or insertion to the muscle, just a central bunching or firming

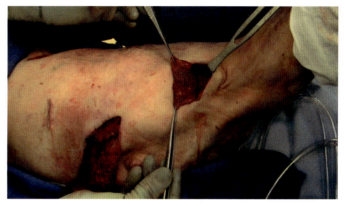

Fig. 19.12 Intraoperative photo demonstrating complete division of the humeral insertion of the latissimus muscle.

of the muscle. Moreover, we find that complete division of the insertion minimizes the axillary bulge that is sometimes seen after flap transposition.[51] We do feel that it is important to either divide the insertion completely or divide the nerve in order to avoid a disconjugate "pulling" sensation.

Flap transposition and inset

Depending on the lateral extent of the mastectomy defect, the mastectomy space may be inadvertently entered during dissection of the lateral muscle. This should be avoided when possible, and suture repair may be necessary if the space is entered too far caudally. The flap should be transposed through a subcutaneous tunnel high in the axilla to avoid a prominent axillary bulge (Figs. 19.13–19.14) (see Video 19.5 ▶). Once the flap is transposed, the muscle is secured at the anterior axillary line with interrupted 2-0 polydioxanone sutures to prevent lateral migration of the flap as well as displacement of the expander/implant to the axillary space. This maneuver also prevents excessive tension on the vascular pedicle when the humeral insertion of the latissimus muscle is completely divided.

The inset of the flap is dictated by the preoperative skin paddle markings, the location of the breast skin resection, and the need for muscular coverage of the associated implant (see Video 19.6 ▶). For immediate reconstruction of a modified radical mastectomy, a transverse mid-back incision is often useful, as this provides muscular coverage both above and below the skin paddle, which is often placed in the mid-breast (Fig. 19.15). When this skin paddle is transposed and the muscle secured medially to cover the prosthesis, there is a tendency for the medial skin paddle to be oriented superiorly. If necessary, the skin can be elevated off of the underlying flap at the level of the subcutaneous tissues to rotate the medial aspect into the proper location (Fig. 19.16). With immediate reconstruction following

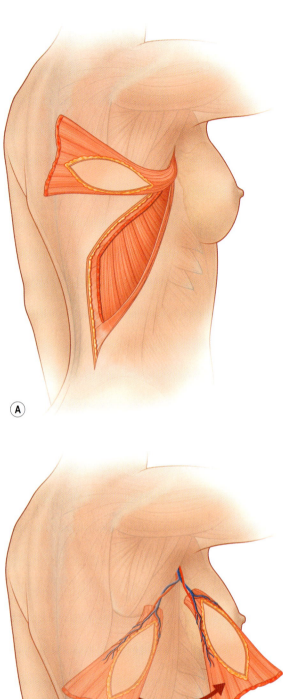

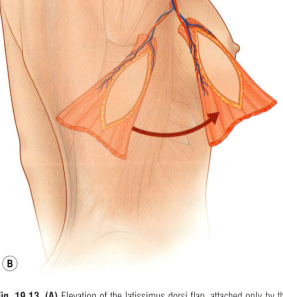

Fig. 19.13 (A) Elevation of the latissimus dorsi flap, attached only by the humeral insertion. **(B)** After division of the humeral insertion, the flap is transposed anteriorly through a subcutaneous tunnel high in the axilla.

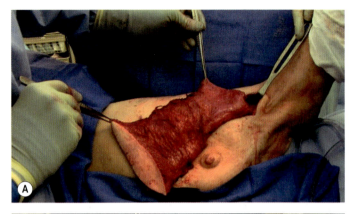

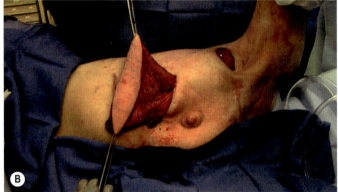

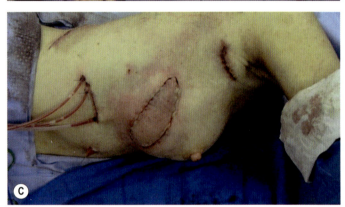

Fig. 19.14 (A) Flap transposed through axillary counter incision. **(B)** Transposition of flap through mastectomy space. **(C)** Final inset of latissimus muscle and skin paddle.

skin-sparing mastectomy, an areolar-sized cutaneous circle will be preserved and the remainder of the skin island will be de-epithelialized (Fig. 19.17). In this instance the authors score the de-epithelialized dermis surrounding the areolar skin paddle to provide an edge to inset the mastectomy flaps and minimize indentation at the periphery of the areola.

When reconstruction is combined with the use of a tissue expander or implant, the authors find it more efficient to leave the pectoralis muscle down, attached to the chest wall, and inset the latissimus flap to its superficial surface. Tabbed expanders are used and secured in place, followed by interrupted 2-0 polydioxanone sutures to define the dimensions of the breast

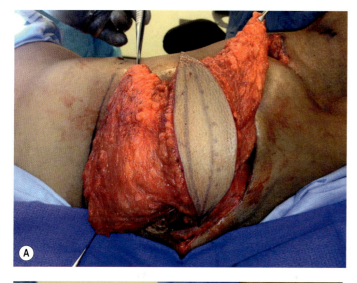

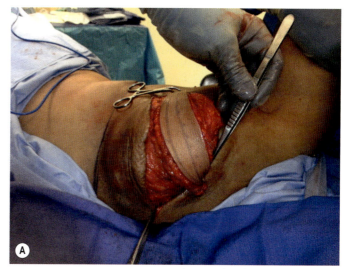

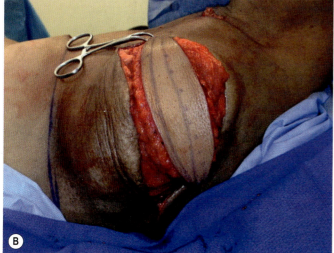

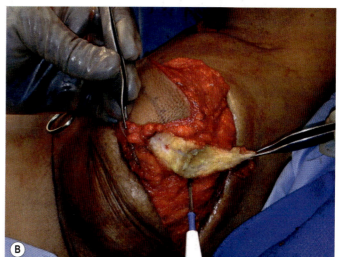

Fig. 19.15 **(A)** Mid-transverse skin paddle, showing muscle bulk above and below the skin paddle. **(B)** Flap inset, showing coverage of the inferior and superior expander with latissimus muscle.

pocket. Securing the flap superiorly helps to provide additional upper pole fullness to the reconstructed breast and provides some camouflage of the transition from the chest wall to the breast prosthesis.

In the case of unilateral reconstructions, we have found that the use of tabbed tissue expanders have allowed us to accurately place the prosthesis and inset the flap with the patient in the lateral decubitus position, eliminating one position change and making the operation significantly more efficient.[25] An assistant closes the back while the latissimus flap is inset into the mastectomy space.

At this point, once the muscle is sutured in place, we will fill the expander to the desired level. We have found that waiting until the flap is inset completely is prohibitive due to the thickness of the back skin overlying the integrated expander port. Moreover, the thin latissimus muscle makes palpation of the fill port simple

Fig. 19.16 Adjustment of the medial skin paddle. **(A)** Flap *in situ* after transposition and muscle inset. **(B)** Elevation of the medial corner of the skin paddle. **(C)** Final inset.

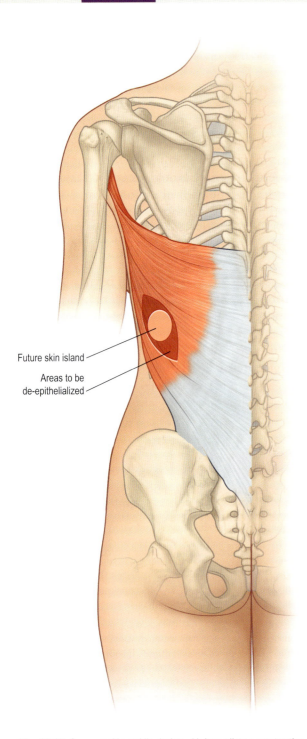

Future skin island

Areas to be
de-epithelialized

Fig. 19.17 Common skin paddle design with immediate reconstruction of a skin-sparing mastectomy.

and minimizes the potential for iatrogenic implant puncture.

In delayed reconstruction, a larger skin paddle will generally be required and is usually placed at the inferior pole of the breast to release contracted tissues and provide a degree of natural ptosis. This can be achieved with a low transverse skin paddle, which places the bulk of the latissimus muscle above the skin paddle, where it can cover the breast prosthesis. If necessary, a

fleur-de-lis skin paddle can be designed, which allows incisional release of the contracted lower pole breast skin and provides a skin paddle extension to insert into this defect (Fig. 19.18).[52]

Bilateral reconstruction

In the case of immediate reconstruction following bilateral mastectomy, hemostasis is confirmed in the mastectomy space before temporarily closing with staples and an adhesive dressing (Ioban or Tegaderm). The patient is then placed in the prone position, and dissection is carried out as outlined above.

It is worth noting that the anterior border of the latissimus flap tends to be farther anterior than anticipated in the prone position, and care should be taken to harvest the muscle in its entirety. Attention to the direction of the muscle fibers and noting the level of the lumbar perforators can prevent accidental elevation of the serratus anterior (serratus muscle fibers run in a perpendicular direction, and the serratus muscle is just caudal to the level of the perforating vessels) or incomplete inclusion of the latissimus muscle. Once each flap is dissected and remains attached only by its pedicle, the flaps are "buried" in the axilla, taking note of their orientation, and the back incisions closed over the flaps in standard fashion, as described above. The patient is then repositioned supine and the flaps retrieved through the mastectomy cavity. It is very important to verify that the flap is transposed in such a way that the pedicle is not twisted or kinked. The flaps are inset with or without a breast prosthesis, as described above. Of particular importance is ensuring symmetric placement of the tissue expanders prior to flap inset. The authors utilize tabbed expanders and transpose the points of fixation to the overlying skin to ensure side-to-side symmetry.[25]

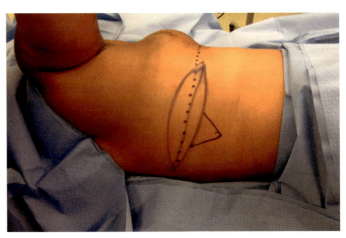

Fig. 19.18 *Fleur-de-lis* skin paddle design with inferior extension designed to interpose in an area of incisional lower pole release.

Donor site closure

The back incision is closed in a layered fashion over two 7 mm or 10 mm flat drains placed to bulb suction. Scarpa's fascia is reapproximated using 0-polydioxanone (PDS) sutures or a single #2 Quill. The skin is closed in layers, with interrupted 3-0 PDS or Vicryl sutures in the dermis, followed by a running subcuticular 3-0 PDS or Monocryl. Steri-Strips are applied to the incision, which is then covered by Telfa and Tegaderm.

Postoperative expansion

Once the incisions are healed, usually within two weeks, serial expansions are begun until the desired size is achieved. The tissues are then allowed to settle for a period of 4–6 weeks before the patient is brought to the operating room for an expander to implant exchange. This is done through the previous incision, and the latissimus muscle is split along the direction of its fibers. At this point, any minor asymmetries or adjustments to the implant pocket can be addressed. The nipple areolar complex can be reconstructed in this or another setting.

Surgical variations

Advances in the understanding of the blood supply to the latissimus dorsi muscle and the overlying skin have lead to the development of surgical variations of this flap to minimize morbidity, namely the extended latissimus,[53] the split latissimus,[54] and the muscle-sparing latissimus dorsi flap.[55]

Extended latissimus flap

Patients with larger breasts or those who desire completely autologous breast reconstruction and are not candidates for abdominal-based tissue transfer can be treated with an extended latissimus flap. One design utilizes a three-pointed skin paddle, designed to capture the largest amount of available soft tissues (Fig. 19.18).[27,52,56] The design of the incision allows a well-concealed donor site scar and minimizes dog-ear formation.[52] While excellent aesthetic results can be achieved,[52,53] it should be noted that the rates of seroma are increased, particularly in obese patients.[53]

Muscle-sparing techniques

In an effort to reduce the donor site morbidity associated with harvest of a latissimus dorsi flap, Angrigiani described the thoracodorsal artery perforator flap in 1995, allowing a skin paddle of 25×15 cm to be elevated without incorporating any of the underlying latissimus muscle.[57] Due to a high rate of flap loss in their experience, Schwabegger and colleagues introduced the muscle-sparing latissimus flap, which included a small strip of latissimus muscle to increase the vascularity of the overlying skin paddle.[58] A disadvantage of this technique was the use of a vertically oriented skin paddle, which later led to the development of the pedicled muscle-sparing latissimus dorsi musculocutaneous flap, described by Saint-Cyr et al. in 2009 (Fig. 19.19).[55] With this technique, the skin paddle is not dependent on a specific perforator and can be designed in any orientation along the axis of the descending branch of the thoracodorsal artery.[55]

Intraoperatively, the thoracodorsal artery and the location of its bifurcation into the transverse and descending branches are identified with a Doppler probe. The bifurcation point is found an average of 5.1 cm from the posterior axillary fold[55] and 2.2 cm from the lateral edge of the muscle.[58] The skin paddle is designed to capture the largest amount of back soft tissue, with the lateral edge of the skin paddle extending 1–2 cm lateral to the anterior border of the latissimus muscle to capture perforators from the descending branch of the thoracodorsal artery. The superior skin flap is elevated first, only above the descending branch of the thoracodorsal vessel. The superior skin is draped over the proposed skin excision to confirm primary closure before committing to the skin paddle design. Next, the inferior skin flap is elevated, again taking care to only elevate the skin above the descending branch. This key maneuver helps to minimize soft-tissue dissection and postoperative seroma formation.[55] The latissimus muscle is then split vertically along its fibers beginning caudally, staying 1 cm medial to the descending branch, up to the point of its bifurcation. The flap is then transposed through an axillary tunnel in standard fashion.

Using this technique, Saint-Cyr reported no seromas or hematomas in twenty-four patients; no significant differences in shoulder range of motion, vertical reach, or strength; low postoperative disability scores as measured by the DASH (Disabilities of the Arm, Shoulder, and Hand) score; and high levels of patient satisfaction.[55]

Endoscopic-assisted reconstruction with latissimus dorsi (EARLi)

The latissimus flap, as classically described, utilizes a large skin incision on the back and may or may not include a skin paddle.[3] In an effort to minimize donor morbidity, some authors have described "mini" latissimus flaps.[59,60] An additional technique that can be

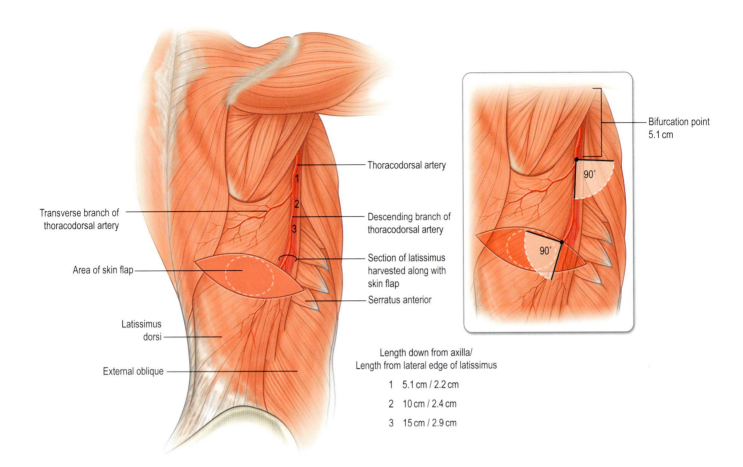

Fig. 19.19 Relevant anatomy and design of the muscle-sparing latissimus dorsi flap based on the descending branch of the thoracodorsal artery, as described by Saint-Cyr *et al*. Limited undermining of skin flaps is used to minimize seroma formation and limit donor site morbidity. *(Redrawn from Saint-Cyr M, Nagarkar P, Schaverien M, et al. The pedicled descending branch muscle-sparing latissimus dorsi flap for breast reconstruction.* Plast Reconstr Surg. *2009;123:13–24.)*

applied for women undergoing BCT who wish to minimize scar burden on the donor site is an endoscopic-assisted harvest and transposition of the muscle only to fill a partial breast defect. This technique, described at the authors' institution in 1994 by the senior author (NAF), has been in use for more than twenty years and has become the authors' preferred method of reconstruction in this patient population. This procedure, which uses a much smaller incision and less traumatic tissue dissection, has allowed many patients the benefits of faster recovery, with decreased postoperative pain and improved cosmesis.[61] With indications for BCT expanding to include larger tumors, more and more breast parenchyma is resected, and many women will require flap reconstruction for an aesthetically pleasing result.[3,62]

This procedure is well suited for women who require resection of 20–30% of their breast volume and is ideal for resections in the upper outer quadrant of the breast, where most cancers occur. This procedure is always performed in a delayed fashion, once the final pathologic margins are known. This can be as early as three days following lumpectomy but should not be delayed more than three weeks to avoid scar contracture that may require release and skin paddle replacement. The contraindications to an EARLi procedure are the same as those for a standard latissimus flap, including known or potential damage to the vascular pedicle.

The patient is positioned, prepped, and draped in the same fashion as a unilateral latissimus flap reconstruction, with the ipsilateral arm prepped into the field so that it can be manipulated during the procedure to maximize visualization. The procedure is carried out using modified laparoscopic instruments (Fig. 19.20) with the primary surgeon facing the patient's chest and the assistant facing the patient's back. The donor site is then infused with tumescent solution in a plane superficial to the latissimus muscle to facilitate intraoperative hemostasis. The lumpectomy defect is then opened and its size approximated using a laparotomy pad (Fig. 19.21) while the epinephrine in the tumescent solution is taking effect.

A curvilinear incision is made at the inferior aspect of the axillary hairline, which must be large enough to

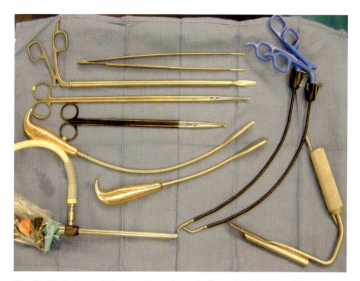

Fig. 19.20 Instrumentation used in endoscopically assisted harvest of the latissimus dorsi muscle.

accommodate the surgeon's hand. Typically, our incisions measure approximately 9 cm. The dissection begins with identification of the thoracodorsal vascular pedicle (Fig. 19.22). In order to avoid the risk of avulsion and to allow full movement of the muscle, the serratus branch and any vascular tributaries supplying the serratus anterior muscle must be clipped and transected. It is critical during this part of the procedure that the thoracodorsal pedicle be unequivocally identified.

After the thoracodorsal pedicle has been identified, the deep surface of the muscle is dissected free using a combination of monopolar electrocautery and blunt dissection. Once space has been created, the surgeon's hand is introduced to ensure the proper plane of dissection and to facilitate blunt dissection beneath the latissimus muscle. A retractor with an endoscope is inserted, and the dissection of the deep surface of the muscle is

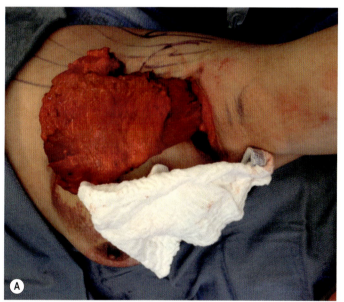

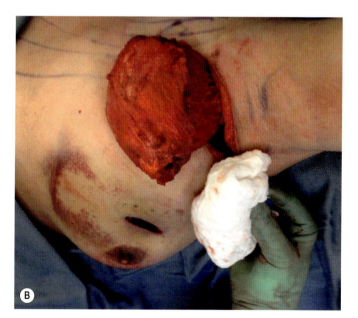

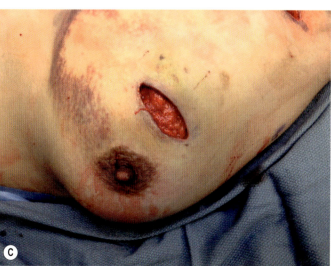

Fig. 19.21 A laparotomy pad may be used to approximate the configuration and size of the latissimus dorsi muscle. The lumpectomy defect in this case was estimated to be roughly the size of a single laparotomy pad. **(A)** Spread out in the pretransposed configuration. **(B)** Balled up to simulate the inset configuration and size similarity to one laparotomy pad. **(C)** Final inset, demonstrating adequate soft-tissue volume to reconstruct the lumpectomy defect.

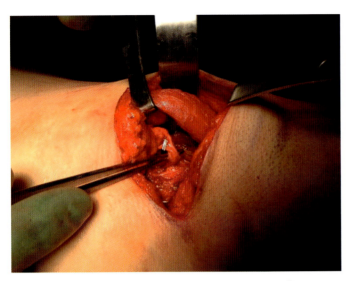

Fig. 19.22 Identification of the thoracodorsal neurovascular pedicle. The serratus branch has been clipped in this photograph.

completed. Care must be taken to properly clip or cauterize the lumbar perforators encountered near the dorsal midline. The authors find that marking the site of these lumbar perforators on the overlying back skin greatly facilitates final hemostasis (Fig. 19.23).

Once the deep dissection is complete, the next step is to dissect on the superficial surface of the muscle. The first 5–6 cm of this dissection represents the part of the muscle that will ultimately be tunneled through the axilla, where extra bulk is not desirable. After freeing 5–6 cm, the plane of dissection changes to the sub-Scarpa's layer to maximize flap volume where it will be needed to fill the lumpectomy defect.

At this point, the remaining muscular attachments are freed using a combination of direct visualization and "tactile guidance", whereby the surgeon places one

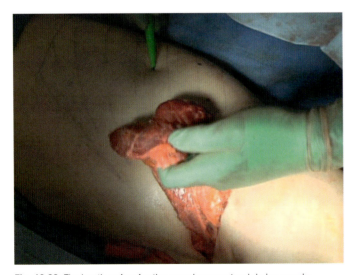

Fig. 19.23 The location of perforating vessels encountered during muscle dissection is marked on the overlying skin to help ensure adequate hemostasis prior to donor site closure.

hand through the incision and grasps the muscle at the point where it must be divided, then cuts just beyond his or her fingertips with the endoscopic scissors. Freeing the most inferior attachments is the most challenging part of the procedure. Once complete, the tendinous humeral insertion is divided using monopolar electrocautery, which fully mobilizes the muscle. An axillary tunnel is then created to the breast defect and the flap transposed into place and loosely secured with absorbable sutures. Endoscopic instruments are then used to cauterize any vessels identified, specifically lumbar perforators noted during flap harvest. It is noteworthy that these vessels may not be actively bleeding due to the epinephrine in the tumescent solution. Careful attention must be paid to ensure all vessels are adequately cauterized or clipped. Once adequate hemostasis is achieved, two 7 mm flat drains are placed in the back donor site and one in the breast, and the incisions are closed in standard fashion. Typical operating time is between two and three hours.

Secondary procedures

Common secondary surgical procedures following latissimus flap breast reconstruction include exchange of tissue expander for permanent implant, donor site revisions, reconstruction of the nipple areolar complex, and procedures on the contralateral breast to improve overall symmetry. Nipple areolar reconstruction and contralateral breast surgery are beyond the scope of this chapter.

Expander to implant exchange

In most cases, a tissue expander is placed at the time of the latissimus flap operation, although direct-to-implant reconstructions have been described.[43,44] The expander pocket is approached through the previous mastectomy incision, with longitudinal splitting of the latissimus muscle fibers to expose the expander. At this time, capsulotomy or other pocket revision procedures can be performed before placement of the final implant. If desired, the skin paddle of the flap can be modified to a more anatomic, areolar shape if the mastectomy flaps are sufficiently mobile, which may improve the final aesthetic appearance of the reconstruction.

Donor site revisions

Depending on the amount of breast skin removed during the mastectomy, the size of the latissimus flap skin paddle will vary greatly. With large skin paddles, the donor site may be closed under excessive tension that may lead to delayed wound healing, dog-ear formation, and widening of the final scar. The donor site responds well to scar revision once the skin tension has relaxed, and dog-ear revision can be performed in the office or in conjunction with secondary procedures on an as-needed basis.

Postoperative management

All patients have two 7 mm or 10 mm closed-suction drains placed in the flap donor site and one or two drains in the mastectomy space. These drains are left in place until the total output from each is 30 cc or less per 24-hour period. An elastic bandage may be gently wrapped circumferentially around the upper torso for comfort and gentle compression, but care must be exercised not to excessively compress the vascular pedicle or flap. All patients receive mechanical and chemoprophylaxis for prevention of venous thromboembolism, and early ambulation is encouraged. The average length of stay is 1–2 days in the hospital.

Dressings are removed prior to discharge (24–48 hours postoperatively), at which time patients may begin showering. Ambulation and activities of daily living, including personal hygiene tasks, are encouraged immediately. More strenuous activities are resumed later, typically 4–6 weeks postoperatively.

Complications

Donor site morbidity

The most common complications associated with the latissimus dorsi flap are related to the donor site. Specifically, donor site seroma formation is particularly problematic, with published rates ranging from 3.9% to 79%.[63,64] Often, these are managed on an outpatient basis with needle aspiration; however, on rare occasions, a persistent seroma may require surgical debridement of the seroma cavity and long-term closed suction drainage. The risk of seroma may be increased with the extended latissimus dorsi flap.[65]

When very large skin paddles are used, the donor site closure may be placed under excessive tension that can lead to delayed wound healing, contour irregularity, and scar widening. Fortunately, these complications are usually minor and can be corrected with minor, secondary procedures.

The latissimus dorsi muscle forms the roof of the superior lumbar triangle. During flap harvest, inadvertent injury to the aponeurosis of the internal oblique and transversus abdominis muscles, which form the floor of this triangle, can lead to lumbar herniation. While this complication is rare, it is important to consider, as

surgical intervention is usually required to repair the hernia and avoid serious complications.[50]

Lastly, in addition to several other roles, the latissimus dorsi is an important adductor of the arm and internal rotator of the shoulder. Harvest of this flap can lead to shoulder weakness, stiffness, and loss of mobility. These complications should be discussed with patients preoperatively; however, in most patients who are not elite athletes or bodybuilders, the loss of strength and range of motion is negligible and responds well to postoperative physical therapy.[66,67]

Complication rates are, expectedly, commensurate with the level of dissection and tissue harvest. Higher rates of seroma are seen in extended latissimus flaps, with conflicting data on the impact of obesity on seroma formation.[53,65,68] In a recent study directly comparing outcomes between the two, the extended latissimus dorsi flap showed significantly higher rates of seroma (muscle-sparing latissimus vs extended latissimus flaps, the rates of seroma were 62.2% vs. 5.6%), limitation of shoulder movement (75.7% vs. 25%), and asymmetry than the muscle-sparing latissimus dorsi flap.[69]

Flap loss

The latissimus dorsi flap has a robust axial blood supply and reliable skin territory, making significant flap loss unusual. This complication is almost universally associated with injury to the vascular pedicle during flap dissection or twisting/kinking of the pedicle during flap transposition. It is therefore very important to understand the orientation of the pedicle before and after tunneling through the axilla to avoid iatrogenic flap loss. Partial flap loss has been reported with rates as high as 7% but is seen more commonly with the extended latissimus flap.[70]

Implant-related complications

In cases where a latissimus dorsi flap is used in conjunction with a tissue expander or implant, the risks of prosthetic use are added to the risk profile of the flap, including implant extrusion, rupture, periprosthetic infection, and capsular contracture.[71] Furthermore, implant migration into the axilla has been reported.[72] This complication is easily avoided by securing the lateral flap to the chest wall to close the communication between the mastectomy cavity and the flap donor site.[72] Furthermore, the use of tabbed tissue expanders can prevent or reduce the incidence of this complication.[25]

Individualized risk assessment

The development of large-scale, multi-institutional databases has allowed a recent emphasis on individualizing

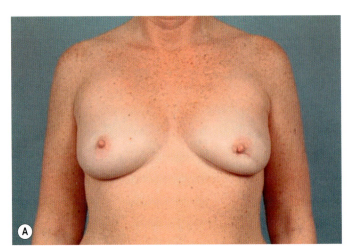
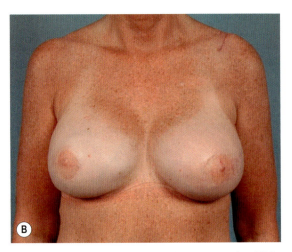

Fig. 19.24 A 48-year-old female who underwent bilateral skin-sparing mastectomy after left lumpectomy and bilateral latissimus flap reconstruction. **(A)** Preoperative appearance. **(B)** Postoperative appearance following bilateral latissimus flap reconstruction with 550 cc Moderate Plus silicone gel implants and nipple/areolar reconstruction and tattooing. *(Photos courtesy of Dr. John Y.S. Kim.)*

risk assessment through statistical modeling. Recently, one of the authors (JYSK) developed the Breast Reconstruction Risk Assessment Score (BRA Score) using widely available resources, like the American Society of Plastic Surgeons Tracking Operations and Outcomes for Plastic Surgeons (TOPS) and the American College of Surgeons National Surgical Quality Improvement Program (NSQIP) databases. This tool aims to provide individualized and quantifiable risk assessment for patients undergoing breast reconstruction in an effort to better inform surgical decision-making and manage patient expectations (see Fig. 14.2).[64]

Outcomes

In a recent review of the American College of Surgeons National Surgical Improvement Program (NSQIP)

database, latissimus flaps accounted for nearly one third of all breast reconstructions (32.7%), and 30 day complication rates were lower than pedicled TRAM and free flap reconstructions.[2] Specifically, rates of flap failure, surgical site infection, and overall complications were lowest in patients undergoing latissimus flap breast reconstruction. Several studies have demonstrated the reliability of the latissimus flap with low rates of flap-related complications and high levels of patient satisfaction.[7,19,27,29,31,48,51,55,68,72,73] Clinical examples are shown in Figs. 19.24–19.27.

Conclusion

In conclusion, the latissimus dorsi flap is an anatomically reliable, technically straightforward option for breast reconstruction with generally fewer complications than

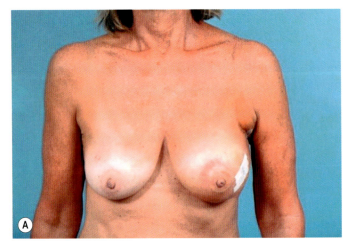
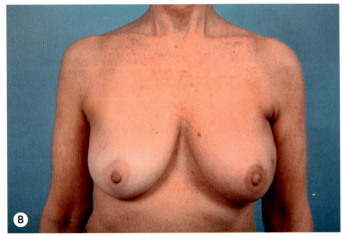

Fig. 19.25 A 54-year-old female with left lumpectomy defect who underwent endoscopic-assisted reconstruction with latissimus dorsi (EARLi) procedure for left breast volume augmentation. **(A)** Following left lumpectomy. **(B)** Following reconstruction with muscle-only latissimus flap. *(Photos courtesy of Dr. John Y.S. Kim.)*

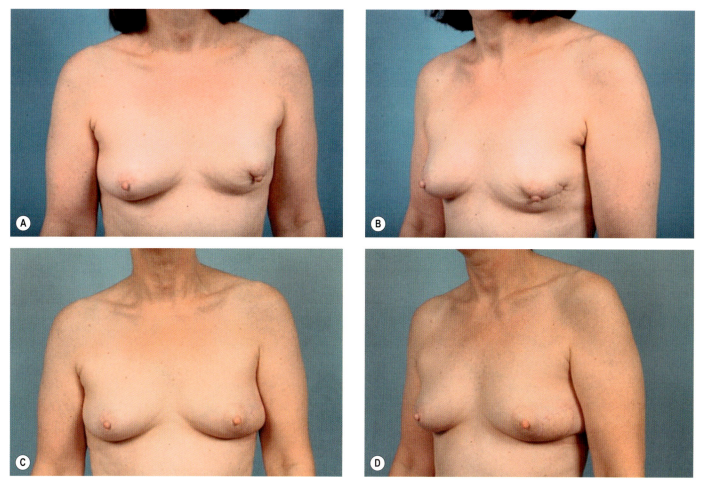

Fig. 19.26 A 54-year-old female who presented following left lumpectomy and radiation therapy. **(A)** Preoperative anteroposterior (AP) view. **(B)** Preoperative oblique view. **(C)** AP view following latissimus flap reconstruction with inferolateral skin paddle designed to release constricted breast skin. **(D)** Postoperative oblique view. *(Photos courtesy of Dr. John Y.S. Kim.)*

other autologous techniques. Moreover, there are variants of the latissimus flap – including minimally invasive muscle harvest techniques and the extended version – which can diversify its utility for both primary and secondary lumpectomy and mastectomy defects. In an era of outcomes-based reimbursement and healthcare cost containment, this combination of utility, ease, and relative cost-efficacy will ensure continued use of varying permutations of the latissimus flap in breast reconstruction.

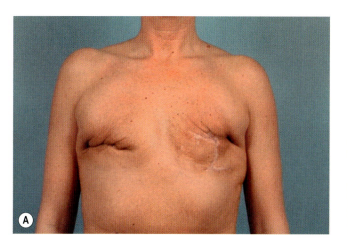
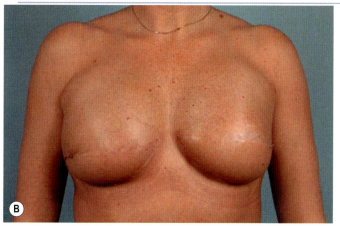

Fig. 19.27 A 47-year-old female who presented following failed bilateral prosthetic-based reconstruction. **(A)** Preoperative appearance. **(B)** Following bilateral latissimus flap reconstruction and expander to implant exchange (nipple/areolar reconstruction was deferred per patient preference). *(Photos courtesy of Dr. John Y.S. Kim.)*

Access the complete reference list online at **http://www.expertconsult.com**

19. Hammond DC. Latissimus dorsi flap breast reconstruction. *Clin Plast Surg.* 2007;34:75–82, abstract vi–vii. *Dr. Hammond describes his extensive experience with the latissimus flap and the technical modifications he has made over time to improve outcomes andaesthetics. He demonstrates that impressive results can be achieved with these modifications and improvements in the design of breast prostheses.*

26. Fisher J, Bostwick J 3rd, Powell RW. Latissimus dorsi blood supply after thoracodorsal vessel division: the serratus collateral. *Plast Reconstr Surg.* 1983;72:502–511.

31. Delay E, Gounot N, Bouillot A, et al. Autologous latissimus breast reconstruction: a 3-year clinical experience with 100 patients. *Plast Reconstr Surg.* 1998;102:1461–1478. *Delay et al. demonstrate their technique for latissimus dorsi flap breast reconstruction and reported on results and complications. Patient satisfaction was high. Postoperative complications included partial necrosis (1%), total necrosis (1%), and seroma (79%). Seroma was noted to occur more regularly in obese patients.*

39. Disa JJ, Cordeiro PG, Heerdt AH, et al. Skin-sparing mastectomy and immediate autologous tissue reconstruction after whole-breast irradiation. *Plast Reconstr Surg.* 2003;111:118–124.

46. Hammond DC, Simon AM, Khuthaila DK, et al. Latissimus dorsi flap salvage of the partially failed TRAM flap breast reconstruction. *Plast Reconstr Surg.* 2007;120:382–389.

48. Spear SL, Boehmler JH, Taylor NS, Prada C. The role of the latissimus dorsi flap in reconstruction of the irradiated breast. *Plast Reconstr Surg.* 2007;119:1–9, discussion 10–11. *The authors describe their 10-year experience using the latissimus dorsi flap in prosthetic reconstruction of irradiated breasts. Twenty-eight patients were identified, 18 of whom had a latissimus flap at the time of expander placement and* 10 of whom underwent secondary latissimus flap reconstruction. No patients developed capsular contracture, and overall patient satisfaction was very high (8.8/10). The authors conclude that latissimus flaps can be combined with prosthetic reconstruction to produce a cosmetically-pleasing result in the previously irradiated breast.

53. Chang DW, Youssef A, Cha S, Reece GP. Autologous breast reconstruction with the extended latissimus dorsi flap. *Plast Reconstr Surg.* 2002;110:751–759, discussion 760–761. *The authors in this study present their clinical series of 75 extended latissimus dorsi flaps for purely autologous breast reconstruction. In this series of 67 patients, 28% developed flap-related complications and 38.7% developed donor site complications. Overall, donor site seroma was the most common complications (25.3%), and the authors conclude that obese patients are at higher risk of developing this complication.*

55. Saint-Cyr M, Nagarkar P, Schaverien M, et al. The pedicled descending branch muscle-sparing latissimus dorsi flap for breast reconstruction. *Plast Reconstr Surg.* 2009;123:13–24. *Saint-Cyr et al. present a series of 24 muscle-sparing latissimus flaps in 20 patient and report on outcomes, complications, and functional disability compared with the nonoperated side. The technique for the pedicled muscle-sparing latissimus flap is also presented. There were no postoperative seromas reported in this series and only one case of partial flap necrosis. When comparing the operated and nonoperated sides, no statistically significant functional differences were detected using the DASH questionnaire.*

67. Russell RC, Pribaz J, Zook EG, et al. Functional evaluation of latissimus dorsi donor site. *Plast Reconstr Surg.* 1986;78:336–344.

73. Pacella SJ, Vogel JE, Locke MB, Codner MA. Aesthetic and technical refinements in latissimus dorsi implant breast reconstruction: a 15-year experience. *Aesthet Surg J.* 2011;31:190–199.

20.1

Introduction to abdominally based free flaps

Maurice Y. Nahabedian

Access video lecture content for this chapter online at expertconsult.com

Breast reconstruction using autologous tissue provides an option for women that is natural, lasts forever, and often provides body-contouring advantages. There are several anatomic regions of the body that can be used including the abdomen, posterior thorax, gluteal region, and thigh. The abdomen is the most commonly considered donor site for a variety of reasons that include sufficient quantity to reconstruct a breast, abdominoplasty type closure, and patient desire. Flaps derived from the abdomen can be based on a pedicle or as a free tissue transfer. Advantages of abdominal free flaps include the ability to optimally position the flap on the chest wall; typically abdominally based free tissue transfer has become the most common form of breast reconstruction.

The evolution of breast reconstruction using abdominal tissue dates back to 1979, when Holmström described a free tissue transfer technique using the abdominal skin and fat.[1] However, this operation was overshadowed primarily because of the work of Carl Hartrampf et al. who described the pedicle TRAM (transverse rectus abdominis musculocutaneous) flap in 1982.[2] The pedicle TRAM flap revolutionized the state-of-the-art for breast reconstruction because it did not require microvascular techniques, it provided an alternative to prosthetic devices and the latissimus dorsi flap, as well as improved abdominal aesthetics. Although the aesthetic outcomes related to the breast were usually excellent, concerns regarding the donor site gradually became an issue due to loss of strength and occasional contour abnormalities. In most cases, the entire rectus abdominis muscle was harvested because the vascularity to the TRAM flap was derived from the perforators emanating from the

superior epigastric artery and vein that traversed through the rectus abdominis muscle. The role of the muscle was essentially that of a conduit for perfusion and occasionally provided volume. While a few surgeons were preserving the continuity of the rectus abdominis muscle, most were elevating the entire length and width, placing the patients at increased risk for weakness and contour abnormality. The use of prosthetic materials to reinforce the abdominal wall was effective; however, the loss of strength could not be overcome, especially when both rectus abdominis muscles were harvested for unilateral or bilateral reconstruction.

The free TRAM did not become a universally accepted option until 1989, when Grotting et al. compared the free TRAM flap to the conventional TRAM flap (see Chapter 20.4).[3] With this flap, the same adipocutaneous territory could be used; however, the vascularity was derived from the inferior epigastric artery and vein rather than the superior epigastric artery and vein. The inferiorly based vessels traversed a shorter length, had a larger caliber, and were not associated with choke vessels, all of which could potentially enhance the perfusion to the flap. Although the free TRAM was still a musculocutaneous flap, less muscle and fascia was removed compared with the pedicle TRAM that served to minimize compromising the anterior abdominal wall. The flap could be harvested with varying degrees of muscle sparing (MS) that included sparing the medial and lateral segments (MS-2) and the medial or lateral segments (MS-1). In some cases, the entire width of the muscle could be harvested (MS-0). Functionally, the MS-0 free TRAM was similar to the pedicle TRAM flap because the continuity of the rectus abdominis muscle was lost. Thus, the era of free tissue transfer for autologous breast reconstruction began.

In 1994, Allen and Treece[4] described the DIEP (deep inferior epigastric perforator) flap for breast reconstruction (see Chapter 20.2). The DIEP flap was similar to the free TRAM, in that it utilized the same adipocutaneous territory and the same vascularity. The principal difference was that the rectus abdominis muscle was preserved in its entirety, thus reducing the likelihood of abdominal weakness or contour abnormality.[5] Although the muscle is preserved, the anterior rectus sheath is incised and a myotomy is performed in order to dissect the inferior epigastric artery and vein. Complexities associated with the DIEP flap include selection of the proper perforator(s) and determination of the perforasomes. There is a plethora of perforators of varying caliber with variable perfusion capacity. The ability to perform a DIEP flap has been facilitated using preoperative technology such as magnetic resonance angiography or computerized tomographic angiography to identify the location and caliber of the dominant perforators. Intraoperative technologies such as fluorescent angiography can provide important information regarding tissue perfusion.

The superficial inferior epigastric artery (SIEA) flap is not technically a perforator flap because the blood supply does not perforate a muscle; rather it is an adipocutaneous flap based on an entirely different blood supply (see Chapter 20.3).[6] This flap was initially described by Grotting in 1991[7] and has the distinct advantage over the other free and pedicle abdominally based flaps, in that it does not require an incision in the anterior rectus sheath or a myotomy in the rectus abdominis muscle. The advantages of this flap are that it is a true abdominoplasty flap and does not violate the integrity of the anterior abdominal wall. The disadvantages of this flap are that the superficial inferior epigastric artery and vein are not usable in approximately 50% of patients and that the perfusion capacity of the flap is generally restricted to zones 1 and 2.

Since the initial descriptions of these three microvascular flaps for breast reconstruction, controversies have existed as to which is best or preferred. The debates are focused over flap perfusion and abdominal morbidity. It can be argued that the free TRAM has the best perfusion because it typically includes the greatest number of perforators. However, the free TRAM by definition includes a segment of the rectus abdominis muscle whereas the others do not. Thus, the questions that arise are whether there is a functional difference between the free TRAM, DIEP, and SIEA flaps, whether this difference is amplified with bilateral reconstruction compared with unilateral reconstructions, and whether differences in perfusion results in differences in fat necrosis, reoperation rates, or total flap failure. The following chapters will address the specifics of all three flaps to improve the readers understanding of the risks and benefits of microvascular breast reconstruction using the abdomen as the donor site.

References

1. Holmström H. The free abdominoplasty flap and its use in breast reconstruction. *Scand J Plast Reconstr Surg.* 1979;13:423–427. *This is the first paper describing the free abdominoplasty flap for breast reconstruction. Failures and successes are reviewed as well as angiographic studies.*

2. Hartrampf CR, Scheflan M, Black PW. Breast reconstruction with a transverse abdominal island flap. *Plast Reconstr Surg.* 1982;69:216–225. *This is the original manuscript describing the pedicle TRAM for breast reconstruction. The anatomy and surgical technique is highlighted.*

3. Grotting JC, Urist MM, Maddox WA, et al. Conventional TRAM flap versus free microsurgical TRAM flap for immediate breast reconstruction. *Plast Reconstr Surg.* 1989;83:828–841. *This paper compares the pedicle and free TRAM flaps for breast reconstruction. The free TRAM compared favorably to the pedicle TRAM in terms of complications, operating time, blood loss, hospitalization, and functional return.*

4. Allen RJ, Treece P. Deep inferior epigastric perforator flap for breast reconstruction. *Ann Plast Surg.* 1994;32:32–38. *This is the original paper describing the DIEP flap for breast reconstruction. A total of 15 flaps were used based on 1, 2, or 3 perforators.*

5. Koshima I, Soeda S. Inferior epigastric artery skin flaps without rectus abdominis muscle. *Br J Plast Surg.* 1989;42:645–648. *The DIEP flap is described without harvesting the rectus abdominis muscle. The authors demonstrate that a single perforator is capable of perfusing an entire flap.*

6. Arnez ZM, Khan U, Pogorelec D, et al. Breast reconstruction using the free superficial inferior epigastric artery (SIEA) flap. *Br J Plast Surg.* 1999;52:276–279. *This paper reviews the authors' experience with five flaps based on the superficial system. The authors describe the anatomy and technique for flap harvest.*

7. Grotting JC. The free abdominoplasty flap for immediate breast reconstruction. *Ann Plast Surg.* 1991;27:351–354. *The free abdominoplasty flap is described demonstrating that muscle does not have to be harvested with a flap to achieve successful outcomes.*

20.2

The deep inferior epigastric artery perforator (DIEAP) flap

Philip N. Blondeel, Colin M. Morrison, and Robert J. Allen, Sr

Access video and video lecture content for this chapter online at expertconsult.com

SYNOPSIS

- The deep inferior epigastric artery perforator (DIEAP) flap provides a large volume of soft, malleable tissue that resembles the natural consistency of the breast.
- DIEAP flap dissection is comparable with conventional myocutaneous free flap surgery, once the initial learning curve is overcome.
- The main advantage of the DIEAP flap is preservation of full rectus abdominis muscle function with less donor site morbidity.
- In experienced hands, the DIEAP flap loss rate is less than 1%.
- The DIEAP flap is the perforator flap of choice for autologous breast reconstruction.

 Access the Historical Perspective section online at
http://www.expertconsult.com

Introduction

Perforator flaps have become increasingly popular in recent years. They are at the top of the reconstructive ladder and are considered an advancement of musculocutaneous and fasciocutaneous flaps. Passive muscle and fascial carriers are no longer required to ensure flap vascularity, and by virtue of their composition, perforator flaps permit excellent "like for like" tissue replacement with minimal aesthetic or functional donor morbidity. Perforator flaps are usually thin, pliable, easily moldable flaps that are well suited to resurfacing work. They are also ideal for reconstructing pliable structures such as the tongue or for molding complex contours in the head and neck region. Perforator flaps

with large amounts of subcutaneous fat are ideal for reconstructing the breast.

A perforator flap is defined as a flap of skin and subcutaneous tissue, which is supplied by an isolated perforator vessel. Perforators pass from their source vessel to the skin surface either through or between the deep tissues (mostly muscle). Any vessel that traverses through muscle before perforating the outer layer of the deep fascia to supply the overlying skin is termed a "myocutaneous perforator". A vessel that traverses through septum, i.e., between the muscle bellies, is designated a "septocutaneous perforator".

Evolution of perforator flaps has been intimately related to growing knowledge of the blood supply to the skin and the history of musculocutaneous and fasciocutaneous flap development.

The deep inferior epigastric artery perforator (DIEAP) flap arose as a refinement of the conventional myocutaneous lower abdominal flap. The myocutaneous perforators of the inferior epigastric vessels were described[1] soon after the first transverse rectus abdominis myocutaneous (TRAM) flap was performed for breast reconstruction by Holmström and Robbins.[2,3] In the mid-1980s, following Taylor's landmark work on the vascular territory of the deep inferior epigastric artery, it became apparent that the lower abdominal flap could be perfused solely by a large periumbilical perforating vessel. That assumption was confirmed in 1989, when Koshima and Soeda[4] published two cases of "inferior epigastric skin flaps without rectus abdominis muscle".

Initially the DIEAP flap met with animosity from many in the surgical community, as it challenged conventional teaching and was thought to be unsafe.

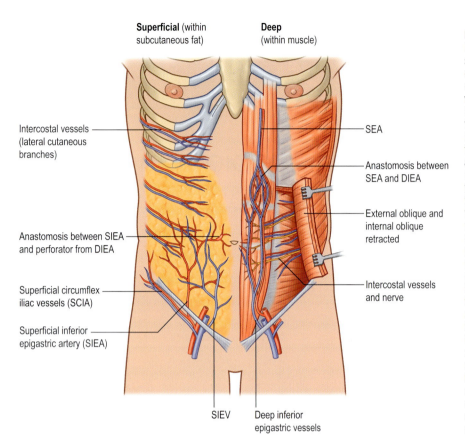

Superficial (within subcutaneous fat)

Deep (within muscle)

Intercostal vessels (lateral cutaneous branches)

Anastomosis between SIEA and perforator from DIEA

Superficial circumflex iliac vessels (SCIA)

Superficial inferior epigastric artery (SIEA)

SEA

Anastomosis between SEA and DIEA

External oblique and internal oblique retracted

Intercostal vessels and nerve

SIEV   Deep inferior epigastric vessels

Fig. 20.2.1 The vascular anatomy of the lower abdomen. In the right hemi-abdomen, the skin is removed down to the superficial inferior epigastric vessels. The artery with its common veins, and the superficial inferior epigastric vein can be found medial to the superficial circumflex iliac vessels. Around the umbilicus, the perforators of the deep inferior epigastric system connect with arteries and veins of the superficial system. The anterior branches of the intercostal arteries and veins move anterior and distally from their origin at the midaxillary line. Variable anastomoses between these different vessels make up for a complex and intense random network between the skin and the deep fascia. On the left side of the abdomen, the deep fascia of the rectus abdominis muscle is removed and the fascia of the external and internal oblique have been retracted. The deep inferior epigastric artery and vein pass deep to the lateral board of rectus abdominis as they move more cranially and enter into the rectus abdominis a few centimeters higher. Segmental branches of the deep inferior epigastric system connect with the anterior branch of the intercostal artery and veins (particularly the lateral branch of the deep inferior epigastric artery). The anterior intercostal nerves run together with the segmental branches and branch into sensory branches that run with the perforators into the subcutaneous tissues and motor branches that run medial and distally in the rectus abdominis muscle. More cranially, the deep inferior epigastric vessels anastomose in the diffuse network throughout the muscle with the superior epigastric artery. DIEA, deep inferior epigastric artery; SEA, superior epigastric artery; SCIA, superficial circumflex iliac artery; SIEA, superficial inferior epigastric artery; SIEV, superficial inferior epigastric vein.

However, we are now in an era where DIEAP flaps are routinely performed in plastic surgery units throughout the world.[5]

With an increased emphasis on optimizing the aesthetic result and minimizing donor site morbidity, in the authors' opinion, the DIEAP flap is the current gold standard in breast reconstruction.

Basic science/anatomy

The deep inferior epigastric artery perforator (DIEAP) flap

The deep inferior epigastric artery arises from the external iliac, immediately above the inguinal ligament. It curves forward in the subperitoneal tissue and then ascends obliquely along the medial margin of the abdominal inguinal ring. Continuing its course upward, it pierces the transversalis fascia, passing in front of the linea semicircularis, ascending between the rectus abdominis and the posterior lamella of its sheath.

The deep inferior epigastric artery finally divides into numerous branches, which anastomose, above the umbilicus, with the superior epigastric branch of the internal thoracic artery and with the lower intercostal arteries (Figs. 20.2.1 & 20.2.2).

The anatomy of the deep inferior epigastric artery system is very variable.[15,16] The average pedicle length is 10.3 cm, and the average vessel diameter is 3.6 mm. Normally, the deep inferior epigastric artery divides into two branches, with a dominant lateral branch (54%). However, if the deep inferior epigastric artery does not divide, the vessel has a central course (28%) with multiple small branches to the muscle and centrally located perforators. If the medial branch is dominant (18%),

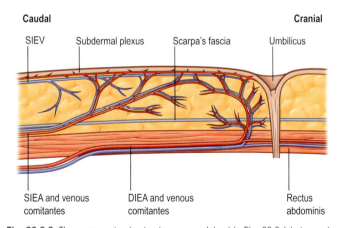

Caudal

Cranial

SIEV   Subdermal plexus   Scarpa's fascia   Umbilicus

SIEA and venous comitantes   DIEA and venous comitantes   Rectus abdominis

Fig. 20.2.2 The same anatomic structures as explained in Fig. 20.2.1 but seen in a paramedian sagittal view. SIEA - superficial inferior epigastric artery; DIEA - deep inferior epigastric artery; SCIA - superficial circumflex iliac artery; SEA - superior epigastric artery; SIEV - superficial inferior epigastric vein

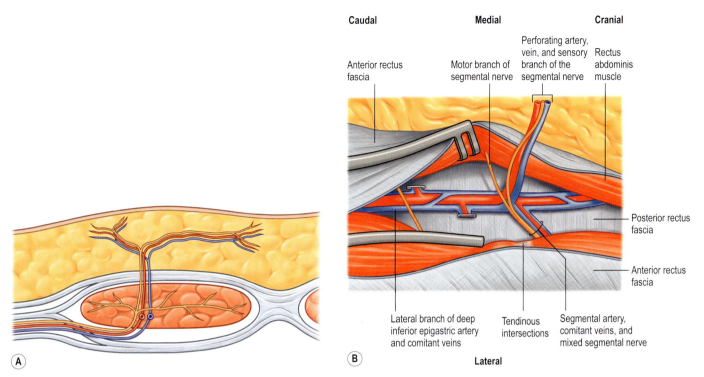

Fig. 20.2.3 (A,B) The anatomy of the intercostal nerves. The mixed intercostal nerves run below the fascia of the internal oblique and predominantly enter the rectus abdominis muscle at its posterior surface at the level of the lateral branch of the deep inferior epigastric artery. They follow the intercostal and segmental vessels and mostly pass over the submuscular or intramuscular part of the lateral branch of the deep inferior epigastric artery. At that point, it splits into two motor branches, one lateral and one medial, and additionally into a pure sensory nerve that accompanies the perforating artery and vein.

flow appears to be significantly lower than in a central system or in patients with a dominant lateral branch.[17]

Blondeel *et al.*[17] found between two and eight large (>0.5 mm) perforators on each side of the midline. The majority of these perforators emerged from the anterior rectus fascia in a paramedian rectangular area 2 cm cranial and 6 cm caudal to the umbilicus and between 1 and 6 cm lateral to the umbilicus. Anatomic symmetry was hardly ever encountered. The closer a perforator is to the midline, the better the blood supply to the least vascularized part of the flap across the midline, as one choke vessel less has to be transgressed. However, the lateral perforators are often dominant and easier to dissect because they run more perpendicularly through the muscle. The sensory nerve that runs with these perforating vessels is also often much larger (Fig. 20.2.3). The medial perforators provide better perfusion of the flap, but they have a longer intramuscular course, requiring more elaborate dissection with extensive longitudinal splitting of the muscle. An alternative is to extend the design of the flap to include more tissue from the flank. If one is uncertain as to whether or not enough volume can be transferred, the perforators can be dissected on both sides (Siamese flap).[6]

Preference is also given to perforators that pass through the rectus abdominis muscle at the level of the tendinous intersections. At this point, the perforators

are frequently large and have few muscular side branches. The distance from the subcutaneous fat to the deep inferior epigastric vessels is also shorter, simplifying this most delicate part of the dissection.[18]

As a result, the design of a DIEAP flap is made over the most centrally located, dominant perforator, lateral or medial, as long as sufficient abdominal subcutaneous fat tissue is available and the least vascularized part of the flap across the midline can be discarded (Fig. 20.2.4). At the origin of the perforator, several nerves are encountered (see Fig. 20.2.3). Although there is no constant anatomy, mixed segmental nerves run underneath or through the muscle from laterally and split into a sensate nerve running with the perforator into the flap and a motor nerve crossing on top of the deep inferior epigastric vessels distal to the bifurcation of the perforator, into the medial part of the rectus abdominis muscle.[19] One should always expect and anticipate a variety of anatomic differences.

The superficial inferior epigastric artery (SIEA) originates 2–3 cm below the inguinal ligament directly from the common femoral artery (17%) or from a common origin with the superficial circumflex iliac artery (48%). It then passes superiorly and laterally in the femoral triangle lying deep to Scarpa's fascia and crosses the inguinal ligament at the midpoint between the anterior superior iliac spine and the pubic tubercle. Above the

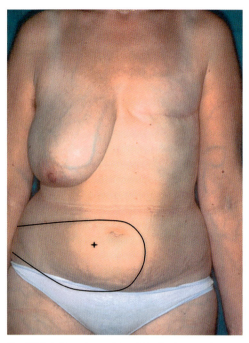

Fig. 20.2.4 Once the position of the dominant perforator is located on the abdomen, the flap is centered over this perforator. The incision on the abdomen is symmetrical on both sides, but the least vascularized part of the flap will be discarded.

inguinal ligament, the SIEA pierces Scarpa's fascia and lies in the superficial subcutaneous tissue. During its course, the SIEA lies deep to and parallel to the superficial inferior epigastric vein. The vein drains directly into the saphenous bulb.[20]

The SIEA is seen as a direct perforator to the skin while the perforators of the deep system are considered indirect perforators (Fig. 20.2.5). Of all vessels, it is important to choose the largest, most dominant

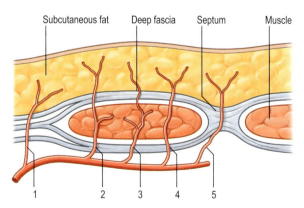

Fig. 20.2.5 The different types of perforators that can be found at the lower abdominal wall. (1) The branches of the superficial inferior epigastric artery are direct perforators that vascularize the subcutaneous fat and skin after perforating the deep and superficial fascia. All other perforators are indirect perforators; (2) perforators that have a predominant vascularization of the subcutaneous fat tissue and skin with few muscular branches; (3) perforators that branch off of side branches that have a predominant goal of nourishing the muscle; (4) perforators that pass through the rectus abdominis muscle without branching; (5) perforators that pass through the septum or around the rectus abdominis muscle with the sole purpose of vascularizing the subcutaneous tissues.

perforator destined to vascularize the fat and skin that has few or no side branches to the muscle.

The superficial inferior epigastric vein is the largest vein draining the skin paddle of the DIEAP flap. It is located below the dermal plexus but above Scarpa's fascia, midway between the anterior superior iliac spine and the pubic symphysis. Harvesting an elliptical skin island transects this vein, redirecting the venous drainage through the smaller perforating veins. Connections between the superficial epigastric vein and the deep inferior epigastric system exist in every patient, but substantial medial branches crossing the midline have been found to be absent in 36% of cases.[21,22] In these flaps, venous connections are only present through the subdermal capillary network. This explains why the portion of a flap farthest from the midline may suffer from venous congestion and why the presence of this problem is so variable and unpredictable.

The lymphatic drainage of the DIEAP flap can be divided into a superficial and a deep system. The superficial collectors are located directly underneath the reticular dermis. Deep cuts performed during de-epithelialization may injure this system. The superficial collectors drain to the superficial lymph nodes in the groin. The deep system drains the deep structures of the abdominal wall, i.e., the muscles and fascia and is located in close proximity to the arteries and veins. Careful dissection of the vascular pedicle avoids iatrogenic damage to this lymphatic system. The deep system drains to the inferior epigastric artery and then to the deep iliac nodes.[23]

Recipient vessels

The internal mammary artery and its accompanying veins are the first choice for DIEAP flap breast reconstruction.[10,12,24] Its central position on the chest wall facilitates microsurgery and offers the most flexibility during breast shaping. The vessels are easy to dissect and are usually protected from radiotherapy damage. In a number of irradiated vessels perivascular fibrosis can be encountered. Chest wall inflammation, following infected implant removal or extreme capsular fibrosis, can sometimes cause severe perivascular scarring.

Although the artery is usually of sufficient caliber, the size of the veins is very variable. In most cases, the veins on the left side of the chest wall are smaller than those on the right side. For this reason, the authors prefer to dissect the vessels at the level of the left third or fourth rib, but at the level of the fourth rib on the right side. A small segment of cartilage can be removed together with some intercostal muscles, both cranially and caudally (Fig. 20.2.6). This provides sufficient exposure of

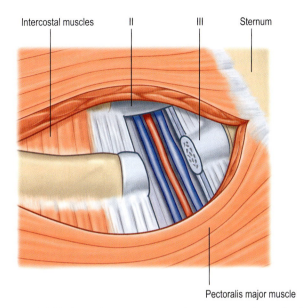

Intercostal muscles | II | III | Sternum

Pectoralis major muscle

Fig. 20.2.6 The internal mammary artery and two common veins on the right side after removing a small part of the costal cartilage of the third rib.

the vessels and adequate recipient vessel length. One can also limit the dissection and exposure to the removal of only the intercostal muscles. Wider exposure can be obtained by nibbling away the lower border of the superior rib and the upper border of the inferior rib.

At the level of the second and third intercostal space, large perforators sometimes emerge from between the intercostal muscles to perforate the medial part of the pectoralis major muscle. The size of these vessels is variable, and it is estimated that they can only be used as recipient vessels for free flaps in about 5–10% of cases. These vessels can be identified and evaluated above and below the pectoralis during preparation of the recipient site. If no adequate perforators are found, the internal mammary artery and the accompanying veins are then prepared.[25]

Patient presentation

When designing a DIEAP flap, the main factor is the amount of viable tissue that can be harvested on a particular perforator. The most accurate indicator of this is preoperative localization of the dominant source of blood inflow by duplex Doppler or computed tomography (CT) imaging. In addition to defining the "safe" flap territory, these techniques provide a degree of reassurance by avoiding intraoperative surprises, and considerably reduce operative time. A reduction of operative costs significantly decreases the overall expense of the reconstructive procedure.

More recently, magnetic resonance angiography has shown promise in the imaging of perforators. In

addition to producing accurate and detailed images, there is no radiation exposure,[26] unlike CT imaging.

Besides this imaging, the conventional preoperative work-up includes blood work, oncologic screening, and additional tests for concomitant diseases if necessary.

Ultrasound evaluation of perforator vessels

This is performed with a color Doppler, which employs a combination of grayscale and color Doppler imaging. This modality has 100% positive predictive value and few false-negatives.[27]

Grayscale imaging shows the anatomic detail of fixed points, axial vessels, and perforating branches. The addition of color Doppler allows identification of blood flow, direction (towards or away from the probe), pattern of flow (i.e., venous or arterial), and finally a measure of blood flow velocity.[28–31]

The disadvantages of color duplex lie in its lack of anatomic detail and operator dependence. It requires a detailed knowledge of 3D vascular anatomy, as well as expertise in the handling of the devise. While it provides dynamic information about blood flow, this may lead to a false sense of security because humeral and nervous stimuli can affect the microcirculation and cause fluctuations in vessel flow. Hence, flow rates do not always correlate with the size of the perforator.

In addition to preoperative imaging, it is possible to use a unidirectional hand-held pencil probe for identification of superficial vessels in the operating theatre. The perforators identified can be marked on the patient's skin to allow accurate flap design and aid intraoperative dissection. This is a simple and inexpensive technique, which provides a useful intraoperative adjunct.[32] There can, however, be false-negative and false-positive signals as a result of interference from axial vessels or perforators that run parallel to the fascia, before entering their suprafascial course.

CT imaging

Multidetector-row helical CT is a recent innovation that permits rapid delineation of an anatomic area of interest, giving excellent resolution and low artifact rating. It takes less than 10 min to perform and is well tolerated by patients. This has become the modality of choice for the identification of abdominal wall perforators.[33–35] The use of magnetic resonance imaging (MRI) to avoid the high X-ray dose is promising but still needs further refinement.[36]

The scanning is performed in conjunction with intravenous contrast medium and allows evaluation of the donor and recipient vessels. Information collected includes the exact location and intramuscular course of

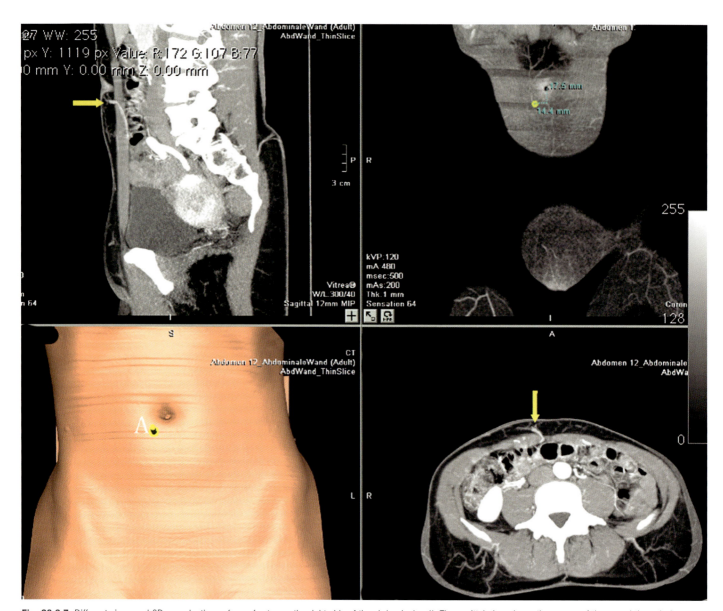

Fig. 20.2.7 Different views and 3D reproductions of a perforator on the right side of the abdominal wall. The sagittal view shows the course of the vessel through the rectus abdominis muscle. The location of the perforator is described in relation to the umbilicus.

vessels from their origin, the caliber of the perforators, and also identifies the dominant vessel. Delineation of the relative dominance of the deep and superficial systems allows the surgeon to consider different options preoperatively. Not only can this modality be used to select suitable patients preoperatively but also operative times are reduced by a mean of 21%, with the obvious associated cost benefits.[37]

The disadvantages of multidetector-row helical CT lie in the X-ray dosage and use of intravenous contrast media, with the resultant risk of anaphylaxis. The X-ray dose, albeit significant, is less than a conventional liver CT scan and can be combined with staging investigations to reduce the overall exposure. Interpretation of the images can be done before and during surgery by the surgeon him/herself and correlated to intraoperative findings (Figs. 20.2.7 & 20.2.8).

Patient selection

Patients eligible for an autologous breast reconstruction with a DIEAP or SIEA flap are mainly those with sufficient lower abdominal subcutaneous fat tissue. In Western society, many women are good candidates, but cultural differences can apply. For example, Asian women are generally slimmer and may prefer other donor sites such as the anterolateral thigh area. The lower abdomen is, however, first preference for autologous breast reconstruction. Only in very slender women, or in cases where scarring of the abdominal wall

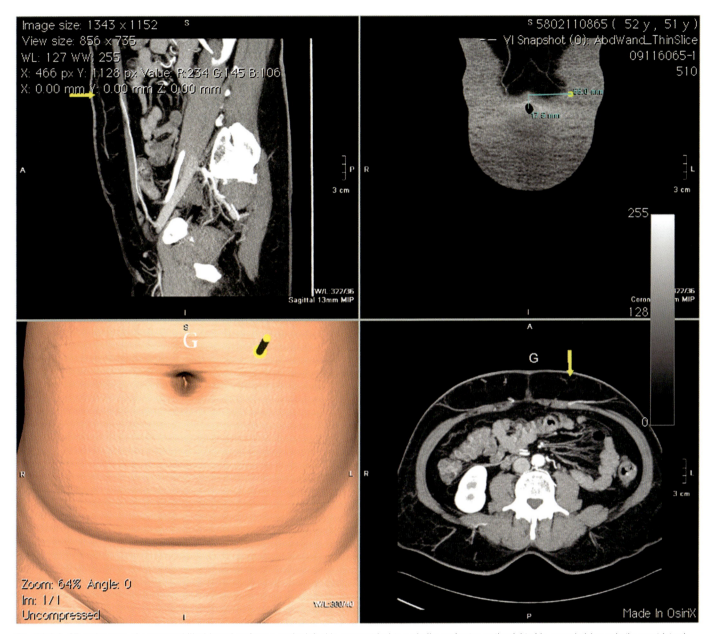

Fig. 20.2.8 CT-angiograms of a supraumbilical lateral perforator on the left side, symmetrical to a similar perforator on the right side, vascularizing only the most lateral parts of the lower abdomen. The sagittal view shows a relatively easy dissection as the vessel penetrates directly in the muscle, but choosing this perforator means that tissue beyond the midline will not be vascularized.

endangers the normal blood circulation of the free flap or the abdominoplasty flap, secondary options, such as gluteal perforator flaps or internal thigh flaps, are considered. Pedicled latissimus dorsi or thoracodorsal artery perforator flaps in combination with an implant are further down the reconstructive ladder and implant basic techniques are avoided if possible.

Severe obesity, uncontrolled diabetes, debilitating cardiovascular disease, and uncontrollable coagulopathies are the most frequent examples of absolute contraindications to DIEP flap reconstruction. Smokers and unmotivated patients are advised to postpone their surgery if oncologically possible. Implant reconstruction is only recommended in patients with a poor prognosis or those with a limited life span because of age or concurrent disease. In addition, patients objecting to donor site scars, those refusing complex surgery, or those unable to accept the possible microsurgical complications are seen as candidates for implant-based surgery.

Surgical technique

Preoperative marking

For this surgical technique,[38] the patient is marked in a standing position. A fusiform skin island is drawn on the abdomen, similar to the one used for breast reconstruction with a free TRAM flap, but the bulk of the flap is centered over the selected perforator. Although the size and shape may vary slightly, the borders of a DIEAP flap are generally located at the level of the suprapubic crease, the umbilicus, and both anterior superior iliac spines, but the flap may be extended laterally to the midaxillary lines.

A DIEAP flap generally measures 12–15 cm in height and 30–45 cm in width. However, the tension of the donor site following closure should be estimated, as this ultimately limits the size of the flap that can be harvested. A horizontal line is drawn just above the umbilicus and another one marked 12–15 cm below this. At a level 2 cm below the umbilicus, the lateral limits of the flap are marked 15–23 cm on either side of the midline. The amount of subcutaneous fat present in the flanks is assessed, as this can be included in the flap if required (Fig. 20.2.9A). All the outer markings are connected by a continuous line placed in natural skin creases.

Operative procedure (see Video 20.2.1 ◉)

The patient is placed in a supine position with the arms positioned beside the trunk. If available, imaging data is drawn on the patient's abdomen using a 1 cm grid system based on the umbilicus. Two intravenous lines, an indwelling urinary catheter, and antithrombotic stockings are applied. A warming blanket is used to keep the patients core body temperature at 37°C. The proposed incision lines are infiltrated with a dilute solution of local anesthetic and adrenaline (40 mL 1% xylocaine with 1/100000 adrenaline in 40 mL sterile water), except in the region of the superficial epigastric veins. Three separate stab incisions are then placed around the umbilicus and connected with the aid of skin hooks. The umbilicus is incised circumferentially down to the fascia. While making the inferior incision, care is taken to preserve the superficial epigastric veins. If the venous drainage of the flap is insufficient or thrombosis of the perforating vein(s) occurs after the anastomosis, the superficial epigastric veins can be used as an additional venous conduit. Two or three veins may be present, but they commonly unite further down the abdominal wall. The veins are dissected over a length of 2–3 cm and ligated with clips to make them easily retrievable later, if needed. If the caliber of the superficial epigastric artery is noted to be large enough, a similar skin island to the DIEAP flap can be harvested on these two vessels. The incisions are continued down to the fascia. Beveling is avoided unless extra volume is required, as this may later lead to a depressed scar in the lower abdomen. Laterally however, the flap may be beveled to include more fat and reduce residual "dog-ears".

Dissection of the vascular pedicle of a DIEAP flap can be divided into three different technical stages: suprafascial, intramuscular, and submuscular. The most demanding stage is the intramuscular dissection of the vascular pedicle.

Suprafascial dissection

Dissection begins laterally in the flanks and progresses medially with the aid of cutting and coagulating diathermy. The skin and subcutaneous fat are lifted off the external oblique fascia up to the lateral border of the rectus abdominis muscle. At this point, dissection proceeds more cautiously as the perforators are identified. Gentle traction on the flap helps provide good exposure of the vessels. Again, if imaging data is available, the dissection can progress rapidly to the preselected perforator, with ligation of the more laterally placed perforators (Fig. 20.2.9B). If only a unidirectional Doppler probe was used, one can try to visualize as many perforators as possible before selecting the largest one. This method needs some expertise, can be time-consuming, and does not allow evaluation of all the medial perforators.

If the caliber of one vessel is estimated to be insufficient, an adjacent perforator located on the same vertical line can also be dissected. The abdominal wall muscles must be relaxed at all times and the perforating vessels kept moist with normal saline. No antispasmodic agents are routinely used. When dissecting a perforator from the lateral side, it is important to realize that a side branch may be located more medially. Extra care must be taken when dissecting the full circumference of a vessel, but complete dissection helps prevent vessel damage when raising the flap from the contralateral side (Fig. 20.2.9C,D).

The anterior rectus fascia is then incised with a pair of scissors following the direction of the rectus abdominis muscle fibers at the rim of the tiny gap in the fascia through which the perforating vessel passes (Fig. 20.2.9E). If more than one perforator is dissected, the different gaps can be connected with each other. A small cuff of fascia may be left around the perforator if the vessel is small or if the surgeon feels more comfortable doing so.

Lifting the fascia helps mobilize the perforator, which can be freed by blunt dissection, gently pushing away the loose connective tissue. The perforator can be adherent to the deep surface of the anterior rectus fascia for a variable distance before it plunges into the muscle. The division of the fascia is continued superiorly for a distance of 3–4 cm and inferiorly to the lateral border of the rectus abdominis muscle in an oblique line towards the inguinal ligament (Fig. 20.2.9F). At this point, the direction of the division of the fascia is changed into the direction of the fibers of the external oblique muscle. This avoids a continuous area of weakness of the lower abdominal wall, as closure of the fascia is performed on top of the rectus abdominis muscle. Two separate incisions, one around the perforator and one over the deep inferior epigastric vessels at the lower lateral border of the rectus muscle, can also be performed.

It is advisable to fully complete the dissection of the DIEAP flap on one side before progressing to the other.

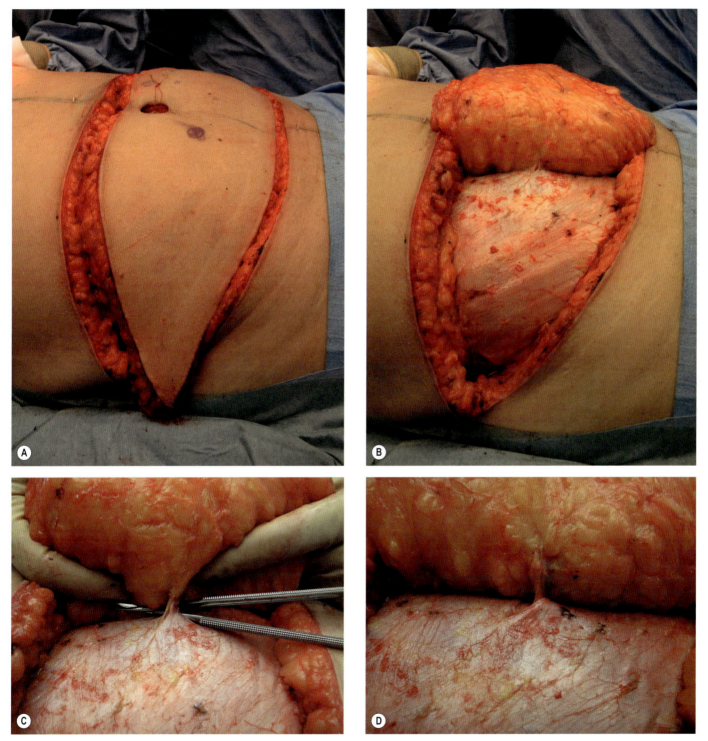

Fig. 20.2.9 **(A)** Incision of skin and subcutaneous tissue is extended towards the flanks if additional tissue is needed. The dominant perforator on the right side is marked with an 'x' on the flap. **(B)** The flap is elevated from lateral to medial until the area around the preoperatively marked perforator is reached. Undermining is then continued proximal and distal to the perforator. **(C)** Undermining continues around the perforator for a distance of about 2 cm. Lifting up the subcutaneous tissue is easier at this point when the deep fascia is still closed. **(D)** Access to the perivascular loose connective tissue is found by incising the gap in the deep fascia and the tissues surrounding the vessels. *Continued*

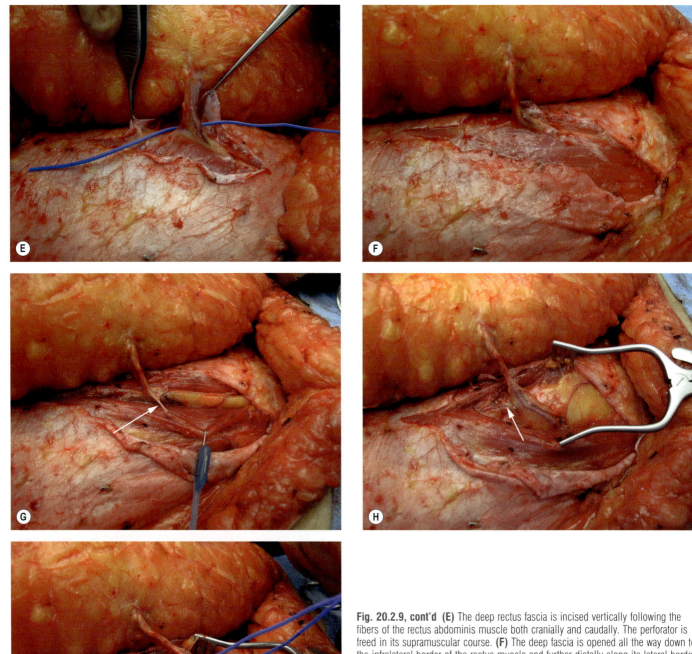

Fig. 20.2.9, cont'd **(E)** The deep rectus fascia is incised vertically following the fibers of the rectus abdominis muscle both cranially and caudally. The perforator is freed in its supramuscular course. **(F)** The deep fascia is opened all the way down to the infralateral border of the rectus muscle and further distally along its lateral border to create exposure of the deep inferior epigastric artery and vein. **(G)** The rectus abdominis muscle is split following the muscle fibers until the posterior fascia or the peritoneum can be seen. Sensory nerves coming from lateral and following the perforator can be transected. Motor nerves are left intact (white arrow). **(H)** Wide exposure is achieved with a self-retaining retractor. A bloodless field allows perfect control of the dissection. The main branch of the deep inferior epigastric artery and its veins is clipped distal to the perforator (white arrow). **(I)** Once the entire course of the perforator and the main vessel is clear, the posterior part of the perforator and the main vessel is dissected off the surrounding tissues. The distal part of the deep inferior epigastric vessels can be dissected either through the same incision through the rectus muscle or from laterally by pulling the rectus muscle medially.

This allows a "life boat" in the form of a contralateral DIEAP flap or TRAM flap to be performed if the perforator is inadvertently damaged. It is important to emphasize that the vessels must be protected at all stages and complete muscle relaxation is necessary until donor site closure is obtained. As dissection progresses,

the DIEAP flap should be secured to the abdominal wall with the aid of staples.

Intramuscular dissection

The rectus abdominis muscle should be split in a longitudinal direction in the perimysial plane through which the perforating vessel traverses. Splitting the muscle fibers makes dissection easier as the vessel becomes larger (Fig. 20.2.9G). The perforator is again liberated by blunt dissection, staying close to the vessel at all times, as it remains covered by a thin layer of loose connective tissue. As a general rule, if resistance to dissection is encountered, a side branch or a nerve will be identified. Different muscular branches must be ligated with care, and hemoclips are placed 1–2 mm away from the main vessel so that if one inadvertently comes off, it can easily be replaced. This technique avoids damage and spasm of the main perforating vessel. Placing a vessel loop around the vascular pedicle allows additional retraction without any unnecessary tension being placed on the vessel. Using bipolar coagulating diathermy and small hemoclips, one continues to ligate all the side branches until the origin of the perforator on the major branch of the deep inferior epigastric vessel is reached at the posterior surface of the rectus abdominis muscle (Fig. 20.2.9H).

If two perforators have been selected, the rectus abdominis muscle must be widely separated. If the perforators run in two adjacent perimysial planes, the fibers may have to be cut. However, transection of large parts of the rectus abdominis muscle or division at the level where a motor nerve crosses from the lateral to the medial side should be avoided.

Submuscular dissection

The lateral border of the rectus abdominis is raised using non-crushing tissue forceps. Special care is taken not to injure the mixed segmental nerves entering the muscle laterally. The sensory nerve branch can be dissected by epineural splitting.[19] In this way, an additional 5–9 cm can be obtained, facilitating neural suturing at the recipient site. If possible, all the motor branches are left intact. However, in cases where a motor branch runs between two perforators, then this nerve has to be cut. Once the flap is harvested, it can be re-sutured.

Between the mixed segmental nerves, the plane posterior to the rectus abdominis muscle is opened, exposing the main deep inferior epigastric vessel. Side branches of the main stem are ligated, and the dissection is continued by retracting the rectus abdominis muscle medially until the proximal part of the pedicle is completely liberated. The length of the pedicle can be tailored to meet the needs of different recipient sites or the demands of the shape of the flap (Fig. 20.2.9I). The more distal the perforator is located in the flap, the further the deep inferior epigastric vessels need to be dissected into the groin. Frequently however, the pedicle can be transected at the lateral border of the rectus abdominis muscle. At this level, there is sufficient

pedicle diameter and length to enable a safe microsurgical anastomosis.

If one is certain that the blood flow through the deep inferior epigastric vessel is sufficient (an ultrasonic flow meter can be used), the remainder of the flap can be raised. In cases of midline scars, or when a large flap is needed, the same vascular dissection can be performed on the contralateral side. Otherwise, all the remaining perforators are ligated, the umbilicus is released and the entire skin flap is raised. The pedicle is finally transected when the recipient vessels have been prepared. A hemoclip can be placed on the lateral comitant vein to help orientate the pedicle.

After division of the pedicle, the flap is turned over and the vessels placed carefully onto its undersurface. One has to be meticulous about the position of the pedicle, as it tends to rotate very easily, especially if only one perforator has been harvested. The flap is then weighed, photographed, and transferred. The ischemia time is noted. The flap is placed on moist gauze at the recipient site to prevent desiccation and again stapled to the surrounding skin for security. The flap may be rotated to facilitate microsurgery, provided a note of this is made and the rotation reversed at the end of the procedure.

Hints and tips

Ten golden rules in perforator flap surgery

1. *Map the perforators preoperatively*: identify the most dominant vessels on each side.
2. *Start dissection on one side of the flap*: leave the contralateral side intact until you have finished the entire dissection of the pedicle.
3. *Preserve every perforator until you encounter a larger one*: discard only the smaller ones that you are sure you will not use. Select one or two perforators with the largest diameter that correspond with your preoperative mapping.
4. *Consider the best location of the perforator within the flap*: the more centrally located, the better blood flow to the outer parts of the flap.
5. *Consider the easiest dissection through the muscle*: long intramuscular dissections are more tedious, increase the risk of damaging the vessels, and are more time-consuming.
6. *Dissect close to the vessels*, remaining within the perivascular loose connective tissue, thereby guaranteeing a bloodless field.
7. *Ensure wide exposure* by splitting the rectus muscle along its fibers (avoid digging a small hole).
8. *Carefully ligate every side-branch* at a distance of about 2 mm away from the main pedicle.
9. *Avoid traction on the perforator*: intima rupture is a frequent cause of unexplained clotting of the perforator.
10. *Transect the other perforators after the entire pedicle is dissected*.

Closure of the donor site and fashioning of the umbilicus

As no fascia has been resected, primary tension-free closure of the fascia with a running, non-absorbable 1-0 suture is always possible. The upper skin flap is undermined using cutting diathermy to the level of the xiphoid and costal margin. Two suction drains are placed at the upper and lower margins of the skin flaps and brought out suprapubically on each side of the midline. The lower border of the umbilicus is marked on the anterior abdominal wall at the level of the anterior superior iliac spines and a 2 cm vertical line is drawn above this point. Only a vertical incision is performed. The anterior abdominal wall is extensively thinned at the site of the new umbilicus by trimming of the subcutaneous fat. The umbilicus is then passed through the defect and inset with an interrupted 4-0 absorbable sutures.

The operating table is put in a flexed position to facilitate closure of the anterior abdominal wall. Scarpa's fascia is approximated with interrupted 1-0 absorbable sutures with particular attention being paid to medial advancement of the wound edges to reduce the dog-ears in the flanks. Finally, interrupted 3-0 sutures are placed intradermally to evert the skin edges and a skin adhesive is applied. No further abdominal dressing is used.

Shaping of the DIEAP flap in secondary autologous breast reconstruction

A systematic approach is applied to create easy and reproducible results in shaping of autologous tissue by using the "3-step principle"[11,12] producing a 3D structure from a flat piece of abdominal fat, and skin is broken down into three essential steps: (1) redefining and recreating the basis and borders of the footprint of the breast (the interface of the posterior surface of the breast gland and the thorax) at the right location on the chest wall (Fig. 20.2.10); (2) molding the flap into a tear drop-shaped conus on top of the footprint by means of specific suturing (Fig. 20.2.11); and (3) repositioning the skin envelope (Fig. 20.2.12) over the conus with the correct tension (Fig. 20.2.13).

The breast footprint

Any previous scars or severely damaged tissue that lies over the footprint of the new breast are excised. In modified radical mastectomy cases, the new inframammary fold is incised to a depth of approximately 1 cm to allow easy suturing of the DIEAP flap. While the position of the borders of the new footprint mirror the position of the contralateral footprint, the new inframammary fold position needs to be placed 2–3 cm higher

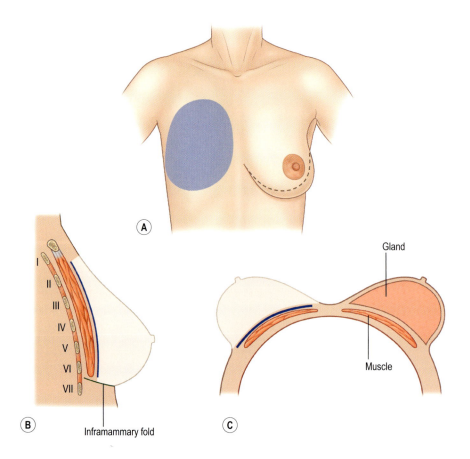

Fig. 20.2.10 (A) Coronal; **(B)** sagittal; and **(C)** transverse view of the footprint of the breast.

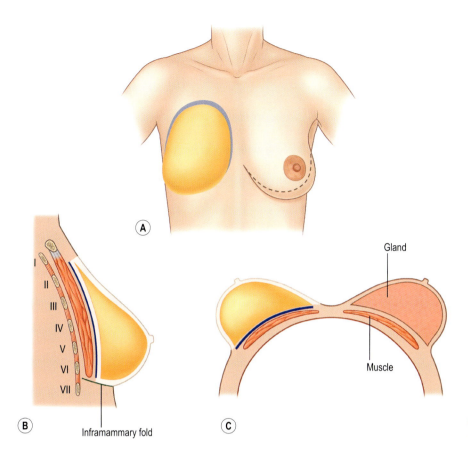

Fig. 20.2.11 (A) Coronal; **(B)** sagittal; and **(C)** transverse view of the conus of the breast.

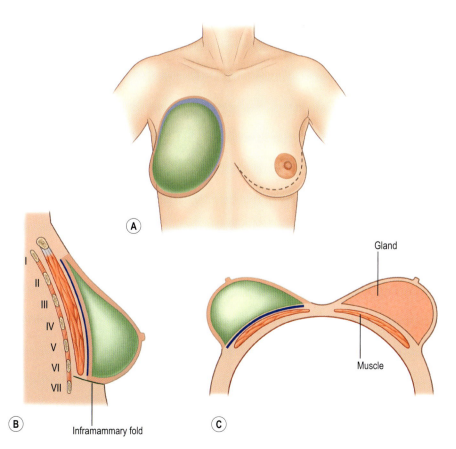

Fig. 20.2.12 (A) Coronal; **(B)** sagittal; and **(C)** transverse view of the envelope of the breast.

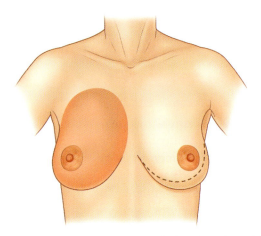

Fig. 20.2.13 The nipple areolar complex is an integral part of the envelope of the breast.

than the contralateral inframammary fold depending on the laxity of the mastectomy flap skin and tension exerted on the abdominoplasty flap closure later in the procedure. The skin in between the mastectomy scar and the inframammary fold is de-epithelialized. In this way, a layer of 1–2 cm of fat in the lower part of the breast is preserved, improving projection. The skin edges of the upper mastectomy flap are thinned down to the dermis for the first 5 mm and then progressively trimmed to obtain a seamless transition into the upper skin edge of the DIEAP flap. The upper mastectomy flap is then undermined on the lateral, cranial, and medial borders of the breast footprint to subsequently accommodate the flap.

In cases of primary breast reconstruction, the edges of the footprint are assumed to be intact. If for oncologic reasons the edges of the footprint need to be undermined or resected, these borders will need to be repaired before transferring the flap.

The breast conus

The authors prefer to use the contralateral DIEAP flap in cases of delayed breast reconstruction. The flap is rotated through 180° prior to transfer, and shaping begins after the anastomosis has been completed (Fig. 20.2.14A).

A wedge of skin is removed around the site of the umbilicus and closed in two layers. This simple maneuver gathers more volume in the lower half of the flap. The more skin that is removed, the more projection that can be achieved, but it does result in compression of the subdermal plexus in this area.

The tendon of the pectoralis major muscle is then identified. The tip of the DIEAP flap is fixed just below the pectoralis tendon by suturing Scarpa's fascia to the pectoralis fascia 2–3 cm medial to the lateral pectoral

muscle border. This first key suture recreates the anterior axillary fold (Fig. 20.2.14B).

The lateral edge of the flap is then stapled to the most lateral part of the inframammary fold under slight tension to avoid excessive lateral fullness (see Fig. 20.2.14B). The transition from the lateral pectoral border into the lateral portion of the flap also recreates a natural lazy-S shape along the lateral border of the breast. The exact position of the second key suture is determined by moving the flap along the inframammary fold while assessing the lazy-S contour. It is always better to have minimal fullness in this location at the time of reconstruction, as the flap will shift laterally and distally in the postoperative period.

Medial to the second key suture, in the midclavicular line, the skin of the flap is then bunched up (Fig. 20.2.14C). This, together with the triangular skin resection around the umbilicus, dramatically increases flap projection. It also helps create a sharp angle between the skin of the flap and the abdominal skin below the inframammary fold.

The third key suture is placed at the medial end of the inframammary fold. The flap is not bunched in this location to avoid overfilling of the inferomedial quadrant of the new breast. However, one should be cautious, as if the flap is not placed medially enough, it can be difficult to achieve sufficient cleavage.

Two important components are then assessed: a volume estimation of the DIEAP flap compared with the contralateral breast; and the poorly vascularized tissue in the flap that needs to be resected (previously zone IV, see Fig. 20.2.14C). The latter can be accomplished either by visual inspection of the skin, or by carving into the dermal plexus with a Bistouri in the most distal corner. Tissues that show mixed arterial and venous bleeding can be kept. When a DIEAP flap with an ipsilateral pedicle is used, poorly vascularized tissue is removed before placing the first key suture. The authors recommend making the reconstructed breast 5–10% larger than the contralateral side, anticipating a postoperative reduction in swelling.

The medial part of the flap is then rounded off, providing a smooth transition into the presternal region. Overfilling of the superomedial regions of the breast is also recommended (Fig. 20.2.14D), as gravity will be pulling the flap caudally over the ensuing 6 months. Excessive fat can be removed later, whereas a depression in this area can be very disturbing for the patient.

The breast envelope

Once the final volume of the flap is determined, one can make a rough estimate of how much skin overlying the

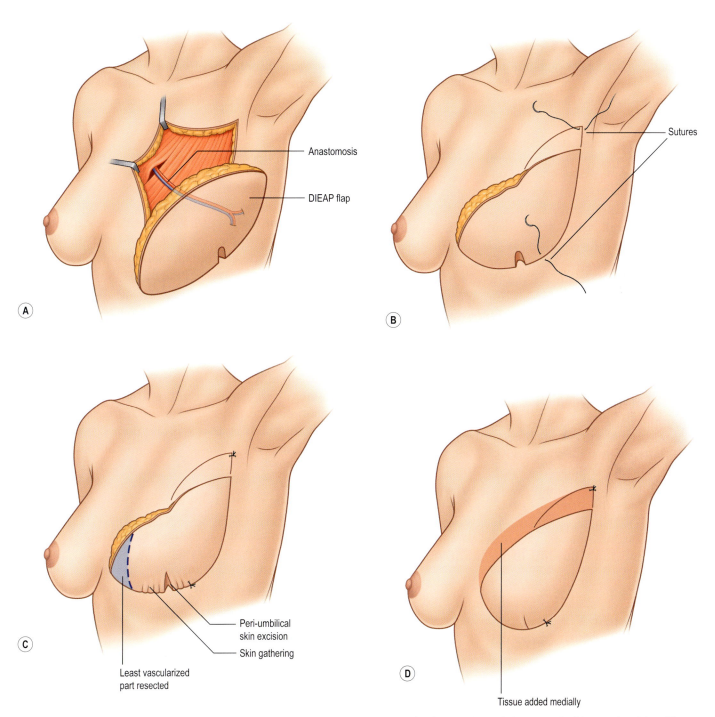

Fig. 20.2.14 **(A)** The deep inferior epigastric artery perforator (DIEAP) flap is turned 180° after performing the microsurgical anastomosis of the vessels and then **(B)** sutured with two key sutures to the pectoral fascia at the anterior axillary fold and the lateral part of the new inframammary fold making sure to avoid any fullness of the inferolateral quadrant of the new breast. **(C)** A triangular excision of skin around the umbilical area and gathering of the skin at the inframammary fold around the midclavicular line will create projection of the flap and a sharp angle between the lower part of the breast and the abdominal wall. **(D)** The least vascularized part of the flap is then resected making sure to preserve enough tissue to fill the upper medial quadrant of the breast.

DIEAP flap will be required. The flap can be pushed up into the pocket or pulled down, leaving more or less vertical skin height, respectively, on the skin paddle of the flap. The more skin left, the more ptosis can be achieved. Also, the more skin resected in the lateral part of the flap, the more the flap will be pushed medially. Once again, the clinical and aesthetic assessment of the contralateral breast is key in fine-tuning the shape of the DIEAP flap. Finally, the upper part of the skin paddle covered by the mastectomy flap is de-epithelialized.

Postoperative care

The postoperative care is simplified as the function of the rectus muscle is preserved. Preserving the integrity of the muscle also significantly decreases postoperative abdominal wall pain, facilitates rehabilitation, and therefore reduces hospitalization time.

Flap monitoring is mainly clinical. Frequency of evaluation is hourly during the first 24 h, 2-hourly in the second 24 h, and every 4 h during the following 2 days. Adhesive thermometer-strips are stuck to the skin island of the flap and the high sternal region. Differences of more than 2°C are reported to the physician on-call. In addition to temperature, color, consistency of the flap, and capillary refill are registered on a specific microsurgical follow-up sheet. Unidirectional Doppler flowmetry and other more sophisticated devices are not used, as they can produce false-positive signals.[39,40]

Patients are mobilized within 24 h after removing the urinary catheter. Systemic antibiotics are given for 24 h. Except for daily subcutaneous prophylactic doses of low-molecular heparin, no other anticoagulants are given. Besides paracetamol as pain relief and anti-inflammatory, no other drugs are given unless a specific medical condition requires it. Drinking starts 12 h postoperatively. Drains are left for 3–7 days depending on their daily output. Dressing changes are not necessary with the use of skin adhesives. A sterile towel covers the breast(s) and the abdomen to keep the flap warm for the first 5 days. After that, a soft and elastic bra is adjusted. No compressive garments are applied.

Outcomes, prognosis, and complications

The dissection of a DIEAP flap has a steep learning curve, involving a specific technique. Dissection is performed close to the perforating vessels in the plane of loose connective tissue surrounding the pedicle, allowing side branches and crossing nerves to be easily identified and preserved. Dissection through other planes will cause excessive bleeding and slow the surgeon down. Two golden rules apply to any type of perforator flap surgery: a bloodless field and wide exposure of the vessels. A common mistake made is to follow the perforator vessels into a deep hole. Muscle, septum, and other tissues through which the perforators travel should be opened widely to get a clear view and help deal with any bleeding encountered.

A number of technical considerations are important in the planning and execution of the dissection. The wrong choice of perforator can have disastrous complications. With the help of imaging and direct intra-operative visualization, the most dominant perforator can be identified. Unusual courses of perforators such as those rounding the medial or lateral edge of the rectus abdominis muscle must be taken into account. Dominance of the superficial system should be recognized at the beginning of flap harvest, at the time of incision of the lower edge of the flap.

During dissection of the pedicle overstretching of the vessels should be avoided. The use of vessel loops is limited to the actual dissection and should not be left in place as they accidentally can come under traction in a later phase of the operation.

Ligation of side branches should be performed at a distance of 2–3 mm away from the pedicle. When a vascular clip or a ligating suture is placed too close to the main pedicle, it can interrupt the arterial or venous flow. Care should be taken during the motor nerve dissection. Excessive traction or crushing of the nerve can permanently affect its function.

In case of a free flap, torsion of the pedicle can easily occur during transfer of the flap. Exact orientation with the help of vascular clips can avoid this problem. Following anastomosis, kinking of the pedicle can be avoided by placing the pedicle in smooth curves once the shaping has finished. During the shaping of the flap, excessive defatting can lead to areas of partial flap necrosis or fat necrosis.[41] Delayed defatting using liposuction is a safer procedure. Poorly vascularized areas should be resected during the initial procedure to reduce the amount of postoperative complications.

In inexperienced hands, the DIEAP flap dissection will require a longer operating time than a conventional myocutaneous flap. After a number of cases, operating time will fall back and be comparable with myocutaneous flap harvesting, or even shorter if a limited pedicle length is needed.

Abdominal scarring is probably the most important risk factor for raising a DIEAP flap. It can cause major problems during the dissection of the perforators and the epigastric vessels. Intramuscular scarring is not

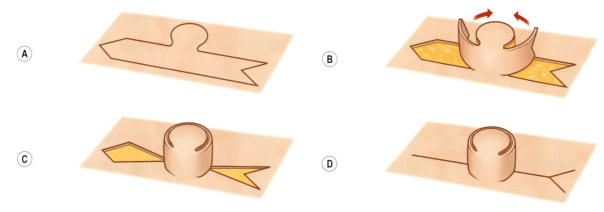

Fig. 20.2.15 (A–D) The modified CV-flap technique for nipple reconstruction.

always diagnosed on preoperative ultrasound and can spread out farther than suspected from the place and length of a previous incision.

Smoking is considered a relative contraindication to raising a DIEAP flap. The authors' impression is that the area most distant from the vascular pedicle of smokers is not well perfused, with prolonged vascular spasm. Additionally, wound healing problems and wound infections have been observed more frequently in smokers. Smokers who request elective, delayed reconstructions are asked to stop smoking at least 3 months before becoming a candidate for surgery. This is an additional way to test the motivation of the patient. An unmotivated patient or poor general medical health are the only absolute contraindications to DIEAP flap breast reconstruction.[38,42,43]

Secondary procedures

The free flap transfer and initial shaping is just the first step in achieving a full and natural breast reconstruction. Following the principles of a sculptor, the authors try to create a breast in the first stage that is slightly bigger than the desired volume but resembles the final result as closely as possible. Obtaining a definite result in one procedure is impossible. As removing tissues is so much easier than adding, specific areas of the flap can be aspirated or resected during the second operation 6 months later to achieve symmetry, which is the final goal of this procedure. If more tissue is needed, the flap can be augmented by lipofilling in specific spots to improve the shape or throughout the flap if pure volume augmentation is necessary. Augmentation by implants is possible as well but performed less and less as results of lipofilling become more predictable and successful. Nipple reconstruction is performed using the modified CV flap (Fig. 20.2.15). Scar revisions and adjustments of the borders of the footprint can easily be performed.

During the second operation, the contralateral breast can also be corrected in case of unilateral reconstruction. Any preferred technique of breast augmentation, reduction, or mastopexy can be performed as long as symmetry of shape and volume can be achieved.

Finally, bilateral tattooing of the nipple areolar complex is performed under local anesthesia. Even if the contralateral breast has not been operated on, the nipple areolar complex is tattooed to obtain a perfect color match and create an optical effect of camouflaging the reconstruction.

Primary reconstructions will always yield better aesthetic results than secondary or tertiary reconstructions as the natural footprint and skin envelope remain intact, especially if postoperative radiotherapy is avoided. If the conus is properly shaped during the first procedure, secondary procedures can be less complex and less frequent. For that reason, prophylactic mastectomies are performed more routinely today as a risk-reducing operation in hereditary breast cancer for BRCA-1 and -2 mutations (Fig. 20.2.16) or for oncologic reasons (i.e., invasive lobular carcinoma). Prophylactic mastectomy and immediate breast reconstruction without adjuvant radiotherapy should also be considered instead of a wide segmentectomy combined with aggressive radiotherapy, as this can lead to significant deformity of the breast mound.

Secondary (Fig. 20.2.17) and specifically tertiary (implant crippled or failed previous autologous attempts) reconstruction is more complex, as it involves correction and adjustment of all three essential parts of the "3-step" principle. Applying this principle, however, allows the surgeon to not only analyze the problem but also provides an opportunity to develop a clear preoperative strategy. In tertiary reconstructions, the surgeon is often left with no other choice but to remove all previous tissue, implants, and scarring and to start the entire reconstructive process again.

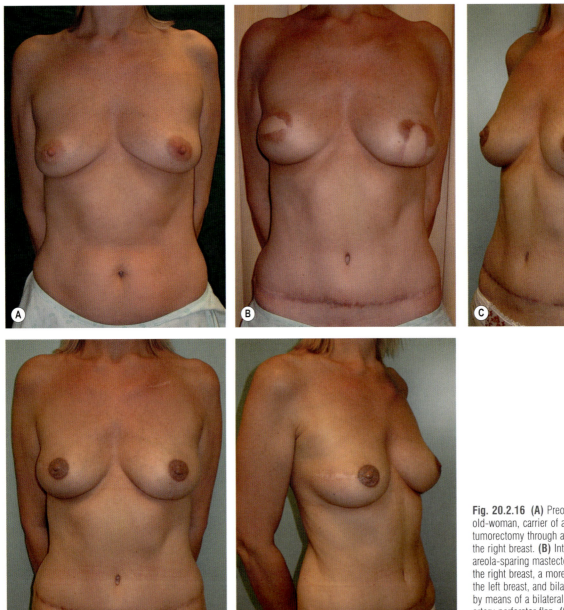

Fig. 20.2.16 (A) Preoperative image of a 46-year-old-woman, carrier of a BRCA-2 mutation, following tumorectomy through a horizontal racquet incision at the right breast. **(B)** Intermediate phase after bilateral areola-sparing mastectomy, using the same scar on the right breast, a more conventional vertical scar on the left breast, and bilateral autologous reconstruction by means of a bilateral free deep inferior epigastric artery perforator flap. **(C–E)** At 2-year-postoperative after bilateral nipple reconstruction using the interposed skin island of the flap and bilateral tattoo.

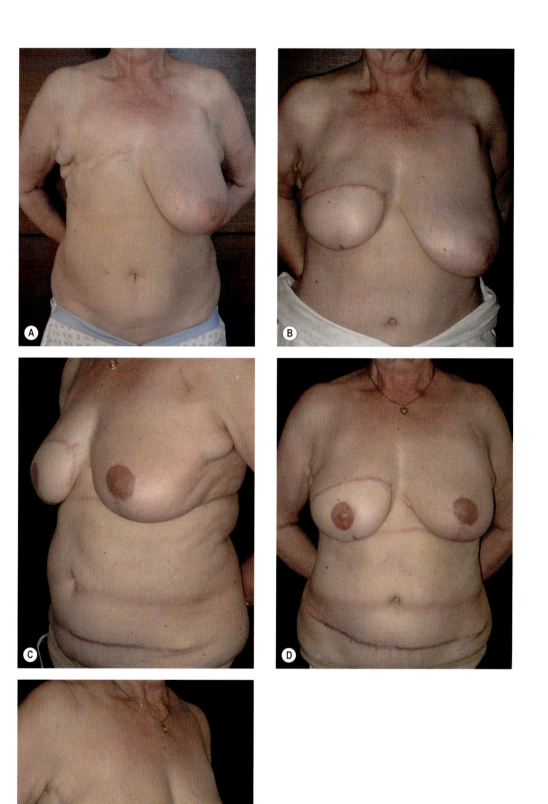

Fig. 20.2.17 (A) Preoperative image of a 62-year-old woman following modified radical mastectomy of the right breast with breast hypertrophy/ptosis of the left breast. **(B)** Intermediate phase after secondary autologous breast reconstruction by means of a unilateral free deep inferior epigastric artery perforator flap. **(C–E)** Final result, 1 year postoperatively, after right nipple reconstruction (and later tattoo) and left breast reduction.

⊕ Access the complete reference list online at   **http://www.expertconsult.com**

4. Koshima I, Soeda S. Inferior epigastric artery skin flaps without rectus abdominis muscle. *Br J Plast Surg.* 1989;42:645–648. *The rectus abdominis musculocutaneous flap has many advantages, but its disadvantages are also well-known. These are the possibility of abdominal herniation and, in certain situations, its bulk. To overcome these problems, an inferior epigastric artery skin flap without rectus abdominis muscle, pedicled on the muscle perforators and the proximal inferior deep epigastric artery, was used. A large flap without muscle can survive on a single muscle perforator.*

5. Reid AW, Szpalski C, Sheppard NN, et al. An international comparison of reimbursement for DIEAP flap breast reconstruction. *J Plast Reconstr Aesthet Surg.* 2015;68:1529–1535. *Results demonstrate that DIEAP flap breast reconstruction is inconsistently funded. Unfortunately, it appears that the current reimbursement offered by many countries may dissuade institutions and surgeons from offering this procedure. However, substantial evidence exists supporting the cost-effectiveness of perforator flaps for breast reconstruction and the long-term clinical benefits make this investment of time and money essential.*

8. Allen RJ, Treece P. Deep inferior epigastric perforator flap for breast reconstruction. *Ann Plast Surg.* 1994;32:32–38.

9. Blondeel PN, Boeckx WD. Refinements in free flap breast reconstruction: the free bilateral deep inferior epigastric perforator flap anastomosed to the internal mammary artery. *Br J Plast Surg.* 1994;47:495–501. *Besides the enormous advantages of reconstructing the amputated breast by means of a conventional TRAM flap, the main disadvantage remains the elevation of small (free TRAM) or larger (pedicled TRAM) parts of the rectus abdominis muscle. In order to overcome this disadvantage, the free deep inferior epigastric perforator (DIEP) skin flap has recently been used for breast mound reconstruction, with excellent clinical results. After achieving favorable results with eight unilateral DIEP-flaps, the authors were challenged by an abdomen with a midline laparotomy scar. By dissecting a bilateral DIEP flap and making adjacent anastomoses to the internal mammary artery, we were able to achieve sufficient flap mobility for easy free flap positioning and breast shaping. Intraoperative segmental nerve stimulation, postoperative functional abdominal wall tests, and CT-scan examination showed normal abdominal muscle activity. On the basis of a case report, the technical considerations and advantages of anastomosing the bipedicled DIEP flap to the internal mammary artery are discussed.*

10. Blondeel PN. One hundred free DIEP flap breast reconstructions: a personal experience. *Br J Plast Surg.* 1999;52:104–111. *This study summarizes the prospectively gathered data of 100 free DIEP flaps used for breast reconstruction in 87 patients. Primary reconstructions were done in 35% of the patients. Well-known risk factors for free flap breast reconstruction were present: smokers 23%, obesity 25%, abdominal scarring 28%, and previous radiotherapy 45%. Mean operating time was 6 h 12 min for unilateral reconstruction and mean hospital stay was 7.9 days. These data indicate that the free DIEP flap is a new but reliable and safe technique for autologous breast reconstruction. This flap offers the patient the same advantages as the TRAM flap and discards the most important disadvantages of the myocutaneous flap by preserving the continuity of the rectus muscle.*

11. Blondeel PN, Hijawi J, Depypere H, et al. Shaping the breast in aesthetic and reconstructive breast surgery: an easy three-step principle. *Plast Reconstr Surg.* 2009;123:455–462.

12. Blondeel PN, Hijawi J, Depypere H, et al. Shaping the breast in aesthetic and reconstructive breast surgery: an easy three-step principle. Part II. Breast reconstruction after total mastectomy. *Plast Reconstr Surg.* 2009;123:794–805. *This is Part II of four parts describing the 3-step principle being applied in reconstructive and aesthetic breast surgery. Part I explains how to analyze a problematic breast by*

understanding the three main anatomic features of a breast and how they interact: the footprint, the conus of the breast, and the skin envelope. This part describes how one can optimize his/her results with breast reconstructions after complete mastectomy. For both primary and secondary reconstructions, the authors explain how to analyze the postmastectomy breast and the deformed chest wall before giving step-by-step guidelines on how to rebuild the entire breast with either autologous tissue or implants. The differences in shaping unilateral or bilateral breast reconstructions with autologous tissue are clarified. Regardless of timing or method of reconstruction, it is shown that by breaking down the surgical strategy in three easy (anatomic) steps, the reconstructive surgeon is able to provide more aesthetically pleasing and reproducible results.*

20. Taylor GI, Daniel RK. The anatomy of several free flap donor sites. *Plast Reconstr Surg.* 1975;56:243–253.

25. Al-Dhamin A, Bissell MB, Prasad V, et al. The use of retrograde limb of internal mammary vein in autologous breast reconstruction with DIEAP flap: anatomical and clinical study. *Ann Plast Surg.* 2014;72:281–284. *It is also worth noting that the retrograde limb of the internal mammary vein seems to be a safe second recipient vein in DIEAP flap reconstruction.*

37. Uppal RS, Casaer B, Van Landuyt K, et al. The efficacy of preoperative mapping of perforators in reducing operative times and complications in perforator flap breast reconstruction. *J Plast Reconstr Aesthet Surg.* 2009;62:859–864.

39. Lie KH, Barker AS, Ashton MW. A classification system for partial and complete DIEP flap necrosis based on a review of 17,096 DIEP flaps in 693 articles including analysis of 152 total flap failures. *Plast Reconstr Surg.* 2013;132:1401–1408. *In documented DIEAP flap losses, 40% involved venous problems, 28% arterial, and 21% were mechanical (pedicle kinking, hematoma).*

40. Wormald JC, Wade RG, Figus A. The increased risk of adverse outcomes in bilateral deep inferior epigastric artery perforator flap breast reconstruction compared to unilateral reconstruction: a systematic review and meta-analysis. *J Plast Reconstr Aesthet Surg.* 2014;67:143–156. *A systematic review of the literature has also confirmed that bilateral DIEP flap breast reconstruction is associated with a significantly higher risk of total flap failure compared with unilateral DIEP flap breast reconstruction.*

41. Bozikov K, Arnez T, Hertl K, et al. Fat necrosis in free DIEAP flaps: incidence, risk, and predictor factors. *Ann Plast Surg.* 2009;63:138–142. *DIEAP flaps harvested on a single perforator, obese patients with a body mass index ≥30, and revision operations all have significantly higher amounts of fat necrosis.*

43. Massey MF, Spiegel AJ, Levine JL, et al. Perforator flaps: recent experience, current trends, and future directions based on 3974 microsurgical breast reconstructions. *Plast Reconstr Surg.* 2009;124:737–751. *Perforator flap breast reconstruction is an accepted surgical option for breast cancer patients electing to restore their body image after mastectomy. Since the introduction of the deep inferior epigastric perforator flap, microsurgical techniques have evolved to support a 99% success rate for a variety of flaps with donor sites that include the abdomen, buttock, thigh, and trunk. Recent experience highlights the perforator flap as a proven solution for patients who have experienced failed breast implant-based reconstructions or those requiring irradiation. Current trends suggest an application of these techniques in patients previously felt to be unacceptable surgical candidates, with a focus on safety, aesthetics, and increased sensitization. Future challenges include the propagation of these reconstructive techniques into the hands of future plastic surgeons with a focus on the development of septocutaneous flaps and vascularized lymph node transfers for the treatment of lymphedema.*

20.3

Superficial inferior epigastric artery (SIEA) flap

Julie Park, Deana S. Shenaq, and David H. Song

Access video lecture content for this chapter online at expertconsult.com

SYNOPSIS

- The superficial inferior epigastric artery (SIEA) flap has the least donor site morbidity of the flaps available from the lower abdomen for autologous tissue breast reconstruction.
- SIEA-specific challenges include short pedicles, vessel size mismatch, and the propensity for arterial spasm.
- Preoperative, intraoperative, and postoperative strategies are described.

 Access the Historical Perspective section online at
http://www.expertconsult.com

Introduction

The use of the lower abdominal tissue for autologous breast reconstruction has been as a gold standard since Hartrampf popularized the rotational transverse rectus abdominis myocutaneous (TRAM) flap.[1] Advances in microsurgical technique have heralded an evolution whereby flap perfusion is optimized while donor site morbidity is minimized. This progression is well illustrated by the free TRAM, muscle-sparing free TRAM (MS-fTRAM), and deep inferior epigastric perforator (DIEP) flap. While all of these flaps compromise essentially the same island of lower abdominal skin and subcutaneous fat, each iteration further minimizes donor site morbidity. The superficial inferior epigastric artery (SIEA) has the least donor site morbidity and is the most muscle-sparing as the dissection is completely subcutaneous and does not violate the fascia.

This chapter will discuss anatomy and dissection technique. Challenges particular to the SIEA flap include vessel size mismatch, short pedicles, and the tendency towards arterial spasm. Preoperative, intraoperative, and postoperative prevention strategies will be described.

Patient selection

When assessing a patient preoperatively for the SIEA flap, the same criteria applies as when determining the suitability of a patient for a DIEP or free TRAM flap. The patient needs sufficient redundant lower abdominal skin and fat in order to approximate final desired breast volume and allow for a primary donor site closure analogous to an abdominoplasty. Specific to the SIEA flap, perfusion across the midline of the abdomen, although reported, is not reliable.[8] Therefore, if the patient requires more than a hemi-abdomen for either skin or volume to reconstruct the breast, it is not advised to plan on using the SIEA flap. The exception to this is when a bilateral hemi-abdominal flap is planned for a unilateral reconstruction, such as a stacked flap (Fig. 20.3.1).[9–11] In these cases, the use of the SIEA, if available, is an excellent method to reduce donor site morbidity.

Preoperative vascular imaging such as computed tomography angiography (CTA) or magnetic resonance angiography may be used to assess the deep and superficial vascular systems.[12–14] However, this is not essential, and a reliable intraoperative algorithm will be described below.

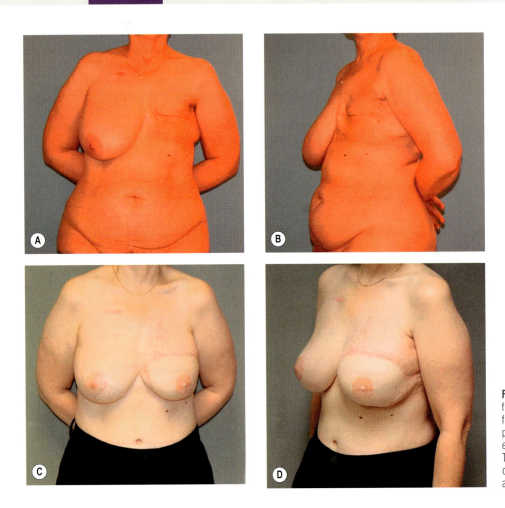

Fig. 20.3.1 (A–D) The use of the SIEA with a DIEP flap for a unilateral reconstruction with a bilateral flap. In this case a bilateral flap was required to provide adequate skin to reconstruct the breast envelope as well as subcutaneous fat for volume. The patient underwent a staged secondary contralateral small reduction for symmetry as well as nipple reconstruction.

Surgical technique

Patient marking

Patient marking is similar to that of the DIEP and free TRAM flaps. A major difference is the location of the transverse ellipse. Some surgeons center the transverse ellipse around the umbilicus to capture periumbilical perforators. To optimize the SIEA flap as an option, it is recommended to lower the incision to encounter the SIEA at a larger caliber. The periumbilical perforators can still be captured if caution is taken with the dissection through the subcutaneous tissues.

Intraoperative technique

The patient is positioned and draped in the same manner of a DIEP or free TRAM flap. When making the superior incision, the majority of the periumbilical perforators can still be preserved even with a more inferior skin paddle with careful dissection through the subcutaneous fat. After sharply incising the superior incision, the dermis is incised with cautery while obtaining hemostasis. After the dermis is released, the tissues open up approximately 1–1.5 cm. Dissection of the subcutaneous

fat at the superior edge of the incision, rather than the middle, will provide approximately 1 cm of extra tissue to protect DIEP perforators (Fig. 20.3.2).

The lower incision is made judiciously as the superior inferior epigastric vein can be very superficial in some patients. The superior inferior epigastric vein (SIEV) is typically found by marking the distance from the pubic symphysis to the anterior superior iliac spine (ASIS) into thirds. It is typically at the area approximately one-third lateral from the pubic symphysis. The SIEA location is more variable. The artery can travel directly lateral to the vein. Alternatively, it can be deeper, just below Scarpa's layer. The SIEA can also travel separately, approximately 3 cm lateral to the SIEV. In this position, it travels with two venae comitantes (Fig. 20.3.3). The venae comitantes can sometimes be of such large caliber that they can be used instead of the SIEV. Alternatively, sometimes the venous perfusion depends on the venae comitantes in addition to SIEV. Rozen *et al.* studied CTA imaging in 200 patients and found that in 40% of cases, there was a medial and lateral SIEV branch, which arose from different trunks altogether; and thus, the authors advocate that both trunks be used to facilitate venous drainage in these instances.[15] Temporarily occluding the veins with Acland clamps and assessing flap perfusion is the

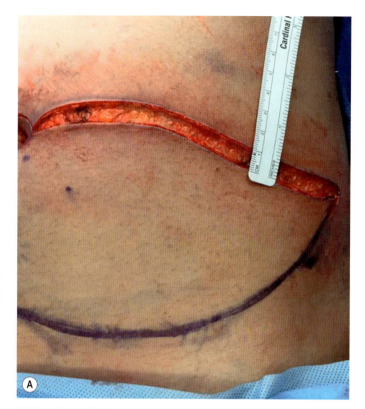

authors' preferred method to establish the necessary venous drainage of the flap (Fig. 20.3.4). It is important to note that the anatomy of the SIEA and SIEV is not necessarily symmetric on both sides of the abdomen.

Many papers have used SIEA caliber as a criterion for suitability of flap use.[15–17] However, in our experience, if the SIEA is palpable at the incision and the SIEV is ≥1.5 cm, the SIEA flap can be utilized even if the SIEA artery is <1 mm.[18] We have found that further dissection towards the femoral artery almost always yields a larger diameter vessel when the SIEA is palpable at the lower abdominal incision.

Intraoperative algorithm for lower abdominal flap choice

A simple intraoperative algorithm is used to determine which lower abdominal flap is used. Preoperative imaging is not necessary. If the SIEV is present and equal to or greater than 1.5 cm, then the SIEA is assessed. If the SIEA is palpable and a hemi-abdomen is sufficient for reconstruction, then a SIEA flap is used. If the SIEA is not present or palpable, then the DIEP perforators are assessed. If there is a dominant DIEP perforator, then a DIEP is performed. If there is not, then the location of the existing perforators is assessed and either a muscle-sparing free TRAM or, rarely, a free TRAM is performed.

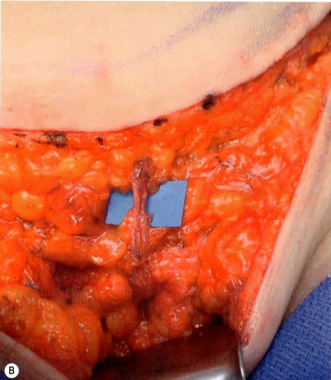

Fig. 20.3.2 (A) After dermis has been incised, the tissues open up approximately 1–1.5 cm. The subcutaneous dissection is carried out at the edge of the superior margin instead of the center of the tissues. **(B)** This results in a cuff of subcutaneous fat that protects any superiorly based deep inferior epigastric perforators.

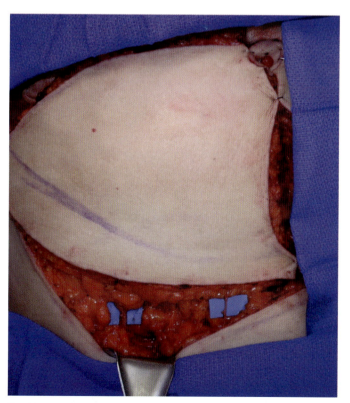

Fig. 20.3.3 Relationship of the superficial inferior epigastric artery (SIEA) to the superior inferior epigastric vein (SIEV). The SIEA can travel along side of the SIEV or lateral to the SIEV with two venae comitantes.

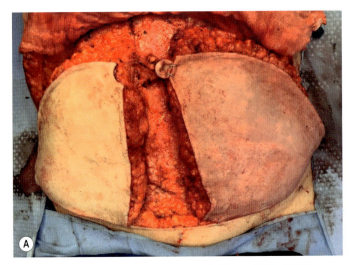

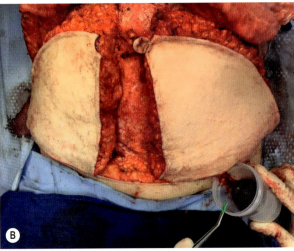

Fig. 20.3.4 (A) Acland clamps on the superior inferior epigastric vein (SIEV) reveal the dependence of this deep inferior epigastric perforator flap on the superficial system for venous drainage. **(B)** Once the clamps are removed, the SIEV is drained, and the flap no longer appears congested. The reliability of specific perforators can be assessed by clamping individual vessels assessing changes in flap perfusion.

If the SIEV is present, but not the SIEA, the SIEV is preserved in consideration for possible venous supercharging of the flap.

Harvesting the SIEA

Once the decision to pursue an SIEA flap is made, the pedicle is dissected. In order to protect from traction injury to the artery and prevent spasm, we recommend non-circumferential dissection of the pedicle initially and focus only on the anterior dissection of the SIEA. This is important because a gentle cephalad traction of the flap coupled with a vertical retraction on the lower groin skin will give optimal access for pedicle dissection. The SIEV can now be easily and quickly dissected to femoral vein. Initially, the SIEA will travel caudally as well. However, prior to entering the femoral sheath, it makes a sharp turn superomedially. To maximize

pedicle length, fully opening the cribriform fascia to expose the SIEA at its origin is essential. Buchel *et al.* advocate that pedicle length should be twice the thickness of the flap.[18] Any branches at this distal level are clipped long for potential use if spatulation is required at branch points to address vessel mismatch.

At this point, we have still not performed any posterior dissection, and therefore, the pedicle remains protected by posterior tissue and less likely to spasm. Once the anterior dissection is complete along the full length of the vessel, we carefully dissect the posterior surface of the arterial pedicle. If concomitant vascular lymph node transfer is not planned, harvesting the fat and lymph nodes that surround the SIEA is avoided. Once the pedicle dissection is completed, the flap is essentially ready for harvest after clipping any DIEP perforators. Because of the SIEA's short pedicle, it is recommended to de-epithelialize the majority of the flap *in situ* on the abdomen to avoid injury to the anastomosis. This is particularly important for larger flaps with a small aperture following skin-sparing mastectomy.

Recipient vessels

Typically the internal mammary artery (IMA) and vein or the perforating branches emanating from the internal mammary vessels are used for recipient vessels. To simplify the anastomosis and maximize recipient vessel length, it is imperative to clear the tissues completely in the intercostal space above and below the harvested rib. Approximately 4 cm of length can typically be prepared. As the surgeon becomes more familiar and comfortable with the flap, shorter recipient vessel length or a rib-sparing technique for access to the internal mammary vessels can be used.

If present, the internal mammary perforators off the second or third rib provide an excellent size match for the SIEA and SIEV.[19–22] Good communication with the breast surgeon is important to preserve these vessels.

Anastomosis

Because of the short SIEA pedicle, the anastomosis is often vertically oriented rather than horizontal. The complexity is compounded by size mismatch of the pedicle and recipient vessels. A surgeon can get more experience with short pedicle anastomosis to the internal mammary vessels by practicing rib-sparing techniques with the DIEP flap.

The use of a venous coupler can facilitate the venous anastomosis given the size mismatch and short pedicle. There are a couple of caveats to the use of a venous coupler. If the surgeon is not already adept with the coupler, then a hand-sewn anastomosis is preferable.

Redoing a venous coupler can result in loss of almost a centimeter of vessel length, which typically cannot be afforded with the SIEA flap. Additionally, when the recipient vein is less than 2 mm in diameter, it is generally advocated to avoid using the venous coupler. Another scenario to avoid using the venous coupler is when the recipient vein is less than 2 mm in diameter. The SIEV is typically large, sometimes with diameters up to 4 mm or greater. It also has a very thick vessel wall compared the DIEP vein and recipient veins. When forced to use a venous coupler less than 2 mm, the redundancy of the thick SIEV in the small aperture of the coupler ring can cause occlusion.[23] In these cases, it is better to hand suture the anastomosis.

To address arterial size mismatch, we recommend making a backcut on the anti-mesenteric side of the vessel. Alternatively, if there were any distal branches, the pedicle could be spatulated at a branch point to increase vessel diameter (Fig. 20.3.5). The arterial anastomosis is hand sewn with interrupted 9-0 nylon sutures under surgical microscopic magnification. Early on in our practice, we exclusively performed non-rib-sparing dissections to access the IMA or IMA perforator but now commonly use rib-sparing techniques.

Inset

When insetting the SIEA flap, care must be taken given the shorter pedicle length, especially with an immediate reconstruction following a skin-sparing mastectomy that provides only a small aperture. The authors recommend holding the superomedial mastectomy skin with one hand and insetting the flap in the superomedial direction first, which removes tension off the pedicle. The remainder of the mastectomy skin can then be carefully draped around the flap. In a patient undergoing completion mastectomy following previous lumpectomy and radiation therapy, the mastectomy skin can be less compliant. Thus, in this scenario, incising the mastectomy skin at 6 o'clock (exact location depending on the size of the flap) may facilitate inset without pedicle disruption. As mentioned previously, the authors recommend performing the majority of the de-epithelialization on the abdomen to avoid the need to deliver the flap through a small space, which places more traction on the pedicle. If the flap must be de-epithelialized on the chest, the surgeon should heed caution again in the situation of a skin-sparing mastectomy with a small aperture. The mastectomy skin coupled with short pedicle length can disrupt the anastomosis.

Avoidance of tension on the pedicle is important to minimize arterial spasm. The mastectomy skin envelope to flap relationship must be evaluated. If the flap is relatively small in a large skin envelope, consider (1) a vertical reduction for a better match; (2) anchoring sutures from the flap to the chest wall; and (3) an external support such as a surgical bra that is fitted carefully to prevent compression while giving inferior and lateral support.

It is also important to remember the superficial nature of the SIEA when de-epithelializing, insetting, and securing the flap, as to avoid injuring the pedicle as it courses through the flap.

Postoperative care

Care for the SIEA flap is similar to the postoperative care for the DIEP flap and other free tissue reconstructions of the breast. Most surgeons follow a postoperative pathway. At the authors' institution, patients leave the operating room with a tissue oximetry monitor attached to the flap and are transferred to the flap unit after a 6-hour period of flap monitoring in the post-anesthesia care unit. The flap is monitored for color, temperature, capillary refill, turgor, arterial signal with hand-held Doppler, and hourly continuous tissue oximetry. Incentive spirometry and chemical and mechanical DVT prophylaxis are initiated. Patients are kept NPO for approximately the first 24 hours, although if the patient and flap are doing well by the next morning, the diet is advanced after evaluation on morning rounds. The Foley catheter is removed and the patient is written to get out of bed to chair and ambulate later in the day.

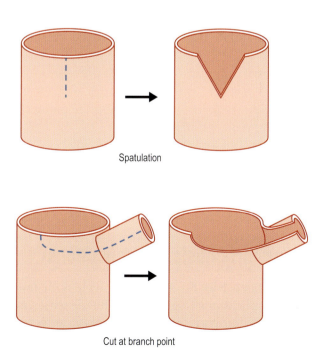

Spatulation

Cut at branch point

Fig. 20.3.5 Spatulation of the vessels can aid with size mismatch between recipient artery and the superficial inferior epigastric artery.

Postoperative day two is spent with continuation of ambulation and converting all pain control to oral medications. Patients are discharged on postoperative day three.

Specific consideration to the postoperative monitoring of the SIEA flap revolves around arterial spasm. Ptosis of the flap can cause stretch on both the venous and arterial anastomosis. Arterial spasm, in addition to resulting in an absent Doppler signal and a cool, pale flap, is often manifested on tissue oximetry as a steady drop of 15–20 points and leveling off, even at levels that may otherwise seem normal, whereas in venous compromise the oxygen saturation continues to drop, often to levels below 30%. Therefore, the *trend* in tissue oximetry rather than just the absolute value is important to prompt flap evaluation.

Maneuvers to avoid arterial vasospasm include controlling pain and anxiety, warming the patient, and preventing dehydration with intravenous fluids. Mechanical measures to help prevent spasm revolve around keeping the flap stable, such as using a surgical bra in those patients with a loose mastectomy skin envelope.

If a patient's flap does go into spasm, often external measures can be tried initially. If the patient has not been wearing a bra, a surgical bra is placed to give support. Medications are adjusted to treated pain, and anti- anxiolytics are added if the patient exhibits anxiety. Calcium channel blockers can be tried if the blood pressure will tolerate it. If the spasm does not break on its own after these measures, operative exploration is warranted. Of course, if there is any surgical concern, such as a difficult anastomosis and the index of suspicion is higher, operative re-exploration is always indicated.

Pitfalls and techniques to avoid them

The main pitfalls of the SIEA flap focus on the predilection of the artery to spasm, vessel size mismatch, and short pedicle. Throughout the chapter, we have discussed strategies to avoid these and will highlight them here.

- Lower the abdominal incision to encounter the SIEA at a larger caliber
- Perform the anterior dissection first rather than circumferential dissection of the artery to protect the artery from vasospasm
- Dissect the artery completely to the femoral artery
- Avoid unnecessary peri-arterial lymph node harvest to increase pedicle length
- De-epithelialize the flap on the abdomen

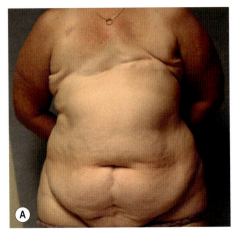
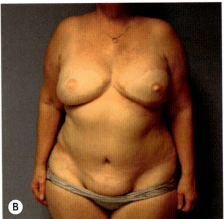

Fig. 20.3.6 (A,B) A patient who underwent bilateral skin-sparing mastectomy with immediate reconstruction with bilateral superficial inferior epigastric artery flaps. She had bilateral immediate autologous reconstructions with abdominal donor site morbidity analogous to an abdominoplasty.

- Maximize recipient vessel length
- Backcut or spatulate the SIEA for improved vessel mismatch
- Careful external support of the flap to prevent ptosis
- Postoperative care focused on warming the patient and reducing pain and anxiety.

We recommend caution in patients who are heavy and active smokers, not so much out of concern for fat necrosis, but for increased vasospasm risk. Intraoperatively, papaverine is particularly useful to address any arterial spasm.

Outcomes, prognosis, complications

Patients who have had SIEA flaps do well with few donor site complications (Fig. 20.3.6). The decreases in donor site morbidity correlate to the decrease in rectus muscle harvested.[21,22,24,25] Anecdotally, in our practice we have observed decreased postoperative pain and time to ambulation. There are no risks of hernia or bulge since the rectus fascia and motor nerves to the rectus muscles are not disturbed. If, during the dissection, one harvests lymph nodes with the flap or does not adequately clip lymphatics, there is a risk for lymphatic leaks and potentially lymphedema, although rare.

Secondary procedures

Staged secondary procedures are the same as any abdominally based autologous tissue breast reconstruction.

🌐 Access the complete reference list online at **http://www.expertconsult.com**

15. Rozen WM, Chubb D, Whitaker IS, Ashton MW. The importance of the superficial venous anatomy of the abdominal wall in planning a superficial inferior epigastric artery (SIEA) flap: case report and clinical study. *Microsurgery.* 2011;31:454–457. *This case report and review of CTA data demonstrates the variability in the number as well as source of regional drainage of SIEV trunks, and advocates that all separate trunks should be maximally dissected in the event that multiple venous anastomoses are needed to optimize drainage in SIEA free flaps. In 40% of cases illustrated in this anatomical study, two SIEV branches arose from different trunks altogether, and the authors advocate that both trunks be used in these instances.*

16. Chevray PM. Breast reconstruction with superficial inferior epigastric artery flaps: a prospective comparison with TRAM and DIEP flaps. *Plast Reconstr Surg.* 2004;114:1077–1083, discussion 1084–1085. *Chevray conducted a prospective study on the reliability and outcomes of SIEA vs. TRAM and DIEP flaps for breast reconstruction, and found that the SIEA flap was usable in 30% of cases. There was a higher rate of reoperation with SIEA flaps, which he attributed to smaller pedicle diameter (1.5 mm or smaller) and significant size mismatch with recipient vessels.*

17. Spiegel AJ, Khan FN. An intraoperative algorithm for use of the SIEA flap for breast reconstruction. *Plast Reconstr Surg.* 2007;120:1450–1459. *This is one of the first reports suggesting an intraoperative algorithm for SIEA flap selection, which advocates for utilization of this flap if arterial caliber is >1.5 mm with a palpable pulse. Although our criteria for SIEA flap selection is only a palpable pulse, this paper set the stage for future studies with higher numbers of patients.*

20. Dorafshar AH, Januszyk M, Song DH. Anatomical and technical tips for use of the superficial inferior epigastric artery (SIEA) flap in breast reconstructive surgery. *J Reconstr Microsurg.* 2010;26:381–389. *This paper set forth a simple approach to harvest of the SIEA flap and demonstrated that favorable results could be achieved with even smaller caliber vessels (average arterial pedicle diameter in this series was 0.96 mm).*

20.4

The free TRAM flap

Maurice Y. Nahabedian

 Access video lecture content for this chapter online at expertconsult.com

SYNOPSIS

- The free transverse rectus abdominis myocutaneous (TRAM) can be classified as a muscle-sparing flap that includes the medial and lateral segments of the rectus abdominis muscle (MS-2), the medial or lateral segments (MS-1), or the full width (MS-0).
- The free TRAM has a reliable and predictable blood supply based off the inferior epigastric artery and vein.
- Functional outcomes of the muscle-sparing free TRAM and deep inferior epigastric perforator flap (DIEP) flap are equivalent.
- Preoperative and intraoperative imaging studies can predict the vascular architecture and perfusion patterns.
- The free TRAM may provide more predictable outcomes in obese and morbidly obese patients compared with the DIEP flap.
- Free TRAM can result in excellent aesthetic outcomes with low complication rates.

Introduction

The abdomen is the most common donor site for autologous breast reconstruction. There are various flaps that are derived from the abdomen including the pedicle TRAM, free TRAM, DIEP, and the superficial inferior epigastric artery flap (SIEA). The evolution of these flaps has been based on improving breast aesthetics and reducing abdominal morbidity. Breast aesthetics are related to volume of abdominal tissue, ability to optimally position the flap on the chest wall, properly shape the flap, and ensure adequate vascular inflow and outflow to optimize perfusion. Donor aesthetics are related to adequate closure of the abdominal soft tissues, continuity and innervation of the rectus abdominis muscles, and maximal preservation of the anterior rectus sheath. The relative risk ratio of these flaps with respect to breast outcome is highest with the SIEA flap followed by the DIEP flap, free TRAM flap, and pedicle TRAM flaps. The relative risk ratio with respect to donor or abdominal outcome is highest with the pedicle TRAM flap followed by the free TRAM, DIEP flap, and the SIEA flap.

The free TRAM flap has been a prominent method of breast reconstruction using autologous tissue since the early 1990s. Advantages of the free TRAM compared with alternative flaps are ultimately related to predictability and reproducibility. This is because the blood supply to the free TRAM is optimized based on the larger caliber deep inferior epigastric perforator vessels as well as inclusion of multiple perforators. In addition, the continuity and innervation of the rectus abdominis muscles are usually preserved with minimal violation of the anterior rectus sheath.

Basic science/anatomy

Patients should have a sufficient quantity of abdominal skin and subcutaneous fat in order to reconstruct a breast. The fat is separated into a subcutaneous and a subscarpal layer separated by Scarpa's fascia. The thickness of these layers varies from 2–8 cm. The anterior rectus sheath is comprised of the aponeurosis of the external and internal oblique muscles and characterized as an interwoven collagen lattice. It is considered the principal support structure for the anterior abdominal wall. Disruption or attenuation of the lattice without proper closure can result in bulge or hernia. There is a loose areolar layer of tissue over the anterior sheath that contains a plexus of vessels that should be preserved to ensure vascularity and viability following the operation.

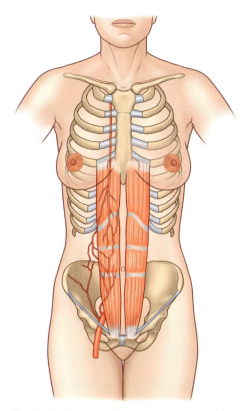

Fig. 20.4.1 Vascular anatomy of the rectus abdominis muscle.

The rectus abdominis muscle is a type 3 muscle that is perfused by the superior and inferior deep epigastric vessels (Fig. 20.4.1). It is segmentally innervated at various levels throughout its length. The free TRAM flap receives its blood supply from the deep inferior epigastric artery and vein, as well as the perforating branches traversing through the anterior rectus sheath. The intramuscular course of the deep inferior epigastric vessels is complex and classified as type 1, 2, or 3 based on the number of dominant branching patterns. The number of perforators emanating from these vessels is variable with the preponderance of perforators located in the periumbilical region. The intercostal motor nerves typically innervate the muscle along the posterior surface at the junction of the lateral and central segment. Proper function of the rectus abdominis muscle requires that these motor nerves remain intact because each nerve controls a different arc of muscle flexion. The intramuscular course of these motor nerves may cross over the dominant source vessels supplying the flap. Sensory nerves are identified along the surface of the anterior rectus sheath and traverse through the subcutaneous layer to the skin.

Classification of free TRAM flaps

Classification of the abdominal flaps is based on the degree of muscle preservation (Table 20.4.1 and Fig. 20.4.2). Preservation of the rectus abdominis muscle is based on subdivision into three vertical segments: medial, central, and lateral.[1,2] Preservation of the entire muscle is classified as an MS-3 (DIEP) flap. Preservation of the medial and lateral segment is classified as an MS-2 (muscle-sparing TRAM) flap (Fig. 20.4.3). Preservation of the lateral or medial segment is classified as an MS-1 (muscle-sparing TRAM) flap (Fig. 20.4.4). A modification of this particular classification is based on whether the medial (M) or lateral (L) segment of the rectus abdominis muscle is preserved. If the medial and central segments of the muscle are harvested with the flap, the free TRAM would be classified as an MS-1L, signifying that the lateral segment was preserved. Sacrifice of the entire width of the muscle is classified as an MS-0 (TRAM) flap (Fig. 20.4.5). MS-1 and MS-2 flaps will preserve the continuity of the rectus abdominis muscle and therefore provide varying degrees of muscle function.

The zones of the free TRAM flap are the same as the zones of all abdominally based flaps and are comprised of four segments (Fig. 20.4.6). Zone 1 represents the adipocutaneous territory over the dominant blood supply. Zone 2 is based on unilateral or bilateral flaps. With unilateral flaps, zone 2 is opposite the midline. Zone 3 is lateral to zone 1, and zone 4 is lateral to zone 3. With bilateral flaps, zone 2 is lateral to zone 1 and zone 3 and 4 do not exist.

Current concepts with free flap breast reconstruction

When considering autologous breast reconstruction with a free TRAM flap, an appreciation of ideal breast aesthetics is important. This incorporates three essential elements: the breast footprint, skin envelope, and conus. This three-step principalization of breast reconstruction was described by Phillip Blondeel and is the basis for achieving ideal breast aesthetics.[3,4] The footprint is unique for each woman and defined and fixed for each breast (Fig. 20.4.7). The borders of the footprint include the clavicle, lateral edge of the sternum, anterior axillary line, and the inframammary fold. It is important to

Table 20.4.1 The classification and definition of the various abdominally based free flaps	
Muscle-sparing technique	**Definition (rectus abdominis)**
MS-0	Full width, partial length
MS-1	Preservation of lateral segment
MS-2	Preservation of lateral and medial segment
MS-3 (DIEP)	Preservation of entire muscle

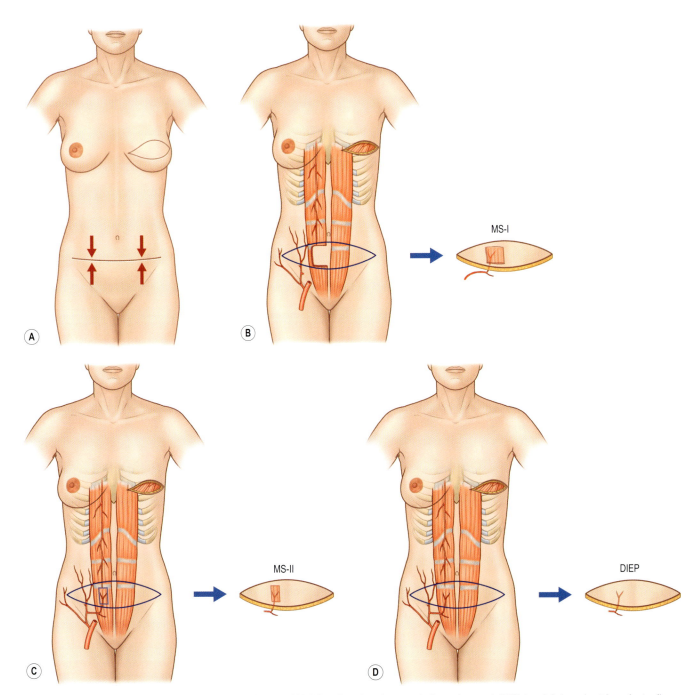

Fig. 20.4.2 (A–D) Schematic illustrations of the MS-1, MS-2, and MS-3 flaps based on the amount of muscle spared. DIEP, deep inferior epigastric perforator flap.

appreciate that the footprint is stable and does not change with weight gain or loss. The footprint represents the foundation for the conus. The conus is representative of the 3D shape, volume, projection, and contour of the breast (Fig. 20.4.8). This will vary with weight gain or loss. The conus is typically characterized with a lower pole prominence. In general, ideal breast proportion is based on the ratio of the distance along the breast meridian with separation into upper and lower distances based on the location of the nipple areolar complex. Ideally, the upper to lower pole ratio is 45:55. The final component is the skin envelope (Fig.

20.4.9). In the setting of immediate reconstruction, the quality and quantity of skin is important. Skin quality is affected by previous surgery, radiation, scar, and vascularity. With immediate reconstruction, it is important to ensure that the flap volume approximates the skin envelope volume. With delayed reconstruction, this is not a factor because the shape of the breast is determined by the amount of skin and fat from the flap, as well as the useable skin from the chest.

Plastic surgeons typically learn the fundamentals of breast shaping during residency or fellowship. This is usually achieved with the apprentice or mentorship

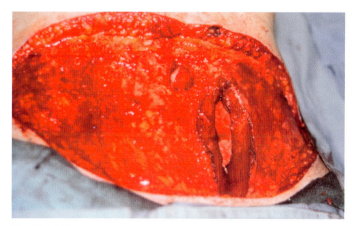

Fig. 20.4.3 The rectus abdominis muscle following harvest on an MS-2 free TRAM flap.

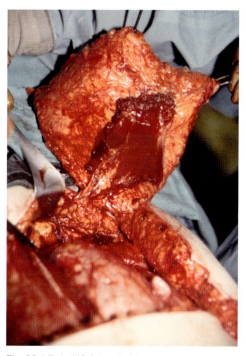

Fig. 20.4.5 An MS-0 free TRAM flap incorporating the full width of the rectus abdominis muscle.

model. Initially the technical aspects of the operation are the most important and require mastery; however, with surgical maturation, the aesthetic aspects become as important, and the artistry of breast reconstruction comes to fruition. The ultimate goal is to create symmetry, proportion, and contour. When positioning a free TRAM flap on the chest wall, the width and height of the tissues should match the desired footprint of the breast. The natural shape or cone of the breast should be appreciated to estimate the amount of skin that will be required to achieve ideal proportions. The relationship of the torso to the breast is assessed to reconstruct a breast that will be appropriate for the patient's frame and body habitus.

Patient selection

Patients who are considered for breast reconstruction with the free TRAM in the immediate setting are usually those diagnosed with breast cancer or at high risk for

developing breast cancer. Some patients will present following a mastectomy and are interested in delayed reconstruction. These patients may have had prior radiation therapy or complications related to prosthetic reconstruction. To be considered a good candidate for a free TRAM flap, patients should have sufficient tissue in the lower abdomen to create a breast that will meet expectations.

Proper patient selection and good outcomes are intimately related.[5,6] Although many women may express an interest in autologous breast reconstruction, not all

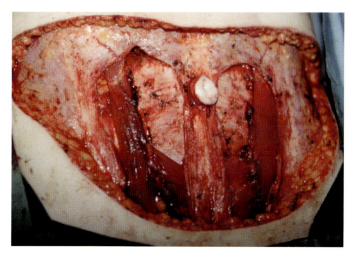

Fig. 20.4.4 The rectus abdominis muscle following harvest of an MS-1 free TRAM flap.

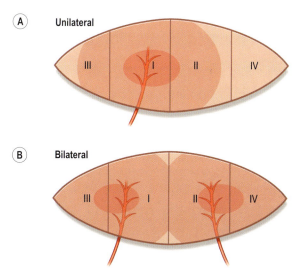

Fig. 20.4.6 The standard zones of the free TRAM flap based on the proximity of the primary blood supply. The unilateral and bilateral variations are shown.

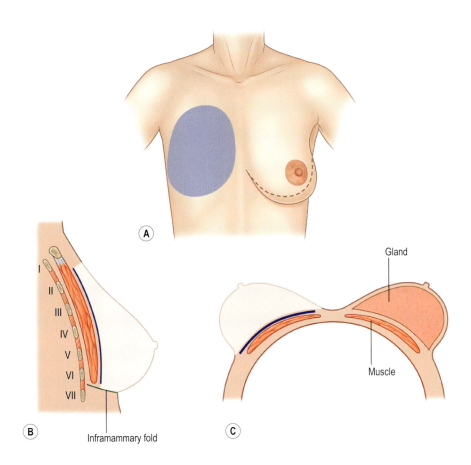

Fig. 20.4.7 The footprint of the breast is illustrated in **(A)** coronal; **(B)** sagittal; and **(C)** transverse views.

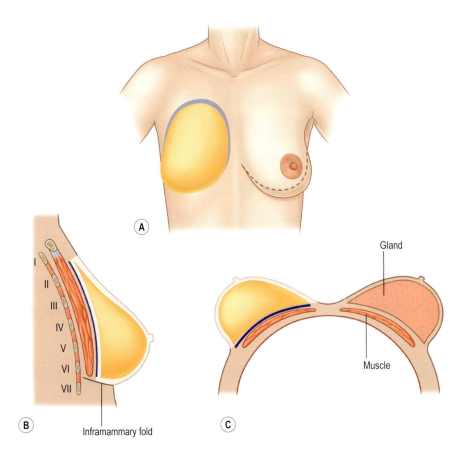

Fig. 20.4.8 The conus of the breast is illustrated in **(A)** coronal; **(B)** sagittal; and **(C)** transverse views.

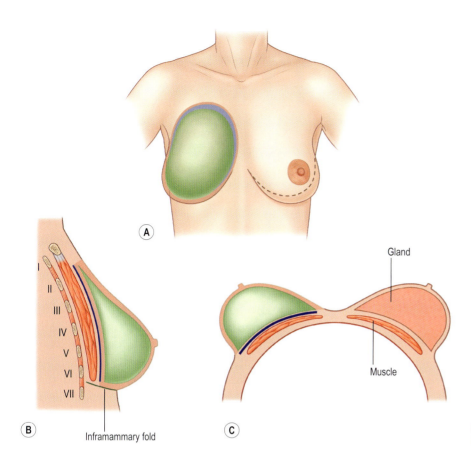

Fig. 20.4.9 The skin envelope of the breast is illustrated in **(A)** coronal; **(B)** sagittal; and **(C)** transverse views.

will be candidates. Current demographics suggest that the number of women interested in bilateral and nipple-sparing mastectomy for therapeutic and prophylactic purposes is increasing.[7] When considering a free TRAM flap, it is important to assess the breast and donor site characteristics, tumor parameters, need for adjuvant therapies, and general health. Ideal candidates for a free TRAM include women with sufficient abdominal tissue, good health status, and low ASA score. Candidacy for free TRAM reconstruction may be precluded because of poorly-controlled medical comorbidities, extremes of body habitus, or a desire for a quick and simple procedure. Preoperative conditions such as diabetes mellitus, hypertension, and cardiac disease must be optimized.[6,8,9] Tobacco use is strictly discouraged.

Physical examination includes the breast, donor site, presence of scars, quality of tissue, as well as measurements including the base width of the breast and the location of the nipple areolar complex.[3,4,6,10] The footprint of the breast is appreciated and serves as a template for the new breast mound. The most important physical requirement is a sufficient quantity of skin and fat to reconstruct a breast with the appropriate volume. Although a woman may be slender with a paucity of abdominal fat, she may still be a candidate for an abdominal flap if the breast volume requirements are

low. In women who are overweight or obese, an abdominal flap is not precluded; however, the flap should be tailored to sustain the perfusion requirement and to minimize the incidence of fat necrosis. In unilateral cases, the volume of the flap may be less than required for symmetry. In this situation, options include a contralateral reduction mammaplasty or mastopexy as well as an ipsilateral implant insertion. The abdomen is usually not considered when there are abdominal scars that will preclude incorporating zones of tissue needed for the reconstruction or when morbidly obese (Table 20.4.2). Paramedian abdominal incisions are usually a contraindication to performing a free TRAM because of the high likelihood of injury to the dominant perforators and source vessel.

Adjuvant therapy such as radiation is an important consideration and can affect the timing of free TRAM flap reconstruction.[11–13] There is controversy regarding the timing of autologous breast reconstruction in relation to radiation therapy. Some surgeons feel that immediate reconstruction with a free TRAM followed by radiation therapy may result in irreversible changes to the flap such as fibrosis, shrinkage, and abnormal contour. Other surgeons feel that the likelihood of this is low and advocate for immediate autologous reconstruction followed by radiation. In general, when the

Table 20.4.2 The effect of prior abdominal incisions on the vascularity of the abdominal flaps

Scar	n	SIEA disruption	DIEA disruption	Perforator disruption
Laparoscopy	20	None	None	None
Open appendectomy	20	All (ipsilateral)	None (ipsilateral)	Medial row of DIEA
Pfannenstiel	35	Medial branch (30/35)	None	NR
Paramedian	3	All (ipsilateral)	All (ipsilateral)	All (ipsilateral)
Open choly	1	None	None	None
Midline	17	None	None	Crossover

(Reproduced with permission from Rozen W, et al. *Clinical Anatomy.* 2009;22:815–823.)

likelihood of radiation therapy exceeds 50%, the delayed-immediate approach using a tissue expander is considered. Conversion to an autologous microvascular reconstruction is performed 6–12 months following radiation. This time interval is recommended because of the perivascular inflammation that may be present along the recipient vessels following radiation therapy.

The topic of complications is discussed and reviewed with all women.[14–24] Following free TRAM flap reconstruction, success rates typically range from 97% to 99%. Factors related to anastomotic or flap failure includes vascular thrombosis, poor vessel quality, and iatrogenic injury. The risk of an abdominal bulge following a free TRAM flap ranges from 3–5% following a unilateral and 5–7% following a bilateral reconstruction. This is related to various factors that include the amount of anterior rectus sheath excised, residual muscle innervation, and the use of mesh reinforcement. The use of a synthetic mesh to reinforce the closure is sometimes used at the initial operation and may be necessary for the correction of an abdominal bulge.

The decision to perform a DIEP or free TRAM flap is based on an intraoperative assessment of the perforators, flap volume, and abdominal characteristics (Table 20.4.3). It is critical to ensure that the location and caliber of the perforating vessels are sufficient to safely perfuse the required flap volume. In the event that the perforators are deemed inadequate, a muscle-sparing free TRAM is usually performed to capture more perforators. It is explained during the initial consultation that most outcome studies have demonstrated no clinically relevant functional difference between the free TRAM and DIEP flaps (Table 20.4.4). Patients are told that a unilateral free TRAM flap may take 4–6 h and a bilateral free TRAM may take 6–8 h to complete; however, these times are variable and based on surgeon and hospital experience. Patients are usually hospitalized for 3 days following free TRAM reconstruction and instructed to refrain from strenuous activity for 6 weeks.

Patient markings

Patients are marked in the standing position (Figs. 20.4.10 & 20.4.11). The breast markings include the sternal midline and the inframammary folds bilaterally. The mastectomy incisions depend on whether mastectomy is skin-sparing or nipple-sparing as well as whether the reconstruction is immediate or delayed. With delayed reconstruction, the prior mastectomy scar

Table 20.4.3 Personal algorithm for abdominal flap selection based on flap volume, number of perforators, and abdominal lipodystrophy

Factor	Free TRAM	DIEP	SIEA
Breast volume requirement			
<800 cc	±	+	±
>800 cc	+	±	−
Abdominal fat			
Mild–moderate	±	+	±
Severe	+	±	−
Perforators >1.5 mm			
0	+	−	−
>1	±	+	±

Table 20.4.4 Adverse events comparing the free TRAM to the DIEP flap

Factor	DIEP (%)	Free TRAM (%)
Fat necrosis	7.30	7.10
Venous congestion	4.50	2.70
Flap failure	2.70	1.80
Abdominal bulge		
Unilateral	4.50	5
Bilateral	6.50	21
Sit-ups		
Unilateral	100	97
Bilateral	95	83

(Reproduced with permission from: Nahabedian MY, et al. *Plast Reconstr Surg.* 2005;115:436.)

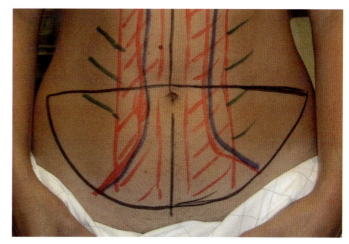

Fig. 20.4.12 Illustrated preoperative marking of a free TRAM flap (black) demonstrating the rectus abdominis muscle (red), intercostal innervation (green), and the inferior epigastric artery (red) and vein (blue).

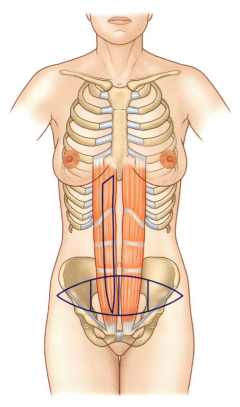

Fig. 20.4.10 The standard elliptical marking of the free TRAM flap with the vascular zones.

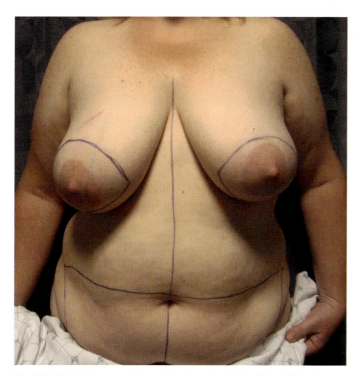

Fig. 20.4.11 Actual preoperative marking of a patient that will have bilateral skin-sparing mastectomies and a bilateral free TRAM flap.

is usually delineated. With immediate reconstruction in the setting of skin-sparing mastectomy, the areolar border is delineated. With immediate reconstruction in the setting of nipple-sparing, it is the author's preference to use a laterally based incision that extends to the lateral edge of the areola. On occasion, the incision may be extended through the areola or around the areolar border by 90–180 degrees. This provides excellent exposure for the mastectomy and the exposure of the internal mammary artery and vein. Some surgeons prefer an inframammary incision for the mastectomy and for access to the recipient vessels.

Important markings for the free TRAM flap include the anterior superior iliac spine (ASIS), midline, and proposed incisions (Fig. 20.4.12). The midline of the abdomen from the xiphoid to the pubic bone is delineated. The proposed upper and lower transverse incisions are delineated and communicated laterally at the ASIS. The proposed lower abdominal incision is an approximation. The final location is determined intraoperatively when the patient is flexed about 30° to ensure that the abdomen can be closed. Sometimes the proposed incision has to be elevated above the pubic hairline in order to ensure closure of the abdomen. The design of the free TRAM flap should incorporate the aesthetic units of the abdomen such that the final scar will be positioned as low as possible extending superolaterally towards the ASIS.

Recipient vessels

Recipient vessels for the free TRAM flap include the internal mammary and the thoracodorsal artery and vein.[25,26] Anatomic studies of the internal mammary vessels at the level of the 4th rib have demonstrated a diameter of 0.99–2.55 mm for the artery and

0.64–4.45 mm for the vein. The diameter of the thoracodorsal vessels ranges from 1.5 to 3.0 mm for the artery and 2.5 to 4.5 mm for the vein. Blood flow rates of the inferior epigastric, internal mammary, and thoracodorsal arteries have been evaluated with flow rates of 11 mL/min (range, 5–17), 25 mL/min (range, 15–35), and 5 mL/min (range, 2–8), respectively. Studies have demonstrated that either vessel is suitable for microvascular anastomosis and that success rates using the internal mammary or thoracodorsal vessels range from 97% to 99%.[25]

The mastectomy skin flaps

In cases of immediate breast reconstruction, the quality of the mastectomy will impact the quality of the reconstruction.[27] Mastectomies are performed using either skin-sparing techniques or nipple areolar sparing techniques. With both approaches, the vascularity of the remaining mastectomy skin flaps must be maintained. Incisional approaches for the mastectomy may be apical, inframammary, or lateral areolar (Fig. 20.4.13). When there has been extensive undermining of the mastectomy flaps, the natural borders are re-established by suturing the inframammary and lateral mammary folds back to the chest wall. If the vascularity of the mastectomy skin flaps is compromised, the edges are excised until normal bleeding is observed. The use of fluorescent angiography can assist the surgeon with the decision-making process regarding tissue perfusion.[28] With all of these approaches, free TRAM reconstruction can be performed with excellent aesthetic outcomes.

An important and sometimes overlooked aspect of achieving ideal breast aesthetics is to make the necessary adjustments to the skin envelope following mastectomy in the setting of immediate reconstruction.[27,29] In the setting of a skin-sparing mastectomy with excess skin, it should be debrided to fit the flap. When the excision pattern is periareolar, the circular excision pattern can be further excised and adjusted to fit the desired skin paddle of the flap with a purse-string suture technique. An alternative option is to partially inset the flap medially and then excise the lateral mastectomy skin such that a laterally based "lollipop" pattern is created. With nipple-sparing mastectomy, it is important to ensure that enough donor tissue is present to fill the skin envelope.

In women considering delayed reconstruction with a free TRAM, there are several factors to consider.[30–33] When radiation therapy has been completed prior to the reconstruction, adequate time must elapse to allow the tissues and vascularity to recover. This is typically 6–12 months. In patients who will receive radiation therapy following reconstruction, consideration to the type of reconstruction being performed is important. Known long-term consequences of radiation are fat atrophy and distortion. To eliminate these effects, many reconstructive surgeons have adopted the delayed-immediate approach as a means to avoid radiation damage to the flap. With this technique, a subpectoral tissue expander is placed immediately following the mastectomy and becomes the target for the radiation. Following radiation, the device is removed and replaced with autologous tissue. Most tissue expanders are placed totally or partially behind the pectoralis major muscle. When these devices are removed, the pectoralis major muscle should be returned to its normal position on the chest wall such that the flap is positioned on top of the muscle. This will optimize aesthetics and prevent animation or distortion

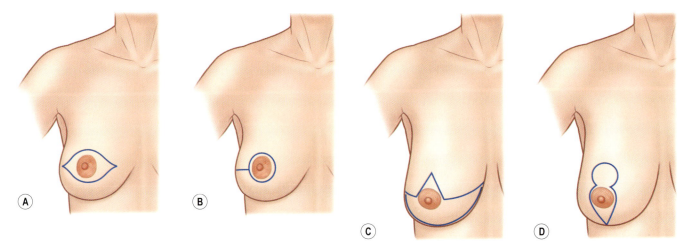

Fig. 20.4.13 Mastectomy planning. **(A)** A standard mastectomy incision via an ellipse that is oriented either obliquely or transversely. **(B)** A skin-sparing mastectomy via periareolar incision which may be supplemented with an extension for better access to the tail and axilla. **(C)** A Wise pattern mastectomy or **(D)** vertical reduction pattern – both are useful for macromastia in which the reconstruction will be smaller than the preoperative state.

with contraction of the pectoralis major muscle. Severely radiated tissues that have been damaged or fibrotic are usually excised. In these cases, the inferior edge of the flap usually becomes the upper aspect of the inframammary fold.

The free TRAM flap

The free TRAM is considered by many plastic surgeons to be the most reliable of the free tissue transfer procedures for breast reconstruction because it has excellent blood supply, does not require a meticulous intramuscular dissection, and is usually easier to harvest. Although a DIEP flap may be the primary choice for many surgeons and patients, a free TRAM flap is considered when the quality of perforators is deemed inadequate for a DIEP flap (<1.5 mm in diameter) or when the flap volume requirements exceed 800 g (see Table 20.4.3). When considering the spectrum of free TRAM flaps, a muscle-sparing free TRAM (MS-1 or MS-2) is performed in the majority of cases. The MS-0 variant is rarely performed because it disrupts the continuity of the rectus abdominis muscle. The advantage of the free TRAM flaps over the DIEP flap is that multiple perforators can be included that may minimize the incidence of fat necrosis or vascular compromise.

The decision regarding whether to perform a free TRAM or DIEP flap is ultimately based on the presence and quality of the abdominal wall perforating vessels.[5,18] Knowledge of these perforators can be assessed either pre- or intraoperatively (Table 20.4.5). Preoperative assessment of perforators is usually obtained using computerized tomography (CT) or magnetic resonance (MR) angiography.[34,35] With either modality, the location and caliber of the perforating vessel or vessels, as well as the intramuscular course of the source vessel, can be adequately determined. The advantage of these imaging modalities is that the "guesswork" as to whether a perforator is present or suitable is essentially eliminated and the harvesting of a DIEP flap can be more reliably performed. In addition, the CT or MR angiogram can alert the surgeon as to the subfascial course of the

perforator. In the event that these imaging studies are inconclusive or the intraoperative assessment does not correlate with the preoperative imaging studies, a free TRAM can be considered

Surgical technique

Preparing for surgery

Following the markings, patients are transported to the operating room and placed in the supine position under general endotracheal anesthesia. Pneumatic compression devices are applied to both legs, and a Foley catheter is inserted. All patients receive a dose of intravenous antibiotics before making the incision. The anesthesiologist is asked to avoid vasoconstricting medication because of the risk of vascular spasm and flap failure. Fluid resuscitation with crystalloid, colloid, or blood is preferred. Muscle relaxation is necessary in all patients to safely dissect the free TRAM flap. The operation is performed using loupe magnifying glasses for the flap dissection. An operating microscope is preferred for the microvascular anastomosis.

Harvesting the flaps

Following the initial upper abdominal incision, the dissection proceeds to the anterior rectus sheath (Fig. 20.4.14A). The anterior rectus sheath is a vascularized lattice of collagen fibers that should be preserved as much as possible. It is important to note that sensory nerves usually pass through the fascia as neurovascular bundles en route to the skin. These nerves should be identified and divided. Clipping these sensory nerves should be avoided to prevent a painful neuroma. Once a network or island of perforators is visualized on the anterior sheath, it is outlined and incised (Fig. 20.4.14B). The dimensions of the fascial excision typically range 1–2 cm in width and 2–4 cm in length. Incising the anterior rectus sheath is not without consequence, as it disrupts the normal lattice of fibers that is considered one of the primary support systems of the anterior abdominal wall. Under normal

Table 20.4.5 Comparison of the various imaging modalities with respect to radiation exposure, contrast requirements, caliber assessment, location, course, flow, and accuracy

Test	Radiation	Contrast	Caliber	Location	Flow	Course	Accuracy
Doppler	No	No	No	Yes	No	No	Low
Color duplex	No	No	No	Yes	Yes	No	Moderate
CTA	Yes	Yes	Yes	Yes	No	Yes	High
MRA	No	Yes	Yes	Yes	No	Yes	High

circumstances, as intra-abdominal pressure increases, the lattice will tighten to maintain contour. It is important to preserve as much of the anterior rectus sheath as possible and to adequately close all layers during the closing phase.

In contrast to the DIEP flap dissection, the anterior rectus sheath is elevated off the surface of the rectus abdominis muscle medially and laterally. The muscle is undermined, and the location of the inferior epigastric artery is visualized and palpated. This maneuver will facilitate the dissection of the free TRAM and minimize the chance of injury to the perforators or primary source vessel. The rectus abdominis muscle is divided along the desired segments using a fine-tip mosquito clamp and an electrocautery device. When the perforators are located in the central segment of the rectus abdominis muscle, a MS-2 free TRAM is harvested. When the perforators are predominately over the medial or lateral

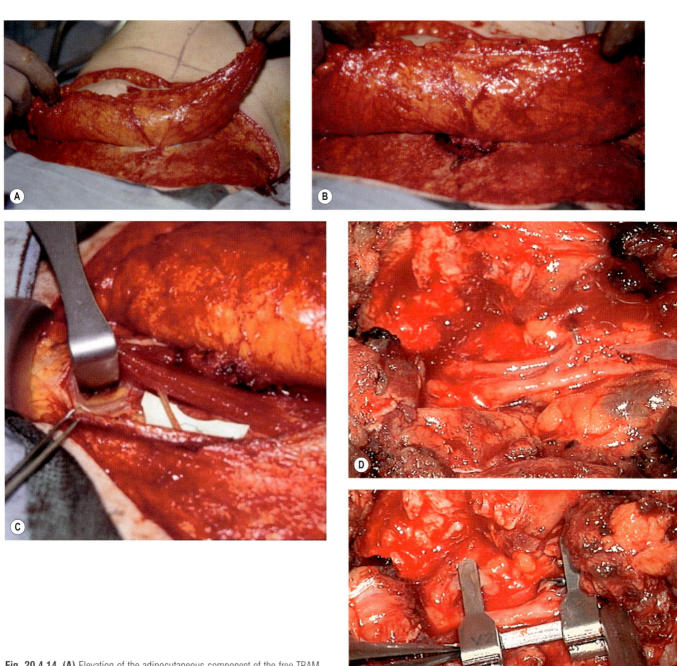

Fig. 20.4.14 **(A)** Elevation of the adipocutaneous component of the free TRAM being elevated off of the anterior rectus sheath extending to an island of perforators. **(B)** The fascial incision around the island of perforators. **(C)** Preservation of the lateral intercostal innervation to the rectus abdominis muscle. **(D)** The internal mammary artery and vein are prepared as the recipient vessels. **(E)** The double approximating vascular clamps are applied to the internal mammary and inferior epigastric veins in preparation for the anastomosis.

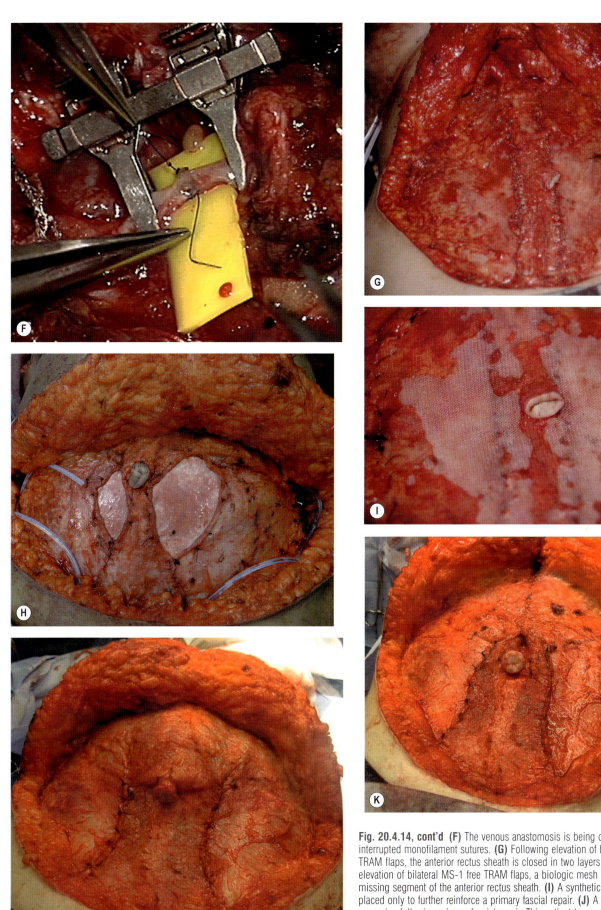

Fig. 20.4.14, cont'd **(F)** The venous anastomosis is being completed with interrupted monofilament sutures. **(G)** Following elevation of bilateral MS-2 free TRAM flaps, the anterior rectus sheath is closed in two layers. **(H)** Following elevation of bilateral MS-1 free TRAM flaps, a biologic mesh is used to replace the missing segment of the anterior rectus sheath. **(I)** A synthetic mesh is occasional placed only to further reinforce a primary fascial repair. **(J)** A contour abnormality may arise following primary fascial repair. This patient has a rectus diastasis with bulging of the upper abdomen. **(K)** Following plication, normal contour of the abdomen is restored.

Continued

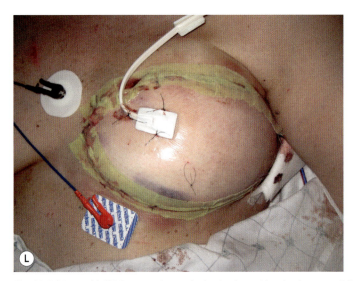

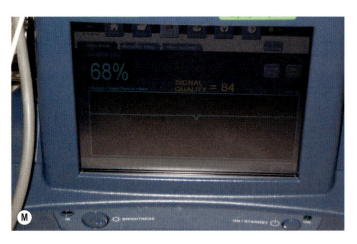

Fig. 20.4.14, cont'd (L) Postoperative monitoring is often achieved using a near infrared spectroscopy probe. **(M)** The unit displays the transcutaneous oxygen saturation (68%) in a time-dependent fashion and the signal quality strength (84%).

aspect of the muscle, then an MS-1 free TRAM is harvested. The lateral intercostal innervation is preserved when possible to ensure muscle contractility (Fig. 20.4.14C). Each of these flaps requires a myotomy or segmental excision of muscle. There are crossover motor nerve branches that will be encountered. These nerves are usually divided sharply without clips to permit axonal sprouting and neurotization of the medial segment of the rectus abdominis.

Maximal preservation of the rectus abdominis muscle and the anterior rectus sheath will usually improve functional outcomes related to the anterior abdominal wall. All variations of myotomy or myomectomy of the rectus abdominis will limit the contractility of the muscle because the contractile sarcomeres are replaced by scar. Loss of continuity of the muscle (MS-0 free TRAM) will result in a non-functional muscle; therefore MS-3, MS-2, and MS-1 flaps are preferred.[1,2,22–24] Limiting the amount of anterior rectus sheath excision will minimize contour abnormalities of the abdomen.

Microsurgery

Following exposure of the recipient vessels and elevation of the flap, the microscope is positioned along the patient (Fig. 20.4.14D). In some cases where the recipient and donor vessels are large (>2.5 mm), surgical loupes can be considered. Prior to division of the free TRAM flap from its source, 3000–5000 units of heparin is administered intravenously. The loose adventitia is cleared from the donor and recipient vessels under the microscope. In some patients a venae comitans is present. The distal recipient vessels are clipped. The microvascular clamps are placed on the donor and

recipient vessels, properly aligned, and divided (Fig. 20.4.14E). The lumen is irrigated with a dilute heparin solution. The anastomosis is completed using 8-0 sutures placed in an interrupted manner or continuous manner (Fig. 20.4.14F). Many surgeons prefer to use a vascular coupler for the venous anastomosis and to hand sew the artery. Following completion of the anastomosis, a Doppler is used to assess arterial and venous patency. The cutaneous Doppler location is marked with a suture for postoperative monitoring.

Closing the abdomen

Abdominal closure requires proper technique, attention to detail, and appropriate use of supplemental materials when necessary.[36–39] It is important to approximate the medial and lateral segments of muscle when an MS-2 or MS-3 flap has been performed to minimize the incidence of lateralization of the muscle that may occur with contraction and intra-abdominal pressure. Proper closure of the anterior rectus sheath is the most important predictive aspect of outcome. With the MS-3 flap, fascial approximation is performed using an absorbable or non-absorbable monofilament suture placed in an interrupted figure-of-8 fashion (Fig. 20.4.14G). All lamellae of the anterior sheath are closed to ensure stability. A second row of sutures is placed in a running, continuous fashion for additional reinforcement. Mesh reinforcement is rarely necessary except when the fascia is weak or tears with suture placement. When an MS-0, MS-1, or MS-2 free TRAM flap has been performed, primary fascial closure without mesh is possible when there is enough laxity or redundancy of the fascia. In situations where it is not, the use of a biologic or synthetic mesh may be necessary (Fig. 20.4.14H,I). The purpose of the mesh is to minimize tension on the fascial closure and to decrease the likelihood of dehiscence or attenuation. The mesh can be placed as an inlay when there is a fascial deficit and as an onlay when the fascial closure needs additional reinforcement. The use of a mesh has been necessary in approximately 10% of patients.

Following fascial closure, additional plication of the superior or midline fascia is considered to achieve ideal contour. With unilateral breast reconstruction, contralateral plication can balance and flatten the anterior abdominal wall and will centralize the umbilicus. With bilateral reconstructions, the supraumbilical fascia is often plicated along the midline to prevent an upper abdominal bulge (Fig. 20.4.14J,K). These sutures are usually monofilament and also placed in a figure-of-8 fashion. Infraumbilical midline sutures are also sometimes useful to achieve ideal contour.

Skin closure is the final stage of abdominal closure and includes the umbilicus and the incisions. The insetting of the umbilicus is an important step to achieve ideal abdominal aesthetics. Various skin incision patterns are possible that include circular, oval, and 'U' designs. A technique that has demonstrated success is the 2-dermal flap umbilical transposition flap.[40] With this technique, the umbilicus is invaginated to shorten the umbilical stalk and yields a very natural appearance. Skin closure is always performed in three layers including Scarpa's fascia, dermis, and epidermis. Closure of Scarpa's layer is important to prevent separation of the fat resulting in an involuted scar. When closing in obese women, the subscarpal fat may be excessive and require excision. This layer is often less vascularized than the subcutaneous fat located above Scarpa's fascia. The thickness of the upper and lower adipocutaneous layers of the abdominal wall should be similar to prevent any step-off deformity. The slight depression of the midline anterior abdominal wall can be recreated by excision of a few millimeters of fat along the midline of the adipose layer. This maneuver will provide a more natural abdominal contour. Monofilament sutures are used for the dermis and subcuticular layers. Lateral "dog-ears" should be identified at time of closure and addressed. This will lengthen the abdominal incision but improve overall abdominal contour. Two closed suction drains are always used to minimize the occurrence of a fluid collection.

Flap insetting

When insetting the free TRAM flap following a unilateral or bilateral reconstruction, it is recommended to flex the patient approximately 45° to assess the position, symmetry, contour, and projection of the breast.[3,4,29,41] In cases of a skin-sparing mastectomy, the skin territory to be exteriorized is delineated and the remainder of the flap is de-epithelialized. When a nipple-sparing mastectomy has been performed, a Doppler is used to identify an arteriovenous signal and delineated with a 2 cm circle. The remainder of the flap is de-epithelialized, and the skin paddle is exteriorized. The vascular pedicle must be visualized with insetting to ensure that it is not twisted or kinked. With delayed reconstruction, the lower mastectomy skin is usually excised or de-epithelialized and the inferior edge of the autologous flap is used to recreate the inframammary fold.

Shaping the free TRAM flap

There are several shaping advantages using free flaps for breast reconstruction when compared with pedicle flaps.[3,4,29] Pedicle flaps are tethered to the donor site muscle that often limits proper positioning of the flap. The free TRAM, however, permits optimal positioning on the chest wall because it is not tethered. With bilateral reconstruction, the abdominal donor tissue is bisected at the midline. The weight of the mastectomy specimen is less relevant because the volume of flap is fixed and limited to the hemi-abdomen. The medial edge of the flap (zone 2) is usually positioned along the sternal border, and the lateral aspect of the flap is positioned on the lateral chest wall. Suturing of the flap to the chest wall is sometimes necessary with immediate reconstruction, especially when the footprint of the old breast is larger than the footprint of the flap. These absorbable sutures can be placed superomedially, inferomedially, and laterally. With delayed reconstruction, the dimensions of the created subcutaneous pocket are usually made to match that of the flap, so internal suturing is usually not necessary.

With a unilateral reconstruction, the goal is to achieve symmetry with the opposite breast. Assessment of patient expectations is critical because it is important to know if the opposite breast will be reduced, augmented, or left as is. The opposite breast is sometimes used as a template for the reconstruction, especially if the volume of the free TRAM is sufficient to match the volume of the breast. Typically with a unilateral reconstruction, zones 1–3 and sometimes zone 4 are utilized, depending on the amount of tissue required and the perfusion characteristics of the flap. Because there is more tissue available for the unilateral flap (zones 1–3) compared with the bilateral flap (zones 1–2), shaping options are increased. The flap can be folded in a conical fashion or it can be folded laterally such that apical portion (zone

2) of the flap is tucked under zone 1, with zone 3 of the flap being positioned along the sternal border. With both maneuvers, the goal is to provide better projection and contour. Suturing the flap laterally is usually necessary, and suturing the flap along the medial border is occasionally necessary.

Another aspect of shaping depends on the location of the recipient vessels. When the anastomosis is to the internal mammary vessels, the flap can be positioned anywhere on the chest wall. When the anastomosis is to the thoracodorsal vessels, the flap may not reach the medial border because the thoracodorsal vessels are laterally based. This is less likely with unilateral reconstruction because of the inclusion of zone 3; however, with bilateral flap reconstruction, a medial deficiency may be noted. Thus, one advantage of the internal mammary recipient vessels is that there is ample length of the vascular pedicle such that the flap can be positioned, shaped, and contoured without impediments.

Postoperative care

Following the operation, patients are transported to the recovery room where diligent monitoring is performed. Patients will typically be monitored using a hand held Doppler and a near infrared spectrometer (Fig. 20.4.14L,M). Other monitoring methods include capillary refill, turgor, color, and temperature. Flap monitoring occurs every 15 min for the first 4 h, hourly for the next 20 h, and then every 2–4 h for the next 48 h. Patients are typically started on aspirin 325 mg daily for 2 weeks. Heparin is administered intraoperatively but not postoperatively.

Outcomes, prognosis, and complications

The free TRAM is capable of achieving excellent aesthetic outcomes that are reproducible and predictable. Because of the excellent vascularity, fat and partial necrosis is uncommon. In addition, greater volumes of fat can be perfused because of the different perforators perfusing different angiosomes. Abdominal outcomes are maintained from a functional and aesthetic perspective (see Table 20.4.4). The ability to perform sit-ups is higher following unilateral free TRAM flap reconstruction compared with bilateral. Fig. 20.4.15A–D illustrates a woman following bilateral skin-sparing mastectomy and immediate reconstruction with MS-2 free TRAM flaps. Fig. 20.4.15E–H shows another woman following bilateral skin-sparing mastectomy and immediate reconstruction with an MS-1 free TRAM flap.

Complications

Factors that may increase the risk of flap failure can be divided into two groups: those that are within the control of the surgeon and those that are not. Factors that can be controlled by the surgeon are often related to meticulous technique, knowledge of the relevant anatomy, and attention to detail. Flap failure is the most serious complication and can be due to arterial or venous factors (Fig. 20.4.16). Venous occlusion due to clot, kinking, or twisting of the vascular pedicle is the most common and characterized by a flap that becomes congested, edematous, and tense (Fig. 20.4.17). Arterial occlusion is less common and may be due to the same factors but is characterized by a flap that is pale, ashen, and soft (Fig. 20.4.18). Both situations require a return to the operating room.

Operative exploration requires a return to the operating room where the flap sutures are removed and the flap is exteriorized. The anastomosis and vascular pedicle are inspected. With venous occlusion, the vein is tense and dilated and may be filled with clotted blood. In some cases, the pedicle may have a kink or twist and realignment of the pedicle is all that is needed to restore circulation. When the etiology is a true thrombosis, management includes takedown of the anastomosis, embolectomy of the venous limb, and irrigation of the lumen with heparin. If clot is suspected in the flap or the muscle, thrombolytic therapy is indicated. Success with this technique depends on the elapsed time interval and is more effective when occlusion has been less than 2 h. If the flap demonstrates sluggish venous outflow, medicinal leech therapy can be considered following exploration.

With arterial occlusion, there is no pulse and the veins are usually flat. The anastomosis is taken down and inspected for thrombin clot or intimal damage. In some cases, the vessels are trimmed and the anastomosis is performed again. When there is persistent disruption of flow, vascular spasm, or a clotting disorder is suspected, 4% lidocaine or papaverine HCl may be used along the adventitia of the vessel to promote vasodilation. If the flap is deemed unsalvageable, then it is removed and sometimes replaced with a tissue expander.

There are other factors that can also influence the success of microvascular breast reconstruction. Advanced patient age and its relationship to microvascular success have demonstrated success rates similar to non-elderly patients and range from 97% to 99%.[42,43] ASA status and length of the operation are significant predictors of postoperative morbidity.[42] Clinical studies related to glycemic status have demonstrated that patients with diabetes mellitus are not at increased risk for flap failure, abnormal healing of the anastomosis, or intolerance to an ischemic challenge, as long as a euglycemic state is maintained in the preoperative period.[9] Hemoglobin A_{1c} levels >7 are associated with increased complications such as delayed healing, incisional dehiscence, and infection. Connective tissue disorders such as lupus and psoriatic arthritis are often thought to

increase complications following breast reconstruction; however, studies have demonstrated that perioperative complication rates are similar to patients without connective tissue disorders.[44]

There are other factors that can lead to partial or total flap failure.[8,14,19,20] Inadequate outflow of the internal mammary system can lead to venous congestion,

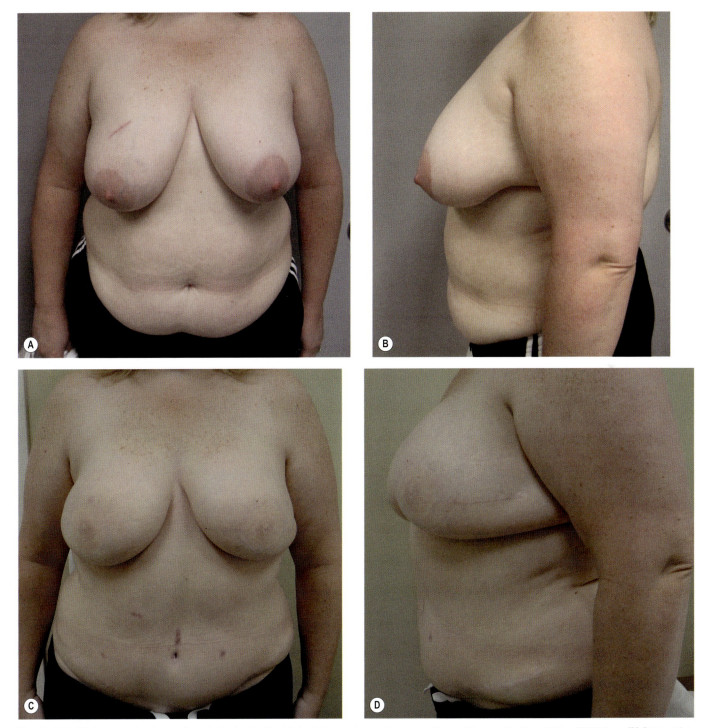

Fig. 20.4.15 (A) A preoperative image of a patient scheduled for bilateral skin-sparing mastectomy and immediate reconstruction with free TRAM flaps. **(B)** Preoperative left lateral view. **(C)** Postoperative view of the breast and abdomen following the bilateral MS-2 free TRAM flaps, at the 2-year follow-up. **(D)** Postoperative left lateral view at the 2-year follow-up.

Continued

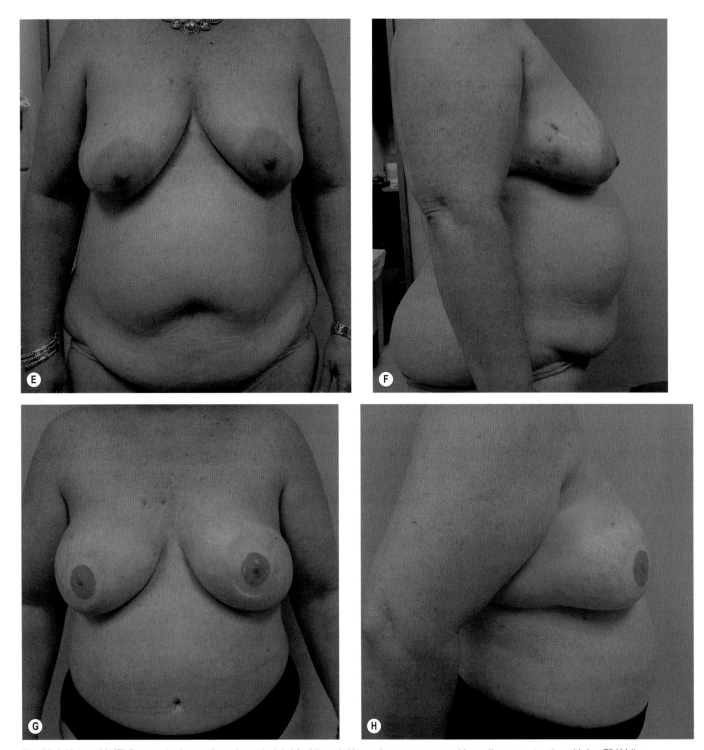

Fig. 20.4.15, cont'd **(E)** Preoperative image of a patient scheduled for bilateral skin-sparing mastectomy and immediate reconstruction with free TRAM flaps.
(F) Preoperative right lateral view. **(G)** Postoperative view of the breast and abdomen following the bilateral MS-2 free TRAM flaps at the 1.5-year follow-up.
(H) Postoperative right lateral view at the 1.5-year follow-up.

partial necrosis, fat necrosis, or total flap failure. Radiation damage to the recipient vessels can be the source of progressive inflammation and lead to vascular thrombosis. Some women will have undiagnosed hypercoagulability states and form clots at the anastomoses. Postoperative bleeding and hematoma formation can result in flap failure. In the author's experience, anastomotic failure is usually due to venous occlusion and is responsible for return to the operating room and flap necrosis in the majority of cases. Two factors commonly associated with anastomotic and flap failure are delayed reconstruction and postoperative hematoma.

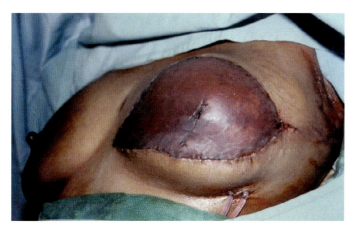

Fig. 20.4.16 Severe venous congestion of a flap demonstrating total flap failure.

Donor site complications include, but are not limited to, contour abnormalities, complex scars, delayed healing, seroma, pain, and infection.[1,2,21–24] Contour abnormalities include abdominal bulge and hernia and with the free TRAM occur more often with bilateral reconstruction (Fig. 20.4.19). Abdominal hernia is rare, and abdominal bulge occurs in the vast majority of cases. The incidence ranges from 3–10% for unilateral cases and 5–15% for bilateral cases. Abdominal fluid collections such as a hematoma or seroma are rare and typically occur in 1–2% of cases. Delayed healing may include incisional necrosis or dehiscence, umbilical necrosis, or soft tissue and fat necrosis (Fig. 20.4.20). This can be the result of prior abdominal incisions, obesity, poor perfusion, excessive tension, or patient comorbidities. Chronic pain may be the result of neuroma formation due to hemoclips placed on the sensory nerves or nerve entrapment.

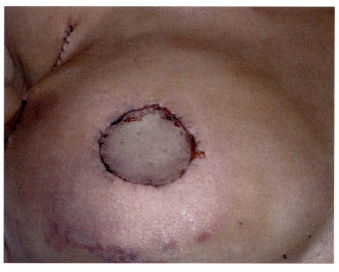

Fig. 20.4.18 Arterial occlusion of a flap demonstrating the pale and ashen color requiring operative exploration.

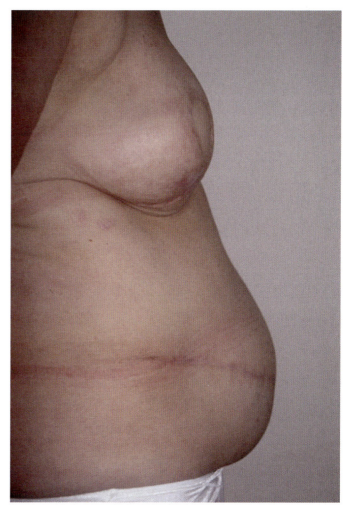

Fig. 20.4.19 Postoperative abdominal bulge is demonstrated following a bilateral free TRAM flap.

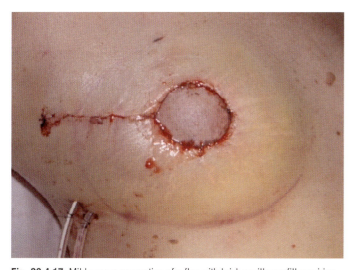

Fig. 20.4.17 Mild venous congestion of a flap with brisk capillary refill requiring operative exploration.

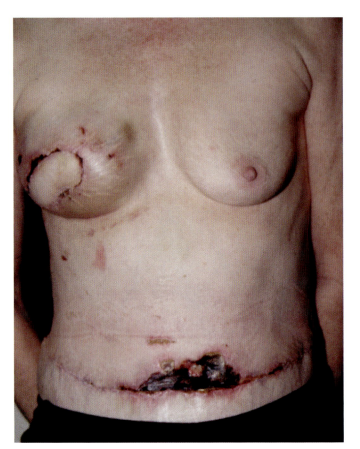

Fig. 20.4.20 Delayed healing and skin necrosis of the abdominal skin in a patient using tobacco products.

Secondary procedures

Secondary revisions are often necessary following autologous reconstruction with the free TRAM as well as most autologous flaps.[11,17,38] This may be to restore volume, contour, and position and include both flaps in the setting of a bilateral reconstruction as well as the ipsilateral and contralateral breast in the setting of a unilateral reconstruction. Various techniques are available for the reconstructed breast including soft-tissue recontouring, fat grafting, burying the flap, and implant placement. Achieving symmetry with the contralateral or non-reconstructed breast can be accomplished via augmentation, mastopexy, or reduction mammaplasty.

The reconstructed breast

The most common method of revision is by direct excision of skin and fat as well as tissue rearrangement.[15,29] The goal may be to reduce the volume, improve the shape, reposition the breast on the chest wall, or to better define the inframammary or lateral mammary folds. The technique of autologous fat grafting to correct contour deformities and to improve skin quality

is a common method that has achieved success. The placement of fat along the breast and chest wall is an excellent method to improve contour in the upper and medial pole of the breast (Fig. 20.4.21). Fat grafting has also been used in radiated breasts where skin damage or volume deficiency is present. The ability of fat and stem cells to regenerate, hydrate, and revascularize damaged skin is well accepted. When reconstruction with a free TRAM results in a breast that is too ptotic, the technique of burying the flap has demonstrated success. The skin territory of the flap is outlined with an elliptical extension and de-epithelialized. The mastectomy skin flaps are undermined superiorly and inferiorly and then re-approximated. Fig. 20.4.22 illustrates a woman with secondarily buried bilateral free TRAM flaps.

For the reconstructed breast that is deficient in volume, two methods of correction are commonly employed.[45–47] The first is to fat graft the parenchyma of the flap, and the second is to place a small implant under the flap. Fat grafting using a small cannula has been effective when placed within the flap itself. Volumes of 100–200 cc are possible because the tissues are soft and supple. When an implant is used to augment flap volume, it is usually saline and ranges in volume from 80 to 125 cc. This is because there is usually scar tissue present that prevents excessive fill volumes initially. In women with a history of chest wall radiation, the device is placed in the prepectoral position; whereas in women without a history of radiation therapy, the device is placed is the subpectoral position. Radiated patients typically have a fibrotic pectoralis major muscle that may increase the incidence of capsular contracture or device malposition.

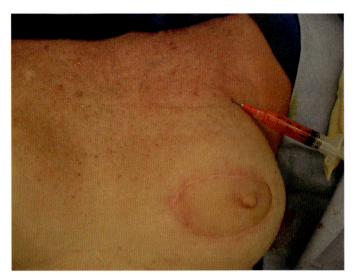

Fig. 20.4.21 The technique of fat grafting is illustrated as a means of secondary contouring of the flap.

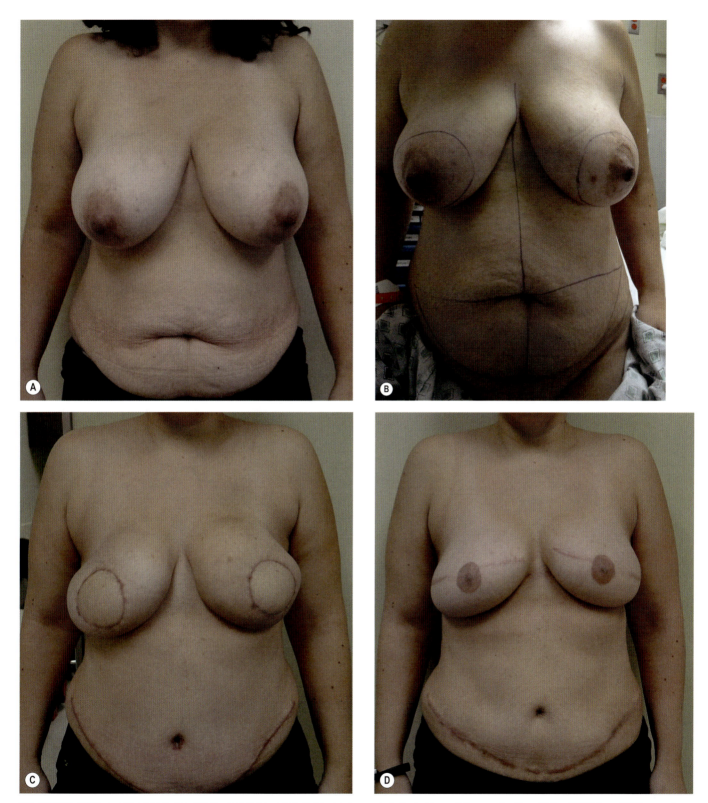

Fig. 20.4.22 (A) Preoperative image of a patient scheduled for bilateral skin-sparing mastectomy and immediate reconstruction with free TRAM flaps. **(B)** Preoperative markings are illustrated for the skin-sparing mastectomy and the flap. **(C)** Postoperative image following an MS-2 bilateral MS-2 free TRAM flap. The patient has bilateral breast ptosis. **(D)** Postoperative image following excision of the skin territory of the flap in an elliptical fashion with undermining of the mastectomy skin flaps and primary closure. Nipple areolar reconstruction has been completed; 1-year follow-up.

Nipple reconstruction is usually the final procedure that is performed. Common methods of nipple areolar reconstruction include various local flaps that include the CV, star, and skate flaps. These are usually performed at the time of secondary procedures. Areolar tattooing is usually performed 3 months following the nipple reconstruction. Nipple reconstruction is usually not advised in women who have had radiation to the free TRAM flap. Many women are choosing to have 3D nipple areolar tattooing performed.

The non-reconstructed breast

In unilateral reconstructions, the non-reconstructed breast is sometimes modified to achieve symmetry.[15,48] Options include unilateral augmentation with an implant, mastopexy, or reduction mammaplasty. Implant selections is facilitated by volumetric analysis using 3D imaging. Standard breast augmentation methods are used. When breast volumes are similar but the natural breast is ptotic, a mastopexy is sometimes performed. This is usually via a periareolar or circumvertical approach; however, in some cases, the inverted-T technique is performed. When the reconstructed breast is smaller than the natural breast, reduction mammaplasty is considered. This can be performed using a variety of techniques that include short scars when the difference is mild to moderate, as well as inverted-T scars when the difference is moderate to severe.

Correcting postoperative abdominal abnormalities

There are several postoperative abnormalities that can occur, and these include abdominal bulge, abdominal hernia, persistent pain, delayed healing, and chronic fluid collection.[1,2,11,17,21,36,37] Many of these can be managed conservatively; however, operative intervention is sometimes necessary. The first step is to address the patient concerns by performing a history and physical examination. Areas of abnormal contour, pain, induration, fluid, and delayed healing are noted. Abnormal contour may be secondary to edema, excess skin, and fascial compromise. It is important to differentiate between a bulge and hernia. A hernia will have a true facial defect that can be palpated, whereas a bulge will not. Pain is usually self-limiting but sometimes chronic due to neuroma formation. Fluid collections are rare but may be secondary to seroma or hematoma.

Abdominal bulge

An abdominal bulge is most often due to attenuation of the anterior rectus sheath. It can be exacerbated by

absence, weakness, or denervation of the rectus abdominis muscle. Imaging studies are usually not necessary with a bulge. With the free TRAM flaps, the bulge is usually located in the lower abdomen and is usually on the side of the flap harvest. When preparing for repair, the area of the bulge is delineated with the patient standing. During the operation, the lower transverse incision is opened and the upper adipocutaneous layer elevated. The bulge is identified and plicated in two vertical layers using a non-absorbable monofilament suture in a figure-of-8 fashion, as well as a continuous suture. The use of a synthetic mesh is usually considered to further reinforce the anterior abdominal wall and typically extends from the costal margin superiorly, the pubic region inferiorly, and the anterior axillary lines laterally. The sutures are usually absorbable monofilament and placed around the periphery of the mesh and centrally to anchor it to the anterior rectus sheath.

Abdominal hernia

The repair of a true hernia differs from that of the bulge (Figs. 20.4.23 & 20.4.24). Given that there is a facial defect, the repair mirrors that of a ventral incisional hernia with the main difference being that the rectus abdominis muscle is altered. The initial phase of the repair includes defining the fascial edges of the defect, followed by excision of the hernia sac. An intra-abdominal approach to the repair is required. Mesh

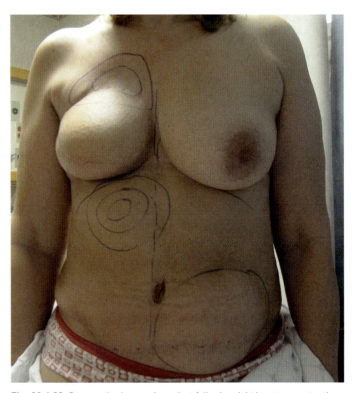

Fig. 20.4.23 Preoperative image of a patient following right breast reconstruction with a free TRAM flap with a left abdominal contour abnormality.

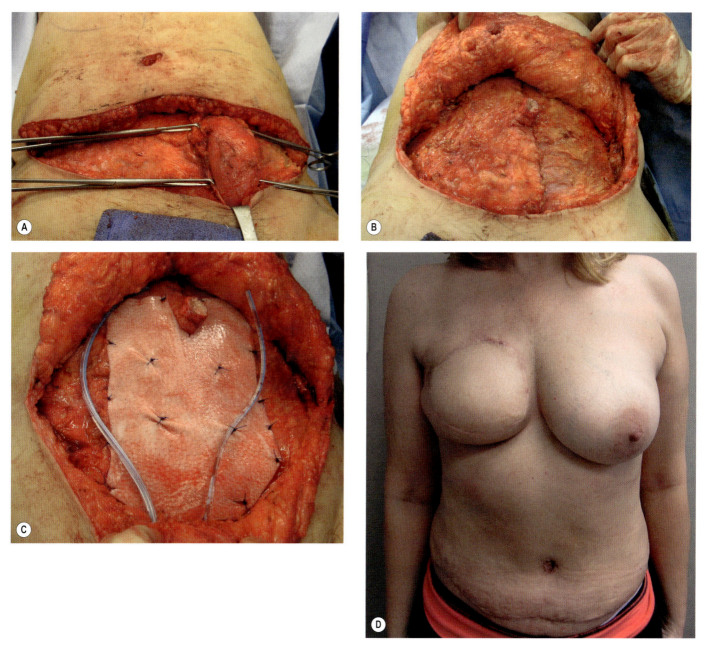

Fig. 20.4.24 **(A)** Intraoperative image of a left fascial defect consistent with an abdominal hernia. **(B)** The hernia sac is excised, and the remaining layers of the anterior rectus sheath are closed in 2-layers. **(C)** A biologic mesh is placed in an onlay fashion to further reinforce the abdominal wall. **(D)** Postoperative view of the abdomen at the 3-month follow-up.

reinforcement is often necessary and can be used as an underlay or onlay fashion. Both synthetic and biologic meshes can be considered. Underlay and onlay mesh should span as much of the anterior abdominal wall as possible. Absorbable monofilament sutures are usually used to anchor the mesh to its surface. The fascial edges are re-approximated when possible using non-absorbable monofilament sutures in an interrupted figure-of-8 fashion followed by a running continuous suture placed along the linea alba. In complex situations associated with recurrence and loss of domain, the use of tissue expanders can be considered to repair a true hernia.

Pain

Chronic pain following abdominal flap reconstruction may be due to scar formation along the anterior rectus sheath or a neuroma.[17] Neuromas usually occur following placement of a surgical clip that has been placed along a sensory branch of the intercostal neurovascular bundle as it traverses through the anterior rectus sheath to the adipocutaneous layer. Other etiologies may include entrapment of the ilioinguinal and iliohypogastric nerves as well as the use of an onlay synthetic mesh. Conservative management is usually recommended for the first 6 months because most of these symptoms are self-limiting. Surgical management is often recommended when the pain persists beyond 6 months and interferes with activities of daily living. Specific management techniques include excision of the neuroma with burial of the nerve stump into the underlying muscle, as well as partial or total removal of synthetic mesh when responsible.

Fluid collections

Fluid collections following abdominal flap reconstruction can occur and may be due to premature drain removal, damage to the loose areolar layer of the anterior rectus sheath, and body habitus. Seroma is the most common followed by hematoma. Many of these fluid collections are small and self-limiting; however, when large and persistent, intervention is usually recommended. Invasive maneuvers include office procedures such as serial aspiration or by placing an indwelling catheter via interventional radiology. Operative evacuation may be considered when refractory to conventional maneuvers.

Conclusion

The free TRAM flap is an excellent option for autologous reconstruction in properly selected patients. The vascularity and perfusion characteristics are predictable and capable of sustaining large flap volumes. The flap can be elevated with variable amounts of the rectus abdominis muscle and classified as MS-0, 1, or 2. Success rates for the free TRAM range from 97% to 99%. Its utility in the setting of skin- and nipple-sparing mastectomy is excellent, and its complication profile is acceptably low. Donor site morbidity is low, and patients usually retain almost all of their preoperative function. Aesthetic outcomes can be excellent and rival those of the other abdominal flaps.

🌐 Access the complete reference list online at   **http://www.expertconsult.com**

5. Nahabedian MY, Momen B, Galdino G, et al. Breast reconstruction with the free TRAM or DIEP flap: patient selection, choice of flap, and outcome. *Plast Reconstr Surg.* 2002;110:466–475. *The authors review their early experience with 163 free TRAM or DIEP flap breast reconstructions performed on 135 women. Selection of the free TRAM or DIEP flap should be made on the basis of patient weight, quantity of abdominal fat, and breast volume requirement, and on the number, caliber, and location of the perforating vessel. Adverse events were similar for the two groups.*

10. Hseih F, Kumiponjera D, Malata CM. An algorithmic approach to abdominal flap breast reconstruction in patients with pre-existing scars: results from a single surgeon's experience. *J Plast Reconstr Aesthet Surg.* 2009;62:1650–1660. *The authors review their experience with pre-existing abdominal scars in 30 patients scheduled for TRAM flaps demonstrating that pre-existing scars are not an absolute contraindication to abdominal flap breast reconstruction. They provide an algorithm for decision-making.*

11. Nahabedian MY. Factors to consider in breast reconstruction. *Womens Health (Lond).* 2015;11:325–342. *This paper reviews essential elements for all types of breast reconstruction with an emphasis on patient selection, reconstructive technique, and outcomes.*

21. Chang E, Chang E, Soto-Miranda MA, et al. Comprehensive analysis of donor-site morbidity in abdominally based free flap breast reconstruction. *Plast Reconstr Surg.* 2013;132:1383–1391. *The authors review 89 of 1507 patients who developed an abdominal bulge/hernia following free abdominal flaps. Contour abnormalities were more likely to occur following full width muscle harvest. There was no difference between MS free TRAM and DIEP patients in the unilateral or bilateral setting.*

23. Nelson JA, Guo Y, Sonnad SS, et al. A comparison between DIEP and muscle-sparing free TRAM flaps in breast reconstruction: a single surgeon's recent experience. *Plast Reconstr Surg.* 2010;126:1428–1435. *The authors review their early outcomes in 144 patients following DIEP or free TRAM flap breast reconstruction, demonstrating that the choice of flap should be made intraoperatively, based on anatomic findings on a patient-by-patient basis.*

31. Mirzabeigi MN, Smartt JM, Nelson JA, et al. An assessment of the risks and benefits of immediate autologous breast reconstruction in patients undergoing postmastectomy radiation therapy. *Ann Plast Surg.* 2013;71:149–155. *This study reviews outcomes in 407 women following autologous reconstruction and radiation therapy. There was a higher incidence of fat necrosis and volume loss in the radiation cohort. Other adverse events were not increased.*

36. Mennie JC, Mohanna PN, O'Donoghue JM, et al. Donor-site hernia repair in abdominal flap breast reconstruction: a population-based cohort study of 7929 patients. *Plast Reconstr Surg.* 2015;136:1–9. *This study reviews hernia rate in 7929 women who had a DIEP or TRAM flap breast reconstruction. The hernia repair rate was 2.45% after 3 years. Mean time to hernia repair following a DIEP or TRAM flap was 17.7 months. The only independent risk factor for hernia repair was age greater than 60 years.*

39. Patel KM, Shuck J, Hung R, et al. Reinforcement of the abdominal wall following breast reconstruction with abdominal flaps: a comparison of synthetic and biologic mesh. *Plast Reconstr Surg.* 2014;133:700–707. *This study reviews 818 patients that had synthetic mesh (n-61) or biological mesh (n-36) to reinforce the abdominal wall. Overall complication rates for the synthetic and biologic cohorts were 6.5% and 5.5%, respectively. Both meshes behave similarly for abdominal reinforcement.*

45. Kaoutzanis C, Xin M, Ballard TN, et al. Autologous fat grafting after breast reconstruction in postmastectomy patients: complications, biopsy rates, and locoregional cancer recurrence rates. *Ann Plast Surg.* 2016;76:270–275. *The authors review 108 women and 167 reconstructions following autologous fat grafting for revision. A total of 53 (31.7%) breasts underwent imaging after autologous fat grafting. Suspicious findings requiring biopsy were noted in four (2.4%) breasts, and clinically palpable masses combined with suspicious imaging findings requiring biopsy occurred in four (2.4%) breasts.*

48. Nahabedian MY. Managing the opposite breast: contralateral symmetry procedures. *Cancer J.* 2008;14:258–263. *A review of various options for managing the contralateral breast following breast reconstruction is provided.*

21.1

Introduction to alternative free flaps for breast reconstruction

Maurice Y. Nahabedian

Gluteal flaps

Many surgeons consider the gluteal free flaps to be among the most complex flaps for the microsurgeon (see Chapter 21.2).[1-4] Gluteal flaps can be raised with or without the gluteus maximus muscle. There are two perforator flaps that are derived from this region that include the superior (SGAP) and inferior (IGAP) gluteal artery perforator flaps. Gluteal flaps can be performed in women with a variety of body types, ranging from short to tall and thin to obese.

For some surgeons, the gluteal flaps are the second choice following the abdomen. Preoperative imaging with computed tomography (CT) or magnetic resonance imaging is useful to identify the caliber and position of the perforating vessels. The superior gluteal vessels are located above the piriformis muscle within the greater sciatic foramen, and the inferior gluteal vessels are located below the piriformis muscle within the lesser sciatic foramen. The vascular pedicle of these flaps is typically shorter and the vessel caliber is thinner than the free transverse rectus abdominis myocutaneous or deep inferior epigastric artery perforator flaps. Gluteal flaps are usually less voluminous than flaps from the abdominal region and range from 300 to 600 g. Following closure, the scars are located along the upper gluteal region (SGAP) or along the infragluteal crease (IGAP).

Medial thigh flaps

The medial thigh donor site provides another alternative donor site and has demonstrated success for breast reconstruction (see Chapter 21.3).[5-7] Flaps such as the transverse upper gracilis (TUG), diagonal upper gracilis (DUG), and transverse musculocutaneous gracilis (TMG) have been described. For some surgeons, the medial thigh is the preferred second choice when the abdomen is not suitable because the vascular pedicle is more predictable based on length and caliber. The caliber of the gracilis vascular pedicle ranges from 1.5 to 2.5 mm. The volume of these medial thigh flaps ranges from 150 to 550 cc.

Candidates for medial thigh flaps include women with insufficient abdomen skin and fat, who prefer not to use the abdomen, and have a moderate amount of skin and fat in the medial thigh. Other indications include bilateral reconstructions in which the mastectomy volume approximates the volume of the medial thigh or meets the expectation of the patient. DUG and TUG flaps are similar except that the orientation of the flap is oblique and posterior and parallel to Langer's lines.[8] The reason for this modification is to minimize disruption to the superficial lymphatic vessels and to conceal the incision when viewed from the frontal and lateral side. Potential adverse events associated with the TUG flaps include postoperative lymphedema, complex scarring, and thigh distortion.

Posterior thigh flaps

The PAP flap is becoming the preferred second option for many surgeons.[9,10] This flap is based off the profunda femoris artery and vein that has several associated perforators within the posterior compartment of the thigh (see Chapter 21.4). This flap is often considered as an alternative to the abdomen and ideally suited for small to moderate sized breasts with lipodystrophy in the posterior thigh territory. The weight of this flap ranges from 250 to 700 g. The advantages of this flap over gluteal flaps and medial thigh flaps are that lymphedema risk is minimal, pedicle length is increased, and gluteal contour is not affected.

The following three chapters describe the indications, technical aspects, and outcomes associated with all of these alternative flaps for breast reconstruction. All are capable of providing excellent outcomes in properly selected patients.

References

1. Ahmadzadeh R, Bergeron L, Tang M, et al. The superior and inferior gluteal artery perforator flaps. *Plast Reconstr Surg.* 2007;120:1551–1556. *This study describes the anatomic basis for these flaps based on perforator length and caliber. The flaps can be used as pedicle or free tissue transfer for a variety of indications.*

2. Allen RJ, Levine JL, Granzow JW. The in-the-crease inferior gluteal artery perforator flap for breast reconstruction. *Plast Reconstr Surg.* 2006;118:333–339. *The authors describe using the inferior gluteal artery in 59 patients. The flap results in a well concealed scar, can be extended as needed, not associated with sciatic nerve injury, and is an excellent alternative to the abdominal donor site.*

3. Guerra AB, Metzinger SE, Bidros RS, et al. Breast reconstruction with gluteal artery perforator flaps: a critical analysis of 142 flaps. *Ann Plast Surg.* 2004;52:118–125. *The authors describe the evolution of gluteal flaps for breast reconstruction. They report on their 9-year experience with this flap and describe important refinements, advantages, disadvantages, and lessons learned.*

4. Granzow JW, Levine JL, Chiu ES, et al. Breast reconstruction with gluteal artery perforator flaps. *J Plast Reconstr Aesthet Surg.*

5. Schoeller T, Huemer GM, Wechselberger G. The transverse musculocutaneous gracilis flap for breast reconstruction: guidelines for flap and patient selection. *Plast Reconstr Surg.* 2008;122:29–38. *A retrospective review of 111 patients and 154 TMG flaps for breast reconstruction. Based on excellent outcomes, the authors feel that this flap may surpass the abdomen as a primary donor site.*

6. Vega SJ, Sandeen SN, Bossert RP, et al. Gracilis myocutaneous free flap in autologous breast reconstruction. *Plast Reconstr Surg.* 2009;124:1400–1409. *The authors review their experience with 27 gracilis flaps for breast reconstruction. Outcomes included a flap success rate of 100% with an average operating time of 4.9 h for unilateral and 6.7 h for bilateral flaps.*

7. Fansa H, Schirmer S, Warnecke IC, et al. The transverse myocutaneous gracilis muscle flap: a fast and reliable method for breast reconstruction. *Plast Reconstr Surg.* 2008;122:1326–1333. *The authors describe their experience with the TMG flap in 32 patients. Mean operating time was 3.7 h for unilateral and 5.4 h for bilateral cases. The vascular pedicle is constant, and the soft tissue component resembles native breast.*

8. Dayan E, Smith ML, Sultan M, et al. The diagonal upper gracilis (DUG) flap: a safe and improved alternative to the TUG flap. *Plast Reconstr Surg.* 2013;132:33–34. *This abstract describes the diagonal upper gracilis flap. The advantages are that the scar is better concealed and the risk of lymphatic disruption is minimized.*

9. Allen RJ, Haddock NT, Ahn CY, et al. Breast reconstruction with the profunda artery perforator flap. *Plast Reconstr Surg.* 2012;129:16e–23e. *The authors review their experience with 27 PAP flaps. The skin paddle measures 27×7 cm on average, and the vascular pedicle is 7–3 in length. This flap represents another excellent alternative to the abdominal donor site.*

10. Haddock NT, Greaney P, Otterburn D, et al. Predicting perforator location on preoperative imaging for the profunda artery perforator flap. *Microsurgery.* 2012;32:507–511. *CT angiography was performed on 40 patients scheduled for PAP flap breast reconstruction. Preoperative imaging was found to correlate with observed perforators in all PAP flaps. Flap survival was 100% in 35 cases.*

The authors describe the technique of harvesting SGAP and IGAP flaps and demonstrate that these flaps are safe and reliable for breast reconstruction.

21.2

Gluteal free flaps for breast reconstruction

Matthew D. Goodwin, Jaime Flores, and Bernard W. Chang

Access video content for this chapter online at expertconsult.com

SYNOPSIS

- Free flap breast reconstruction has advanced in the last 15 years, especially in the development of perforator flap reconstruction, and numerous donor sites have been identified based on reliable and identifiable perforating blood vessels.
- The mainstay of donor sites remains the abdomen; however, not all patients are candidates for deep inferior epigastric artery perforator (DIEP) flap or superficial inferior epigastric artery (SIEA) reconstructions due to lack of tissue or previous surgery.
- The gluteal region remains a good secondary source of tissue for breast reconstruction in most patients, including thin patients. These flaps usually provide excellent projection and volume for breast reconstruction. The blood supply is very well defined with fairly reliable perforators being always present.
- The difficulty remains in the dissection of these perforators to their source at the superior gluteal artery or inferior gluteal artery as well as limitations in pedicle length and vessel mismatch with recipient vessels.
- Numerous branches also exist prior to gluteal flap source vessels, which are typically a better size match distal to these branches for the internal mammary vessels.

Introduction

Free flap breast reconstruction has advanced significantly in the last 15 years, especially in the development of perforator flap reconstruction. Numerous donor sites have been identified based on reliable and identifiable perforating blood vessels. The mainstay of donor sites remains the abdomen; however, not all patients are candidates for DIEP flap or SIEA reconstructions due to lack of tissue or previous surgery. The gluteal region remains a good secondary source of tissue for breast reconstruction in most patients who are not candidates for

reconstruction from the abdomen (i.e., paucity of tissue, previous abdominal surgery including failed transverse rectus abdominis myocutaneous (TRAM) or DIEP flap reconstruction, or incisions or scarring that have affected the blood supply to the abdomen) or have failed implant reconstruction. These flaps usually provide excellent projection and volume for breast reconstruction. Sufficient gluteal tissue is usually present, even in very thin patients, depending on how much tissue is required for reconstruction. The blood supply is very well defined with fairly reliable perforators being present. Gluteal tissue may be harvested based on the superior gluteal artery (SGAP) or the inferior gluteal artery (IGAP). The difficulty remains in the dissection of these perforators to their source at the SGAP or IGAP as well as the limitations in pedicle length and vessel mismatch with recipient vessels. Numerous branches also exist prior to gluteal flap source vessels which are typically a better size match for the internal mammary vessels. This chapter reviews the anatomy, surgical planning, and execution of the dissection of gluteal flaps.

Gluteal tissue for autogenous breast reconstruction was first introduced by Fujino et al. (1975)[1] for patients with congenital aplasia of the breast. Shaw,[2] Codner, and Nahai[3] popularized the gluteal myocutaneous flaps (both superior and inferior gluteal flaps), noting the disadvantage of a short pedicle necessitating vein grafts. Koshima et al. (1993)[4] described the SGAP flap for pedicled reconstruction of sacral pressure sores. Allen and Tucker[5] in 1995 first reported the technique of SGAP flap breast reconstruction. Since then, gluteal flaps have become an increasingly utilized method of breast reconstruction in microsurgery even for bilateral reconstruction.[6] Yet, many breast microsurgeons still do not perform the procedure due to lack of experience with the technique and the availability of more familiar alternatives (e.g., TRAM, DIEP, latissimus dorsi).

While technically demanding, the anatomy of the superior gluteal donor site consistently has adequate tissue and vessels for microsurgical transfer on a consistent basis.

Plastic surgeons with good microsurgical experience should be able to safely and consistently perform this procedure. Beyond the abdominal tissue donor site, options for breast reconstruction from other autogenous donor sites (e.g., latissimus dorsi, anterolateral thigh) often require an implant to obtain enough volume for symmetry. Other donor sites are also available but often have less donor tissue present or less consistent anatomy and smaller vessels (e.g., profunda artery perforator, transverse upper gracilis). Gluteal flap breast reconstruction should be considered a part of any complete breast reconstructive surgeon's microsurgical armamentarium.

Indications and contraindications

- Usually secondary choice to DIEP flap reconstruction
- Most patients are eligible candidates
- Avoid in obese patients due to shorter pedicle length and bulk of flap
- May be indicated for immediate or delayed reconstruction
- Consider expanding skin for delayed reconstruction if skin too tight or radiated
- Bilateral reconstruction can be performed at once or each side in two separate operations
- Avoid internal mammary recipient vessels in patients with cardiac history or strong family history of cardiac disease.

Indications

Candidates for gluteal flap breast reconstruction may include patients electing autogenous breast reconstruction but who do not desire implant reconstruction, or if the abdominal donor site is unavailable due to previous surgery, failed abdominal free flap, or those who are too thin. Implant reconstruction is also less desirable in patients who have undergone previous chest wall radiation, failed previous reconstruction, or due to patient preference. In the authors' practice, gluteal flap reconstruction may be offered to all patients electing autogenous reconstruction; however, it is usually a secondary choice if DIEP flap reconstruction is available. The DIEP flap is usually more popular for donor site cosmetic reasons. Advantages of the gluteal flap include no risk of hernia; good projection; sufficient tissue in thin patients; and a donor site that is relatively well hidden. This practice's preference is usually the SGAP flap over the IGAP flap, mainly because of the better scar donor site location, which may be more easily hidden under clothing.

Contraindications

Relative contraindications typically include patients of poor general medical health, for whom prolonged surgery and general anesthetic would expose them to excess risk. Patients who are likely to require radiation are usually delayed until after radiation treatment to avoid radiation damage to the flap, which may cause atrophy and scarring of the tissues and aesthetic changes in breast shape. Obesity and tobacco use are usually not exclusionary criteria in this practice; however, the patient is counseled that risk of flap failure, either complete or partial, is greater. The authors have found a significantly increased rate of flap failure in patients with a body mass index greater than 30; therefore SGAP reconstruction is not recommend for this population. The increased risk in this population is related to logistics of flap positioning during microsurgical anastomosis (i.e., increased flap thickness and a relatively short pedicle). The only absolute contraindication is if there is inadequate tissue or previous surgery or trauma to either the donor or recipient sites that would make the operation too difficult or impossible to perform.

Disadvantages of the gluteal flap include longer operative times (6–8 h minimum) than the DIEP flap; potential for vessel mismatch; shorter pedicle length; thinner donor site veins; more technical skills required for flap dissection and anastomoses; and a lower success rate than with the DIEP flap. The main disadvantage of the IGAP flap is dissection adjacent to the sciatic nerve, which can result in transient sciatica due to swelling around the sciatic nerve.

Patient selection

In the authors' practice, lower abdominal perforators (DIEP and SIEA) and the SGAP are our most commonly used flaps for autogenous breast reconstruction. All patients are examined carefully for sufficient donor site tissue in these locations and for the possibility of implant reconstruction. Concomitant variables are assessed including skin tightness, radiation changes, and any other relevant medical issues. Patient education is important as is assessing the patient's understanding of the processes involved in all types of reconstruction. Ultimately, the patients are given all options that are reasonable, with their potential risks and complications, and the patient may choose the method of reconstruction that they feel comfortable with. Special consideration is given to bilateral reconstruction if SGAP or IGAP breast reconstruction is chosen. If only one experienced microsurgeon is available, bilateral reconstruction is usually staged several months apart due to the complexity and length of the procedure. If two microsurgeons are available, bilateral gluteal flap reconstruction may be possible with only a moderate increase in operating room time, since simultaneous flap harvest may be performed.

Preoperative history and considerations

A thorough preoperative history and physical exam is necessary prior to surgery due to the length of surgery and to help avoid complications. In patients who are newly diagnosed, the type of tumor is important, as well as the potential for locoregional or distant spread. These factors may directly impact the outcome if radiation therapy is needed, or if there is a high likelihood of local recurrence. Some patients may have already undergone preoperative adjuvant chemotherapy or previous radiation therapy. In patients who are having delayed reconstruction, prior radiation to the chest wall or tight, thin skin may necessitate pre-flap tissue expansion. Other risk factors need to be assessed including smoking history, age, diabetes, and other general health issues such as cardiac or pulmonary problems. Past medical history and physical exam are performed with attention paid to the donor and recipient sites for evidence of previous surgery or trauma that may complicate the surgery.

The patient is examined with regard to the donor site, as well as the contralateral breast to assess for symmetry. Ptotic or large contralateral breasts may require a mastopexy or reduction for balancing during second stage surgery. In rare cases, the patient may have a smaller breast on the contralateral side that they wish to have augmented. This needs to be discussed carefully with the surgical oncologist and the patient before being pursued. The gluteal region is assessed for adequate tissue by palpation. The tissue that is utilized for the SGAP is over the greater sciatic foramen, which can be palpated and is oriented in an oblique fashion (see Surgical technique section, below). Inferior gluteal tissue may be utilized and can be harvested "in-the-crease" or above.

Patient education is very important and should be employed with numerous modalities (e.g., consultation,

video, brochure, etc.). It is important to fully inform the patient so that they may know what to expect; this is especially important with regard to possible flap failure or the inability to do reconstruction intraoperatively. Secondary options, if they exist, should be planned ahead of time and may be possible with the initial surgery if the gluteal flap is not feasible at surgery (i.e., inadequate recipient vessels). Each stage of the reconstruction with timing should be explained as well as the in-hospital stay. Patients need to be advised ahead of time to avoid positions in the postoperative period that may cause kinking of the vascular pedicle.

Preoperative computed tomography angiography for perforator mapping

Although preoperative perforator imaging is not utilized in the authors' practice, it can be a useful modality for mapping out perforators prior to surgery if it is available. The authors have found the perforators to be uniformly present for gluteal flap reconstruction, and they are located with a hand-held Doppler. In addition, this avoids added radiation exposure to the patient and lowers costs involved with the reconstruction.

Operative approach

Overview

The operation begins with the patient in the supine position for preparation of the recipient mastectomy defect and the internal mammary vessels. The internal mammary vessels are usually exposed at the level of the 3rd medial rib cartilage but may be utilized at the 4th or 5th cartilage. If a large internal mammary space is available, dissection may be performed in the interspace without cartilage removal, but this is not usually done. If a large internal mammary perforator is present, this can also be used. If previous internal mammary vessel dissection has been performed, the vessels may still be used one level up, or the distal portion of the internal mammary vessels may possibly be used. In cases where internal mammary vessels are not available due to radiation or previous surgery, a vein loop may be created to the thoracodorsal vessels with a saphenous vein graft, which may be used for the gluteal flap.

The patient is then placed in the prone position for unilateral or bilateral flap harvest. After flap harvest, the flap vessels are prepared with microscopic visualization on a side-table, while the donor site is being closed. The patient is then placed back in the supine position for arterial and venous anastomosis, followed by contouring and insetting of the flap.

Basic science/anatomy

Perforator flap reconstruction relies on blood supply to the skin and fat emanating from the perforating vessels, which travel between underlying muscle fibers, in some cases, as intermuscular vessels. These vessels are dissected out as a pedicle through the muscle fibers down to their origin and terminate in the overlying skin and fat. This pedicle is divided and re-anastomosed to recipient vessels at the site of reconstruction as a free tissue transfer.

The primary recipient vessel choice for SGAP reconstruction is the internal mammary artery and vein. In the authors' experience, the internal mammary vessels are almost always available, even after failed DIEP reconstruction, since the thoracodorsal vessels are the preferred recipient vessels for DIEP flaps. Alternatively, if the internal mammary vessels have already been used, dissection may be performed one rib space further cephalad. The second rib cartilage is easily palpated for reference, and the third cartilage is usually removed medially through a split in the pectoral muscle. Occasionally, the 4th or 5th rib cartilage may be used. The internal mammary vessels are located fairly medially. Each respective internal mammary artery (IMA) originates from the first part of the subclavian artery and descends behind the costal cartilages 1–1.5 cm lateral to the sternum with numerous branches to the intercostals and perforators to the overlying breast tissue and skin. It ultimately splits to supply the musculophrenic and superior epigastric arteries at the level of the 6th costal cartilage. At the level of the 3rd costal cartilage the IMA diameter is approximately 2–3 mm in diameter and is usually accompanied by 1–2 venae comitantes which drain into the respective brachiocephalic veins. Internal mammary vein diameter typically ranges from 2.5–3.5 mm.

Alternative recipient vessels include the thoracodorsal vessels but are less ideal given the short flap pedicle length of the SGAP. Cephalic vein turndown from the shoulder may be used as a venous backup or for additional venous drainage if necessary and is identified between the clavicular and sternal head of the pectoralis major muscle. It can be dissected distal into the upper arm through several small counter incisions.

The superior gluteal artery and vein emanate from the pelvis through the greater sciatic foramen above the piriformis muscle, just under the subgluteal fat pad. Several large branches exist at this level traveling along the periosteum and into the overlying muscle. The main vessels and several small branches typically lie against the periosteum, making dissection difficult. Some surgeons have referred to this region as "Medusa's Head" due to the number of branches and to the risk of

following the wrong vessel. Numerous perforating branches from the superior gluteal artery and venae comitantes supply the superior buttock tissue and skin, although usually one or two are dominant. The pedicle length is typically between 6 and 8 cm. Several cadaveric anatomic studies of the vascular anatomy for the SGAP flap have found perforator diameter to range from 0.9 to 1.5 mm.[7,8]

The inferior gluteal artery and vein emanates from the anterior division of the internal iliac artery and vein and also exits the pelvis through the greater sciatic foramen above the piriformis. The artery travels adjacent to the sciatic nerve beneath the gluteus muscle. Dissection is not always necessary to this level. The perforator tends to travel more obliquely, and therefore a slightly longer pedicle may be obtained (7–10 cm).

Surgical technique

Recipient site markings

The outline of the breast for immediate reconstruction should be marked in the standing upright position with special reference to the medial, lateral, and inframammary crease (Fig. 21.2.1). These landmarks are especially important if these areas are disrupted by the surgical oncologist and need to be anchored at flap inset. If previous reconstruction or a mastectomy has been performed and a delayed reconstruction is planned, appropriate borders are marked, based on judgement, using the contralateral breast if available, as a guide. Previous scars are marked to make safe skin flaps. The 3rd costal cartilage is palpated and marked.

Donor site markings

The SGAP flap design should be centered over the main perforators of the superior gluteal artery (Fig. 21.2.2). These can be found by palpating the greater sciatic foramen and are confirmed by a hand-held Doppler, with the patient prepped or in the preoperative area with the patient prone (Figs. 21.2.3–21.2.5). The flap markings should then be adjusted with these Dopplered points as the central portion of the flap. The dominant perforators usually lie a few centimeters below the upper edge of the greater sciatic foramen. The axis of the flap is slightly oblique or may be more horizontally oriented. The medial extension of the flap design is usually located several centimeters below the upper portion of the midgluteal crease and may be curved down to avoid a dogear. The width of the flap is usually between 8 and 12 cm and may be closed with slight undermining.

IGAP flap design begins with the lower border of the flap in the gluteal crease, and the upper edge of the flap may be outlined after Doppler confirmation of

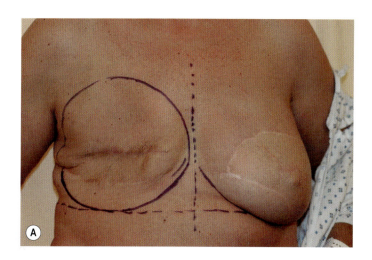

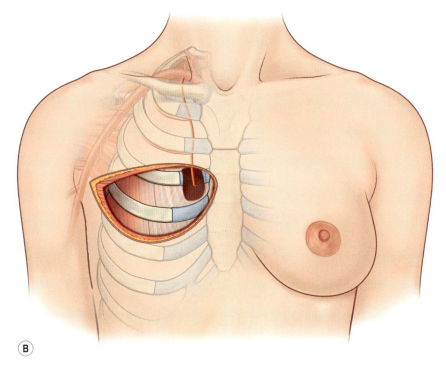

Fig. 21.2.1 (A,B) The outline of the breast for immediate reconstruction should be marked in the standing upright position with special reference to the medial, lateral, and inframammary crease. The preferred location for exposure of the internal mammary artery and vein is the 3rd interspace.

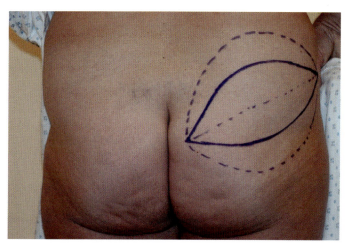

Fig. 21.2.2 The superior gluteal artery perforator flap design should be centered over the main perforators of the superior gluteal artery.

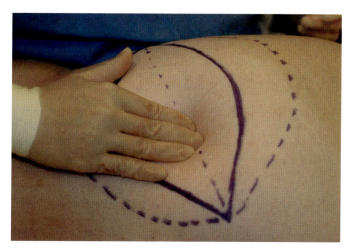

Fig. 21.2.3 The main perforators of the superior gluteal artery can be found by palpating the greater sciatic foramen and are confirmed by a hand-held Doppler with the patient prepped or in the preoperative area with the patient prone.

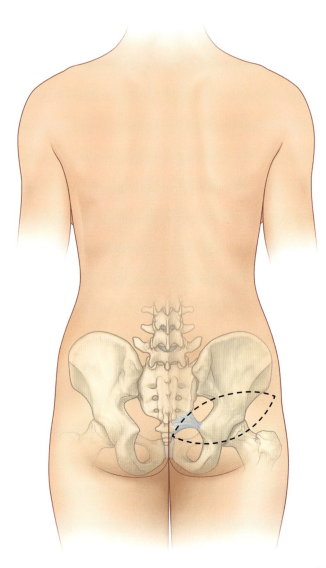

Fig. 21.2.4 The main perforators of the superior gluteal artery can be found by palpating the greater sciatic foramen and are confirmed by a hand-held Doppler with the patient prepped or in the preoperative area with the patient prone.

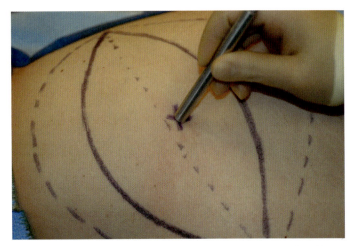

Fig. 21.2.5 The main perforators of the superior gluteal artery can be found by palpating the greater sciatic foramen and are confirmed by a hand-held Doppler with the patient prepped or in the preoperative area with the patient prone.

perforators above the lower flap margin. The width of the flap is usually between 8 and 12 cm.

Recipient site preparation

The patient is prepped and draped in the supine position. This may have been done prior to mastectomy by the oncologic breast surgeon. If a previous reconstruction has been performed, remaining tissue or implant material is removed. A capsulectomy is performed if capsular tissue is present. The recipient bed is assessed for areas where the breast borders may have been violated by the resection. These can be re-established with interrupted 3-0 Vicryl sutures. The 3rd costal cartilage is then located by palpation in the upper medial quadrant. Dissection by electrocautery is used to split the pectoralis muscle along fibers and expose the costal cartilage. The perichondrium is dissected off by use of

electrocautery and a Freer elevator. Great care must be maintained when under the cartilage because the vessels and the parietal pleural are located immediately posterior. The cartilage is removed by use of a rib-cutter and rongeur up to the edge of the sternum.

The posterior perichondrium is opened laterally with a 15-blade, and a Freer elevator is passed beneath the perichondrium above the internal mammary vessels. The perichondrium is opened longitudinally with scissors and the vessels exposed. Intercostal muscle is divided along the entire interspace between the 2nd and 4th costal cartilages. There will often be some remaining fascia overlying the vessels that can be carefully removed by use of a Freer elevator and Metzenbaum scissors. The vessels themselves are then separated along their extent to facilitate mobility upon ligation prior to anastomosis. Note the quality and caliber of the vessels (Figs. 21.2.6). The recipient site is temporarily closed with staples and a bio-occlusive dressing is placed.

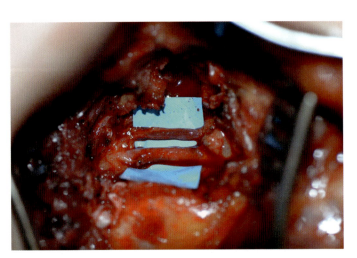

Fig. 21.2.6 Note the quality and caliber of the internal mammary vessels.

Occasionally, IMA perforators can be found that are adequate for recipient vessel anastomosis. This necessitates their having been left following the mastectomy and their having sufficient caliber. This technique, however, can spare the patient significant morbidity from harvest of the rib cartilage and spares the vessels for potential future procedures such as coronary artery bypass.

Donor flap dissection

The patient is then repositioned in the prone position. The patient is re-prepped and draped. Through the use of a hand-held Doppler probe, several arterial perforators may be identified. These usually lie a few centimeters inferior to the marked site of the center of the greater sciatic foramen. If necessary, the flap marking is adjusted so that these perforators lie at the central portion of the flap. The skin is incised, and dissection proceeds with electrocautery (power 30–40 W) beveling away from the flap for improved contour. Dissection continues directly down to the underlying muscle. Flap elevation is performed from the lateral and medial aspect of the flap to identify perforators. Upon encountering the muscle at the lateral edge of the buttock, electrocautery is decreased to begin the careful search for perforators. The iliotibial band of the fascia lata is most lateral. The gluteal fat is lifted off this fascia until the insertion of the gluteus maximus is encountered. This is noted when muscle fibers change from a cephalad-caudal direction to an oblique-downward lateral direction. At this point, the fascia is incised and dissection proceeds directly on the muscle in the subfascial plane taking care to identify and protect potential perforators (Fig. 21.2.7 & 21.2.8). Usually 1–3 potential perforators are discovered. The authors

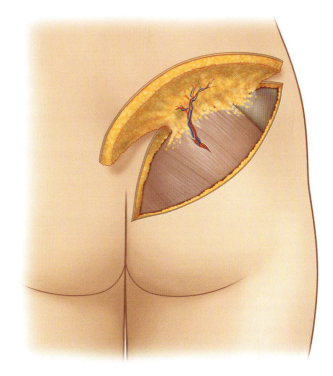

Fig. 21.2.8 The fascia is incised, and schematic illustration depicting the subfacial dissection to isolate the perforator

typically utilize one perforator that has adequate caliber; however, very occasionally two perforators are utilized, especially if they are close together and are lined up in the same muscle split.

Dissection continues through the muscle adjacent to the perforator, with the use of a long hemostatic forcep/clamp (Figs. 21.2.9 & 21.2.10). Vessel clips are used liberally to divide the numerous muscular branches.

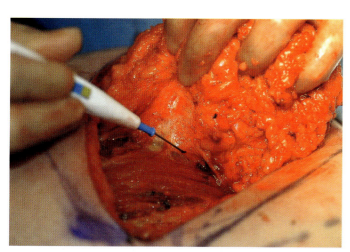

Fig. 21.2.7 The fascia is incised, and intraoperative depiction of the dissection proceeding along the surface of the gluteus maximus muscle

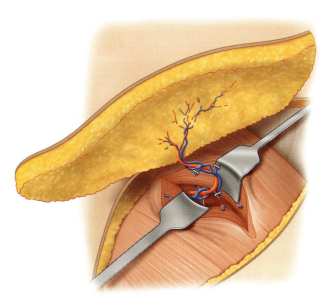

Fig. 21.2.9 Schematic illustration demonstrating the intramuscular dissection of the superior gluteal artery perforator.

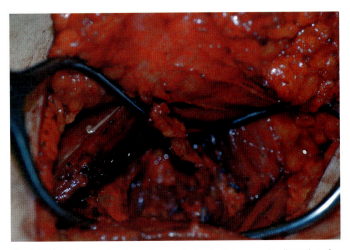

Fig. 21.2.10 Intraoperative image demonstrating the intramuscular dissection of the gluteal artery perforator.

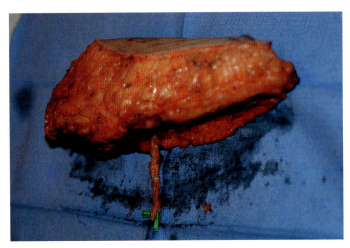

Fig. 21.2.12 Pedicle length typically range at 6–8 cm.

Self-retaining retractors are placed and frequently adjusted to enable sufficient visualization of the deep dissection. For SGAP flaps, the pedicle dissection will usually lead to fascial edges of either the gluteus medius, minimus, or piriformis muscles. These must also be released for several centimeters to allow for adequate visualization (Fig. 21.2.11). As the dissection proceeds deeper beneath these fascial planes, numerous large and small periosteal branches are encountered (Medusa's Head). Care must be taken to examine each branch to avoid damaging the pedicle. It is important not to terminate dissection too early to preserve pedicle length and to have adequate arterial diameter for a good size match to the IMA. Pedicle length typically ranges between 6 and 8 cm (Fig. 21.2.12). At the deepest extent of the dissection, the pedicle lies along the periosteum of the pelvis as it passes through the greater sciatic foramen. As it does so, numerous small branches exist and go under, in, and over the periosteum. Careful

dissection is necessary here to avoid deep bleeding. Once the pedicle is free from the periosteum and branches are divided, the artery and vein are cleaned and sometimes separated (Video 21.2.1 ▶). For IGAP flap dissection, the perforator is dissected in a muscle split in the gluteus maximus and is followed until adequate arterial vessel diameter is found, which is often prior to the greater sciatic foramen. There are less branches encountered in this dissection, and periosteal branches are less often visualized (Video 21.2.2 ▶).

Preparing for pedicle division, it is our practice to give the patient 5000 units of intravenous heparin. At 5 min after giving heparin, the artery and vein are divided with vessel clips and ischemia time is noted. The remaining portion of the flap is dissected off with electrocautery. The flap is then removed from the field and placed onto a side-table for microdissection and separation of the artery and vein within the pedicle with the use of the sterile draped microscope (Fig. 21.2.13).

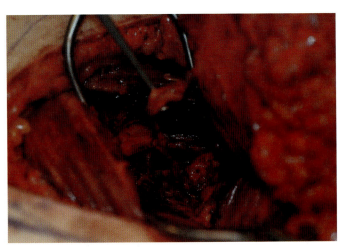

Fig. 21.2.11 The pedicle dissection will usually lead to fascial edges of either the gluteus medius, minimus, or piriformis muscles. These must also be released for several centimeters to allow for adequate visualization.

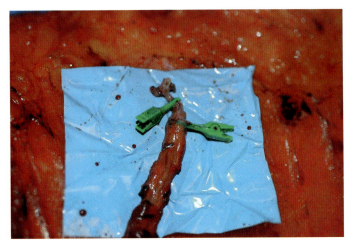

Fig. 21.2.13 The flap is then removed from the field and placed onto a side-table for microdissection and separation of the artery and vein within the pedicle with the use of the sterile draped microscope.

The artery is cleaned first, and a microclamp is applied to the vein. Sterile saline is then infused antegrade in order to dilate the venous system. This facilitates preparing the venous end, which normally is very thin, friable, and floppy. Furthermore, the inside of the vein must be assessed for nearby valves that could create an obstruction. If a valve is noted near the end of the vein, another site proximal to the valve should be selected and prepared.

The donor site is irrigated and assessed for hemostasis. The muscle is closed with interrupted 2-0 Vicryl sutures. A single fluted 15 French drain is placed coming out at the superior lateral end of the wound. The deep fat and Scarpa's fascia are closed with interrupted 2-0 Vicryl sutures. Extra sutures are often placed in the central portion because this is the area of greatest tension. The skin is closed with interrupted 3-0 Vicryl inverted dermal sutures, a running 4-0 Monocryl subcuticular suture, and DermaBond.

Anastomosis and flap inset

Along with operating room staff, the team member that closed the donor site re-preps the patient. The patient is returned to the supine position. The recipient site exposure is obtained with large retractors and sutures to retract the skin.

Once the flap preparation on the side-table is complete, it is brought into the surgical field. It is placed in a surgical towel and secured with towel clips in a manner that facilitates appropriate placement and exposure of the anastomosis. Given the thickness of gluteal flaps, which can impede direct vision of the anastomosis, the authors often elevate the back of the patient to ease visualization. This is where optimized pedicle and recipient vessel length is valuable.

The microscope is placed over the field in a position appropriate for both the microsurgeon and assistant. The pedicle and recipient sites are reassessed, further prepared, and approximated for anastomosis.

The arterial anastomosis proceeds first. The recipient artery is clipped distally. This is usually just above the 4th rib. A double Acland clamp is placed on the proximal side. The artery is divided just proximal to the clip with microscissors. The artery is then assessed for patency and adequate blood pressure by quickly and carefully releasing and then replacing the Acland clamp. The recipient arterial end is then cleaned and freshened. The flap side artery is then placed in the other side of the double Acland clamp, approximating the two arterial sides. Using an 8-0 nylon microsuture in an interrupted fashion, the arterial ends are anastomosed.

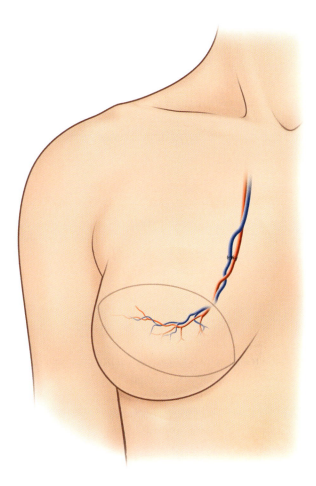

Fig. 21.2.14 The mastectomy skin flaps are trimmed and the gluteal flap skin de-epithelialized as necessary for appropriate inset.

The venous anastomosis is next performed with a venous coupler device (Synovis Micro Companies Alliance, Birmingham, AL; Fig. 21.2.14). A vessel sizer is utilized to choose the appropriate coupler size. The authors usually use coupler sizes ranging from 2.0 to 3.5 mm. A vessel clip is placed on the distal end of the recipient vein usually located just above the 4th rib. A single Acland clamp is placed on the proximal side. The vein is divided just proximal to the clip with microscissors. The recipient side vein end is then cleaned and freshened. The flap side vein is placed in a single Acland clamp. The two venous ends are placed within the coupler holes and secured to the prongs. When ready, the coupler device is activated for anastomosis.

The Acland clamps are removed in the following order: distal vein, proximal vein, distal artery, proximal artery. End of ischemia time is noted. The anastomoses are assessed for patency and for leaks. Occasionally, additional sutures are needed to stop arterial leaks. Mild oozing is monitored for several minutes; this will usually stop. Continued oozing from the venous side will usually require removal and revision of the coupler device.

Once the anastomoses are deemed patent and intact, the path of the pedicle is assessed for potential sites of compression or kinking. The authors will often divide some extra muscle on the edges to prevent compression on the pedicle or create a groove in the muscle with cautery. This is also a good point to ensure recipient site hemostasis.

The retractors are then removed and the flap inset. Take care to avoid over-rotation and stretching of the pedicle. Occasionally, it is useful to place several deep absorbable sutures securing the Scarpa's layer of the flap to the chest wall in order to prevent sliding of the flap that may damage the pedicle. Most often, however, the skin envelope with dermal sutures are used to secure the flap.

A fluted 15 French drain is placed exiting through the skin in the axilla. The drain position should be away from the pedicle.

The mastectomy skin flaps are trimmed and the gluteal flap skin de-epithelialized as necessary for appropriate inset (see Fig. 21.2.15). Care must be taken to avoid an overly tight skin envelope that can compress the flap. A hand-held Doppler probe is used to re-identify the cutaneous arterial perforators. These are marked and the gluteal flap skin paddle designed around them for postoperative monitoring. Alternately, Vioptix, transcutaneous oxygen monitoring for flap monitoring, which may also be connected to WiFi for mobile phone or computer access, can be used.

The skin is closed with interrupted 3-0 Vicryl deep dermal sutures, a running 4-0 Monocryl subcuticular suture, and DermaBond.

The patient is undraped, cleansed, and anesthesia terminated. This marks the end of the operation.

Postoperative care

Immediate

Patients are relieved of general anesthesia and extubated in the operating room upon completion of the operation. They may be transferred to the recovery room or directly to the observation/ICU. The patient typically will spend the first postoperative night in this observation/ICU. The level of care required in this unit must permit hourly patient and flap monitoring. Nursing staff should be aware of signs of flap compromise including color changes, flap temperature, capillary refill times, loss of Doppler pulse, and expanding hematoma. Patients remain on bedrest and nothing per os (NPO) for the first postoperative night. They receive intravenous fluid, antibiotics, and pain control by patient-controlled analgesic (PCA). Postoperative deep venous thrombosis (DVT) prophylaxis should be used routinely with sequential compression devices. Adjuvant DVT prophylaxis (e.g., subcutaneous heparin, enoxaparin, etc.) should be considered, especially in overweight or obese patients.

On postoperative day 1, the patient is transferred to the surgical floor if the flap is assessed as successful. They are begun on a clear diet and advanced as tolerated. Activity may also include transferring to a reclining chair.

On postoperative day 2, the patient's Foley catheter is removed and she may begin ambulating. Pain control is changed to oral pills. Occupational therapy and drain care teaching is employed to prepare the patient for discharge.

On postoperative day 3, if the patient is tolerating food, oral pain control, ambulation, and voiding spontaneously, she may be discharged from the hospital with instructions to follow-up in the clinic 1 week later. Prescriptions for pain control and antibiotics are provided. Furthermore, the patient is instructed to limit activity but may shower. Home nursing care to assist with drain care is often prescribed.

The 1st week follow-up appointment usually consists of drain removal from the breast pocket. The patients return for further follow-up appointments as necessary for removal of the donor site drain and revision planning. As stated above, percutaneous aspiration of seromas is often required.

Long-term care

The intervals between each step are usually 3 months; therefore the entire process can take 6 months to 1 year, or longer if complications occur. Upon completion, the patient should return for yearly follow-up for cancer surveillance. Gluteal flaps will grow and shrink with weight fluctuations and develop progressive ptosis, similar to the contralateral breast. Unlike implant reconstruction, further surgery is usually unnecessary.

Bilateral gluteal flap reconstruction

When the surgical team includes two microsurgeons, simultaneous bilateral SGAP or IGAP reconstruction can be performed safely and with reasonable operative times.[9,10] Each side can be operated on simultaneously for most of the procedure except for when using the microscope for anastomosis. Ideally, each side has its own separate team including assistant, surgical scrub technician, and surgical instruments.

Revisions

Complete gluteal flap reconstruction usually requires three or four procedures on separate visits. These include:

- The initial free flap, as described above.
- Gluteal flap reshaping usually is performed at least 3 months following the initial free flap. This usually involves trimming or removing the remaining skin paddle and softening the edges of the flap to improve breast shape. Occasionally, some liposuction is utilized for shaping and softening areas of fat necrosis. The authors are increasingly utilizing fat grafting for flap enlargement or contour deformities. Often, this is combined with a contralateral breast reduction, mastopexy, or augmentation as necessary to improve symmetry.
- The donor site scar is often revised at this point, with trimming of dog-ears and liposuction of irregularities to improve upper buttock contour. The contralateral buttock is also sometimes treated with liposuction for symmetry.
- Reconstruction of the nipple areolar complex (NAC) can sometimes be performed in the second stage when adequate symmetry between breasts is present. If a procedure for symmetry is required, however, NAC reconstruction should be delayed until a third stage. There are numerous techniques in the literature adequate for NAC reconstruction. The final procedure performed, after all shaping and symmetry procedures are healed, is tattooing of the NAC.

Sensate SGAP flap

Including nervous repair in the SGAP reconstruction has been described for creating a sensate breast reconstruction.[12] Typically 1–2 nerve perforators are repaired to the T4 thoracic nerve branch.

Complications and side effects

The most serious complications in SGAP reconstruction are those similar to all surgeries requiring general anesthesia: myocardial infarction, DVT, pulmonary embolism, possibly even death. SGAP surgery, especially when combined with mastectomy, is prolonged, usually more than 6 h, which raises these risks. Patient selection based on medical history, physical examination, and preoperative testing is paramount for avoiding these disasters.

Flap failure is the most serious complication specific for free flap reconstruction.

Flap failure, partial or complete, can be the result of a multitude of factors. These include:

- Microsurgical technique
- Patient anatomy
- Patient risk factors
- Postoperative care.

For published series of greater than 10 SGAP reconstructions, flap failure rates range from 0% to 7.7%.[10–13]

In the authors' unpublished data of 106 flaps on 90 patients over 7 years, the flap success rate has increased yearly as experience has increased from 88.7% to 96.5%, with an overall success rate of 92.5%.[14]

Even with these listed factors, surgical technique is usually a component of every flap failure, especially complete flap loss. Meticulous microsurgical technique can avoid anastomotic obstruction. Details of technique are, however, beyond the scope of this chapter. Venous occlusion is also responsible for the vast majority of flap failures.[15] The pedicle can be compromised from kinking, stretching, a tight skin closure, or an expanding hematoma or seroma. Attention to detail cannot be overstressed.

Occasionally, patient anatomy prohibits gluteal flap reconstruction. Patients having had radiation may have scarred or thrombosed IMA vessels. Very rarely, patients simply have vessels that are too small for free flap reconstruction.

Patient risk factors including smoking, atherosclerosis, obesity, hypertension, and hypercholesterolemia often negatively impact outcome. These can contribute to partial flap loss. Various blood clotting disorders can also lead to clotted venous pedicles or excessive bleeding.

Postoperative care is important in preserving the integrity of the flap and its perfusion. Excessive motion or inappropriate patient positioning can compromise the flap pedicle. Furthermore, frequent flap monitoring by those knowledgeable on the signs of flap compromise can potentially lead to a failing flap being saved.

Other complications include bleeding, hematoma, seroma, infection, wound breakdown, scarring, pain, and pneumothorax.

How to prevent and manage complications

Bleeding and hematoma are prevented by meticulous hemostasis. An enlarging hematoma can potentially lead to a venous clot when compressing on the pedicle. Expanding flap pocket, change in color of flap or mastectomy skin, tachycardia, and anemia are all signs that should raise suspicion. There should be a low threshold for returning to the operating room for evacuation when present in the immediate postoperative period.

Seroma is a long-term sequela that most often presents at the donor site (>80% SGAP patients). Drains are left in the reconstruction site and donor site until daily drainage drops to less than 30 cc/day consistently. This is usually 1 week at the reconstruction site and 2–3 weeks at the donor site. Despite this, seromas often form at the donor site requiring percutaneous aspiration during follow-up visits. Seromas should not be left to expand without treatment to avoid potential wound breakdown.

Wound infections at either surgical site are rare. Pre- and intraoperative antibiotics should be given routinely in this surgery. The authors also give a short course of postoperative antibiotics. Erythema, swelling, or purulent drainage are signs of infection that should be aggressively treated with antibiotics and/or surgical drainage as necessary.

Wound breakdown typically results from the aforementioned complications. It should be treated with standard local wound care.

As with any surgery, scars are a sequela of every incision. Therefore, the surgeon must balance the need for surgical exposure with the development of scarring. Patients should be educated preoperatively regarding these scars in order to have realistic expectations of the final cosmetic result. Scar revision and treatment of deeper fibrotic scars and fat necrosis are usually performed in the revision stages.

The most acutely painful site in this surgery is typically where the rib cartilage is removed. A PCA usually provides adequate pain control. The authors prefer avoiding the use of non-steroidal anti-inflammatory drugs (e.g., ketorolac) in the immediate postoperative period, from fear of bleeding complications. Patients will often have some degree of splinting; therefore, an incentive spirometer should be utilized routinely to relieve atelectasis. Long-term pain from scarring or pinched nerves is rare but possible and should be treated appropriately.

It is uncommon for patients to develop a symptomatic pneumothorax from the rib cartilage resection. Careful dissection and rib removal should avoid damaging the parietal pleura. If a pneumothorax is suspected, diagnosis can be confirmed with radiographs. A small pneumothorax can often be treated with a small suction tube and immediately closed. More significant lung collapse should be treated with thoracostomy tube suction.

Patient examples

Various patient examples are shown for SGAP and IGAP procedures, in Figs. 21.1.15–21.2.22.

Conclusion

As autogenous tissue has become increasingly utilized for breast reconstruction, surgical techniques have evolved, setting new standards and raising patient expectations. Traditional donor sites for breast reconstruction may not be available, yet the same outcome is still expected. SGAP or IGAP reconstruction is a valuable option for patients that are not candidates for reconstruction using their abdominal tissue. While it is a challenging procedure, it has relatively consistent anatomy and provides excellent results, thus making it an important part of the breast reconstructive surgeon's repertoire.

Text continued on p. 391

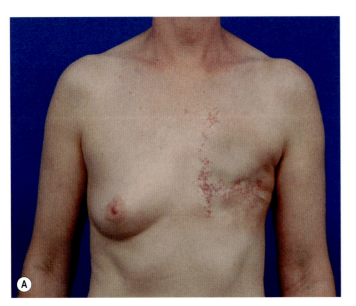 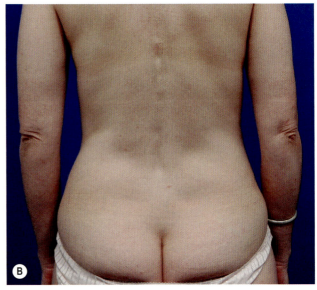

Fig. 21.2.15 (A–D) History of radiation therapy to left chest after mastectomy. Bilateral superior gluteal artery perforator reconstruction.

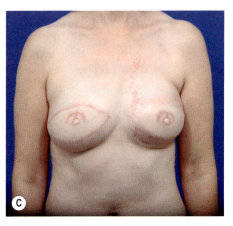
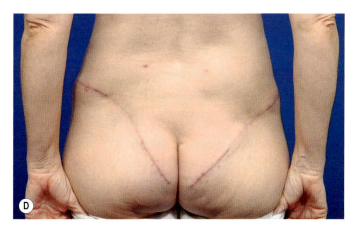

Fig. 21.2.15, cont'd

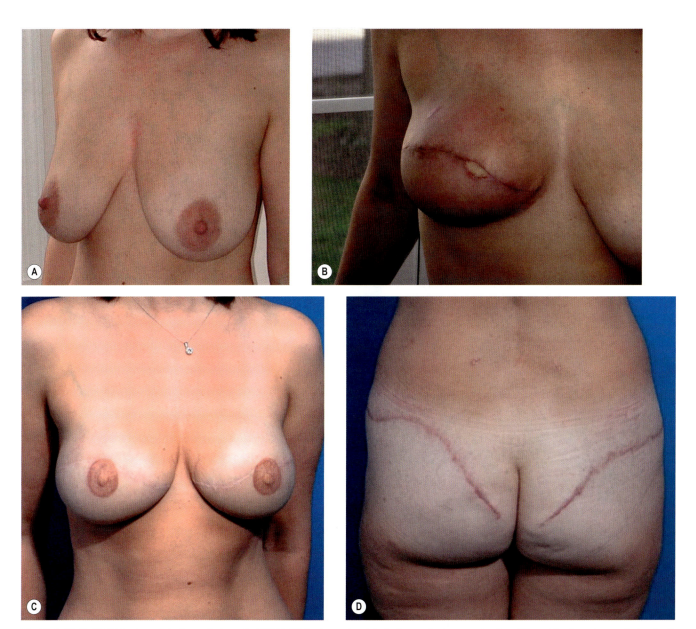

Fig. 21.2.16 (A–D) Bilateral prophylactic mastectomy for BRCA1. Bilateral superior gluteal artery perforator reconstruction. Skin paddle shown for monitoring the flap and final result.

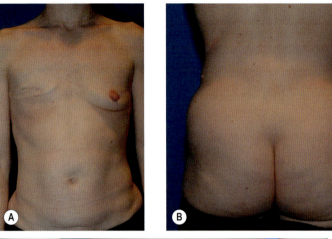

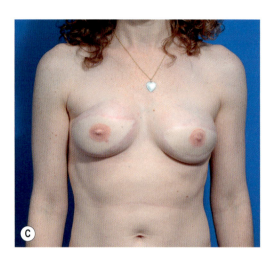

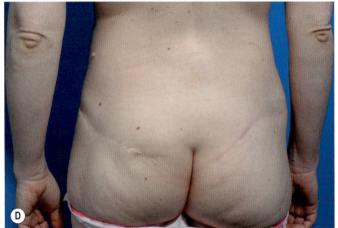

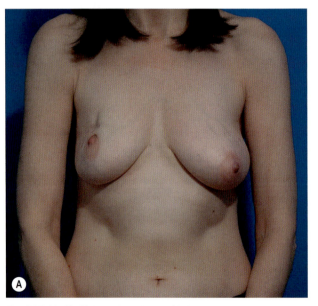

Fig. 21.2.17 (A–D) Delayed right and immediate left superior gluteal artery perforator..

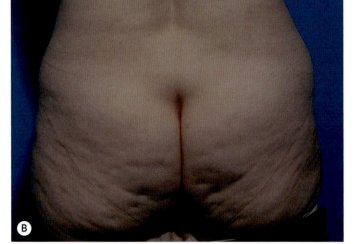

Fig. 21.2.18 (A–D) Immediate bilateral SGAP.

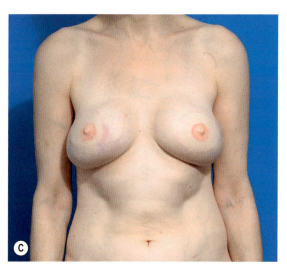

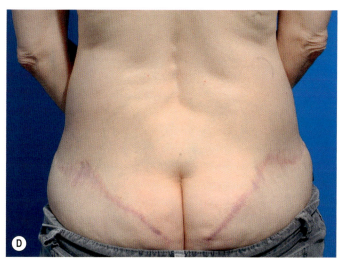

Fig. 21.2.18, cont'd

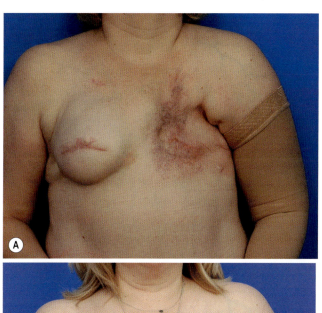

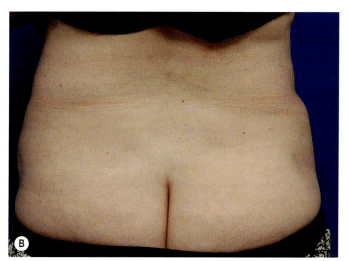

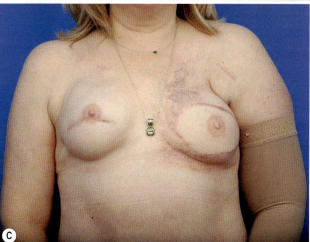

Fig. 21.2.19 (A–C) Left delayed superior gluteal artery perforator with history of radiation therapy and failed deep inferior epigastric artery perforator to internal mammary vessels. Saphenous vein loop to thoracodorsal vessels.

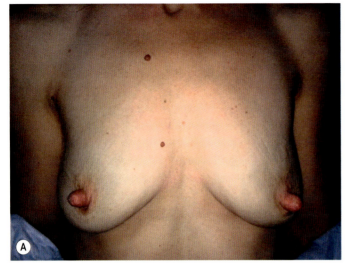

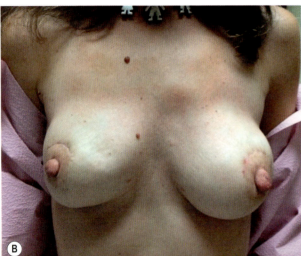

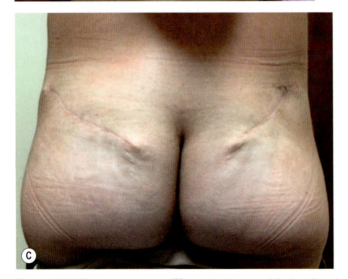

Fig. 21.2.20 **(A)** preoperative image; **(B)** postoperative image following bilateral SGAPs; **(C)** postoperative image of the gluteal donor site.

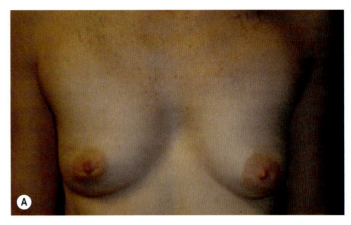

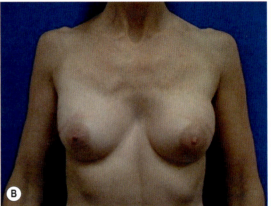

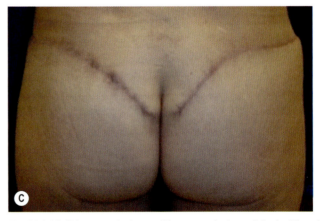

Fig. 21.2.21 **(A)** preoperative image; **(B)** postoperative image following bilateral SGAP flaps; **(C)** postoperative image of the gluteal donor site.

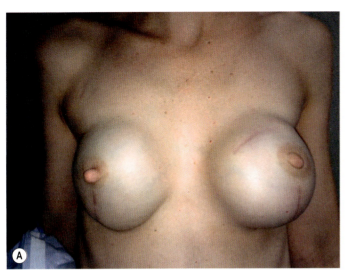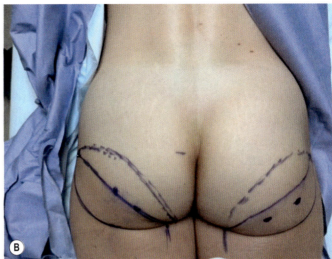

Fig. 21.2.22 (A,B) Bilateral nipple-sparing mastectomy and immediate inferior gluteal artery perforator..

🌐 **Access the complete reference list online at**   **http://www.expertconsult.com**

2. Shaw WW. Superior gluteal free flap breast reconstruction. *Clin Plast Surg.* 1998;25:267–274. *Illustrates some of the early work done on the anatomy of this region and how the SGAP evolved.*

3. Codner MA, Nahai F. The gluteal free flap breast reconstruction: making it work. *Clin Plast Surg.* 1994;21:289–296. *Helpful tips for performing this difficult surgery.*

5. Allen RJ, Tucker C. Superior gluteal artery perforator free flap for breast reconstruction. *Plast Reconstr Surg.* 1995;95:1207–1212. *Good overall review of anatomy and technique for SGAP reconstruction.*

6. Flores JI, Magarakis M, Venkat R, et al. Bilateral simultaneous breast reconstruction with SGAP flaps. *Microsurgery.* 2012;32:344–350. *Another example of how bilateral SGAPS can be accomplished by two skilled microsurgeons.*

7. Mu LH, Yan YP, Luan J, et al. Anatomy study of superior and inferior gluteal artery perforator flap. *Zhonghua Zheng Xing Wai Ke Za Zhi.* 2005;21:278–280. *Helps to understand the vessel anatomy in this region.*

8. Kankaya Y, Ulusoy MG, Oruç M, et al. Perforating arteries of the gluteal region. *Ann Plast Surg.* 2006;56:409–412. *Helps to understand the perforator anatomy of the SAP and IGAP flap.*

10. Della Croce FJ, Sullivan SK. Application of the superior gluteal artery perforator free flap for bilateral simultaneous breast reconstruction. *Plast Reconstr Surg.* 2005;116:87–104. *Not for the average microsurgeon but shows how bilateral gluteal flaps may be performed by two microsurgeons.*

11. Munhoz AM, Ishida LH, Montag E, et al. Perforator flap breast reconstruction using internal mammary perforator branches as a recipient site: an anatomical and clinical analysis. *Plast Reconstr Surg.* 2004;114:62–68. *An alternative for recipient vessels for the SGAP flap.*

15. Nahabedian MY, Momen B, Manson PN. Factors associated with anastomotic failure after microvascular reconstruction of the breast. *Plast Reconstr Surg.* 2004;114:74–82. *Helps to understand the pitfalls of micro-anastomotic failure.*

21.3

Medial thigh flaps for breast reconstruction

Venkat V. Ramakrishnan and Nakul Gamanlal Patel

 Access video content for this chapter online at expertconsult.com

SYNOPSIS

- Autologous free tissue transfer has proved to be an ideal method for breast reconstruction with long-standing aesthetic outcome.
- Many women undergo procedures on their abdomen or would want to avoid surgery that uses the abdomen as a donor site.
- Alternative autologous options include the transverse upper gracilis (TUG) flap.
- Understanding of the anatomy helps with the potential donor site morbidity.
- The TUG flap is not only useful for women with small- to moderate-sized breasts with no available lower abdominal tissue but also occasionally for larger breasts.
- The criticism of this flap has been its short vascular pedicle, limited volume that can be achieved, and the donor site morbidity.

 Access the Historical Perspective section and Fig. 21.3.1 online at

http://www.expertconsult.com

Introduction

The transverse upper gracilis (TUG) flap, also known as the transverse myocutaneous gracilis (TMG) flap, with the variations in flap design, is a useful donor site when abdominal flaps are not an option.

Careful patient selection is essential for optimal breast and donor site outcomes. This flap can be harvested in the supine position, thereby allowing a two-team approach. It provides soft and easily moldable tissue with an early recovery.

Operative considerations focus on minimizing donor site morbidity, ensuring adequate tissue harvest, and contouring of the flap.

More posterior shift of the skin paddle, caudal extension of sub-Scarpa fat, recruitment of posterior thigh fat, preservation of the saphenous vein with the accompanying lymphatics, and limiting the muscle harvest reduce morbidity and allow adequate tissue harvest.

Pleasing breast shape can be achieved by molding the flap in three ways, to match the breast morphology. The use of intercostal perforators as the recipients, adjunctive procedures such as primary lipofilling of the pectoralis or the gracilis muscle, additional flaps, and use of implants increase the applications of the flap. The main criticisms of the TUG flaps are limited volume, short pedicle, and donor site issues.

The variations in skin paddle design including the extended TUG and the diagonal upper gracilis (DUG) flaps are useful variations of this flap.

Basic science/disease process

The gracilis muscle is a type II musculocutaneous flap in the Mathes and Nahai classification.[12] The myocutaneous gracilis flap can be designed with several skin paddle types, and there are numerous acronyms. These include transverse upper gracilis (TUG), transverse myocutaneous gracilis (TMG), diagonal upper gracilis (DUG), vertical upper gracilis (VUG), and bilateral stacked vertical upper gracilis (BUG).[13–16] This chapter will focus on the TUG flap (Fig. 21.3.2).

Anatomical studies have demonstrated that the angiosomes of the upper gracilis muscle lie at 90° to the muscle, hence a transverse skin paddle has been more reliable.[6,17]

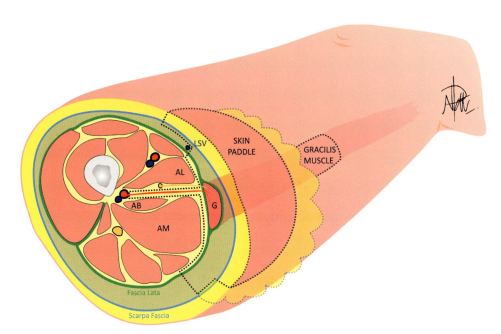

Fig. 21.3.2 The anatomy of the transverse upper gracilis flap with key landmarks. AB, adductor brevis; AL, adductor longus; AM, adductor magnus; G, gracilis; LSV, long saphenous vein. (© *Nakul Patel and Venkat Ramakrishnan.*)

Diagnosis/patient presentation

The common use of the TUG flap is immediate breast reconstruction with a skin-sparing mastectomy approach. The TUG flap with immediate nipple reconstruction lends itself well to this procedure. A smaller proportion of patients presents in a delayed manner with either no reconstruction or complications of their implant-based reconstruction. Lastly, the TUG flap has also been useful in partial breast defect reconstruction or when used in conjunction with implants and another free flap.

In our practice, the TUG flap has replaced the use of latissimus dorsi (LD) musculocutaneous flap for breast reconstruction. The TUG flap provides a skin island comparable to the LD flap. The LD is the largest muscle of the back and carries a reliable skin paddle. The flap can be raised with ease and mitigates the need for microsurgery. All these factors have led to its popularity and widespread use. There has been associated functional impairment and weakness seen in those that have this muscle harvested.[18] In addition, the volume of muscle from the LD decreases with time as it atrophies. These problems are largely addressed with the use of the TUG flap. It provides a similar vascular envelope with another choice of concealed scar.

> **Tip**
>
> • Delayed reconstructions often require more skin, which can be a challenge in comparison to immediate reconstruction following skin-sparing mastectomy (Fig. 21.3.3)

Patient selection

If the abdomen cannot be used as a donor site due to multiple scars or patient preference, autologous reconstruction using the medial thigh can be considered as a second choice.

The typical patient for TUG flap reconstruction is a slim patient with a small to moderate-sized breast in which the abdomen cannot be used (Fig. 21.3.4). The indications of the TUG flap have increased, and many more patients can be considered for a TUG flap; however, additional measures are required with the larger reconstructions, and these are discussed later in the chapter (Figs. 21.3.5–21.3.9).

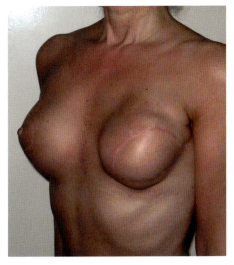

Fig. 21.3.3 Patient with bilateral transverse upper gracilis flap reconstructions – right skin-sparing mastectomy with immediate reconstruction and left delayed reconstruction. (© *Nakul Patel and Venkat Ramakrishnan.*)

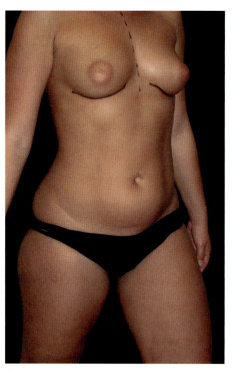

Fig. 21.3.4 Typical patient suitable for transverse upper gracilis flap breast reconstruction with small breasts and no abdominal donor site. (© *Nakul Patel and Venkat Ramakrishnan.*)

Treatment/surgical technique

The patient is marked in the standing position with the donor leg slightly forward. The upper border of the flap is marked a finger-breadth below the thigh–groin junction, and with a pinch test the lower border of the flap

is decided. Typically, the width of the crescent is 7 cm although in those with an excessive laxity up to 12 cm can be taken.[19] The crescent is completed posteriorly reaching the gluteal crease almost to the ischial tuberosity. Fat is recruited beyond the skin island, predominantly from the inferior border medially and posteriorly (Fig. 21.3.10). The original description was to take a cutaneous skin paddle centered over gracilis, but in the authors' experience skewing the flap design more posteriorly helps with fat recruitment, concealing the scar in the medial thigh and infragluteal crease and reduces the possibility of injury to the lymphatic tissues.[20]

Tips

- It is useful to mark the midaxial line of the thigh anteriorly and posteriorly.
- Posteriorly avoid fat recruitment lateral to the midaxial line to avoid damage to the posterior cutaneous nerve of the thigh.
- The upper border of the flap is marked one finger-breadth below the groin–thigh crease both to allow re-suspension of the donor site without distortion of the labia majora and to leave the scar away from the gusset of underwear, which could cause discomfort (see Fig. 21.3.10).

Patient positioning

The patient is positioned supine on the operating table. The whole thigh is prepared and abducted with the hip and knee flexed during the procedure with the

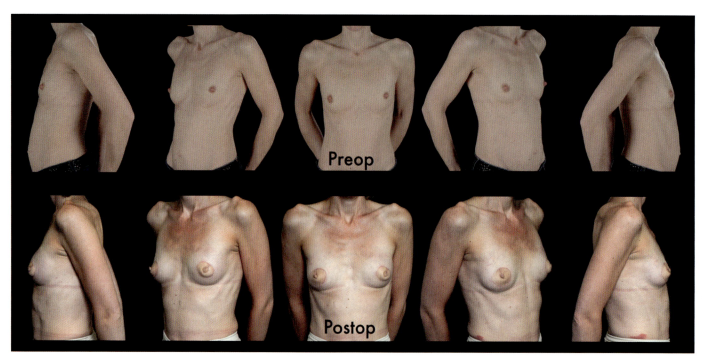

Fig. 21.3.5 No breast volume – pre- and postoperative photographs of a patient with virtually no breast tissue reconstructed with bilateral transverse upper gracilis flaps. (© *Nakul Patel and Venkat Ramakrishnan.*)

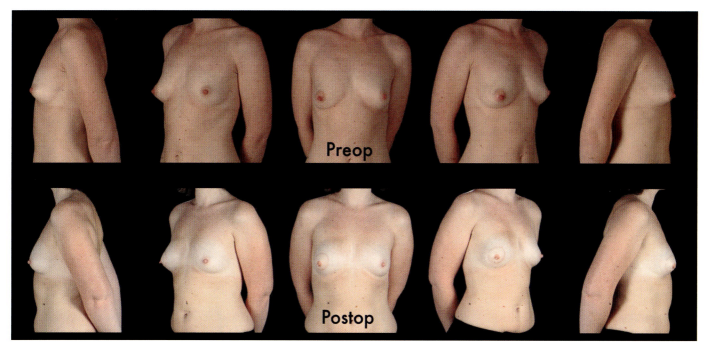

Fig. 21.3.6 Small breast volume – pre- and postoperative photographs of a patient with right breast reconstruction with a transverse upper gracilis flap. (© *Nakul Patel and Venkat Ramakrishnan.*)

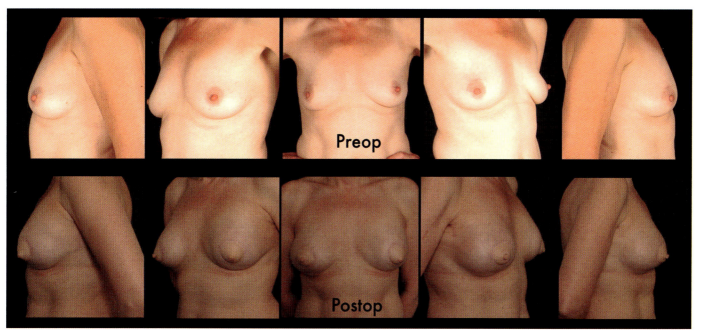

Fig. 21.3.7 Moderate breast volume – pre- and postoperative photographs of a patient with bilateral transverse upper gracilis flaps with implants. (© *Nakul Patel and Venkat Ramakrishnan.*)

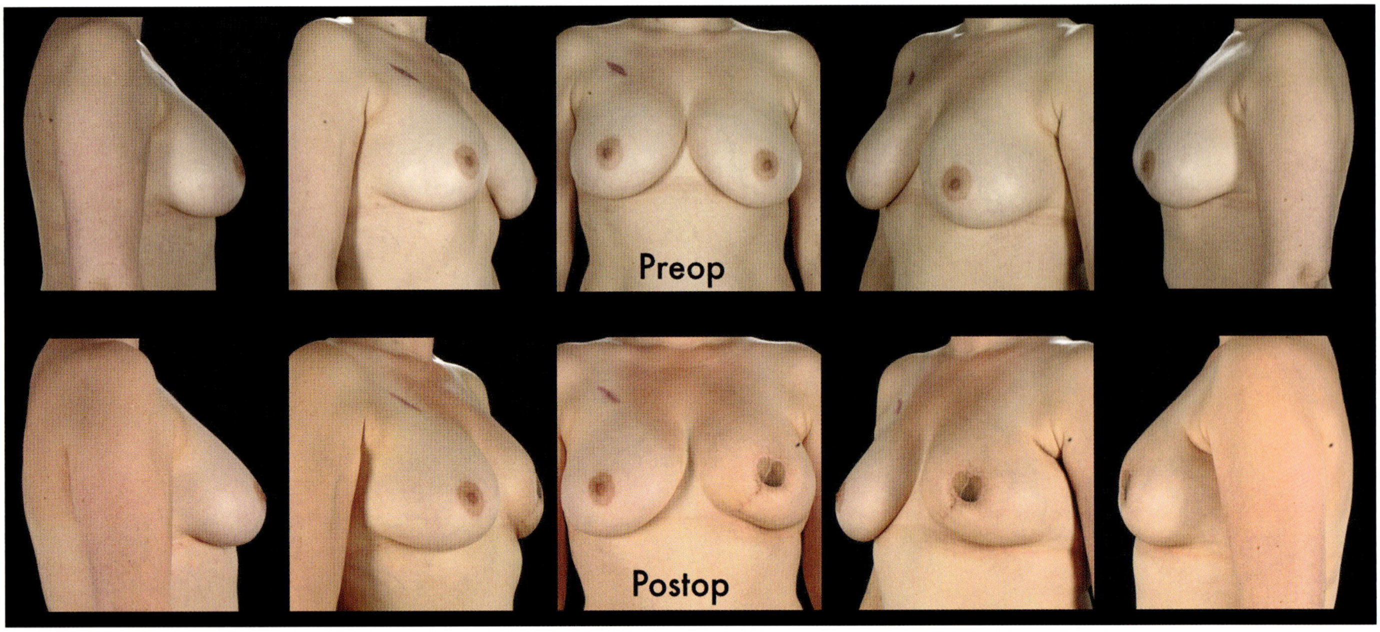

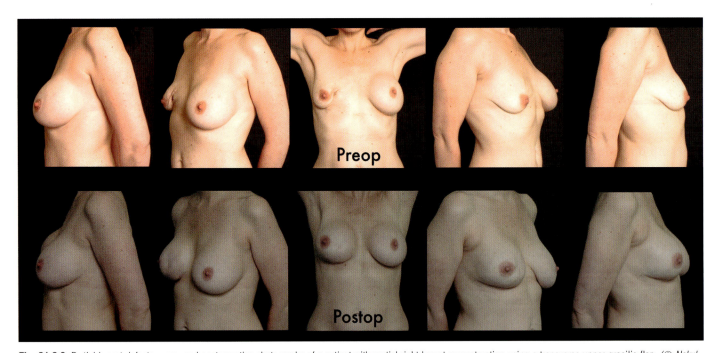

Fig. 21.3.8 Large breast volume – pre- and postoperative photographs of a patient with right breast reconstruction using stacked transverse upper gracilis flaps. (© *Nakul Patel and Venkat Ramakrishnan.*)

Fig. 21.3.9 Partial breast defects – pre- and postoperative photographs of a patient with partial right breast reconstruction using a transverse upper gracilis flap. (© *Nakul Patel and Venkat Ramakrishnan.*)

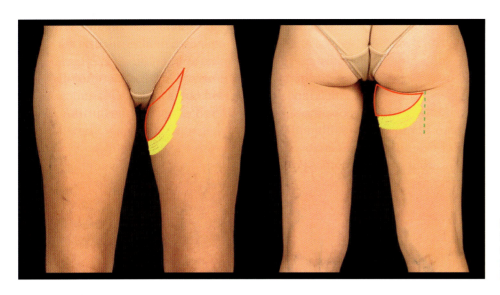

Fig. 21.3.10 Preoperative markings of a transverse upper gracilis flap with a skewed flap design to recruit fat from the inferior border medially and posteriorly. (© *Nakul Patel and Venkat Ramakrishnan.*)

operating surgeon standing on the contralateral side to flap harvest (Fig. 21.3.11).

> **Tip**
>
> • The leg is free-draped such that this can be moved during the procedure to aid harvest and closure of the flap (see Fig. 21.3.11).

Flap harvest

There are certain key points in harvesting this flap safely and efficiently, these including the marking and positioning of the patient, flap design, preservation of structures, dissection technique, and flap inset.

Step 1: caudal incision with fat recruitment

The medial-most bulk of tissue in the upper thigh is composed of adductor longus (anterior two-thirds) and gracilis muscles (posterior one-third). Marking these

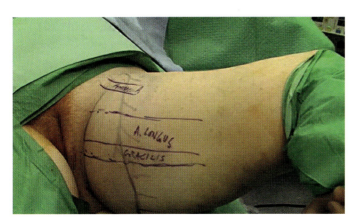

Fig. 21.3.11 Patient is positioned supine with the legs draped freely. (© *Nakul Patel and Venkat Ramakrishnan.*)

muscles will help with orientation during flap harvest. An incision is made along the inferior border of the flap. The fat below the membranous layer of the superficial fascia is recruited to increase the flap volume (Fig. 21.3.12).

> **Tip**
>
> • Even a small increase in volume of fat recruited can have a significant impact overall (i.e., 50 g of extra fat recruitment in a 250 g flap accounts for a 20% increase in the new breast reconstruction).

Step 2: anterior flap elevation (see Videos 21.3.1 and 21.3.2 ⊙)

The anterior flap is raised just above the Scarpa fascia up to the level of the long saphenous vein, leaving it *in situ*. The venae comitantes drain the flap predictably without requiring the long saphenous system. Exclusion of the long saphenous vein makes the dissection quicker and preserves the lymphatics along the vein (Fig. 21.3.13).

> **Tip**
>
> • Avoid transgressing the femoral triangle and lymphatic content, which could theoretically lead to increased risk of seroma, lymphocele, wound breakdown, infection, and potentially lymphedema.

Once the dissection is past the long saphenous vein, the dissection can continue medially in a deeper subfascial plane, through the loose areolar tissue, up to the septum between adductor longus and gracilis. It is within this

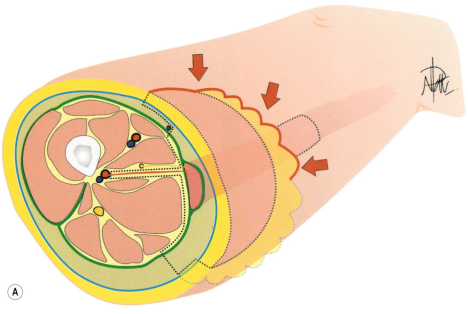

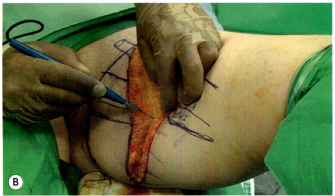

Fig. 21.3.12 Step 1 – caudal incision with fat recruitment. (© *Nakul Patel and Venkat Ramakrishnan.*)

septum that both the vascular and nerve pedicles to gracilis can be found. The key to identification of the medical circumflex femoral vessels is lateral retraction of adductor longus.

> **Tip**
> • The anterior branch of the obturator nerve lies obliquely compared to the vascular pedicle, which is orientated transversely. This is a useful way of identifying the gracilis pedicle (see Fig. 21.3.17).

Step 3: division of distal gracilis

Using blunt dissection, the distal end of the gracilis muscle is freed, and whilst exerting traction, the muscle is divided without the need of a second incision. It is important to ensure adequate hemostasis of the muscle edge as there can be bleeding from the secondary pedicles to the gracilis muscle (Fig. 21.3.14).

> **Tip**
> • The transection of gracilis is through the middle third of the muscle belly with direct vision. Recruitment of the distal half of gracilis does not add much volume to the flap but might lead to bleeding from the secondary pedicles, which may be difficult to visualize and access (see Fig. 21.3.14).

Step 4: elevation of posterior flap

The posterior border of the flap is incised, anterior to the midline of the posterior thigh, with further recruitment of fat in the sub-Scarpa plane, from posterior to anterior. It is critical to ensure that sufficient volume has been harvested as this provides the bulk of the flap volume (Fig. 21.3.15).

> **Tip**
> • Avoiding dissection past the midline of the posterior thigh will prevent injury to the posterior cutaneous nerve of the thigh and secondary painful neuromas and paraesthesia.

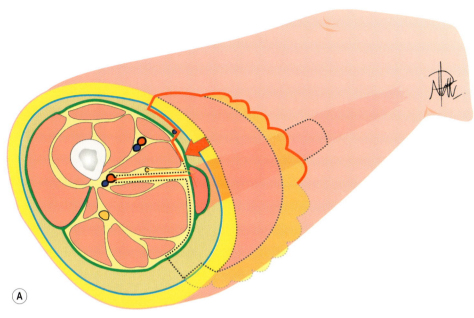

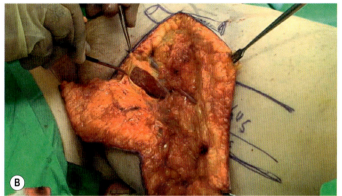

Fig. 21.3.13 Step 2 – anterior flap elevation. (© *Nakul Patel and Venkat Ramakrishnan.*)

Step 5: division of proximal gracilis

As the posterior flap is being raised, ensure that the dissection plane is deep to the gracilis muscle incorporating the investing fascia without trying to identify the musculocutaneous perforators and then lifting away from the adductor musculature. Divide the proximal gracilis from its origin (Fig. 21.3.16).

Step 6: pedicle dissection and flap detachment

Dissect the medial circumflex femoral vessels to the profunda femoris and divide them at the origin to ensure a long pedicle and large caliber vessels.

Although some descriptions of the flap describe identification of musculocutaneous perforators entering the skin paddle, this is not necessary. Instead, by ensuring that the investing fascia of the gracilis muscle is left intact, the flap is more reliable, speed of flap harvest improved, and some difficult dissection is avoided (Fig. 21.3.17).

> **Tip**
>
> - There are often large muscle branches to the adductors, which are worth dissecting out should a double TUG be required.

Step 7: flap molding and inset

The flap is usually molded into a cone shape by bringing the tips of the ellipse together. It will form a peak at the apex, which will be used to make a nipple (Fig. 21.3.18). The appropriate areas are de-epithelialized for flap inset within the skin envelope.

Flap molding and shaping is determined intraoperatively depending on the thickness of the flap and fat distribution within it. In addition, comparison is made to the contralateral breast shape, size, footplate, and glandular tissue distribution. The degree of coning is determined by the width of the breast, such that a half cone or unconed TUG flap could be utilized (Fig. 21.3.19).

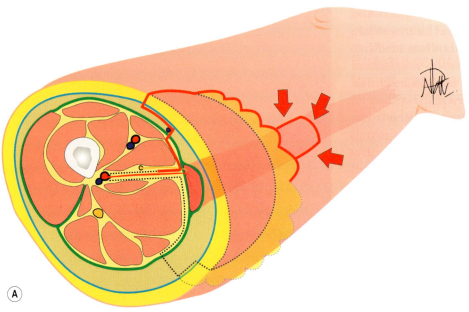

(A)

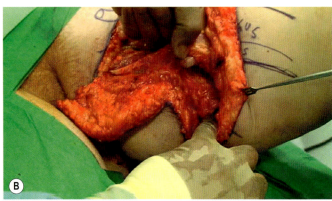

(B)

Fig. 21.3.14 Step 3 – division of distal gracilis. (© *Nakul Patel and Venkat Ramakrishnan.*)

The closure is started posteriorly by flexing the hip and feeding in the standing cone deformity. The leg can then be straightened for the remaining closure. Use a 2-0 vicryl suture for the fascia and an absorbable 3-0 barbed suture closed over a suction drain (Fig. 21.3.20).

Step 8: microsurgery

Because of the relatively short pedicle length and size of medial circumflex femoral vessels, anastomosis to the internal mammary perforators is more convenient. By dissecting deep into the intercostal space, a suitable length of the intercostal perforator in the second, third, or occasionally fourth interspace can be used for comfortable anastomoses. The internal mammary vessels at the fourth interspace tend to be of good size match (Fig. 21.3.21).

Tips

- Use of the intercostal perforators compliments the short pedicle length of the gracilis flap.
- Opportunistic use of the lower perforators allows for more aesthetic lateralization of the breast mound.

Secondary choices include the thoracodorsal system, serratus anterior branches, or the thoracoacromial vessels, which may require interposition vein graft.

Postoperative care

Patients are nursed in a supine position with the head slightly up and knees slightly flexed. Flap observations are undertaken every 15 minutes in recovery and every hour on the ward overnight, with urgent surgical team review if there are any concerns. Patients are able to drink clear fluids the first postoperative night with additional intravenous fluid to maintain urine outputs of greater than 0.5 mL/kg/hr. Forced-air warming blankets (Bair Hugger, 3M) are used to maintain the patient's temperature between 36.5°C and 37.5°C. It normally stays on overnight postoperatively.

Analgesic requirements include regular paracetamol and non-steroidal anti-inflammatories supplemented with OxyContin as required. Postoperative nausea and vomiting are combated with regular cyclizine and breakthrough ondansetron. Patients are also given

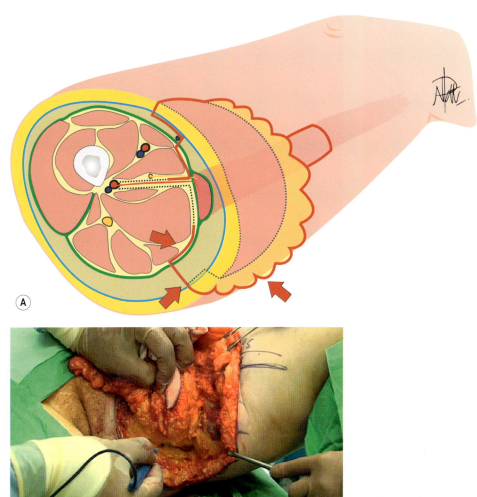

Fig. 21.3.15 Step 4 – elevation of posterior flap. (© *Nakul Patel and Venkat Ramakrishnan.*)

intravenous antibiotics over 48 hours with a further 5 days of oral. Venous thromboembolic prophylaxis is a must for these patients, especially if ambulation is delayed. Routinely all are given a prophylactic dose of low-molecular-weight heparin (such as Clexane 40 mg) from the night before surgery, and then six hours post-operatively and then daily until fully mobilized. Anti-embolic stockings are also used, and patients at higher risk are given intermittent pneumatic compression devices (such as Flowtrons).

The patient should use tight thigh compression garments, which stay on for 4–6 weeks. This provides compression and relaxes the wound. Patients typically are sitting out the next day with some mobilization. They are significantly more mobile the second day with removal of the urinary catheter, followed by drains over the next few days and finally discharged around 4–6 days post-surgery.

The patient is reviewed in a nurse-led breast clinic one week postoperatively and in a consultant clinic 6–8 weeks later. Revision procedures, if required, are considered after three months.

Outcomes, prognosis, and complications

The TUG flap is well-accepted in autologous breast reconstruction. The scar is relativity concealable; flap raise is consistent and vessel caliber sufficient for reliable breast reconstruction (Fig. 21.3.22).[10,14,21]

When comparing the TUG to abdominal flaps, the natural crescent-shaped skin paddle of the TUG lends itself to coning and resembles a natural breast shape compared to a relatively flat abdomen.[10]

The consistency of the TUG flap is similar to the breast tissue, in comparison to the gluteal artery perforator (GAP) flaps. It also allows parallel operating without the need to change the patient's position.

The flap remains a reliable and easy to harvest flap; however, a relatively closely linked flap, the profunda artery perforator (PAP) flap, which is also harvested from the medial thigh, may give the TUG some competition. The scars for this tend to be inferior and slightly more posterior, thereby making them more visible than

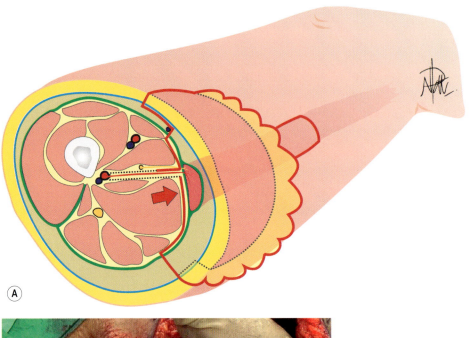

(A)

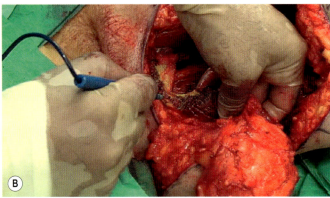

(B)

Fig. 21.3.16 Step 5 – division of proximal gracilis. (© *Nakul Patel and Venkat Ramakrishnan.*)

the TUG. The PAP flap, however, does avoid harvesting muscle and is discussed further in the following chapter (Fig. 21.3.23).[22–27]

The donor site morbidity is minimal in our series although some groups have had higher rates of complications.[28] Locke and colleagues had a 62.5% complication rate within their donor site including sensory disturbance within the medial thigh and poor scar requiring revision. They also noticed deficient flap volume and contour defects. The complication rates have been reduced by those units performing large numbers with the modification of the original description, which includes a skewed flap design, preservation of the long saphenous vein and associated lymphatics, fat recruitment from the inferior margin, and minimal muscle harvest.[29–33] In addition, patient selection remains key to minimizing complications.[19] Schoeller presents a large series of 111 patients with 154 TUG flaps for breast reconstructions. This series has total and partial flap failure rates of 2% each, a fat necrosis rate of 5%, delayed wound healing in 6%, a hematoma rate of 3%, and

transient sensory deficit over the posterior thigh in a third of cases.[19]

The most common drawback of the thigh donor site is the scar, which is not concealable in underwear and swimwear[8] (Fig. 21.3.24). Infection, seroma, and delayed wound healing around the groin are well recognized complications, which may be managed with dressings alone though re-operation to debride and re-suture the wounds may be required in a few cases. All patients should be counseled that some minor delayed healing is possible.[34]

A serious complication that the authors have not seen is the chance of temporary or permanent lymphedema given that the surgical site is over the lymphatics of the groin.

More subtle complications that we have noticed include the abrupt change in color of the groin skin from the donor site and contour change with the lack of medial bulging at the superomedial thigh.

The relatively darker skin of the thigh forms a nice nipple area complex in those patients undergoing

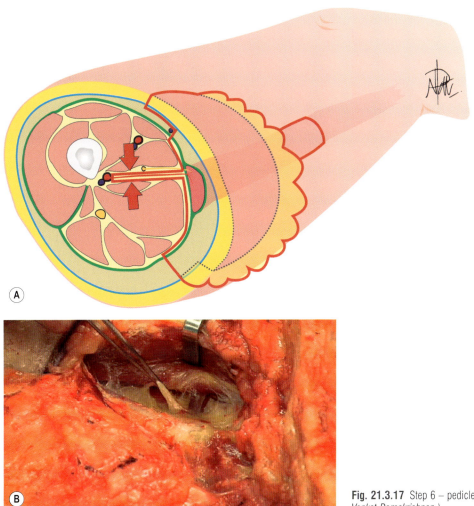

Fig. 21.3.17 Step 6 – pedicle dissection and flap detachment. (© *Nakul Patel and Venkat Ramakrishnan.*)

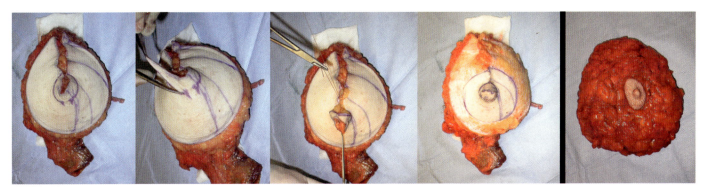

Fig. 21.3.18 Step 7 – full-cone shaping of transverse upper gracilis flap with nipple reconstruction created as "V-shaped" flaps that are inset as folded arms (left) and skin-sparing mastectomy specimen (far right) demonstrates a similar shape to the flap. (© *Nakul Patel and Venkat Ramakrishnan.*)

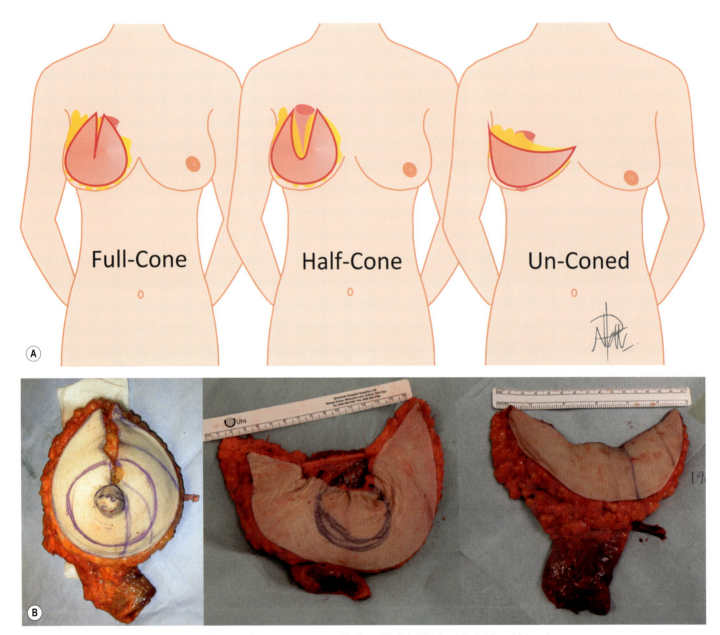

Fig. 21.3.19 Step 7 – full-cone, half-cone, and un-coned transverse upper gracilis flaps. (© *Nakul Patel and Venkat Ramakrishnan.*)

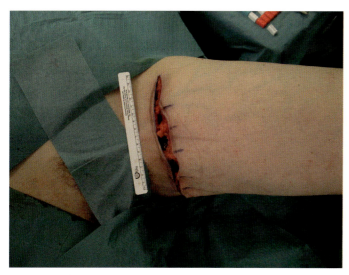

Fig. 21.3.20 Step 7 – closure of the donor site. (© Nakul Patel and Venkat Ramakrishnan.)

immediate skin-sparing mastectomies; however, in delayed cases, the dark skin paddle can be an obvious eyesore on the lighter colored chest.

Secondary procedures – TUG plus...

There are several adjunctive procedures that can enhance the flap and increase its indications in breast reconstruction. The algorithm in Fig. 21.3.25 describes the circumstances in which these additional procedures may be considered.

Lipofilling

Primary lipofilling of the gracilis muscle and pectoralis muscle can be useful for small volume differences. The muscle is an ideal vascular matrix for adipocytes and

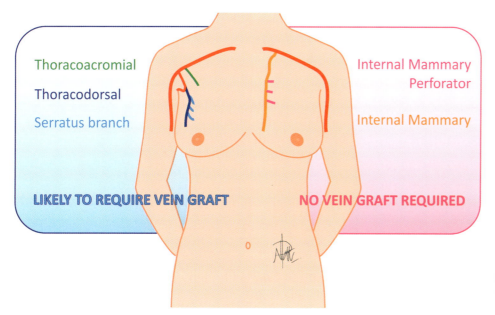

Thoracoacromial

Thoracodorsal

Serratus branch

Internal Mammary Perforator

Internal Mammary

LIKELY TO REQUIRE VEIN GRAFT

NO VEIN GRAFT REQUIRED

Fig. 21.3.21 Step 8 – recipient vessels for microsurgical anastomoses. (© Nakul Patel and Venkat Ramakrishnan.)

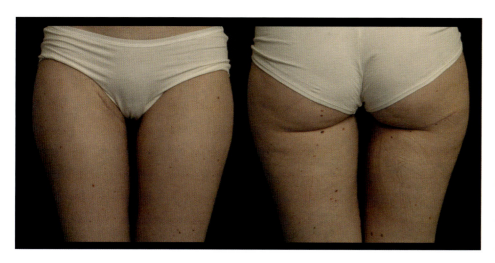

Fig. 21.3.22 Right transverse upper gracilis donor site highlights visible scar and lack of fullness in the upper medial thigh. In comparison to the normal left side, there is minimal change in overall volume and position of the gluteal crease. (© Nakul Patel and Venkat Ramakrishnan.)

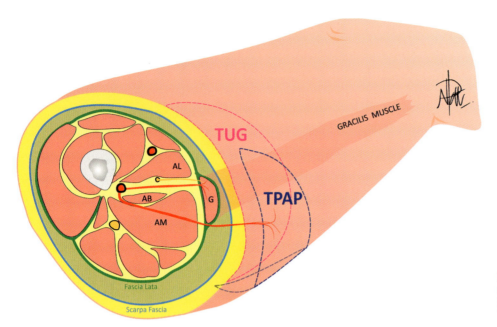

Fig. 21.3.23 Comparison of the transverse upper gracilis and transverse profunda artery perforator flap anatomy and donor sites. (© *Nakul Patel and Venkat Ramakrishnan.*)

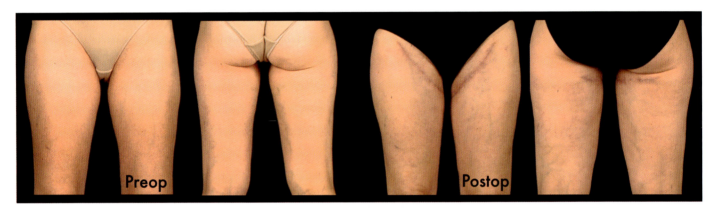

Fig. 21.3.24 Bilateral transverse upper gracilis flap donor site scars. The scars are stretched and have changed the contour of the upper medial thigh. These are visible in typical swimwear. (© *Nakul Patel and Venkat Ramakrishnan.*)

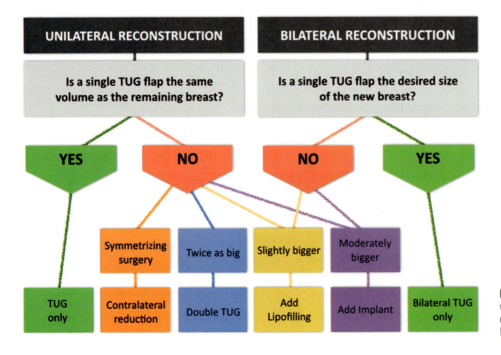

Fig. 21.3.25 Algorithm for additional procedures, which can be considered during the initial operation or at a second stage. (© *Nakul Patel and Venkat Ramakrishnan.*)

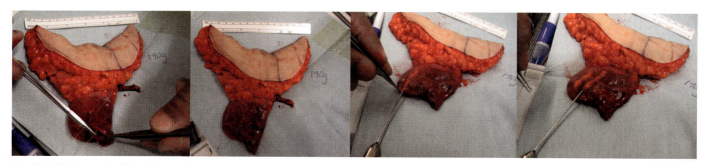

Fig. 21.3.26 Primary lipofilling of the gracilis muscle as a vascular matrix transfer. This requires closure of the epimysium prior to lipofilling into the muscle. (© Nakul Patel and Venkat Ramakrishnan.)

the authors advocate closure of the epimysium at the distal end of the muscle prior to fat transfer (Fig. 21.3.26). The TUG flap can also act as a vascular matrix for effective secondary lipofilling.

Implant

The use of implants under flaps is well described and is an excellent tool for allowing greater flexibility to what can otherwise be achieved.[35] Depending on the size of the device used, moderate to large differences can be addressed with the use of an implant either in the primary or secondary setting. We use implants with a mesh construct to keep the device in place prior to insetting the flap (Fig. 21.3.27).

Two flaps for one breast

Double TUG breast reconstructions are common for the larger breasted patient and are well described.[13,29,33] We

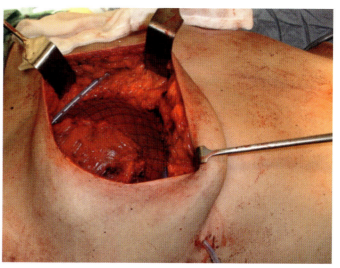

Fig. 21.3.27 Implant placed under a mesh construct to increase the breast volume. (© Nakul Patel and Venkat Ramakrishnan.)

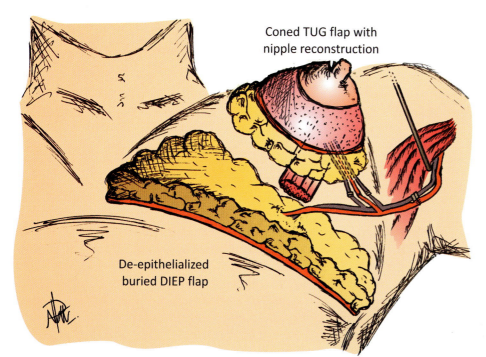

Coned TUG flap with nipple reconstruction

De-epithelialized buried DIEP flap

Fig. 21.3.28 An illustration of typical four-flap breast reconstruction with both transverse upper gracilis and deep inferior epigastric perforator flap stacked reconstructions. (© Nakul Patel and Venkat Ramakrishnan.)

suggest that a yin-yang orientation of the flaps with parallel anastomoses in both the axilla and chest allow optimum breast shape (see Fig. 21.3.7).

Flap-to-flap anastomoses, also known as "in-series anastomoses" of the two flaps, are an option when a sufficient adductor branch of the gracilis pedicle is available. Hunter and colleagues undertook both a clinical and anatomical study of branching patterns from the gracilis pedicle and showed that three-quarters of cases should be suitable for in-series anastomoses.[33]

If significantly more volume is required and the patient prefers a totally autologous reconstruction, TUG with another free flap such as the DIEP can given significant increase to the volume of the breast reconstruction (Fig. 21.3.28).

The TUG flap remains a reliable autologous option for breast reconstruction in those patients where the abdomen is not available. It is a reliable flap with consistent anatomy and potentially acceptable donor site. In combination with other procedures it can be used in those patients with larger breasts.

Bonus images for this chapter can be found online at
http://www.expertconsult.com

Fig. 21.3.1 Timeline for the TUG flap.

Access the complete reference list online at **http://www.expertconsult.com**

2. Orticochea M. The musculo-cutaneous flap method: an immediate and heroic substitute for the method of delay. *Br J Plast Surg.* 1972;25:106–110. *First use of the gracilis musculocutaneous flap to reconstruct an ankle defect.*

3. Harii K, Ohmori K, Sekiguchi J. The free musculocutaneous flap. *Plast Reconstr Surg.* 1976;57:294–303. *First free gracilis musculocutaneous flap presented in canine models, cadaver dissections, and clinical applications for reconstruction of the head and neck and lower extremity.*

9. Arnez ZM, Pogorelec D, Planinsek F, Ahcan U. Breast reconstruction by the free transverse gracilis (TUG) flap. *Br J Plast Surg.* 2004;57:20–26. *First early series of seven free TUG flaps was used for breast reconstruction, of which five were successful.*

10. Schoeller T, Wechselberger G. Breast reconstruction by the free transverse gracilis (TUG) flap. *Br J Plast Surg.* 2004;57:481–482. *Schoeller and Wechselberger described the use of 12 TUG flaps for breast reconstruction that were all successful. It is this work that has led to the popularity for the TUG flap for breast reconstruction.*

22. Hunter JE, Lardi AM, Dower DR, Farhadi J. Evolution from the TUG to PAP flap for breast reconstruction: comparison and refinements of technique. *J Plast Reconstr Aesthet Surg.* 2015;68:960–965. *Describes the evolution of the TUG to the PAP flap, which is in the same region.*

29. Fattah A, Figus A, Mathur B, Ramakrishnan VV. The transverse myocutaneous gracilis flap: technical refinements. *J Plast Reconstr Aesthet Surg.* 2010;63:305–313. *Describes a number of modifications of the original description, which includes a skewed flap design, preservation of the long saphenous vein and associated lymphatics, fat recruitment from the inferior margin, and minimal muscle harvest to reduce complications and ease flap harvest.*

30. Buchel EW, Dalke KR, Hayakawa TE. The transverse upper gracilis flap: efficiencies and design tips. *Can J Plast Surg.* 2013;21:162–166. *Describes reliable and rapid TUG flap harvest and provides a video using only monopolar cautery for the dissection.*

31. Saint-Cyr M, Wong C, Oni G, et al. Modifications to extend the transverse upper gracilis flap in breast reconstruction: clinical series and results. *Plast Reconstr Surg.* 2012;129:24e–36e. *Modifications to increase flap volume by using extended and vertical extended flaps are described in this paper.*

33. Hunter JE, Mackey SP, Boca R, Harris PA. Microvascular modifications to optimize the transverse upper gracilis flap for breast reconstruction. *Plast Reconstr Surg.* 2014;133:1315–1325. *Describes a new classification system for the branching pattern of the TUG flap pedicle to allow flap-to-flap anastomoses in 75 percent of patients.*

21.4

Profunda artery perforator flap for breast reconstruction

James L. Mayo, Z-Hye Lee, and Robert J. Allen Sr

SYNOPSIS

- The profunda artery perforator (PAP) flap is a favorable flap for autologous breast reconstruction leaving a donor scar in the upper medial thigh and inferior gluteal crease.
- Preoperative imaging with magnetic resonance angiography or computed tomography angiography is a useful adjunct in surgical planning and efficiency.
- The dissection of the PAP flap is straightforward through the adductor magnus muscle, providing a mean pedicle length of 10 cm and average flap weight of 360 g.
- The donor site of the PAP flap has been shown to have an acceptable complication profile compared with the deep inferior epigastric perforator (DIEP) flap reconstruction.
- The PAP flap should be strongly considered when the DIEP flap is not an option.

 Access the Historical Perspective section online at
http://www.expertconsult.com

Introduction

Perforator flap breast reconstruction has evolved into a reconstructive modality touting the ability to provide "natural-like" tissue for breast reconstruction with a low morbidity profile. The deep inferior epigastric perforator (DIEP) flap first described for breast reconstruction by Allen in 1992 remains the gold standard.[1] Tissue from the abdomen is harvested based on perforator(s) from the deep inferior epigastric artery sparing the surrounding rectus abdominis muscle leaving the patient with a slimmer midline. Outcome studies have shown this flap to be aesthetically pleasing while providing limited donor site morbidity.[2–7] Algorithms and techniques have evolved from an extensive background of experience and time aimed to perfect DIEP free flap breast reconstruction.[8,9]

While the application of the DIEP for breast reconstruction has spread with aims of further reducing complications and perfecting aesthetics, not uncommonly does a reconstructive surgeon find the abdomen to be either insufficient in volume or contraindicated due to previous surgery. In a review of 20 years performing microsurgical breast reconstruction, the senior author, Dr Allen, has performed DIEP flaps in 66% of his reconstructions, leaving one-third of patients in need of a secondary site. The ideal site would offer an adequate volume of pliable fat and skin with limited donor site morbidity and a fairly well-hidden scar.

The search for the optimal "secondary" flap for microsurgical breast reconstruction has been extensive. Reported flaps have included the superior and inferior gluteal artery perforator (GAP) flaps, transverse upper gracilis (TUG) flaps, lumbar artery perforator flaps, and profunda artery perforator (PAP) flaps.[10–14] After early experience with gluteal flaps, a search for the next flap option was directed to the thighs. The gluteal flaps were successful and remain a viable option for breast reconstruction. However, a difficult dissection and suboptimal efficiency with patient repositioning seen in the SGAP can be burdensome. Also, both GAP flaps occasionally led to donor site contour deformities requiring secondary procedures.[15,16]

The PAP flap offers adequate volume, pliable tissue, and a donor site well hidden within the upper thigh and buttock crease (Fig. 21.4.1). Beginning in 2010, the senior

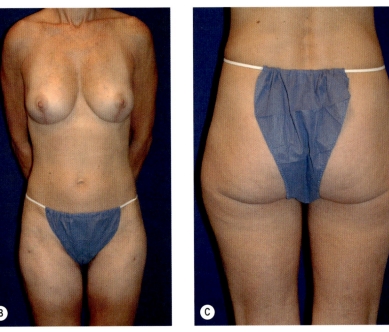

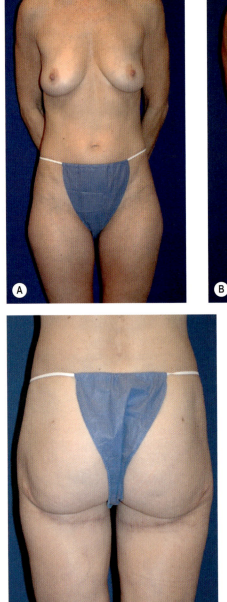

Fig. 21.4.1 Anterior view of a 54-year-old BRCA-positive woman. **(A)** Preoperative and **(B)** postoperative images for bilateral nipple-sparing mastectomies and profunda artery perforator flap reconstruction. **(C,D)** Posteromedial thigh donor site in the 54-year-old woman who underwent bilateral profunda artery perforator free flap breast reconstruction. The upper incision is placed 1–2 cm below the thigh crease but can vary based on location of the key perforator. *(Courtesy of Christina Ahn, MD.)*

author, Dr Allen, has utilized the PAP flap as his second option for perforator-based breast reconstruction performing roughly 200 PAP flaps for breast reconstruction. This chapter discusses the evolution/history of the PAP flap, reviews pertinent anatomy, and details operative technique, followed by outlining outcomes and complications.

Basic science/anatomy

The anatomic vascular basis to the PAP flap has been well documented by both cadaveric and radiographic studies.[20,22–24] The profunda artery arises from the

common femoral artery traveling into the posterior compartment of the thigh prior to branching into a lateral and medial branch. The lateral branch provides perforators to the more lateral/posterior thigh, many of which are septocutaneous perforators. The medial branch travels in the adductor compartment sending musculocutaneous perforators to and through the gracilis and adductors.

The ideal perforators identified for the PAP flap are those found medially piercing the adductor magnus. Utilizing these perforators allows for harvest of the flap with the patient in a supine position and gives ideal pedicle length. Original imaging studies by

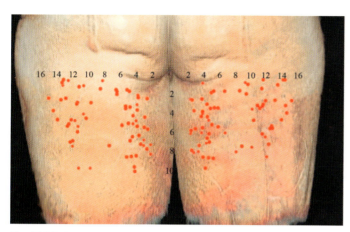

Fig. 21.4.2 Coordinates of significant profunda artery perforators found in a review of 40 preoperative computed tomographic angiographies of the lower extremities. *(Reprinted from: Haddock NT, Greaney P, Otterburn D, et al. Predicting perforator location on preoperative imaging for the profunda artery perforator flap. Microsurgery. 2012;32:507–511.)*

Table 21.4.1 Average location, size, and consistency of medial, lateral, and central profunda artery perforators

	Medial	Central	Lateral
Size	1.9±0.4 mm	1.8±0.4 mm	1.9±0.4 mm
Location			
X-axis	3.8 cm	6.5 cm	12 cm
Y-axis	5 cm	4.1 cm	5 cm
Border muscles	Adductor	Semimembranosus	Biceps
	Magnus		Femoris
		Semitendinosus	Vastus
			Lateralis
Consistency			
Present in thighs	86.0%	32.7%	65.0%

(Reprinted from: Haddock NT, Greaney P, Otterburn D, et al. Predicting perforator location on preoperative imaging for the profunda artery perforator flap. Microsurgery. 2012;32:507–511.)

Allen described a lateral and medial posterior thigh distribution to the PAPs with the majority being 3.8 cm from the midline and 5 cm below the gluteal fold (Fig. 21.4.2).[20] In further CT angiographic studies, DeLong *et al.* confirmed a close to 50/50 distribution between medially and laterally oriented perforators to the posterior thigh originating from the profunda artery.[23] The average pedicle length (10.7 cm) and distance from the gluteal crease (6.19 cm) were similar to previous studies.

In a review of the senior author's (Dr Allen) clinical experience, average flap weight was 367.4 g, reconstructing an average mastectomy weight of 321 g. Flap dimensions averaged 27.2×6.3 cm with an average pedicle length of 10.2 cm. The artery and vein diameters averaged 2.2 mm and 2.8 mm, respectively (Box 21.4.1 and Table 21.4.1).

Patient selection

The ideal patient for PAP flap breast reconstruction is a patient with either a paucity of abdominal tissue or a contraindication to use the abdomen as a donor for breast reconstruction. She should have small- to moderate-sized breasts, or planning for additional volume procedures such as stacking flaps, fat grafting,

or local flaps would be necessary to achieve a higher volume (Fig. 21.4.3).[25–27] As with other autologous flaps, immediate and delayed reconstructions are both applicable. Avoiding radiating the flap is preferable, so those patients identified as being higher risk for needing radiation therapy are delayed. Preoperative imaging allows the identification and localization of the key perforator, which is then identified in the office via hand-held Doppler and marked as described below (Fig. 21.4.4).

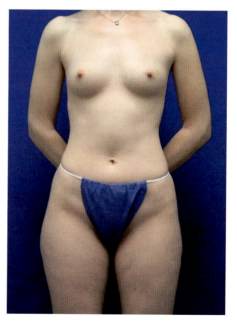

Fig. 21.4.3 The ideal profunda artery perforator flap candidate: thin, relatively small to moderate breast size, paucity of abdominal tissue, with available inner thigh volume.

BOX 21.4.1 **Flap characteristics**

- Average flap weight: 367 g
- Average flap dimensions: 27×6 cm
- Average pedicle length: 10.2 cm
- Average artery diameter: 2.2 mm
- Average vein diameter: 2.8 mm

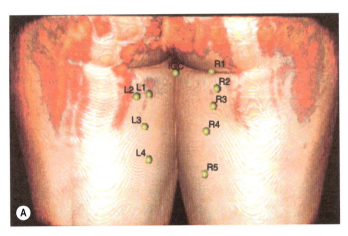

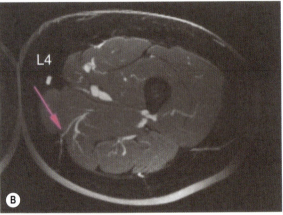

Fig. 21.4.4 (A) Representative preoperative magnetic resonance angiography mapping out the posteromedial profunda artery perforators. **(B)** The perforator (pink arrow) coursing through the adductor magnus posterior to the gracilis muscle. A significant perforator can be found within 8 cm of the upper thigh/gluteal crease.

drawing the upper incision from the adductor longus along the thigh crease posteriorly to the end of the gluteal crease (Fig. 21.4.5). The preoperative magnetic resonance angiography (MRA) or computed tomography angiography (CTA) is reviewed to identify key perforators. The perforator for each PAP flap is identified via hand-held Doppler with the patient in a prone position. The lower incision is placed 6–7 cm at its lowest point. This is drawn to include the key perforator in as much of a concentric placement as possible. If the key medial (adductor magnus) perforator is found to be too low, a perforator can commonly be found more posterolaterally based off a descending branch of the inferior gluteal artery or one of the laterally based profunda perforators (as described in the anatomy section above). The perforator at times is best identified and marked with the patient in the prone position.

In the operating room, the patient is laid supine in a frog-legged position. The lower extremities are fully prepped and draped into the operative field. With the thighs abducted, the flaps are raised in an anterior to posterior direction with the tip of the flap starting just behind the lymphatic-rich groin area bordered by the adductor longus. Superiorly, no beveling of the fat is performed in an effort to leave the ischial fat pad intact. Inferiorly, beveling is performed as necessary, based on volume needs and perforator location.

Once the gracilis is encountered, the fascia is opened vertically over the posterior portion while retracting the

Patient age averages 48 years and body mass index 22.5. The indications for surgery are mainly reconstruction after mastectomy for breast cancer, 59.5%. Other indications include reconstruction after prophylactic mastectomy (35.7%) and congenital breast deformity correction (4.8%). Patient demographics include an 18.8% rate of tobacco use, 18% history of radiation therapy, and 60.4% history of prior abdominal surgery including abdominoplasty, liposuction, hernia repair, and C-section.

Immediate breast reconstruction predominated (52.8%), while reconstruction after failed prior breast reconstruction also remained a significant indication for surgery (38.6%), mostly due to failed implant reconstruction (91.7%). Of the immediate reconstructions, 82.7% were nipple-sparing mastectomies with no incidence of postoperative nipple necrosis.

Surgical technique

The patient is seen in the office the day prior to surgery. The patient is first marked in a standing position

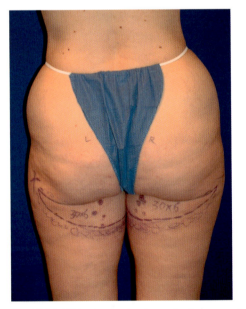

Fig. 21.4.5 Bilateral profunda artery perforator preoperative markings drawn in the office the day prior to surgery. The anterior tip of the flap starts at the insertion of adductor longus. The upper limit of the flap is 1–2 cm below the thigh crease and travels to the posterior extent of the gluteal crease for around 30 cm length. The flap width is typically 6–7 cm. These measurements are general guidelines; incorporating the key perforator in the flap design is paramount.

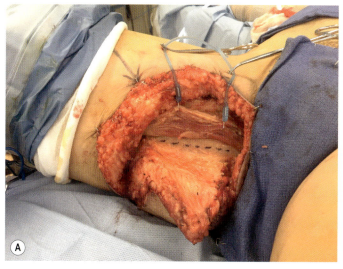

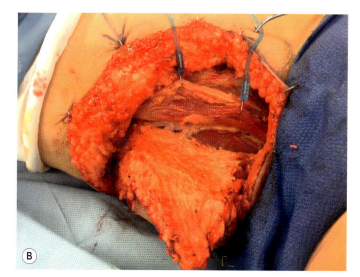

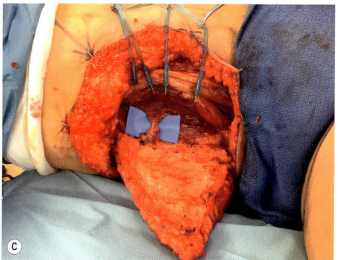

Fig. 21.4.6 Intraoperative images displaying **(A)** elevation anteriorly of the gracilis muscle to expose the adductor magnus fascia; **(B)** incision longitudinally of the adductor magnus fascia in order to proceed posteriorly in a subfascial plane towards identifying the key perforator; and, finally, **(C)** dissecting the key perforator through the adductor magnus muscle to its origin at the profunda artery and vein.

gracilis muscle anteriorly (Fig. 21.4.6). This maneuver exposes the adjacent adductor magnus muscle and allows for dissection through the adductor magnus fascia in an area safe from injuring the adductor perforators. Dissection proceeds along a subadductor magnus fascial plane until the key perforator is identified. The perforator is then dissected through the adductor magnus muscle until entering the fatty plane behind the adductor magnus. Utilizing "fish hook" retractors and self-retaining retractors at either end of the wound aids in perforator dissection. The retractors must be repositioned frequently with attention given to avoiding narrowing of the field, which would create a hole. The perforator can be dissected further to its origin at the profunda vein/artery for added length. A length of 8–12 cm can be reliably harvested.

Once the pedicle is isolated, dissection posteriorly can be performed in a suprafascial plane to decrease the area of fascial resection. The posterior skin incision is then completed with the aid of anteriorly stapling the flap and adduction of the leg. The flap is then fully isolated to its perforator. The pedicle is dissected off the posterior adductor magnus muscle and fully harvested. With experience, the pedicle can be harvested first then dissected off the posterior adductor magnus fascia in a retrograde fashion. The donor site is closed in multiple layers over a closed suction drain.

The flap is then anastomosed in the chest most commonly to the internal mammary vessels, though the thoracodorsal vessels are feasible recipient vessels. The match to the internal mammary vessels is favorable with an average PAP arterial diameter of 2.2 mm and venous diameter of 2.7 mm. The flap is then coned for inset to provide projection, and the pocket is contoured to the flap. When stacked PAP flaps for unilateral reconstruction, a wider base can be obtained without coning by suturing the two flaps together with each flap forming a breast hemisphere. A skin paddle is left for monitoring.

Table 21.4.2 Complications

	(%)
Flap loss	0.5
OR take-back	3
Fat necrosis	7
Donor site seroma	6
Donor site hematoma	2
Donor site infection	2
Lower extremity lymphedema	0

Postoperative care

Patients are sent to the post-anesthesia care unit for 1–2 h postoperatively, followed by transfer to a regular hospital room. Monitoring of the flap is based mainly on clinical exam with hand-held Doppler checks adjunctively every 4 h. Pain management consists of intravenous acetaminophen and per os ibuprofen with intravenous narcotics as needed through the first night after surgery. Patients are up in a chair and ambulating in postoperative day 1. The IV line is also removed the day following surgery, and no routine blood tests are drawn. Patients shower and are, most commonly, discharged on the third postoperative day. Breast drains are removed prior to discharge, and donor site drains are left in place for at least 1 week. A second stage operation is planned for 3 months after surgery and includes removal of the skin island previously left for monitoring; nipple reconstruction if needed; breast flap revision for symmetry; shape and/or size; and possible donor site revision.

Outcomes and complications

A review of 200 PAP flaps for breast reconstruction from 2010–2015 was performed by the authors. Flap success rate was 99.5% after losing one flap. The operating room take-back rate was 3%. The complication profile includes a fat necrosis rate of 7%, seroma 6%, hematoma 1.9%, and donor site infection 1.9%. There were no episodes of lymphedema. Short-term donor site morbidity includes tenderness for 7–14 days from sitting on a toilet seat and discomfort for up to 3 months from sitting on hard surfaces. No long-term sitting or decreased sensation has been reported (Table 21.4.2).

Secondary procedures

All patients undergo secondary procedures at as early as 3 months. To avoid deficient reconstructed breast volume, the senior author is increasingly performing two flap breast reconstruction as the primary procedure. Combinations used include stacked PAP flaps, PAP/DIEP, and PAP/ICAP. Fat grafting is commonly utilized at the second stage. Less than 1% of the time, additional volume is necessary and local flaps (ICAP/TDAP) are performed at the second stage.[28] Also performed at the second stage are skin island removal, nipple reconstruction if necessary, mastopexy, and shaping to achieve the optimal aesthetic result.

Trends/alterations

Variations to the PAP flap have recently evolved, to maximize reconstructive goals, expand candidate selection, and decrease complications. The design of the flap has been configured in a vertical fashion and applied to other areas of reconstruction.[29] This flap has the advantage of choosing from a multitude of PAPs all piercing the adductor magnus while providing a well-healed donor site in a configuration that could produce a lower wound complication profile (Fig. 21.4.7). To date, patients selected for this configuration have been those with moderate obesity presenting the potential for increased donor site wound complications. From a practical standpoint, the flap orientation should be designed to fit a specific patient's perforator anatomy and maximize volume of tissue harvested and closure aesthetics.

In cases requiring a significant additional volume than one flap might offer, stacking flaps can offer this

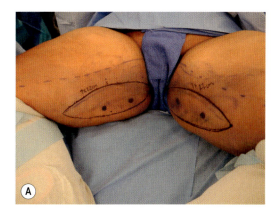

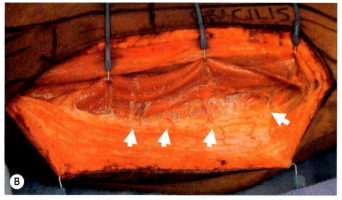

Fig. 21.4.7 (A) Design of the profunda artery perforator flap in a vertical fashion. **(B)** Intraoperative dissection of the vertical profunda artery perforator flap perforators. Numerous perforators are available on which to base the flap.

- Well-hidden donor site scar within upper thigh and buttock crease
- Ability to stack with other flaps

Disadvantages

- Not every patient is a good candidate due to body habitus variations
- Acceptable but not abundant flap volume
- Early donor site discomfort with sitting improved with positioning modifications.

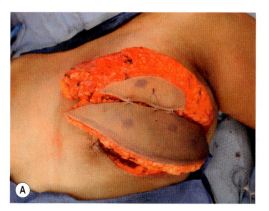

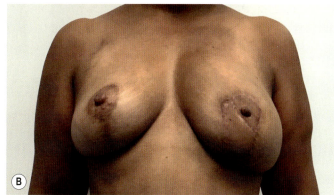

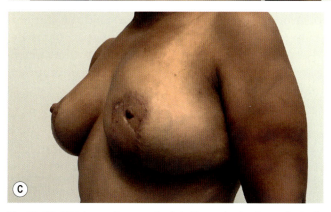

additional volume, as well as a more favorable volume distribution. For unilateral reconstruction in which the abdomen is not available and a single PAP flap is not sufficient, stacked PAP flaps may be performed. This may obviate the need for secondary fat grafting or local flaps (Fig. 21.4.8).[25] In cases of bilateral reconstruction when the abdomen provides insufficient volume, the senior author, Dr Allen, has historically combined DIEP and PAP flaps for superior volume and aesthetics.[30] The combination of the DIEP and PAP flaps utilizes the PAP for inferior pole volume and projection while the DIEP flap provides necessary superior pole volume. Most commonly, one flap is anastomosed to the antegrade internal mammary vessels and the other flap to the retrograde internal mammary vessels. This combination has proven to be both safe and successful.

Advantages and disadvantages

Advantages

- Easy dissection through the adductor magnus muscle
- Reliable perforator with long pedicle (~10 cm)
- Pliable flap tissue optimal for coning to reconstruct the breast

Fig. 21.4.8 (A) Intraoperative example of stacking profunda artery perforator flaps for unilateral breast reconstruction. Specific example is of a stacked vertical PAP flap with antegrade and retrograde internal mammary vessels used as recipient vessels. **(B,C)** Postoperative images of a patient who underwent left unilateral breast reconstruction with stacked vertical profunda artery perforator flaps. The patient, prior to left mastectomy for breast cancer, had a history of bilateral mastopexy and abdominoplasty. Stacking the flaps added the additional volume necessary to provide an aesthetic, symmetric reconstruction.

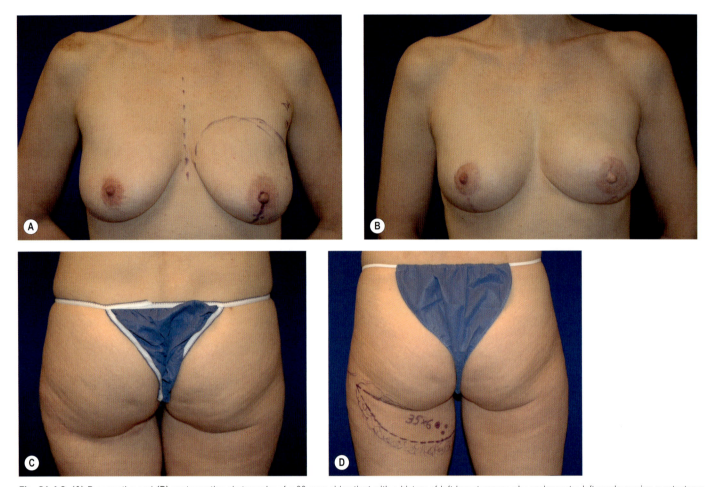

Fig. 21.4.9 **(A)** Preoperative and **(B)** postoperative photographs of a 38-year-old patient with a history of left breast cancer who underwent a left areola sparing mastectomy and profunda artery perforator (PAP) free flap reconstruction. **(C)** Preoperative (superior) and **(D)** postoperative (inferior) photographs of posteromedial thigh donor site in a 38-year-old patient who underwent unilateral PAP free flap breast reconstruction. *(Courtesy of Christina Ahn, MD.)*

Conclusion

With improvements in surgical techniques and an expansion of donor site options, autologous breast reconstruction has evolved into a field of patient-specific reconstruction. The DIEP free flap remains the gold standard but at times has either an unavailable donor site or is insufficient in providing appropriate volume for reconstruction. The PAP flap offers an alternative flap for reconstruction as well as an adjunct to the DIEP in creating an aesthetic breast. With a multitude of configurations to harvest optimal volume and minimize donor site morbidity based on a patient's specific anatomy and the ability to be stacked with an additional flap to offer additional volume or improved aesthetics, the PAP flap represents a safe, effective flap for any microsurgeons free flap armamentarium (Fig. 21.4.9).

🌐 Access the complete reference list online at **http://www.expertconsult.com**

2. Gill PS, Hunt JP, Guerra AB, et al. A 10-year retrospective review of 758 DIEP flaps for breast reconstruction. *Plast Reconstr Surg.* 2004;113:1153–1160. *The authors present one of the largest series of DIEP flaps for breast reconstruction and provides an in-depth analysis of this workhouse flap. Overall complication rate was 20.2% with the donor site complication being 13.6%. Furthermore, the rate of fat necrosis was 12.9% (n=98). They demonstrate that the DIEP flap has reduced donor site morbidity compared with the TRAM flap and has evolved to be the first choice for autologous breast reconstruction.*

13. Saad A, Sadeghi A, Allen RJ. The anatomic basis of the profunda femoris artery perforator flap: a new option for autologous breast reconstruction–a cadaveric and computer tomography angiogram study. *J Reconstr Microsurg.* 2012;28:381–386. *This study examined 10 cadaveric thighs to outline in detail the anatomic basis for the profunda femoris artery perforator flap. They identified key parameters including length of pedicle, vessel diameters, and flap characteristic. The authors show the pedicle to be on average 10.6 cm in length, the diameter of the artery at 2.3 mm, and the vein 2.8 mm. The flap on average measured 28×8 cm and weighed 206 g (100–260 g). This study also examined the CT scans of these cadavers and determined the average location of the perforators (4.4 cm caudal to gluteal crease and 5.1 cm lateral to midline). This was the first study to propose the use of the posterior thigh flap based on the perforators of the profunda femoris artery.*

18. Angrigiani C, Grilli D, Thorne CH. The adductor flap: a new method for transferring posterior and medial thigh skin. *Plast Reconstr Surg.* 2001;107:1725–1731. *The first flaps from the medial thigh*

had been primarily based on the gracilis musculocutaneous unit. This was the first study to delineate an anatomic basis for medial and posterior thigh flap based PAPs through the adductor magnus muscle. They examined 20 cadavers and found reliable cutaneous perforators of the adductor magnus muscle allowing for skin flaps as large as 30×23 cm. They also provided a clinical series of 25 patients in which these adductor flaps were used, 11 of which were microvascular free flaps. Five of the flaps were for resurfacing burn scar contractures and six were for reconstructing lower extremity defects. While they did not use the posterior thigh flap for breast reconstruction, it was the first study to demonstrate that the skin of the medial and posterior thigh region can be successfully transferred based on several different vascular perforators that are reliable and consistent.

21. Allen RJ, Haddock NT, Ahn CY, et al. Breast reconstruction with the profunda artery perforator flap. *Plast Reconstr Surg.* 2012;129: 16e–23e. *This was the largest clinical series to date using the PAP flap for breast reconstruction before our current series. The authors present a series of 27 flaps and demonstrate the reliability of this flap with a long pedicle and sufficient vessel caliber. The average weight of the flap was 385 g (range, 235–695 g), average artery size 2.2 cm, and average vein size 2.8 cm. All PAP flaps were successful with two donor site complications, one seroma, and one hematoma. One important adjustment made during their experience with the first 27 flaps was the transition to a supine frog-leg position from a prone position to avoid intraoperative repositioning. This was the first large clinical series to describe the experience using PAP flap for breast reconstruction.*

22. Haddock NT, Greaney P, Otterburn D, et al. Predicting perforator location on preoperative imaging for the profunda artery perforator flap. *Microsurgery.* 2012;32:507–511. *This radiographic study further delineated the anatomic details of the PAP flap, especially regarding the number, location, and size of the perforators. A review of 40 preoperative posterior thigh CTAs and MRAs demonstrated that suitable PAPs were present in 98.8% of thighs. The most common perforator was medial (in 85.6% of thighs). Based on this study, the current preference in designing PAP flaps is to use a medial perforator, although this study found that the second most common perforator was lateral (present in 65.4% of thighs). Most importantly, preoperative imaging corresponded well to perforators intraoperatively during the pedicle dissection.*

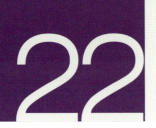

Secondary procedures following autologous reconstruction

Joshua Fosnot and Joseph M. Serletti

SYNOPSIS

- Secondary procedures following autologous reconstruction are common.
- Secondary procedures often follow the same principles of other forms of breast surgery.
- Common procedures include fat grafting, reduction, augmentation, nipple areolar reconstruction and refinement of the skin envelope.
- While uncommon, hernia repair following free TRAM reconstruction is discussed here as it can be a challenge to correct.
- Oftentimes, a single secondary operative procedure can combine all revisions in one and is commonly the last stage of reconstruction.

Access the Historical Perspective section online at
http://www.expertconsult.com

Introduction

Although the pedicled transverse rectus abdominis myocutaneous (TRAM) flap provided a foundation for the burgeoning field of breast reconstruction, the overall contemporary trend has focused on approaches which provide improved aesthetic outcomes while minimizing complications and donor site morbidity. Advances in microsurgical technique have thus led the field toward the utilization of free flaps, which benefit from a more profound blood supply while sacrificing less of the abdominal wall. A spectrum exists which includes the free TRAM, muscle-sparing free TRAM (MsfTRAM), deep inferior epigastric perforator (DIEP) and superficial inferior epigastric artery (SIEA) flaps, all of which utilize the same transverse island of lower abdominal wall skin and soft tissue for the recreation of a breast

mound with varying degrees of abdominal wall intrusion. In addition, non-abdominal-based flaps have gained in popularity such as the transverse upper gracilis (TUG), superficial circumflex iliac perforator (SCIP), or posterior thigh flaps. The free flap can be thought of as importing clay to the sculpting table. In many cases, the initial flap transfer is sufficient to provide an excellent aesthetic result and one which provides longevity. However, it is also very common that revisions are necessary to achieve the optimal outcome and one which is in line with the desires of the critical patient and surgeon. Common techniques employed for revision of the autologous reconstruction are those used quite frequently for other forms of aesthetic breast surgery. These techniques include fat grafting, augmentation, reduction and refinement of the skin envelope. While many of these topics are covered in other chapters in this book, this chapter will focus specifically on their use in autologous reconstruction.

Basic science/disease process

One in eight women will suffer from breast cancer over the course of their lifetime.[22] While certainly not everyone will seek a mastectomy, the frequency of mastectomy is rising nationally. In addition, the prevalence of prophylactic mastectomy has risen as well. Both implant and autologous reconstruction each have their own risks and benefits. While nationally, implant reconstruction remains more common, in certain geographic locations free flap reconstruction has become more accessible and thus relatively commonplace.[23] Both often require secondary procedures; however, autologous revision is usually a short-term undertaking, whereas implant reconstruction requires maintenance of the implants over the course of a woman's lifetime. Revision is not always necessary, but can be indicated for a number of problems. Fortunately, multiple modalities exist to improve the long-term result, which generally speaking are well tolerated by patients and offer excellent, long-lasting results.

Diagnosis/patient presentation

The most important step to take before considering revision of the reconstructed breast is to listen to your patient. After mastectomy and free flap reconstruction, some patients are exhausted and others are eager to proceed. From an aesthetic perspective, some patients are highly critical and others are content with asymmetries that you as a surgeon find unacceptable. Listening to your patient affords the opportunity to make sure surgeon and patient are in agreement on the need for further surgery, determine if further surgery is likely to provide benefit and to refine the surgical plan. Fig. 22.1 provides a general approach to the identification and correction of chest asymmetry discussed in this chapter.

Timing

Consideration of revision typically is entertained at the 3 month mark. Revision should occur once a relatively stable breast mound has been achieved and several months are necessary to get to this point. When radiation is involved, this process takes even longer. The radiated reconstruction benefits from a recovery time of up to 6 months after completion of treatments. This may be almost 9 months after initial reconstruction; however, an adequate delay allows for more specific and refined revision. Waiting also allows patients time to decide what they like and don't like about their reconstruction. Some patients initially are happy with their results, but notice small things bother them in time, while others initially are unhappy and become more accustomed with the reconstruction with time, no longer desiring revision.[24] Lastly, there is no temporal limit to waiting, nor any reason to rush into revision.

Timing of balancing procedures is also important in unilateral reconstruction. While it is tempting to perform a balancing procedure during immediate reconstruction, it is difficult to control all of the variables of performing two different operations from side to side to achieve symmetry. If mild to moderate asymmetries are expected based upon ptosis or volume, we usually delay the balancing procedure until a later date; whereas, if large changes (such as a large reduction) are necessary,

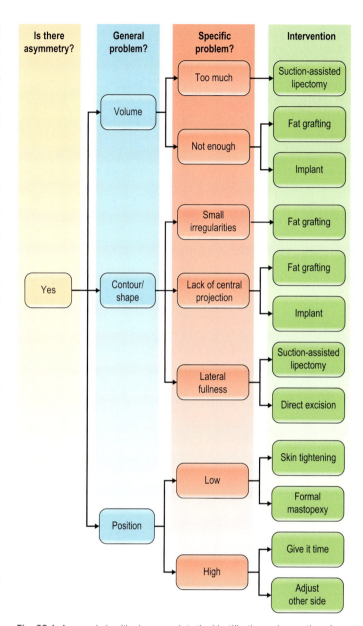

Fig. 22.1 A general algorithmic approach to the identification and correction of breast asymmetry following autologous reconstruction. Oftentimes, multiple issues may coexist, thus necessitating the use of multiple modalities.

these patients may benefit from an immediate balancing approach. This avoids a patient having to live with a large discrepancy for several months. In these cases, however, we recommend telling patients that revision of either the native or reconstructed side may be necessary in the future in order to fine tune symmetry.

Assessing the problem

Volume

It is useful to categorize deformities based upon patient and surgeon observations. Firstly, volume asymmetry is one of the biggest drivers of patient dissatisfaction since bra fitting is a challenge. In unilateral reconstruction, the free flap may be smaller or larger than anticipated; however, even in bilateral reconstruction, volume asymmetry occurs. Treatment of volume differences greatly depends upon patient wishes. Small reductions in a flap can be easily performed with liposuction, whereas large reductions may require a more formal approach with resection. Conversely, augmentation of the contralateral side can be performed with fat grafting or implants. Which side to modify greatly depends upon patient goals.

Contour/shape

Contour irregularities are common following free flap reconstruction. The cause is multifactorial but most commonly is a baseline mismatch in size or shape between the breast tissue removed and the free flap inset. This can be most notable in the upper pole or tail of the reconstructed breast mound where a tapered effect is difficult to achieve primarily. Small areas of fat necrosis can lead to hollowing or frank masses which may require revision. In addition, lack of central projection relative to a natural breast is a common complaint. This is generally due to an inability to completely cone the central mound in a manner similar to a native youthful breast. A free flap (particularly a DIEP without muscle) is often fairly uniform in depth, which can lead to a flat-appearing breast mound. All of these issues can be addressed with fat grafting although on occasion, a small implant centrally can work very well to add central projection. Oftentimes, however, women have chosen autologous reconstruction to avoid the issues associated with implants; thus, staged fat grafting may be a better choice. Fat necrosis can be treated either by direct excision, liposuction or with an aeration technique which will be discussed later in this chapter.

Position

Patients with grade I ptosis are rarely subject to problems with flap position in the postoperative period as long as the mastectomy pocket remains confined to the breast tissue. To avoid problems with position, the mastectomy pocket should be redefined with suturing prior to inset of the flap. If the pocket is not redefined, positioning may be wrong, thus resulting in a need to redefine the inframammary fold (IMF), medial or lateral borders. Simple changes may be amenable to liposuction, but generally speaking, major changes require recreation of the pocket, movement of the flap and redefining of the pocket. As this is not a minor revision, every attempt should be made to avoid this problem to begin with.

More likely, positional problems arise in patients with pre-existing ptosis where skin envelope changes are being made in immediate reconstruction or in delayed reconstruction where the envelope is being recreated. A common issue is a vertical discrepancy related to uneven skin resection from side to side, or vertical discrepancy in unilateral reconstruction where a contralateral balancing procedure is needed. Assessing symmetry and patient satisfaction should be approached similarly to how a surgeon would assess any breast consultation. Similar techniques also can be used to improve vertical positioning such as the vertical mastopexy. Usually, however, these are skin only procedures as opposed to formal parenchymal/pillar procedures. In all cases, but delayed reconstruction in particular, it is important to ensure enough time has passed to allow the envelope to relax and drop before revision.

Donor site

The most common donor site for free flap breast reconstruction is the lower abdomen. While the majority of patients heal well and are happy with their donor site, two common complaints/problems can arise. Delayed wound healing of the central abdomen is unfortunately a fairly common complication likely a result of tension or low grade ischemia related to perfusion and/or comorbidities. While small areas are easily treated with wet to dry dressing changes, sometimes large dehiscence occurs. Debridement and VAC therapy is a useful adjunct; however, early secondary revision and closure has been shown to be safe and perhaps is a faster way to achieve completely closed wounds.[25] Regardless of duration of healing, the tension on this wound can lead to fat necrosis and widened scars. Revision of these scars should be undertaken only after the scar has stabilized and the soft tissue is lax enough to allow for excision and reclosure without any tension.

Dog-ear deformities are not uncommon as well. While every attempt at avoidance should be attempted, sometimes adequate exposure to the far lateral flank at the time of free flap harvest is limited. Dog-ear excision and liposuction of the flanks can help improve lateral contour. Donor site revision can often be performed at the same time as breast mound revision or nipple areolar reconstruction.

Treatment/surgical technique

Fat grafting

The use of fat grafting is quite possibly the most important technique available to revise the reconstructed breast (see Fig. 22.2). An entire chapter is dedicated to fat grafting techniques elsewhere in this book (see Chapter 24); however, some technical points are worth discussing here. The donor site may play a role in graft take as some studies have shown the lower abdomen and inner thighs to be higher in adipose-derived stem cells.[26] These cells are believed to aid in survival; however, other studies have failed to highlight major differences in donor site value.[27–29] The donor site of choice is injected with 1% lidocaine with epinephrine. Fat can be procured using manual aspiration or a formal liposuction device. Larger cannula diameters may yield healthier fat cells.[30] If a liposuction device is employed, it is likely that lower aspiration pressures aid in cell survival, but further research is needed in this area. Preparation of the fat before use is needed to remove fluid, debris and free oil. This can be done using filtration, sedimentation or a centrifugation system can be

employed to spin the fat down. For larger volumes, centrifugation is certainly more practical; however, no one method of preparation has been shown to be the most effective.[31] Several procurement and processing systems are now on the market to make the process more efficient and hopefully offer better results, however this remains to be seen. Research on the quality of the fat based upon site of harvest and methods of procurement is constantly evolving and at this time not convincing that one method far surpasses another.[31]

What is likely the most important factor contributing to long-term survival is the environment in which the fat is placed. Fat should be placed in small aliquots (no more than 0.5 cc per pass) using a multipass technique as described by Coleman. The fat should be placed in multiple planes even if the defect feels superficial. Superficial and deep planes allow for placement of each

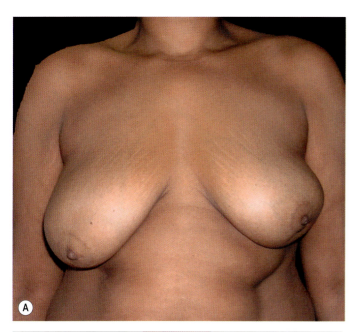

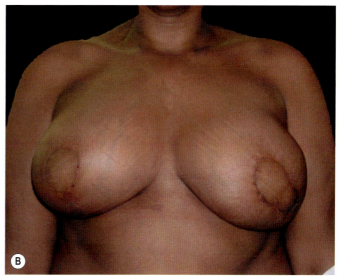

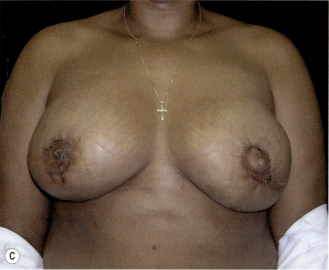

Fig. 22.2 (A) This patient has a history of radiation on the right and underwent bilateral mastectomies with bilateral gluteal artery perforator flap reconstructions. The right side is smaller and higher than the left. **(B)** Following revision with right high volume fat grafting and left refinement of the skin envelope.

pass into its own space. The pectoralis muscle can be injected directly into, as it serves as an excellent recipient site for fat survival. Fat should be injected in multiple directions as well. This technique requires multiple access points. As this can be done through 1-mm access points, scarring should not be a concern. Having a finite mental image of a three-dimensional crosshatch network of lines should be the goal, not simply injecting through convenient locations. When larger volumes are necessary, one must avoid the temptation to try to achieve perfection in one setting. Overfilling leads to lower retention rates[32] and most patients, if educated properly, will understand why staged surgical procedures are necessary and beneficial. Lastly, a radiated bed can still receive fat grafts; however, retention rates are likely lower.[33] Therefore, one should be aware that fat grafting may require more stages or even be ultimately less successful following radiation therapy.

Liposuction

Standard suction-assisted lipectomy can be very useful in not only reducing volume, but blending transition points well (Fig. 22.3). The borders of the flap can feel like a step-off to patients and gentle liposuction can help smooth the edges. In addition, the lateral aspect of the flap can be shaped nicely with liposuction as it transitions to the lateral chest wall. Injection of 1% lidocaine with epinephrine is usually adequate as opposed to tumescence. Regardless of what indication it is being used for, one should be aware that a free flap will quickly lose its volume with SAL; therefore, it is easy to overshoot the goal unless one is careful.

Skin refinement

Refining the skin envelope is not technically challenging; however, achieving the desired effect without adding new scars can be difficult. The most common areas where the envelope needs revision is the lateral breast mound as it transitions to the chest wall. This is particularly true in women who had large ptotic breasts prior to mastectomy. These women would benefit from a Wise pattern skin reduction at the time of mastectomy, but using this approach would compromise mastectomy skin flap perfusion.[34] Thus, the correction is often necessary due to a purposeful cautious approach initially. The correction simply involves excising the lateral dog-ear similarly to the lateral extension of a Wise pattern reduction.

The other common problem of the skin envelope is of undercorrection of the vertical component of a vertical pattern skin reduction at the time of mastectomy. In a standard breast reduction or mastopexy, the vertical component is generally overcorrected. Tension on the

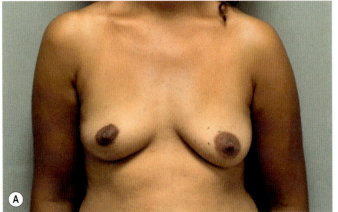

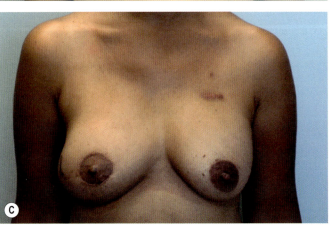

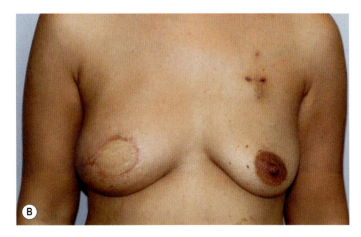

Fig. 22.3 **(A)** Preoperative photo of a patient with left breast cancer planning on bilateral mastectomy. **(B)** Following bilateral DIEP flaps, the patient complained of being too large and of lateral fullness. **(C)** Following revision with nipple areolar reconstruction and suction-assisted lipectomy to reduce volume and lateral fullness. *(Courtesy of Liza Wu, MD, FACS.)*

skin is ameliorated somewhat by pillar sutures; however, this overcorrection relaxes over the next few months. When a vertical pattern is chosen during a mastectomy, one does not have the luxury of overcorrection. Tension on the mastectomy skin flaps can further compromise already tenuous mastectomy skin flaps. Thus, undercorrection of ptosis is common and leads to the necessary revision as a result of purposeful caution. The surgical correction is often fairly straightforward – further excision of the vertical component without changing the position of the nipple areolar complex (NAC).

Implants

While most women choose autologous reconstruction to avoid a prosthetic device, implants can play a specific role in adding overall volume, improving large contour deformities or adding central projection (Fig. 22.4). Implant choice follows the same principles as when used for other indications. In thin patients, form stable implants may have a definitive role to add natural shape. In most circumstances, however, the implants used are less than 250 cc where the difference between a form stable and standard round implant becomes less noticeable. In these cases, round implants may be a better choice due to their softer nature. Saline implants are rarely used. Textured implants may have some benefit in the irradiated field in trying to reduce the risk of capsular contracture.[35,36] In terms of style, small implants have a very narrow footprint regardless of projection. If one is trying to correct an overall volume discrepancy, a lower profile implant may be a good choice to fill out as much width as possible, whereas, if central projection is the main goal, then a higher profile implant may be warranted. In this case, the pocket should be left small so as to avoid implant malposition. From a technical standpoint, we prefer to place implants in a submuscular plane. This avoids any concern about dissecting the pedicle off the muscle, and places the implant into an unoperated tissue plane. When the internal mammary vessels are used for a recipient site, this is usually far enough away from the pocket created to avoid injury. Access to the submuscular plane may be achievable through existing scars, but a standard IMF incision is generally the best approach and one that allows for excellent exposure, ease of dissection and placement of the implant itself.

Fat necrosis

Small areas of fat necrosis can be treated with excision; however, larger volumes or areas in the far upper pole can be difficult to treat with excision without creating obvious contour deformities or new visible scars. Contour deformities from excision can be treated with fat grafting, but this may commit patients to multiple surgeries. An alternative technique can employ either liposuction, ultrasonic liposuction or a power dissector.[37] In this technique, the small cannula is used to drill holes in multiple directions in the area of fat necrosis. This technique is similar to aerating a green on a golf course. These small holes often soften the feel of the necrotic area and may allow for tissue ingrowth which leads to improvement with time.

Balancing mastopexy/reduction

In general, lifting or reduction techniques should follow standard techniques such as vertical or Wise pattern skin resections with standard pedicle design. That being said, one technical pearl is to keep in mind that one is trying to match the reconstructed side, not necessarily perform the standard technique employed elsewhere.

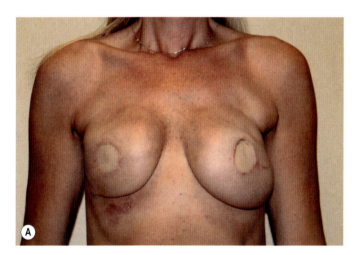

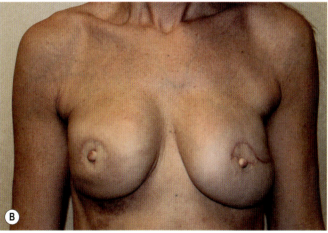

Fig. 22.4 (A) Preoperative photo of a patient with right breast cancer with pre-existing asymmetry. **(B)** Intermediate stage following a right DIEP. The right side is larger, but the patient preferred this side to her native left side. **(C)** Following revision with right nipple areolar reconstruction and a left augmentation with a submuscular implant. She would likely benefit from a left circumareolar mastopexy but she did not want additional scars. She is overall very happy with the volumetric correction.

For instance, a standard vertical mastopexy with a superior pedicle is often performed by tucking the central pillar underneath the NAC to add central projection and create a more coned, youthful breast. Oftentimes a reconstructed breast with a free flap lacks this coned effect. If a patient is happy with the reconstructed side and just wants balance, then avoiding the central coning with the mastopexy is beneficial.

Abdominal donor site hernia

The hernia which can arise in the abdominal donor site is not often addressed in chapters, yet it can be very challenging to correct. Thus, we thought it worth discussing here. The most common site for hernia formation is below the arcuate line. Above this line, the posterior sheath is not violated in the flap harvest, yet still has significant strength leading to little risk of hernia over time. Below the arcuate line, all of the strength layers of the abdominal fascia are anterior to the rectus muscles and thus by definition are all violated in a DIEP/MsfTRAM harvest. The fascia is universally attenuated in these hernias; thus, primary closure of the hernia defect would lead to unsatisfactory repair. Therefore, placement of mesh is a universal tenet. While biologic mesh may play a significant role in contaminated wounds, to date little or no evidence supports their use over permanent mesh in clean wounds, especially given their high cost.[38,39] The authors therefore recommend synthetic permanent mesh. As the hernia defect is commonly under or near the skin incision, placing any underlay with complete fascial coverage allows for a two-layered strength closure as well as complete coverage of the mesh. The hernia is easily approached via the existing transverse scar. The hernia sac is dissected in continuity into the preperitoneal space. This may end up being above or below the rectus muscle – either is acceptable. The mesh is sewn into place in this plane and the fascia is closed over the top. If necessary, release of the external oblique muscles laterally via component separation allows for midline advancement of the fascia.

Postoperative care

In general, no specific postoperative care is necessary following revision. We recommend wearing a supportive brassiere which is not tightly compressive for a few weeks postoperatively. If revision has been coupled with nipple areolar reconstruction (discussed in Chapter 27), then the patient should avoid tight-fitting clothing which compresses the NAR flaps. Almost all revision can be done as an outpatient procedure and we routinely tell patients to expect to be back to work within a week, if not a day or two. Most of the areas treated are lacking in sensation to begin with, which makes the recovery fairly reasonable for the patient. Most importantly, we tell patients to have *patience*. If fat grafting or liposuction were employed, the full effects of these treatments will not be known for a minimum of 3 months. If further dissatisfaction is noted at that time, then further revision may be addressed.

Outcomes, prognosis, and complications

The majority of women require only one revision to complete their reconstruction. Quite commonly, this includes nipple areolar reconstruction. In general, complications are few and far between, but do exist. Fat grafting can, albeit rarely, result in fat cysts or necrosis. This is a result of injecting too much fat into one area. Oil cysts feel firm but can be aspirated to resolution. If frank fat necrosis results from fat grafting, the treatment resorts to that previously described. The most common "complication" of fat grafting would be volume loss or lack of effect. Roughly 50% of the injected volume may be lost with time; thus, multiple sessions of fat grafting may be necessary to achieve a final acceptable result.[31] Volumetric or positional asymmetry can result from over- or undercorrecting the original problem. This would be addressed similarly with another revision. Implant complications are no different than those seen with breast augmentation, although irradiated fields are more likely to experience capsular contracture. Implant infection and extrusion should be treated conservatively.

Secondary procedures

The vast majority of patients are happy after one revision. One major benefit of autologous reconstruction over implant reconstruction is that autologous tissue behaves much more naturally with time. As a result, patients typically become happier with their reconstruction as the years pass.[24] That being said, some patients return for multiple revisions. Planned staged fat grafting is one example which can be predictably necessary and incredibly powerful. When large volumetric changes are required, three to five fat grafting sessions are commonly needed to impact change. When unplanned multiple revisions are sought by a patient, one generally needs to be aware of the curve of diminishing returns. While cancer patients often have a much more reasonable aesthetic goal than the typical cosmetic patient, some patients occasionally have persistent complaints about their results. One should approach these patients with caution, always asking if surgeon and patient both agree on any deformity and if surgery is likely to be successful in correcting the problem. Mastectomy and reconstruction can have a profound effect on self-image and sometimes purposefully drawing out the interval between revisions allows not only for physical evolution of the reconstruction, but psychological adjustment of the patient to the surgery. Lastly, like all surgery, if persistent revision does not yield patient satisfaction, one should never overlook that referral for a second opinion can either offer a fresh approach or, at the very least, peace of mind for the patient that nothing more should be done.

🌐 **Access the complete reference list online at** **http://www.expertconsult.com**

21. Coleman SR, Saboeiro AP. Primary breast augmentation with fat grafting. *Clin Plast Surg.* 2015;42:301–306. *Dr. Coleman is widely considered to be one the pioneers of fat grafting. In this paper, he discusses the use of fat grafting for a wide variety of breast procedures including efficacy, technique and safety.*

24. Hu ES, Pusic AL, Waljee JF, et al. Patient-reported aesthetic satisfaction with breast reconstruction during the long-term survivorship Period. *Plast Reconstr Surg.* 2009;124:1–8. *There is a large body of literature on short-term results of breast reconstruction; however, very little literature is available on the long-term results. This is an excellent paper looking at the difference in satisfaction rates between autologous and alloplastic reconstruction in the long term.*

25. Mirzabeigi MN, Wilson AJ, Fischer JP, et al. Predicting and managing donor-site wound complications in abdominally based free flap breast reconstruction: improved outcomes with early reoperative closure. *Plast Reconstr Surg.* 2015;135:14–23. *This is a large retrospective review of donor site complications using free tissue transfer from the abdomen. It characterizes the donor site complications and quantifies the impact these complications have on the healthcare system. It presents data to support early secondary closure of delayed wound healing and dehiscence.*

28. Rohrich RJ, Sorokin ES, Brown SA. In search of improved fat transfer viability: a quantitative analysis of the role of centrifugation and harvest site. *Plast Reconstr Surg.* 2004;113:391–395, discussion 396–397. *Much controversy exists on the proper technique involved in fat graft harvest, preparation and placement. This article discusses some of the existing data and presents some new data to suggest that many techniques and harvest sites are likely equivalent.*

31. Gabriel A, Champaneria MC, Maxwell GP. Fat grafting and breast reconstruction: tips for ensuring predictability. *Gland Surg.* 2015;4:232–243. *While much of the existing data remains controversial, this article summarizes well many articles which have sought to answer the question as to how to best harvest, process and place fat grafts.*

32. Del Vecchio DA, Del Vecchio SJ. The graft-to-capacity ratio: volumetric planning in large-volume fat transplantation. *Plast Reconstr Surg.* 2014;133:561–569. *This is a well thought out article presenting data on how to think about the volume of fat graft relative to the overlying envelope. The data presented perhaps offers more clarity on the volume of fat necessary to achieve the desired result while minimizing complications.*

34. Lin IC, Bergey M, Sonnad SS, Serletti JM, Wu LC. Management of the ptotic or hypertrophic breast in immediate autologous breast reconstruction: a comparison between the wise and vertical reduction patterns for mastectomy. *Ann Plast Surg.* 2013;70(3):264–270. *Often, the existing skin envelope is mismatched with the volume of the free flap, or there is significant ptosis which requires correction. This article disccuses how to best manage envelope changes at the time of mastectomy.*

36. Liu X, Zhou L, Pan F, et al. Comparison of the postoperative incidence rate of capsular contracture among different breast implants: a cumulative meta-analysis. *PLoS ONE.* 2015;10:e0116071. *This is a metanalysis of the existing data comparing capsular contracture rates using smooth versus textured breast implants. Based upon this article, there is good evidence to support the use of textured implants to lower the risk of developing capsular contracture.*

37. Hassa A, Curtis MS, Colakoglu S, et al. Early results using ultrasound-assisted liposuction as a treatment for fat necrosis in breast reconstruction. *Plast Reconstr Surg.* 2010;126:762–768. *Fat necrosis is an unfortunate complication of autologous reconstruction as it can bother patients tremendously to feel a firm mass after surviving breast cancer. This paper offers evidence to support the use of ultrasound-assisted liposuction to successfully treat these areas and is usually successful in one to two sessions.*

38. Ibrahim AM, Vargas CR, Colakoglu S, et al. Properties of meshes used in hernia repair: a comprehensive review of synthetic and biologic meshes. *J Reconstr Microsurg.* 2015;31:83–94. *This article discusses different types of mesh which can be used for hernia repair. This review article summarizes existing data and discusses the risks and benefits of synthetic versus biologic mesh.*

23.1

Introduction to oncoplastic surgery

Maurice Y. Nahabedian

Introduction

Oncoplastic surgery has become a well-recognized and accepted option for women with breast cancer. Oncoplastic surgery is defined as wide excision of a local tumor using oncologic principles followed by the immediate or staged-immediate correction of the defect using plastic surgical principles, the benefit being that the reconstruction is performed prior to radiation therapy. The feasibility, safety, and efficacy of oncoplastic surgery stems from our improved understanding of the biology of breast cancers, appreciation for quality of life, patient satisfaction, and the wide armamentarium of plastic surgery techniques for correction.

The evolution of oncoplastic surgery can be traced back to the origins of breast-conserving therapy (BCT) for the management of tumors in women that did not want mastectomy. Prior to oncoplastic surgery, BCT frequently resulted in breast distortion and asymmetry that was more notable following radiation therapy, resulting in many patients who were unhappy with the outcomes and desired corrective procedures. Corrective procedures such as reduction mammaplasty, implant insertion, and tissue rearrangement following radiation therapy were frequently associated with higher rates of morbidity that included delayed healing, fat necrosis, and capsular contracture. Often, the ideal treatment was to recreate the lumpectomy defect by excision of the scar and damaged tissue followed by the delayed reconstruction of the defect with a local flap such as the latissimus dorsi.

Oncoplastic surgery differs from standard BCT, in that the margin and volume of excision is typically greater than that of lumpectomy or quadrantectomy. Excision margins typically range from 1 to 2 cm and resection volumes may range from 100 to 300 cm^3. The reconstruction is performed immediately or on a staged-immediate basis using techniques of tissue rearrangement, volume displacement, and volume rearrangement. These will be discussed in greater detail in Chapters 23.2 and 23.3.

Safety and efficacy of oncoplastic surgery

The indications and patient selection criteria are important when considering oncoplastic surgery. This is achieved by adhering to oncologic principles and by applying appropriate plastic surgical techniques for restoration. In order for oncoplastic surgery to be safely and effectively performed, patients should be properly selected and consented for these procedures. They should be informed about local recurrence, long-term survival, donor site considerations, secondary procedures, and effects over time. The application of these principles for the ablative and reconstructive surgeons will facilitate the acceptance and success of oncoplastic surgery.

Safety in oncoplastic surgery requires selection of proper surgical techniques and attention to detail. The importance of obtaining a clear margin is especially important because the consequence of a positive margin following parenchymal reorganization usually includes re-operation, breast distortion, or possible mastectomy. When surgical margins are in question following the initial ablative procedure, a staged-immediate approach can be considered.[1] With this approach, the defect is closed following the ablative procedure without formal reconstruction. The specimen is sent to pathology, and when final pathologic margins are confirmed, definitive reconstruction is performed, usually 1–2 weeks later. The relative risk of a tumor recurrence is 15-fold higher when the surgical margin is not clear.[2] A positive margin is often related to the size of the primary tumor (T3 > T2 > T1) and to histologic subtype (lobular > ductal).[3] Preoperative identification of these women with infiltrating lobular carcinoma who may be at higher risk of a positive surgical margin can sometimes be made via mammography based on the presence of architectural distortion.[4]

Given that larger tumors have an increased likelihood of a positive margin, the benefit of wide excision with a 1–2 cm margin, compared with lumpectomy with a 1–2 mm margin, is recognized. When resection margins are increased, the incidence of a positive margin is reduced when comparing oncoplastic resection to standard quadrantectomy.[5] With oncoplastic tumor excision, glandular resection is increased, histologic margins are wider, the need for re-excision is decreased, and mastectomies are fewer.[6] As a result, immediate reconstruction of the partial mastectomy is usually safe; however, as previously mentioned, when margin status is in question, a delayed approach is usually considered.

Immediate reconstruction of the partial mastectomy deformity

The techniques that are currently used for the reconstruction of the partial mastectomy defect are based on two different concepts: volume displacement and volume replacement. Volume displacement procedures include local tissue rearrangement, reduction mammaplasty, and mastopexy. Volume replacement procedures include local and remote flaps from various regions of the body. The indications for each are different, and various algorithms have been devised to assist with the decision process.[7,8] These options will be described in the following chapters. In most cases, the specific technique is based on breast volume and defect size. In general, women with smaller breasts tend to be considered for volume replacement procedures, e.g., local flap, latissimus dorsi, lateral thoracic flap; whereas, women with larger breasts are better candidates for volume displacement procedures, e.g., adjacent tissue rearrangement, reduction mammaplasty, mastopexy.

Reduction mammaplasty

It is generally accepted that the individual credited with the introduction and popularization of oncoplastic surgery is Melvin J. Silverstein, MD, in 1982, following the excision of a fibroadenoma that was immediately repaired using a reduction mammaplasty approach.[9] Several studies over the years have demonstrated success.[7–11] Various reduction mammaplasty techniques can be used including the short scar or the inverted-T patterns. Pedicle orientation is usually based on the location of the tumor excision. For example, a laterally based defect is usually repaired with a medially based pedicle. Contralateral reduction mammaplasty is usually performed at the same time for symmetry. Outcomes have been favorable, with a 5-year local recurrence rate of 9.4%; a survival rate of 95.7%; and the metastasis-free survival rate of 82.8%.[10] Satisfactory aesthetic outcome was achieved in 82% of women. Complications following oncoplastic reduction mammaplasty include local recurrence, fat necrosis, persistent contour abnormality, delayed healing, loss of nipple sensation/viability, nipple hypopigmentation, complex scar; and breast asymmetry.[12]

Adjacent tissue rearrangement

Adjacent tissue rearrangement is perhaps the most common method by which the partial mastectomy defect is reconstructed because the ablative surgeon is usually able to close the defect using several volume displacement approaches. These techniques are useful in situations where there is ample tissue to achieve closure and minimize distortion. Veronesi et al. introduced the concept of segmental parenchymal wide excision including the overlying skin.[13] These operations were generally performed using a radial approach for tumors that were laterally based. An alternative to the radial approach was the periareolar approach described by Amanti et al.[14] This permitted excisions that resulted in less conspicuous scars. Periareolar incisions could be created circumferentially around the nipple areolar complex and remain relatively inconspicuous. Silverstein introduced the parallelogram pattern and batwing mastopexy.[9] These parallelogram incisions permitted wider excision margins and maintained the natural contour of the breast. The batwing mastopexy is usually used for centrally located tumors near the nipple areolar complex. Clough and colleagues introduced the technique of reduction mastopexy lumpectomy.[10] This technique has been especially useful for tumors located at the lower pole of the breast to minimize inferior displacement of the nipple areolar complex that was typically seen with standard lumpectomy.

Local and remote flaps

Local and remote flaps fall within the domain of volume replacement procedures. These options have been most useful for defects in which volume displacement procedures would not be adequate due to breast volume considerations or extent of resection. There are several options that have been useful. The selection of one technique versus another will depend upon the abilities of the reconstructive surgeon and include pedicle or free musculocutaneous and perforator flaps.

The most commonly used flap for the immediate reconstruction of the partial mastectomy defect has been the latissimus dorsi musculocutaneous flap.[15–17] This flap has been effectively used for deformities of the superior, lateral, and inferior aspects of the breasts. The latissimus dorsi flap can be harvested via a posterolateral thoracic incision or through an endoscope.[17] A variation of the latissimus dorsi flap is miniflap.[15,16] The advantage of the miniflap is that variable amounts of the latissimus dorsi muscle can be harvested based on the volume requirements of the breast. The flap is generally harvested through an extended anterolateral breast incision that is also used for the resection.

Outcomes using the latissimus dorsi flap have been favorable. In a review of 30 patients, Kat et al. demonstrated total flap survival and favorable aesthetic outcomes in all.[18] Losken et al. reviewed their experience using the latissimus dorsi muscle flap harvested endoscopically in 39 women.[15] Donor site morbidities occurred in 12 women (31%) and included a seroma in seven women as well as skin necrosis, lymphedema, dehiscence, hypertrophic scarring, and a persistent sinus tract.

The miniflaps have also demonstrated success. Rainsbury feels that it extends the role of BCT and oncoplastic surgery by enabling reconstruction for defects involving 20–30% of the breast that are located in the central,

upper-inner, and upper-outer quadrant tumors.[17] Gendy et al. used the latissimus dorsi miniflap in 89 women following oncoplastic surgery demonstrating favorable outcomes compared with skin sparing mastectomy and immediate reconstruction.[16] Postoperative complications were fewer (8% vs 14%); surgical interventions were fewer (12% vs 79%); sensory loss of the nipple areolar complex was retained in 98%; restricted activities were fewer (54% vs 73%); and cosmetic outcome was superior (visual analog score: 83.5 vs 72).

The use of perforator flaps for the reconstruction of the partial mastectomy has been receiving increasing attention. There are three flaps that have been used for this purpose: the thoracodorsal artery perforator flap (TDAP); the lateral thoracic flap; and the intercostal perforator flap.[19] The TDAP is an adipocutaneous flap in which the latissimus dorsi muscle is totally spared. The vascularity of the flap is derived from the perforating branches of the thoracodorsal artery and vein. The lateral thoracic flap is a fasciocutaneous flap that is perfused via either the lateral thoracic, axillary, or thoracodorsal artery and vein. The intercostal perforator flap is usually perfused via a perforating intercostal artery and vein that is based along the inferior aspect of the anterior axillary line. These flaps are usually transferred on a vascularized pedicle but may also be transferred as a free tissue transfer.

Clinical experience with these flaps has been encouraging. Levine and Allen have provided an algorithm for perforator flap utilization.[19] The first choice is the TDAP flap followed by the lateral thoracic flap, and finally the intercostal perforator flap. The decision is based on the quality of the vessels during the operative procedure. Munhoz et al. used the lateral thoracic flap in 34 women for partial breast reconstruction.[20] Flap complications included partial necrosis in three (8.8%) that included fat necrosis that developed in two women. Another woman developed an infection. Donor site complications included a seroma in five women (14.7%) and wound dehiscence in three women (8.8%). Patient satisfaction was achieved in 88% of women with a mean follow-up period of 23 months.

⊕ Access the complete reference list online at   http://www.expertconsult.com

1. Patel KM, Hannan C, Gatti M, et al. A head to head comparison of quality of life and aesthetic outcomes following immediate, staged-immediate, and delayed oncoplastic reduction mammaplasty. *Plast Reconstr Surg.* 2011;127:2167–2175. *This paper describes the advantages of waiting 1–2 weeks following the partial mastectomy before definitive reconstruction. This ensures a clear margin and obviates the possibility of mastectomy.*

2. Schnitt SJ, Abner A, Gelman R, et al. The relationship between microscopic margins of resection and the risk of local recurrence in patients treated with breast conserving surgery and radiation therapy. *Cancer.* 1994;74:1746–1751. *One of the first studies to review*

local recurrence associated with extensive intraductal carcinoma managed with local excision and radiotherapy. It was demonstrated that BCT, in all patients with uninvolved margins, was a reasonable option for local control.

4. Moore MM, Borossa G, Imbrie JZ, et al. Association of infiltrating lobular carcinoma with positive surgical margins after breast-conservation therapy. *Ann Surg.* 2000;231:877–882. *This study attempts to assess oncologic safety of lumpectomy based on tumor type. The incidence of positive margins was greater with infiltrating lobular carcinoma compared with the infiltrating ductal carcinoma.*

5. Kaur N, Petit JY, Rietjens M, et al. Comparative study of surgical margins in oncoplastic surgery and quadrantectomy in breast cancer. *Ann Surg Oncol*. 2005;12:539–545. *This study compares 30 patients following quadrantectomy with 30 patients following oncoplastic surgery. It was demonstrated that oncoplastic surgery adds to the oncologic safety of breast-conserving treatment because a larger volume of breast tissue can be excised with a wider negative margin.*

7. Kronowitz SJ, Feledy JA, Hunt KK. Determining the optimal approach to breast reconstruction after partial mastectomy. *Plast Reconstr Surg*. 2006;117:1–11. *The authors compared the results of immediate and delayed oncoplastic procedures using a tissue rearrangement, reduction mammaplasty, and flap techniques. It was demonstrated that immediate repair with tissue rearrangement and reduction had a lower risk of complications and better aesthetic outcomes than immediate repair with a latissimus dorsi flap.*

8. Losken A, Styblo TM, Carlson GW, et al. Management algorithm and outcome evaluation of partial mastectomy defects treated using reduction or mastopexy techniques. *Ann Plast Surg*. 2007;59:235–242. *This manuscript describes a treatment algorithm based on patient selection, diagnosis, tumor margins, and recurrence rates for management of the partial mastectomy defect. Reduction mammaplasty proved to be an excellent option in women with moderate to severe mammary hypertrophy.*

10. Clough KB, Lewis JS, Couturaud B, et al. Oncoplastic techniques allow extensive resections for breast-conserving therapy of breast carcinomas. *Ann Surg*. 2003;237:26–34. *In a prospective study of 101 patients, oncoplastic techniques and contralateral breast surgery allows for an extensive tumor resection resulting in favorable oncologic and aesthetic outcomes. Oncoplastic surgery is useful in extending the indications for breast-conserving therapy.*

13. Veronesi U, Luini A, Galimberti V, et al. Conservation approaches for the management of stage I/II carcinoma of the breast: Milan Cancer Institute trials. *World J Surg*. 1994;18:70–75. *In this study from the Milan Cancer Institute, from 1973 to 1988, the authors demonstrated that reducing the extent of surgery from quadrantectomy to lumpectomy increases the risk of local recurrence by nearly three times, as does withdrawing radiotherapy.*

16. Gendy RK, Able JA, Rainsbury RM. Impact of skin sparing mastectomy with immediate reconstruction and breast sparing reconstruction with miniflaps on the outcomes of oncoplastic breast surgery. *Br J Surg*. 2003;90:433–439. *This study compares 57 skin sparing mastectomy patients with 49 oncoplastic surgery patients demonstrating that oncoplastic surgery with latissimus dorsi miniflaps had more favorable outcomes based on postoperative complications (14% vs 8%); further surgical interventions (12% vs 79%); nipple sensory loss (2% vs 98%); restricted activities (54% vs 73%); and cosmetic outcome by panel assessment.*

19. Levine JL, Soueid NE, Allen RJ. Algorithm for autologous breast reconstruction for partial mastectomy defects. *Plast Reconstr Surg*. 2005;116:762–767. *The authors describe the use of lateral thoracic flaps in the reconstruction of partial mastectomy defects with an emphasis on appropriate patient selection, algorithms, and technique.*

23.2

Partial breast reconstruction using reduction and mastopexy techniques

Albert Losken and Alexandra M. Hart

 Access video content for this chapter online at expertconsult.com

SYNOPSIS

- Breast-conserving therapy increases in popularity, driven by equivalent survival rates, preservation of body image, quality of life, and reduced physiologic morbidity.
- Poor cosmetic results following breast-conserving therapy are not uncommon and are usually due to breast shape, tumor size, tumor location, and postoperative radiation.
- Partial breast reconstruction is indicated whenever the potential for a poor cosmetic result exists, or for patients with tumors in whom a standard lumpectomy would lead to breast deformity or gross asymmetry.

Introduction

Patient presentation/selection

Women with breast cancer who have large or ptotic breasts are at increased risk for poor cosmetic results, and it is often difficult to perform total breast reconstruction on these patients. The emerging popularity of reconstructing the partial mastectomy defect has shown to be beneficial in this patient population.[1] Reduction and mastopexy techniques are ideal, given these patients' breast shape and the relatively large amount of breast tissue left behind after partial resection. This approach has grown in popularity over the last decade and has been proven to be a safe and reliable option for women with breast cancer.[2–5]

Assuming the patient is a candidate for breast-conserving therapy (BCT), the main indication for using oncoplastic reduction techniques is to minimize the potential for a poor cosmetic result. In a subset of women, oncoplastic reduction may also broaden the indication for BCT to include women who were not previously candidates.

The oncoplastic goals are to:
1. Avoid the BCT deformity.
2. Broaden the indications for BCT and avoid mastectomy in certain patients.
3. Maintain shape, symmetry, and improve ptosis.
4. Maximize resection to reduce the local recurrence.

Poor cosmetic results have been reported in up to 20% of women following BCT due to breast shape, tumor size, tumor location, and postoperative radiation (Fig. 23.2.1).[6] Traditionally, women with large breasts have been deemed poor candidates for breast-conserving surgery because of reduced effectiveness, increased complications, and worse cosmetic outcome. The postradiation sequela in women with *macromastia* is significantly worse, leading to poor long-term symmetry. Additionally, radiation-induced fibrosis is thought to be greater in women with larger breasts, given the dosing inhomogeneity.[7,8] Late-radiation fibrosis occurs 36% of the time in patients with larger breasts, compared with 3.6% with smaller breasts. Furthermore, higher doses of radiation therapy are often necessary in women with larger breasts contributing to morbidity and adversely affecting the appearance.

The cosmetic results following BCT in women with large breasts are also reduced.[9] In an early report, Clarke *et al.* have shown excellent results in 100% of women with A cup breasts following BCT, compared with 50% in women with D cup breasts.[10] Women with central or lower quadrant tumors have also been shown to have a worse cosmetic outcome because of *tumor location*, especially when a significant amount of skin is removed.

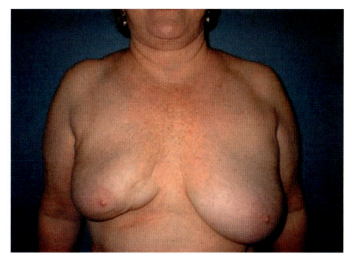

Fig. 23.2.1 A 42-year-old woman who underwent a 20 g resection from the lower inner quadrant. Her resultant breast-conserving therapy deformity demonstrates shape and size distortion 2 years following radiation therapy.

Lower quadrant lumpectomies have been shown to reduce cosmesis by 50% when compared with other quadrants. In the past, central breast tumors close to the areolar have been a contraindication to BCT, but even these are often able to be reconstructed using oncoplastic techniques. The *tumor to breast ratio* is one of the most important factors when predicting the potential for a poor outcome. In general, when more than 20% of the breast is excised with partial mastectomy, the cosmetic result is likely to be unfavorable.[11]

In addition to the aesthetic reasons, there have recently emerged oncologic benefits to choosing the oncoplastic approach. Larger tumors and patients who have received neoadjuvant chemotherapy are now considered reasonable candidates for BCT using the oncoplastic techniques.[3,12,13] Another indication is when the surgeon is concerned about the potential for negative margins with standard resection. In patients who need a *wider excision* based on initial pathology or breast imaging studies, lumpectomies performed in combination with oncoplastic reduction have shown a benefit-to-margin control when compared with standard resection margins (Table 23.2.1).[9,14,15]

Table 23.2.1 Indications for oncoplastic surgery	
Cosmetic reasons	**Oncologic reasons**
High tumor to breast ratio (>20%)	Concern about clear margins
Tumor location: central, inferior, medial	Wide excision required
Macromastia	Poor candidate for mastectomy and reconstruction (i.e., age, breast size)
Large tumor	
Patient desires smaller breasts	
Significant ptosis or breast asymmetry	Patient desires breast-conserving therapy

Surgical technique

The breast reshaping procedures are all reliant upon shrinking the defect into a smaller or lifted breast to improve symmetry and the efficacy of adjuvant radiation therapy. The ideal patient is one where the tumor can be excised within the expected breast reduction specimen. In medium to large or ptotic breasts, sufficient breast parenchyma remains following resection to reshape the mound. Masetti *et al.* describe a 4-step design for oncoplastic operations: (1) planning skin incisions and parenchymal excisions following common reduction/mastopexy templates; (2) parenchymal reshaping after excision; (3) repositioning the nipple; and (4) correction of the contralateral breast for symmetry.[16] The vertical skin pattern is a reasonable option for women with smaller breasts who have a tumor in the lower, medial, or lateral quadrant (Fig. 23.2.2). This is a relatively easy way to start, since the tumor is often resected as part of the medial and lateral pillar creation.

The Wise skin pattern tends to be the most versatile and can be used to reconstruct a partial mastectomy defect anywhere in the breast. The pedicle type necessary for nipple viability depends on the surgeon's preference, the patient's breast size and shape, and the location of the defect. For example, the inferior pedicle can be used in any tumor location except inferior ones (Fig. 23.2.3). Creative pedicle designs can often be used to auto-augment the defect by either using an extended traditional pedicle or by using a secondary de-epithelialized dermoglandular pedicle.

As with all operations, preoperative planning is essential to obtaining a good result. Communication between the two surgical teams is essential. *Well planned preoperative markings* are important. Additionally, reviewing the imaging with the breast surgeon will assist in predicting the location and size of the defect relative to the nipple and skin. Any preoperative asymmetry is also documented to help guide the amount of tissue resected from each breast. Resections are performed within the Wise pattern area to be resected and if possible, without violation of proposed nipple pedicle. After the resection, the cavity is inspected, paying attention to the defect location in relation to the nipple and the remaining breast tissue. Additional cavity samples are then taken for permanent pathology, and the cavity is marked with metallic clips for localization and cancer surveillance. The reconstructive goals include (1) preservation of nipple viability; (2) filling the defect; and (3) reducing and reshaping the breast mound. The nipple and dermoglandular pedicle is created through de-epithelialization and glandular dissection. Once it has been determined how the defect

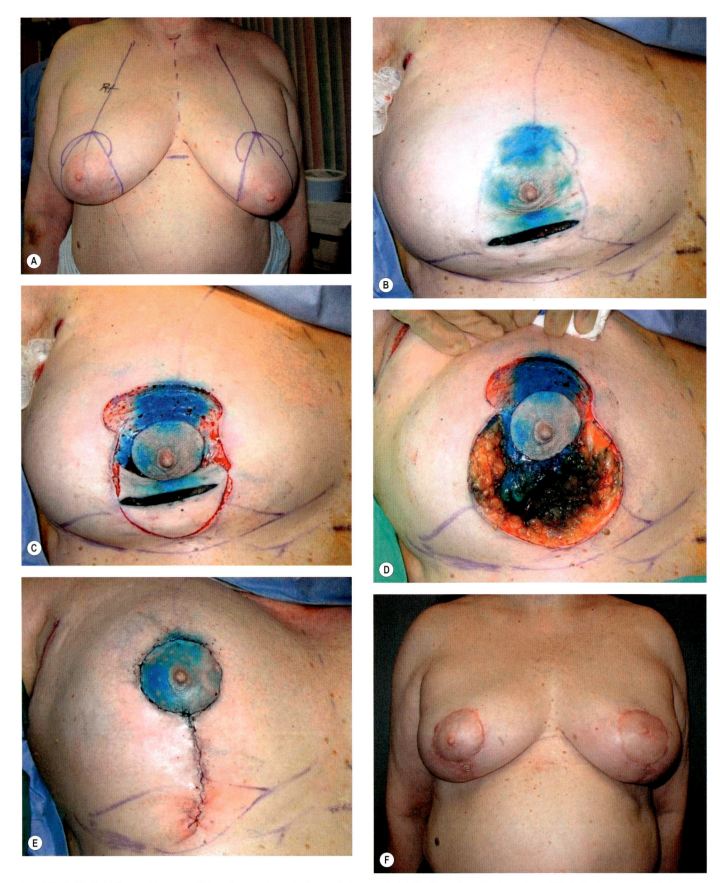

Fig. 23.2.2 (A–F) A 53-year-old woman with breast asymmetry and a lower pole invasive ductal CA. She underwent a lumpectomy (65 g). The tumor was within the reduction specimen, additional tissue was sent (30 g), and a superior pedicle mastopexy was performed. A similar procedure was performed on the contralateral side removing a total of 110 g. Her early result is shown with improvement of symmetry and shape.

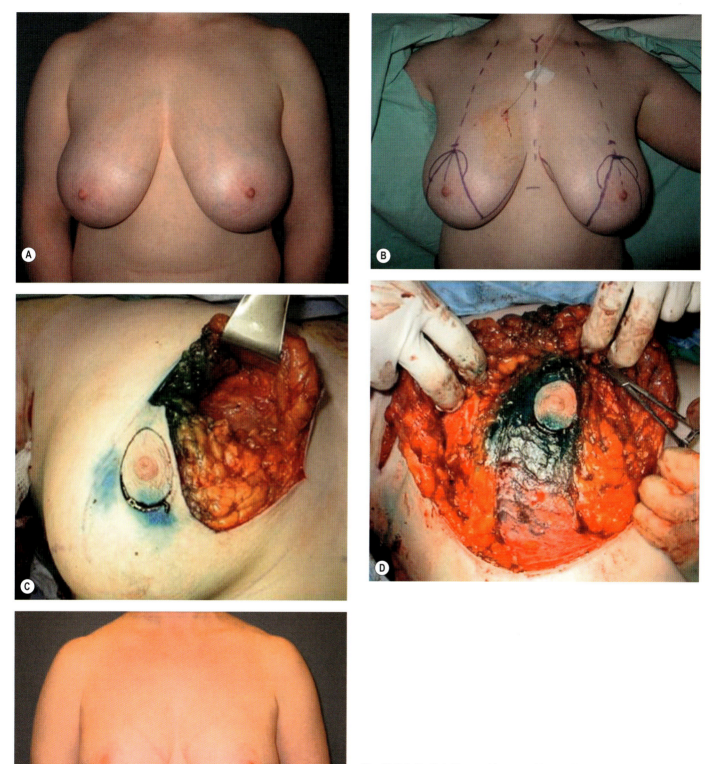

Fig. 23.2.3 (A–E) A 33-year-old woman with stage III breast cancer had a good response to chemotherapy and desired breast conservation. Her tumor location was upper quadrant and, in order to minimize the potential for a poor cosmetic result, she underwent a 100 g lumpectomy with simultaneous bilateral breast reduction. The total volume including specimen on the left was 250 g, and on the right, 150 g. An inferior pedicle was used to reposition the nipple and reconstruct the defect. Her result is shown 1 year following completion of right-sided breast irradiation, with good symmetry.

is going to be filled, the remaining tissue is resected and the breast mound is reshaped. Occasionally, additional dermoglandular or glandular pedicles can be created from tissue that might otherwise have been resected, and rotated to auto-augment the defect.

Lower quadrant tumors in women with larger breasts are ideally suited for the oncoplastic approach. Quadrantectomy-type resections are possible, removing skin and parenchyma from this location, reshaping the breast using a superior or superomedial pedicle. Lower pole tumors in moderate-sized breasts can be excised along with skin as needed in the usual vertical pattern, utilizing a superior pedicle followed by plication of the vertical pillars, and vertical reduction on the contralateral side (see Fig. 23.2.2). *Upper quadrant tumors* can be filled as long as the defect is under the skin (lumpectomy type). Auto-augmentation techniques have become popular to fill the dead space and maintain shape. Inferior or medial pedicles allow for safe excisions in the upper half of the breast without impairing nipple viability, and parenchyma is often rearranged when insufficient tissue remains in the upper pole to maintain the desired fullness. However, when skin is resected in the upper half of the breast, such remodeling techniques are not possible. *Lateral or upper-outer quadrant* defects allow parenchymal remodeling using the superomedial pedicle. These types of reconstructions become difficult when skin is resected with the specimen and are better suited for the lumpectomy type defects. In women with medium-sized ptotic breasts, the superomedial pedicle can be extended down to the inframammary fold as an auto-augmented pedicle. This can then be rotated to fill a lateral volume void. The vertical pillars are then plicated in the usual fashion to maintain shape. If tissue is removed from above the Wise pattern markings, a flap is often required. In women with macromastia, a reduction can still be performed utilizing the inferior pedicle skin to replace missing breast skin even when above the Wise markings.

In the past, *central tumors* have been considered relative contraindications to BCT; however, with the oncoplastic approach in women with macromastia, the tumor and nipple areolar complex can be widely excised and reconstructed using a variety of techniques. The mound can be remodeled in the inverted-T closure pattern, similar to breast amputation reduction techniques. The nipple is then reconstructed later using the reconstruction technique of choice. Another option, if the tumor is located more superiorly or lateral, is to perform a central elliptical excision of skin, nipple, and parenchyma, and mirror image contralateral reduction for symmetry. A third option includes creation of a skin island on a dermatoglandular pedicle to rotate into the central

defect to allow for shape preservation and nipple reconstruction. The breast is marked preoperatively for an inverted-T or a vertical approach, depending on breast size, and the skin island is brought in from inferior or medial (Fig. 23.2.4).

Additional mastopexy options exist for oncoplastic breast conservation.[17] The *donut mastopexy* allows a breast segment to be removed through a periareolar incision and is useful for segmentally distributed cancers in the upper or lateral portion of the breast. The *batwing mastopexy* involves a full-thickness excision of lesions deep within the breast centrally or adjacent to the nipple areolar complex. The two similar half-circle incisions with angled wings on either side of the areolar allow advancement of the fibroglandular tissue to close the defect. A similar mirror image resection is often performed on the opposite side for symmetry. Larger quadrantectomy defects, especially above the nipple, can be incorporated into a batwing mastopexy or elliptical type incision and provide preservation or improvement of shape and elevation of the ptotic breast along with the tumor resection. Since this removes sufficient breast tissue and skin to alter the size of the breast and nipple position, a similar contralateral lift is occasionally required to achieve symmetry.

A contralateral reduction is typically performed for symmetry using a similar technique on all patients at the time of the oncoplastic procedure. Additionally, if the patient is a candidate for BCT and has multiple areas that need to be resected, as long as sufficient tissue remains, remodeling techniques can be used in a similar fashion. The contralateral side is typically kept about 10% smaller in anticipation for radiation fibrosis on the opposite side. A small revision to the opposite breast after completion of radiation therapy is occasionally required (<10%) if asymmetry exists.

Benefits

While initially the driving force behind the use of oncoplastic reduction techniques was improved cosmesis, numerous additional benefits have been documented. The oncoplastic approach has been shown to broaden the indications for BCT in patients with tumors larger than 4 cm, locally advanced cancers, and prior neoadjuvant chemotherapy.[12] Additionally, patients with advanced stage breast cancer can undergo BCT using this technique.

The amount of tissue resected in patients undergoing an oncoplastic reduction is significantly greater. Clough *et al.* have shown that extensive resections are possible with this technique, in over 101 patients with the average specimen weight of 222 g.[3] A recent meta-analysis has

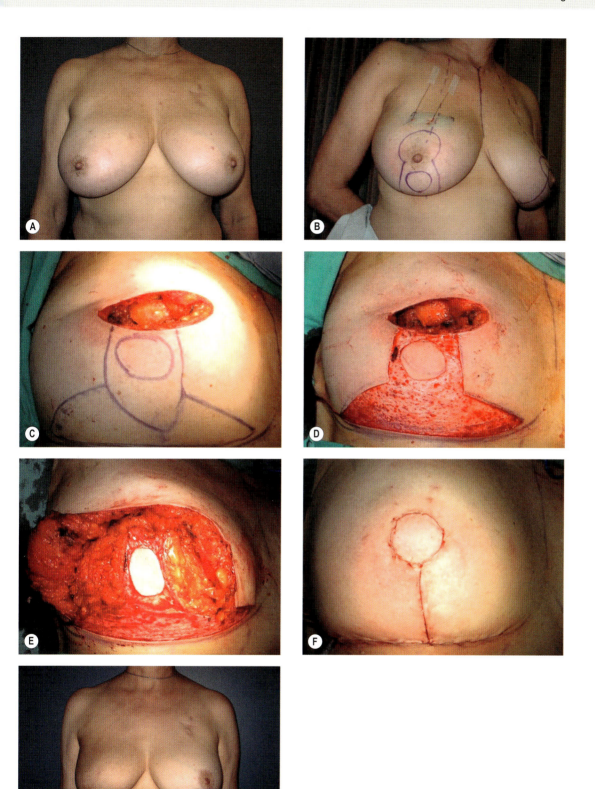

Fig. 23.2.4 (A–G) This patient did not want to undergo skin-sparing mastectomy and reconstruction and, despite having a sub-areolar tumor, elected to have breast preservation. Given the proximity, she had resection of the nipple areolar complex with her partial mastectomy. An inferior pedicle was created leaving a skin island appropriately located for nipple areolar replacement. The result is shown 9 months following completion of radiation therapy just prior to nipple areolar reconstruction.

shown that average resection in these patients is well over 200 g compared with a typical resection of about 50 g when traditional BCT is performed alone.[9] The ability to perform a generous resection often translates into superior margin clearance. Although there is a lack of randomized control data comparing the two groups, the incidence of positive margins in retrospective comparisons is significantly less in the oncoplastic reduction group compared with BCT alone. Kaur et al. performed a prospective trial comparing quadrantectomy alone (n=30) and resection with oncoplastic reconstruction (n=30). They demonstrated that larger resection weights (200 vs 118 g; p=0.16) resulted in fewer close or positive margins (16.7% vs 43.3%; p=0.5) in the oncoplastic group.[15] Furthermore, ductal carcinoma in situ (DCIS) histology was more prevalent in the quadrantectomy alone group and accounted for some of the differences. Giacalone et al. performed a similar prospective comparative study comparing quadrantectomy alone (n=43) and resection with oncoplastic reconstruction (n=31). The authors found margins ≥5 mm in 67% of oncoplastic group versus 42% in the quadrantectomy alone group (p=0.3).[4] Losken et al. demonstrated a lower positive margin rate (24.1% vs 41.0%; p=0.01); fewer surgical re-excisions (12.0% vs 25.9%; p=0.01); and wider margins from the tumor edge (4.3 vs 2.8 mm; p=0.01) when oncoplastic surgery was performed.[14] A recent meta-analysis also found a reduction in the positive margin rate for both invasive and in situ disease from 21% with BCT alone to 12% in oncoplastic excisions.[9] The long-term influence of this on cancer recurrence remains to be seen.

An additional benefit of the oncoplastic approach is the ease of performing a reduction in women with macromastia compared with skin sparing mastectomy (SSM) and immediate reconstruction.[14] Lower breast complication rates (22% vs 50%); no donor site complications; shorter hospital stay (0.87 vs 3.5 days); and fewer additional procedures (2.5 vs 5.8) have been shown following oncoplastic reductions when compared with traditional total reconstruction procedures. Furthermore, results of patient reported outcomes have documented an improved quality of life and self-esteem when the oncoplastic approach is added to BCT.[18] Given the many functional and psychological benefits of a breast reduction, it is not surprising that women who had an oncoplastic reduction also report an increase in their satisfaction with body image, an unexpected increase in their ability to wear sexually provocative clothing, and an unforeseen increase in their partners perception of them as womanly.[19]

The use of this approach also allows additional sampling of ipsilateral and contralateral breast tissue with the ability to occasionally diagnose other breast pathology and potentially reduce cancer risk by removing additional breast tissue.[20]

Timing

The oncoplastic reduction is preferably performed at the time of tumor removal and prior to radiation therapy. It is easier to preserve breast shape during the initial resection than to reconstruct a deformity in an irradiated breast. In the authors' own patients, it has been shown that utilization of oncoplastic reduction techniques prior to radiation therapy results in significantly fewer complications when compared with performing reductions after completion of radiation therapy (21% vs 57%; p<0.001).[21] Similar results (24% vs 50%) have been shown by Kronowitz et al.[22] The main concern with immediate reconstruction is the potential for positive margins requiring re-excision. When there is any concern about margin status, delayed immediate reconstruction is an option (Fig. 23.2.5). This postpones the reconstructive procedure until confirmation of negative margins, giving the benefit of immediate reconstruction with the luxury of negative margins. The disadvantage of this is that it requires two operations. Our institutional preference is to minimize positive margins through patient selection and cavity sampling. Based on our experience of a critical analysis of failed oncoplastic reduction techniques, patients at higher risk for positive margins tend to be women less than 40 years of age with extensive DCIS.[23] Other characteristics that may potentially make it more difficult to obtain negative margins include infiltrating lobular carcinoma, prior chemotherapy, or multicentric disease.

Confirmation of margin status prior to reconstruction may be beneficial for some patients. Preoperative breast imaging (i.e., MRI, ultrasound, or mammography) is often helpful in determining the extent of the disease to guide the necessary resection. Intraoperative cavity sampling is another way to minimize positive margins and the need for re-excision. Sending separate cavity margins at the time of lumpectomy has been shown to significantly reduce the need for re-excision. Using this technique, Cao et al. demonstrated that final margin status was negative in 60% of patients with positive margins on initial resection.[24] Potential factors contributing to the false-positive margin status include seepage of ink into crevices of the specimen promoted by excessive inking, tumor friability promoting displacement of tumor into ink, and manipulation of specimens for radiographs and retraction artifact. Additional intraoperative confirmatory procedures include radiography of the specimen or intraoperative frozen sections for invasive cancer.

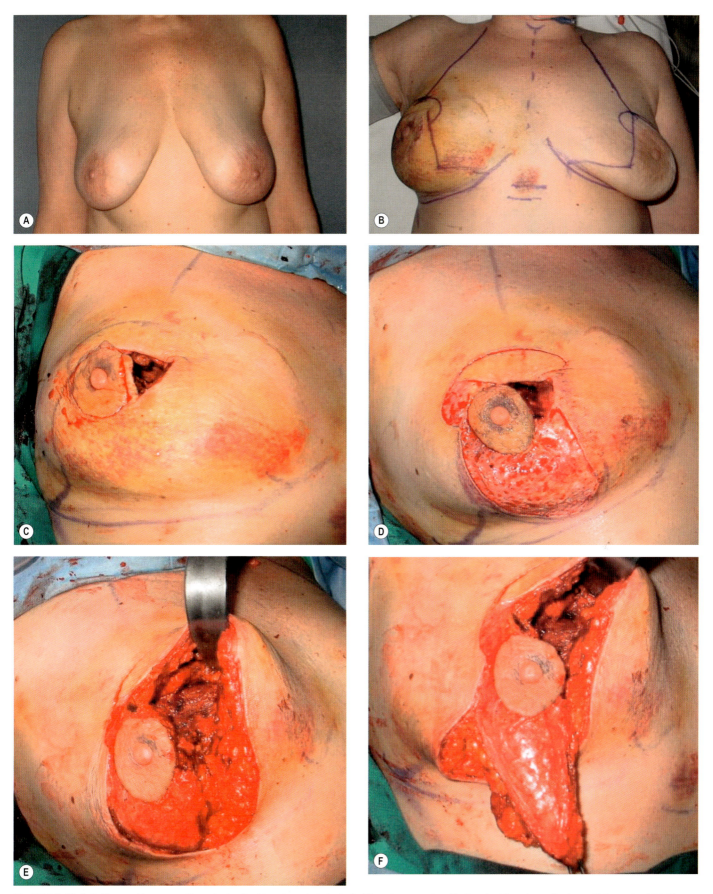

Fig. 23.2.5 (A–I) A 40-year-old woman with moderate-sized breasts and ptosis desired breast preservation. She has ductal carcinoma *in situ* medially on the right. Given oncologic concerns, a decision was made to delay reconstruction until confirmation of clear margins. Her medial defect is demonstrated following 50 g resection. A decision was made to perform a superolateral pedicle extending the pedicle down to the chest wall. This was then rotated into the medial defect, and the medial and lateral pillars were plicated. A contralateral symmetry procedure was performed removing 65 g. The result is shown following radiation therapy with breast edema and size discrepancy. She is then shown 1 year later with good size and symmetry.

Continued

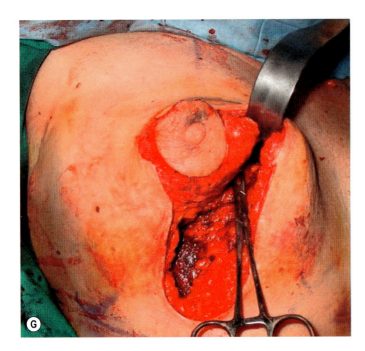

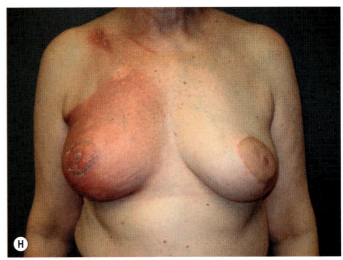

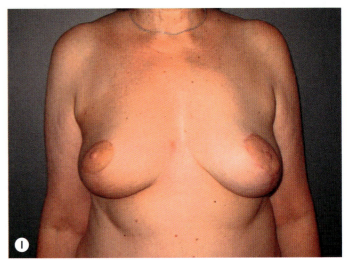

Fig. 23.2.5, cont'd

Management of positive margins

If final pathology reveals positive margins on the tumor specimen and additional parenchyma was not removed from around the tumor site as in remodeling mammaplasty-like techniques, then there are commonly two options: completion mastectomy or re-excision. When margins are positive following oncoplastic techniques that produce wide excisions, the extent of disease will typically dictate that a mastectomy be performed rather than a re-excision. There is little downside to completion mastectomy and reconstruction, as the contralateral symmetry procedure has already been performed (Fig. 23.2.6). Therefore the typical skin removal pattern has also been completed, which will allow for easier reconstruction of a smaller breast. Depending on the patient, re-excision is possible when performed in conjunction with both the breast and reconstructive surgeon, as the cavity architecture might have been altered during the initial surgery. Intraoperative cavity clipping during the original resection

will assist with re-excision, as well as guide postoperative surveillance or the need for radiation boost.

Outcomes

Importantly, complications resulting from oncoplastic techniques should not interfere with the initiation of adjuvant therapy. A meta-analysis demonstrated an average complication rate of 16% in the oncoplastic reduction group. However, there was not a delay in the initiation of adjuvant therapy.[9] Additional procedures will invariably increase complications; however, most of these are minor. Some larger series report complications such as delayed wound healing (3–15%), fat necrosis (3–10%), and infection (1–5%).[18,21,22] In the largest oncoplastic series of 540 patients, the complication rate was also 16%.[5] The authors found the severity of the complications requiring surgical intervention in the oncoplastic groups was approximately 3%. In series of BCT alone, complications are rarely recorded; however, in one

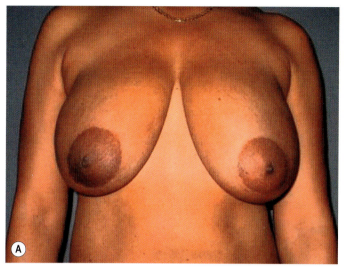

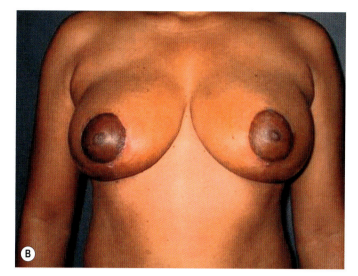

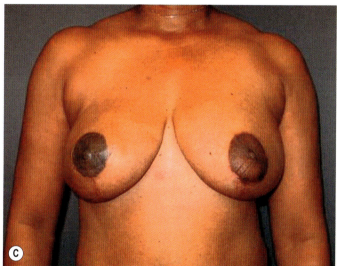

Fig. 23.2.6 (A–C) A 43-year-old woman with right-sided breast cancer who underwent partial reconstruction using the oncoplastic reduction approach. Her lumpectomy margins were clear; however, ductal carcinoma *in situ* was identified in the additional tissue removed during the right reduction. A decision was made to perform a right skin-sparing mastectomy, and she underwent a latissimus dorsi reconstruction with implant.

series of 714 patients with BCT alone, the reported complication rate was 24%.[25] Although potentially higher, studies thus far have failed to show that complications following oncoplastic reduction result in a negative impact on the oncologic management of patients. Appropriate technique and patient selection is required to minimize morbidity when this approach is selected. Late complications requiring additional surgery are usually related to aesthetic outcome, radiation changes, or recurrence.

Improvement in cosmesis is one of the main driving forces behind the increasing use of the oncoplastic approach, and many of the indications for oncoplastic surgery revolve around predicting high-risk patients and minimizing the potential for a poor cosmetic result. Nevertheless, this approach cannot prevent or reverse the effects of radiation therapy. Given that the majority of patient's will receive radiotherapy and the effects will persist, the assessment of shape and symmetry needs to be made in the context of long-term changes following

adjuvant therapy. Iwuchukwu *et al.* reviewed oncoplastic reduction techniques in the literature siting a 5–14% poor cosmetic outcome following these procedures.[26] When aesthetic and patient satisfaction was evaluated in a recent meta-analysis, the overall satisfaction with BCT alone was 80%, compared with 90% when an oncoplastic reduction was performed. Patient dissatisfaction was correlated with postoperative complications and breast asymmetry.[25] Having a 90% satisfaction in the oncoplastic groups is understandable. These are self-selected, high-risk patients for poor cosmetic results, and despite correcting the volume loss secondary to tumor resection with immediate reconstruction, the adverse effects of radiation therapy will still persist but potentially be less obvious.

Local recurrence is an important outcome that needs to be evaluated. Most reviews in the literature are of intermediate follow-up times (longest = 4.5 years), with local recurrence rates varying from 0% to 1.8% per year.[27] Actuarial 5-year local recurrence rates range from 8.5%

to 9.4%. To further evaluate the oncologic outcome, longer-term studies are required. To date, the largest series of 540 consecutive patients from the Institute Curie demonstrated that in women with high tumor-to-breast volume ratios, use of the oncoplastic approach provides good outcomes.[5] The 5-year local recurrence (6.8%) and overall survival rates (92.9%) were acceptable with low complication rates (16%) and good aesthetic results at 1 year (97.7%) and at 5 years (90.3%). In a study of our own patients following oncoplastic reduction, the 5-year ipsilateral breast tumor control rates were 91% for DCIS and 93% for invasive cancer.[28]

Secondary procedures, although not common, are usually performed for size or shape discrepancies long term. While the oncoplastic approach minimizes the potential for poor aesthetic outcomes, the effects of radiation therapy persist and can contribute to changes over time. In most circumstances, waiting at least 1 year following completion of radiation therapy to discuss revisional procedures is advised. Even with resolution of acute radiation changes (i.e., erythema, skin breakdown, burns) and tissue edema, it is important to respect native tissue planes and blood supply, and if possible keep revisions to a minimum, since it is still an irradiated breast, which carries the associated risks.

Surveillance postoperative care

Original concerns with this approach were that increased tissue rearrangement, scarring, and disruption of breast architecture might impair the ability to screen and detect recurrent breast cancer. Although valid, adherence to appropriate surveillance and cross-specialty communication will reduce this issue. The three main tools in postoperative surveillance include the physical examination, radiologic imaging, and tissue sampling. It is important that all members of the team are aware of the various surgical components, since differences in presentation of recurrence might exist depending on the type and technique of reconstruction. In a study at the authors' institution it was demonstrated that following partial breast reconstruction using reduction techniques mammography was just as sensitive as a screening tool when compared with patients with BCT alone.[29] While the qualitative mammographic findings were similar in the two groups over the average 6-year follow-up, there was a slight trend towards longer times to mammographic stability in the oncoplastic reduction group of 25.6 versus 21.2 months in the BCT alone group. This

means it might take the oncoplastic reduction patients slightly longer to reach the point where any change in mammographic findings might be suspicious for malignancy. The clinical significance of this finding remains to be seen. An accurate interpretation of mammography requires familiarity with these temporal changes and mammograms should be compared over time. These data need to be taken into consideration when designing the most appropriate surveillance programs for these patients.

As technology improves, other imaging techniques such as ultrasound and MRI will likely become more popular. Microcalcifications and areas of fat necrosis are easily identified, and no interference in postoperative surveillance has been demonstrated. Although routine tissue sampling is not recommended for screening, any clinical concern necessitates fine-needle aspiration, core-needle biopsy, or surgical biopsy, to rule out malignancy. Patients who undergo partial breast reconstruction may have an increase in the amount of tissue sampling requirements. In the authors' series, 53% in the oncoplastic group compared with 18% in the BCT alone group over an average of 7 years required tissue sampling. In contrast, in a report by Piper *et al.*, an age-matched comparison of women following BCT versus oncoplastic reduction did not show a significant difference in abnormal mammographic findings prompting biopsy or biopsy rates themselves for up to 5 years postoperatively.[30] Although these are typically benign, additional scarring from the reconstruction might raise clinical suspicion, which is why more biopsies are expected in patients who undergo partial breast reconstruction.

Conclusion

The details differ when dealing with lumpectomy versus quadrantectomy defects, or whether a two-team or single surgeon approach is used; however, the principles are the same. The benefits of using the oncoplastic reduction techniques have been well demonstrated and will continue to gain popularity and acceptance in the future. The options for women with breast cancer are numerous, and this provides an additional, and often favorable, choice. Critical evaluations of results measuring functional, oncologic, and aesthetic outcomes are necessary to establish safe and effective practice guidelines to maximize oncologic safety.

1. Losken A, Hamdi M. Partial breast reconstruction: current perspectives. *Plast Reconstr Surg*. 2009;124:722–736.

3. Clough KB, Lewis JS, Couturaud B, et al. Oncoplastic techniques allow extensive resections for breast-conserving therapy of breast carcinomas. *Ann Surg*. 2003;237:26–34.

5. Fitoussi AD, Berry MG, Famà F, et al. Oncoplastic breast surgery for cancer: analysis of 540 consecutive cases [outcomes article]. *Plast Reconstr Surg*. 2010;125:454–462.

6. Matory WE Jr, Wertheimer M, Fitzgerald TJ, et al. Aesthetic results following partial mastectomy and radiation therapy. *Plast Reconstr Surg*. 1990;85:739–746.

9. Losken A, Dugal CS, Styblo TM, et al. A meta-analysis comparing breast conservation therapy alone to the oncoplastic technique. *Ann Plast Surg*. 2014;72:145–149.

12. Regaño S, Hernanz F, Ortega E, et al. Oncoplastic techniques extend breast-conserving surgery to patients with neoadjuvant chemotherapy response unfit for conventional techniques. *World J Surg*. 2009;33:2082–2086.

13. Clough KB, Acosta-Marín V, Nos C, et al. Rates of neoadjuvant chemotherapy and oncoplastic surgery for breast cancer surgery: a French national survey. *Ann Surg Oncol*. 2015;22:3504–3511.

14. Losken A, Pinell-White X, Hart AM, et al. The oncoplastic reduction approach to breast conservation therapy: benefits for margin control. *Aesthet Surg J*. 2014;34:1185–1191.

18. Veiga DF, Veiga-Filho J, Ribeiro LM, et al. Quality-of-life and self-esteem outcomes after oncoplastic breast-conserving surgery. *Plast Reconstr Surg*. 2010;125:811–817.

20. Munhoz AM, Gemperli R, Filassi JR. Occult carcinoma in 866 reduction mammaplasties: preserving the choice of lumpectomy. *Plast Reconstr Surg*. 2011;128:816–818.

22. Kronowitz SJ, Kuerer HM, Buchholz TA, et al. A management algorithm and practical oncoplastic surgical techniques for repairing partial mastectomy defects. *Plast Reconstr Surg*. 2008;122:1631–1647.

29. Losken A, Schaefer TG, Newell M, et al. The impact of partial breast reconstruction using reduction techniques on postoperative cancer surveillance. *Plast Reconstr Surg*. 2009;124:9–17.

23.3

Pedicled and free flaps in oncoplastic surgery

Moustapha Hamdi and Jana Van Thielen

SYNOPSIS

- Breast-conserving therapy (BCT) is applied to most early stages of breast cancer.
- Oncoplastic surgery within a multidisciplinary approach is the gold standard in BCT.
- Using pedicled flaps is indicated in high tumor/breast size ratio.
- Partial breast reconstruction with a pedicled flap is alternative to mastectomy in selected patients.
- Overcorrection is essential when a pedicled flap is used in partial breast reconstruction.
- Perforator or muscle-sparing latissimus dorsi flaps is the first choice of flap surgical technique.
- Fat grafting and contralateral breast remodeling may be required to achieve breast symmetry at long-term follow-up.

 Access the Historical Perspective section online at
http://www.expertconsult.com

Introduction

- Breast-conserving therapy (BCT) with tumor resection and radiotherapy is a valuable component of breast cancer treatment, with an equivalent survival outcome to that of mastectomy.
- Quadrantectomy or partial mastectomy offers wider, safe margins and reduces the rate of local recurrence.
- Partial breast reconstruction is required in most of the cases of quadrantectomy to avoid post BCT-breast deformity.
- Every case requiring partial breast reconstruction should be addressed within a multidisciplinary approach.

- Local flaps are required in partial reconstruction of small-to-moderate size breasts.
- Pedicled perforator flaps provide adequate partial breast reconstruction with minimal donor site morbidity.

Basic science

Partial mastectomy combined with radiotherapy, often referred to as breast-conserving therapy (BCT) followed by breast irradiation, has replaced modified radical mastectomy as the preferred treatment for early stage invasive breast cancer in many patients. The 5-year survival rate of partial mastectomy with radiation is not statistically different when compared with mastectomy alone in patients with stage I or II breast cancer.[5,6] Women diagnosed at early stages of invasive breast cancer have equivalent outcomes when they are treated with lumpectomy and radiation therapy or modified radical mastectomy.[7]

It is interesting to point out that the surgical clearance of pathologic margins has the most significant impact upon local recurrence in patients treated with BCT and RT. The presence of ductal carcinoma *in situ* (DCIS) at the surgical margin is associated with the identification of residual DSIC in 40–82% of re-excised specimens and is correlated with margin widths of 41% at 1 mm, 31% at 1–2 mm, and 0% with 2 mm of clearance.[5] A recent meta-analysis concluded that a margin width was significantly superior to lesser margins.[8]

A further recent meta-analysis by Losken *et al.* showed lower positive margins after oncoplastic surgery (12%)

compared with breast conservative surgery without oncoplastic reconstruction (21%).[9]

The incidence of local recurrence depends upon certain factors, such as the tumor margin, nuclear grade-histology, radiation therapy, and patient age. Most local recurrences occurred at the site of initial tumor excision (57–88%) or in the same breast quadrant (22–28%). In general, during the first 10 years after lumpectomy with radiation, the recurrence rate is 1.4% per year. The treatment of in-breast tumor recurrence in patients is completion mastectomy.[10] Therefore, more radical excision, including the tumor with large surrounding tissue (quadrectomy or partial mastectomy), is recommended; however, it may result in an unacceptable aesthetic outcome.

Partial breast reconstruction has become a preferable option for an increasing number of patients. These techniques allow for local excision with oncologic benefits while avoiding more extensive surgery with higher complications and increased morbidity rates associated with total mastectomy and immediate reconstruction.

This chapter discusses the use of the loco-regional flaps in partial breast reconstruction.

Diagnosis/patient presentation

The decision to undertake a partial mastectomy, or alternatively a total mastectomy, to treat a patient with breast cancer is ultimately an oncologic determination. In cases where the two treatments options are oncologic equivalent, the patient becomes an active participant in the decision-making process in order to maximize their sense of satisfaction with their treatment.

Breast-conserving approaches may be preferable over a total mastectomy in some cases. This is especially true for patients with early stage disease, because the majority of the breast can be preserved and the operation is perceived as less invasive than a mastectomy. Most early-stage cancers (T1 and T2 cancers with or without nodal involvement) are indicated for BCT; however, there are some exceptions. Commonly known reasons for contraindications are patients with a high probability for recurrence, especially those with multicentric disease; those who are pregnant or have collagen vascular disease; or those who have a history of prior radiation therapy.[11] Relative contraindications include patients with a high probability of subsequent cancers (BRCA mutations) and patients who are likely to have a poor cosmetic result, which includes patients with a high tumor/breast ratio, medially-, and inferiorly-based tumors and tumors that require removal of the nipple areolar complex (NAC).

Approximately 10–30% of patients are dissatisfied with the aesthetic result after partial mastectomy with radiation.[12] Although the causes may vary, the factors that motivate patients to seek corrective surgery after partial mastectomy are a volume discrepancy, contour deformity, and nipple malposition.[13] The resection of more than 15–20% of the breast parenchyma in a small-volume (A or B cup) and more than 30% in the larger breast will cause volumetric deformities and bilateral asymmetries. In addition, radiation therapy extenuates the image of the breast, initially causing breast edema and skin erythema and eventually causing parenchyma fibrosis, retraction, skin envelope atrophy, hyperpigmentation, hypopigmentation, and telangiectasia. The long-term final effects of radiation are difficult to predict but seem to stabilize 1–3 years post-radiation.[14,15]

The intention of this chapter is not to extend on the indications of BCT, but to identify the complexity of partial breast reconstruction, to optimize reconstruction planning, and to indicate the importance of the use of local flaps in breast oncoplastic surgery.

Patient selection

The success of this procedure depends on the size of the cancer, the anatomic position, and the volume of resection needed to achieve clear margins in relation to the volume of the breast. Especially in cases of partial breast reconstruction after the excision of wide localized tumors, the value of oncoplastic surgery increases.

The choice of the technique used depends on many factors, including the extent of resection, the time of surgery, the breast size and tumor location, and patient preferences.

Type of reconstruction

There are two basic types of surgery techniques in partial breast reconstruction: volume displacement and volume replacement.

1. *Volume displacement* techniques refer to advancement, rotation, or transposition of large local breast flaps into the smaller created defect, redistributing the volume loss. The dissection involves the advancement of a full-thickness segment of breast fibroglandular tissue to fill the dead space. Volume displacement procedures and surgical scars are optimal when combined with mastopexy-reduction techniques. The tumor is excised within the planned markings of the reduction specimen in medium, large, or ptotic breasts, and the remaining parenchyma is sufficient enough to reshape the breast mound.[16]

2. *Volume replacement* techniques are technically more difficult and are used in small–moderate size breasts or when the tumor/breast ratio is large and the remaining breast tissue is insufficient for the rearrangement and the replacement of the defect. Volume replacement with the use of non-breast local or distant flaps provides both tissue for the filling of the glandular defect and the skin deficiency of the reconstructed breast.[17]

Surgery for volume displacement avoids donor site morbidity but is associated with ischemia of the dermo-glandular pedicle and may require contralateral breast surgery in order to achieve symmetry. The amount of tissue that is obtained for defect coverage and breast reconstruction is limited.

Volume replacement techniques maintain the original size and shape of the breast without the need for any contralateral breast surgery, but are associated with longer operation times, require competent surgical skills, and possible complications in the flap and the donor site.

Timing of reconstruction

Reconstruction of partial mastectomies can either include delayed, immediate, or immediate delayed procedures. In delayed reconstruction, at least 6 months to a year is allowed to elapse after the last radiation therapy session, in order to evaluate the deformities of the breast and plan the appropriate reconstruction modality. In immediate reconstruction, the goal is to perform, co-instantaneously, tumor resection with oncologically appropriate margins and partial breast reconstruction. Immediate delayed partial breast reconstruction is actually a two-stage immediate surgical approach with delayed reconstruction (within a few days) until the results of the pathology report are known and the margins of the tumor excision are determined as sufficient or must be re-excised to clear margins before reconstruction. The final aesthetic outcomes are similar to those with immediate reconstruction.[18]

Immediate breast reconstruction offers many advantages over delayed breast reconstruction, such as a better aesthetic outcome due to the preservation of the 3D breast skin envelope. The aim of immediate reconstruction after BCT is essentially to give better aesthetic results with the same oncologic safety. Our target should be the reshaping of the treated breast with the alteration of the opposite breast for better symmetry, as part of the treatment, when indicated. Immediate reconstruction before radiation therapy is also preferred because the breast can be better manipulated before radiation, with potentially decreased complication rates and improved

aesthetic outcomes. In planning the approach on which method should be used to treat the partial mastectomy defect, the primary decision that must be made is if reparative surgery will be needed after the tumor excision. If oncoplastic surgery is necessary, the next step is to choose the technique. If there is sufficient tissue, reshaping the breast, along with reduction of the opposite breast for symmetry, is usually the best option. If there is not enough tissue left for breast reshaping, tissue must be added. If the defect is not too large, local tissue can be used, with simple techniques, such as rotation or transposition fasciocutaneous flaps from the axillary area or superiorly-based composite flap of skin, subcutaneous fat, and upper pole breast parenchyma. If the defect is too large to be filled by local tissue alone, a loco-regional pedicled or distal pedicled or free flap will be required (Fig. 23.3.1).

Breast and plastic surgeons must have a thorough understanding of breast anatomy, physiology, and the qualities of an aesthetically pleasing breast shape. Surgeons using the oncoplastic approach should consider the aesthetic subunits when planning cosmetic quadrantectomy, resections, and reconstructions.[19] Also, knowledge of the anatomic landmarks, breast proportions, and shape is essential in order to achieve a pleasing outcome.

Preoperative evaluation of the patient and her breasts must be standard and detailed. The examination must include evaluation of breast skin, elasticity, thickness, scars, and any defining marks such as tattoos, stretch marks, contour irregularities, and previous breast surgery should be taken into account when planning BCT. Palpation for masses or abnormalities in the breast parenchyma, nipple inspection, and detailed documentation of breast sensation are integral. Breast shape,

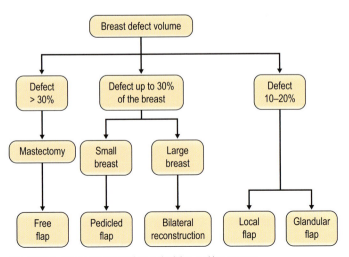

Fig. 23.3.1 Breast reconstruction: a decision-making process.

grade of ptosis, and size are determinants of success in surgical treatment.

The base and width of the breast, the width of the NAC, the height of the nipple, and the distance from the sternal notch, midline, and inframammary crease must be recorded in detail.[19] Any natural breast asymmetry should be pointed out to the patient before surgery. Different body types, skin laxity, and fat distribution are important factors in the decision-making process.

Treatment/surgical techniques

Large defects in large breasts may be treated by converting a partial mastectomy into a reduction mammaplasty. Planning of skin incisions and parenchymal excisions follow templates using reduction mammaplasty and mastopexy techniques. The pattern can be rotated laterally or medially to fit the location of the defect. The choice of pedicle is related to the tumor location and the blood supply of the breast. It is important that skin incisions be planned so that if mastectomy is ultimately required for margin control, the incision site can be comfortably included within the mastectomy skin island.[6,16] Relative contraindications for oncologic reduction mammoplasty are large tumor/breast size ratio. Oncologic reduction mammoplasty should also be used cautiously in patients with DCIS since resection margins are more often positive compared with invasive carcinoma and often leads to re-excision or salvage mastectomy.[20]

When volume replacement is necessary for BCT reconstruction, the decision of which technique will be used is determined mostly by the surgeon's experience and the size of the defect in relation to the size of the remaining breast. The use of non-breast locoregional flaps offer the extra volume needed in large tumor excisions/quadrantectomies for the replacement of the breast volume; however, they can be more demanding procedures and associated with donor site and flap morbidity.

A small lateral defect can be easily covered with a skin rotation flap or a lateral thoracic axial flap. Especially in obese patients (with breast rolls), the lateral thoracic flap is useful. However, most of these fasciocutaneous flaps may be unavailable in the axillary lymph node dissection patients.

The latissimus dorsi muscle or musculocutaneous flaps have been very popular as a method of choice in partial breast reconstruction.[21] However, pedicled perforator flaps have enabled surgeons to replace large defects with minimum donor site morbidity. The advantage of perforator flaps, which are skin and subcutaneous flaps, is that they offer sufficient coverage without sacrificing the muscle and motor innervations and minimize seroma formation rate.

Classification and vascular anatomy of flaps

The latissimus dorsi (LD) flap has a constant anatomy.[22] The blood supply of the latissimus dorsi comes from a terminal branch of the subscapular artery (Fig. 23.3.2). The subscapular artery runs about 5 cm before dividing into the scapular circumflex and thoracodorsal arteries. The thoracodorsal artery is about 2–4 mm in diameter, and it courses along the posterior portion of the axilla for about 8–14 cm before it pierces the latissimus dorsi on its costal surface. The thoracodorsal artery gives off one or two branches to the serratus anterior muscle and one branch to the skin. The basic pattern of the thoracodorsal bundle (artery, nerve, and 1–2 venae comitantes) branching is to bifurcate into a lateral (vertical) and a medial (horizontal) branch. The lateral branch follows a course parallel to the muscle fibers, 1–4 cm medial to the free-lateral border of the muscle, and gives off perforating vessels that supply the skin. The smaller medial branch diverges at an angle of 45° and travels medially. A vigorous blood supply to the muscle is also available at its origin. Perforating vessels from the intercostal and lumbar arteries supply the muscle and overlying skin.[22,23]

The pedicled perforator flaps mostly used in our hands for partial breast reconstruction, classified according to the basic nutrient arteries, and recommended by the "Gent" Consensus update in 2002 are (Fig. 23.3.3)[24]:

- Thoracodorsal artery perforator (TDAP) flap
- Serratus anterior artery perforator (SAAP) flap
- Intercostal artery perforator (ICAP) flap
- Superior epigastric artery perforator (SEAP) flap.

The TDAP flap

The TDAP flap is based on perforators originating from the descending (vertical) or horizontal branches of the thoracodorsal vessels. Anatomic studies on cadavers have reported the presence of 2–3 musculocutaneous perforators from the vertical branch.[25,26] The proximal perforator enters the subcutaneous plane obliquely 8–10 cm distal to the posterior axillary fold and 2–3 cm posterior to the anterior border of the muscle. The second perforator is found 2–4 cm distally to the first one. Occasionally, a direct cutaneous perforator arising from the thoracodorsal vessel passes around the anterior border of the muscle, making flap harvesting easier.

There may not always be a single reliable perforator for the TDAP flap, due to anatomic variations.[27] In these cases, the surgeon must be aware and be prepared to modify the flap dissection intraoperatively, as a muscle-sparing TDAP flap.

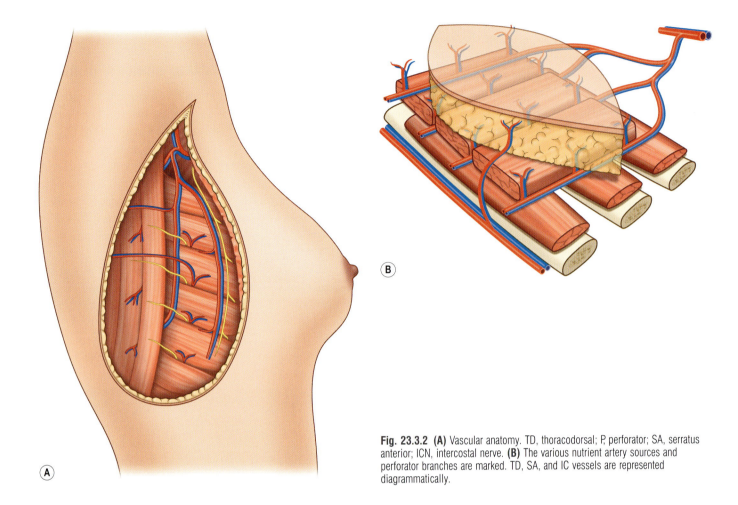

Fig. 23.3.2 (A) Vascular anatomy. TD, thoracodorsal; P, perforator; SA, serratus anterior; ICN, intercostal nerve. **(B)** The various nutrient artery sources and perforator branches are marked. TD, SA, and IC vessels are represented diagrammatically.

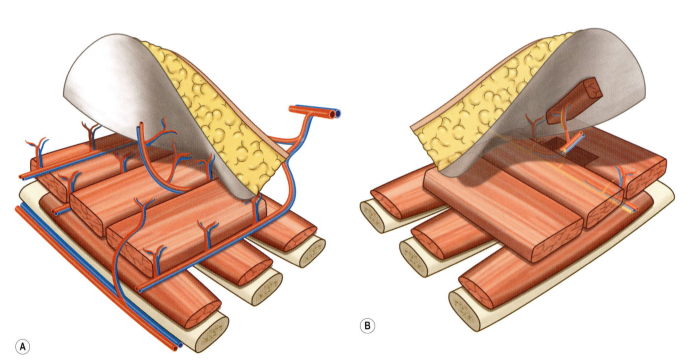

Fig. 23.3.3 Classification of flaps: **(A)** thoracodorsal artery perforator (TDAP) flap; **(B)** TDAP MS-I flap; **(C)** TDAP MS II flap; **(D)** lateral intercostal artery perforator flap; **(E)** serratus anterior artery perforator flap.

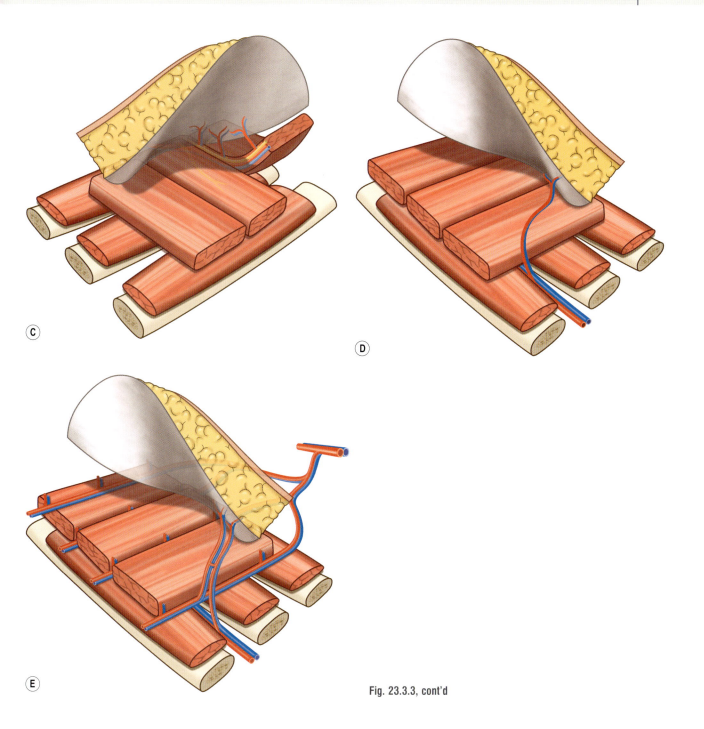

Fig. 23.3.3, cont'd

The TDAP flaps are classified as follows[28]:

- TDAP flap, when no muscle component is included in the flap (Fig. 23.3.3A)
- TDAP-MS-I, where a small segment of muscle (4×2 cm) kept attached to the back of the perforator vessels. The muscle segment protects the perforator from excessive tension and provides more freedom in flap positioning (Fig. 23.3.3B)
- TDAP-MS-II is indicated when multiple but small perforators are encountered. A larger segment, up to 5 cm wide along the anterior border of the latissimus dorsi muscle, together with the descending branch of the thoracodorsal vessels is then included within the flap in order to insure a maximal blood supply to the skin paddle (Fig. 23.3.3C).

The ICAP flap

The ICAP flap is based on perforators, arising from the intercostal vessels. The intercostal vessels form an arcade between the aorta and the internal mammary vessels and divide in four segments: vertebral, intercostal, intermuscular, and rectus segments.[29]

The ICAP flaps are classified as follows:

- The dorsal intercostal artery perforator (DICAP) flap. The flap is based on perforators originating from the vertebral segment of the intercostals vessels
- The lateral intercostal artery perforator (LICAP) flap, based on perforators arising from the intercostal segment (Fig. 23.3.3D)
- The anterior intercostal artery perforator (AICAP) flap. The nutrient perforators of this flap arise from the muscular or rectal segment.

The intercostal segment, which is the longest (12 cm), is very important because it gives 5–7 musculocutaneous perforators.[30]

The LICAP, commonly used in breast surgery, originates from the costal segment of the intercostals vessels. The largest perforator is most frequently found in the 6th intercostal space, 0.8–3.5 cm from the anterior border of the latissimus dorsi muscle.[31] The pedicle has adequate length, allowing the rotation of the flap up to 180° without tension and with no need to extend the dissection into the costal groove. An intercostal nerve may be included in the harvesting as an ICAP-sensate flap.

For small defects, the LICAP is designed on the lateral aspect of the thorax, and for moderate-large defects the distal limit of the skin pad can reach the posterior thoracic region, planned in a fashion similar to the skin pad of a LD flap.[32]

The AICAP flap is outlined over the upper abdomen so that the final scar will be hidden under the brassier strap. The donor site can be closed primarily if it is up to 6 cm wide (preoperative pinch test to be assured), or else in a reversed abdominoplasty fashion. The advantage of AICAP and SEAP flaps is that the patient is prepped in a supine position throughout the whole procedure. These flaps are mostly known for defects in the inferomedial quadrant of the breast.

The SAAP flap

The SAAP flap is based on a connection between the thoracodorsal artery branch to the serratus anterior muscle and the intercostal perforators (Fig. 23.3.3E). It is not a constant perforator (21%).[30] When an appropriately sized perforator is identified in front of the anterior border of the LD, it can be followed back to the nutrient artery, which in this case is the serratus anterior branch by dissecting the pedicle within the fascia and the fibers of the aforementioned muscle.

The SEAP flap

The SEAP flaps are based on perforators arising from either the superficial or the deep branch of the superior epigastric artery, and the perforator flaps are named SSEAP and DSEAP, respectively. As mentioned above, the superior epigastric artery perforator flap has similar indications as the anterior intercostal artery perforator flap[33]; however, it has a longer pedicle that allows it to reach the defect with less tension. Pedicled SEAP flaps should be used only in selected cases, since it excludes the secondary use of abdominal tissue for autologous breast reconstruction (DIEAP, SIEAP, TRAM flaps) if completion mastectomy is later indicated.

Indications for pedicled flaps

The main use for pedicled flaps is partial breast reconstruction (immediate or delayed) when volume replacement is necessary; however, other reasons include:

- Salvage procedure after partial/total free flap loss for breast reconstruction
- Postmastectomy breast reconstruction in combination with implant
- Breast augmentation with autologous tissue
- Shoulder, back, and chest wall defects.

Contraindications of pedicled flaps

The harvesting of a local perforator flap demands expertise of the technique and sufficient knowledge of the anatomy of the area. Less experienced surgeons may choose other reconstructive options to familiarize themselves with perforator flap harvesting, such as the deep inferior epigastric artery perforator, superior gluteal artery perforator flaps, or transverse myocutaneous gracilis flap, because the perforators associated with these flaps are larger and there are more to choose from.

The area of the defect may have limited access, especially when localized in the inferomedial quadrant, and is difficult to be reached by a pedicled perforator flap based on the axillary vessels. However, the AICAP or SEAP flaps are ideal for such defects.

Previous axillary or thoracic surgery with damage to the thoracodorsal pedicle is an ideal candidate for using a LICAP flap, but not for a LD or TDAP flap. Previous scars and radiation injury to the area may also result in the limitation of local pedicled perforator flaps.[28] When breast deformity after partial mastectomy with radiation is severe, the optimum choice is to perform a complete mastectomy and autologous reconstruction with a free flap transfer.

Flap design

Flap choice

Based on the thoracodorsal–serratus, intercostal, or superior epigastric vessels, several pedicle flaps can be raised on perforators in the axillary, back, anterior thoracic, and upper abdominal regions, depending on the location of the desired recipient site, the surgeon's preference, and other anatomic and surgical indications.[34]

The pedicled TDAP flap is ideal for partial breast reconstructions, especially for defects located in the superior or inferolateral quadrants. The LICAP is a good alternative to TDAP flap for lateral and inferior breast defects (Fig. 23.3.4). However, the TDAP flap has a longer pedicle with a greater arc of rotation and reaches most of the breast except for the inferomedial quadrants (Fig. 23.3.5).

Preoperative perforator mapping

Perforator mapping with correct flap design is the keystone in this technique. To localize the thoracodorsal perforators, a unidirectional Doppler (8 Hz) ultrasonography examination is performed for perforator mapping in the planned skin flap area. This device, although quite handy and less costly, has the disadvantage of generating false-negative and false-positive signals and provides less detailed anatomic vessel information. This is due to the misleading background signal from the thoracodorsal vessels, which can be confusing and difficult to distinguish from the perforator signal. To avoid this, the patient is positioned, as in surgery, at a lateral position with 90° of shoulder abduction and 90° of elbow flexion. Also, multidetector (MD) row computed tomography scan can be used with accuracy to localize the perforator (Fig. 23.3.4C).[35]

Markings

The patient is preferably marked the day before surgery. The breast size, tumor size, and location, as well as the final defect size, are estimated. The incisions for the tumor resection are chosen from an oncologic aspect but in the most aesthetically pleasing fashion. The TDAP flap planned for the partial breast reconstruction is designed to include the located perforators (one or more) at the proximal part if feasible, in the directions of relaxed skin lines, the bra line, or even horizontally according to the patient's preference. Skin laxity and fat excess in the lateral thorax and back area are estimated by the pinch test. The size of the flap is determined by the need for defect coverage and is an average of 20×8 cm. The skin drawings are applied at first with the patient in an upright position, and the anterior border of the LD muscle is palpated and marked. Then the patient is placed in a lying position on her side, with the reconstruction side facing upwards, as in surgery, for the perforator mapping and the flap design in the lateral thorax. The skin island is always extended over the anterior border of the

latissimus dorsi to include the premuscular perforators if present. The proximal border of the flap approximates the inframammary fold (Fig. 23.3.4C). If the defect is more medially, the flap is designed more distally, further in the back. The same design is applied for the LICAP, however, the flap is placed more anteriorly, towards the breast. The AICAP or SEAP flaps are usually designed under the inframammary fold along the rib.

Surgical technique

The patient is prepped and positioned in the supine position for the tumor excision (Fig. 23.3.4D,E). After the lumpectomy/quadrectomy at clear margins, clips are placed in the wound bed and left there in order to indicate the area for future radiation therapy. If the plan is to proceed with the TDAP, LICAP, or SAAP flap, the patient is positioned and prepped again in the lateral position, as in typical LD musculocutaneous flap dissection. Otherwise, for the AICAP/SEAP flap, the patient remains in the original position.

The flap harvesting starts with skin incisions. A posterior approach is usually used in the TDAP flap. The surgeon continues dissection down to the LD suprafascial plane, while beveling in favor of the flap, in order to gain as much of extra tissue as possible. Harvesting proceeds from the back towards the axillary region. Further harvesting under loop magnification continues meticulously, until the perforator vessel is visualized (Fig. 23.3.4F). If the perforator is visibly pulsate and adequate in caliber (>0.5 mm), the dissection continues along the perforator course up to the nutrient thoracodorsal pedicle. If a large pedicle length is required, the TD vessels can be dissected up to their subscapular vessel origin and included in the flap. If the perforators have an intramuscular course, dissection is performed in the direction of the muscle fibers and any nerves that come across are carefully preserved (Fig. 23.3.4G). Within the muscle, all the perforator side branches are either ligated or coagulated. If two perforators are found along the same course, they can both be included within the flap, without sacrificing any muscle fibers (Fig. 23.3.4H).

In cases in which the perforators are inadequate in size, the flap harvesting is continued as a muscle-sparing LD flap, by including a small segment of the latissimus dorsi muscle attached to the posterior wall of the perforators. The most important component of a muscle-sparing LD flap is to preserve the innervation to the muscle to avoid compromise of muscle function. This modification is also useful when the flap is intended for the medial breast area, because it protects the perforators from presumed tension.

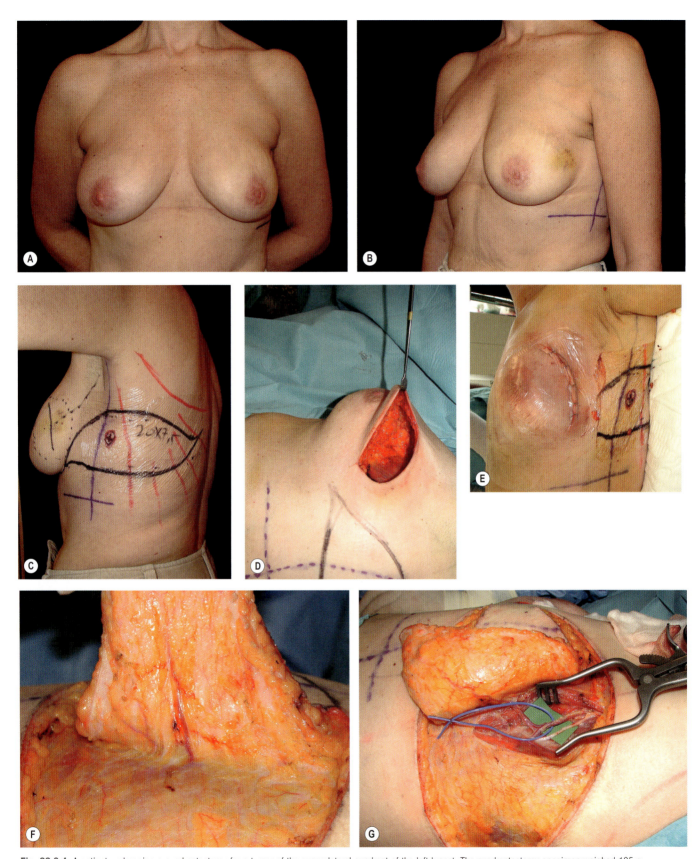

Fig. 23.3.4 A patient undergoing a quadrantectomy for a tumor of the superolateral quadrant of the left breast. The quadrantectomy specimen weighed 195 g. Reconstruction is with a completely de-epithelialized thoracodorsal artery perforator flap based on one perforator. **(A,B)** Preoperative views. **(C)** Flap design. The dominant Doppler was preoperatively located using MDCT. **(D,E)** The quadrantectomy was performed and the skin was closed in order to repositioned the patient. **(F)** A suprafacial dissection was performed until the dominant perforator was encountered. **(G)** The latissimus dorsi muscle is split and the perforator dissected back to the main pedicle.

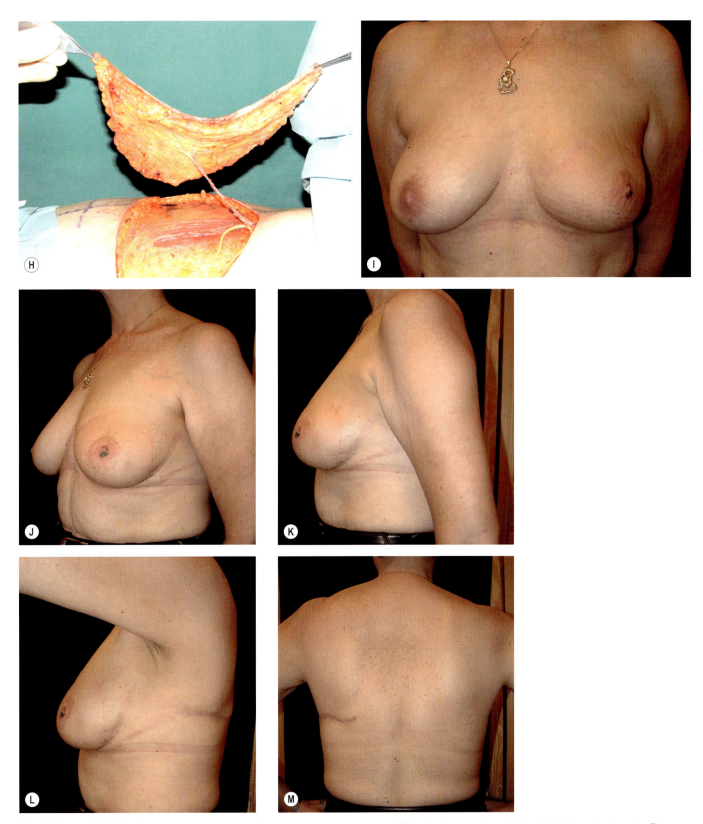

Fig. 23.3.4, cont'd (H) The thoracodorsal artery perforator flap was based on one perforator. **(I)** The flap is passed through the split latissimus dorsi muscle. The thoracodorsal nerve is preserved. **(J–M)** The outcome of the reconstruction and the donor site, 18 months postoperatively.

```
                    ┌──────────────────┐
                    │  Breast defect   │
                    └──────────────────┘
              ┌────────────┼───────────────┐
              ▼            ▼               ▼
    ┌─────────────────┐ ┌──────────────┐ ┌──────────────┐
    │All breast       │ │Lateral       │ │Median        │
    │quadrants,       │ │quadrants     │ │quadrant      │
    │except the median│ │              │ │              │
    │quadrant         │ │              │ │              │
    └─────────────────┘ └──────────────┘ └──────────────┘
              ▼            ▼               ▼
    ┌─────────────────┐ ┌──────────────┐ ┌──────────────┐
    │LD, TDAP,        │ │LD, TDAP, MS I│ │AICAP flap or │
    │MS I or II       │ │or II, LICAP  │ │SEAP flap     │
    │                 │ │or SAAP       │ │              │
    └─────────────────┘ └──────────────┘ └──────────────┘
```

Fig. 23.3.5 Choosing pedicled perforator flaps for partial breast.

The flap harvesting carries on, with the skin incisions continued proximal to the axilla and lateral to the LD and the dissection proceeds anteriorly, until the flap is freed from the donor site tissues and left connected only to the vascular pedicle. The pedicle is carefully passed under a subcutaneous tunnel in the axilla-lateral thoracic area that has been previously prepared to the recipient breast area, avoiding any avulsion of the pedicle (Fig. 23.3.4I). The donor site is sutured in three anatomic layers with a drain in place, and the patient is returned again to the supine position.

Before final closure of the defect, the flap can be partially or totally de-epithelialized (depending on the native skin reservations of the recipient site) and folded accordingly, to give extra projection to the reconstructed breast mount but always in a tension-free manner.

In LICAP flap dissection (Fig. 23.3.6), an anterior approach is performed from the breast side towards the anterior-free border of the LD muscle. Perforator dissection is done within the serratus muscle until its origin from the costal grove. Further dissection is usually not needed.

Postoperative care

Postoperatively, a protocol specific for perforator flap monitoring is implemented. Patients are administered low-molecular-weight heparin during the time of relative immobilization. Patients normally remain in the hospital until the drains are removed, typically 3–5 days. The arm is positioned in 45° abduction. Arm stretching is restricted for 1 week. Physiotherapy is usually initiated after 1 week. Most patients require between 9 and 14 sessions of shoulder physiotherapy. Patients treated for BCT with pedicled perforator flaps have a short rehabilitation course.[6]

Adjuvant irradiation of the breast, if indicated, can be started at 6 weeks' post-reconstruction. However, most patients in our experience receive adjuvant chemotherapy first that typically lasts for 6 months. Chemotherapy when necessary typically starts 3 weeks postoperatively.

Outcomes, prognosis, and complications

Complications

Donor site morbidity after harvesting loco-regional pedicle perforator flaps for partial breast reconstruction is reduced to a minimum. Only a very limited rate of seroma formation has been observed and treated mainly conservatively. Wound dehiscence of the donor site has only been observed when the wound edges are closed under tension. This is another infrequent event and is usually managed with local wound care. Data from a recent study shows a seroma rate of 5.5% in MS TDAP II flaps, compared with no seroma formation in perforator flaps. Other postoperative complications observed were wound dehiscence (4%), infection (2%), and hematoma (2%).[36]

Partial or total flap losses are very rare incidents, and one must exclude coagulopathies or other medical diseases and conditions. Palpable (partial) fat necrosis of the flap has been observed and can be treated, if necessary, by excision and primary closure or reconstruction by a local flap. If necrosis is too extensive, a mastectomy with total breast reconstruction may be indicated.[36]

Unpleasing scars, flap contractures, and volume loss are less rare sequelae and may need secondary surgical treatment. Also, flap reconstruction of breast defect may give a "plugged in" appearance, which seems to slightly improve after radiation therapy. It is hard to predict the long-term outcomes of partial breast reconstruction with pedicled perforator flaps due to the indefinite impact of irradiation to the final result.

Finally, some patients who undergo partial breast reconstruction with a TDAP flap document an initial decrease in forward arm elevation and passive abduction, which recover over time.[37]

Prognosis

Many concerns have been raised about oncologic safety of oncoplastic surgery.

A recent meta-analysis showed that oncoplastic surgery shows to be an oncologically safe procedure, with fewer recurrence rates (4%) compared with breast conservative surgery (7%) alone.[9] After oncoplastic reduction mammoplasty, resection margins are more often negative, and if recurrences occur, they most often occur in the preoperative quadrant of the tumor, and not the location after displacement techniques.[20] As

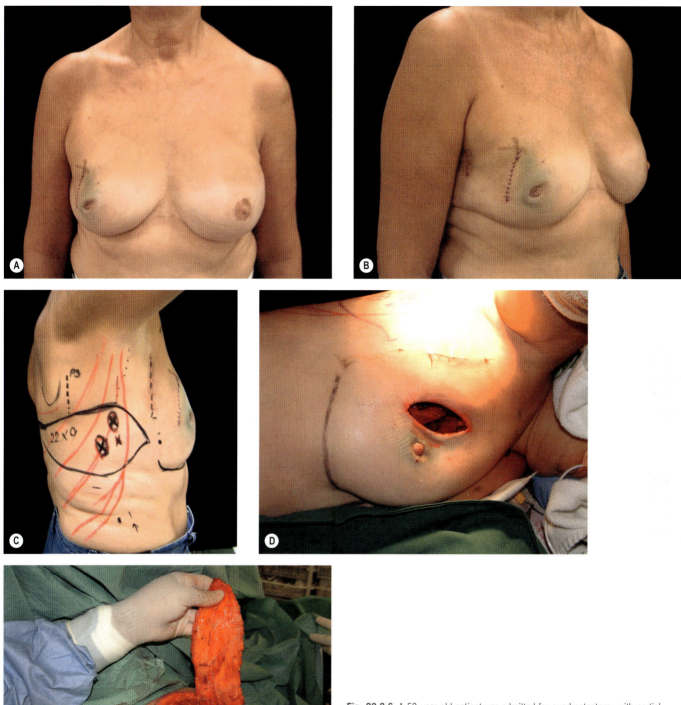

Fig. 23.3.6 A 59-year-old patient was admitted for quadrantectomy with partial breast reconstruction for right breast cancer located at superolateral quadrant. Two years previously, the patient had undergone a mastectomy at the left side with an immediate breast reconstruction using a deep inferior epigastric perforator flap. **(A,B)** Preoperative views. **(C)** A 22×9 cm flap was designed with the mapped perforators. **(D)** The defect after the quadrantectomy. **(E)** A preoperative view shows one intercostal perforator, lateral intercostal artery perforator. The intercostal nerve was also included in the flap. The flap was completely de-epithelialized and folded to fill the defect.

Continued

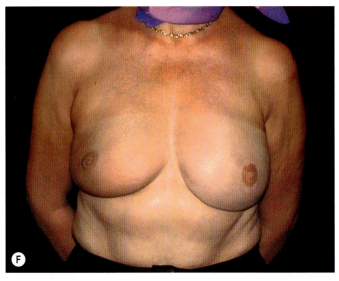

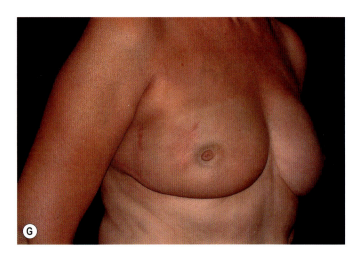

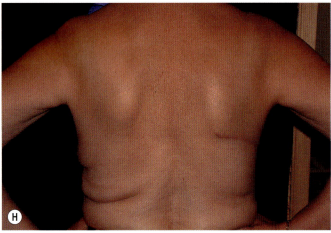

Fig. 23.3.6, cont'd **(F–H)** Postoperative views.

stated earlier, if DCIS is present, oncoplastic techniques should be used cautiously.

Local recurrence rates reported in the literature for oncoplastic surgery vary from 0% to 7% of the patients.[36]

Oncologic follow-up

Oncologic follow-up after oncoplastic procedures remains important. Given the rearrangement of parenchymal tissues, scar tissue or fat necrosis is not uncommon and might be suspicious on several radiologic imaging modalities. Biopsy with fine-needle aspiration, core biopsy, or excisional biopsy may be necessary to rule out tumor recurrence (up to 25%).[38] The addition of breast remodeling procedures does not seem to affect mammographic sensitivity, and qualitative changes are similar to those found following breast conservation therapy alone.[39]

Secondary procedures

Our experience has demonstrated stable long-term outcomes (Fig. 23.3.7). However, one may expect breast asymmetry due to different aging processes between the two breasts. The non-irradiated side may become more ptotic as compared with the radiated side. On the other hand, the irradiated side may show signs of total breast atrophy. When the breast asymmetry becomes obvious, fat grafting alone or with contralateral breast remodeling can be considered.

The use of lipofilling technique, alone or most commonly in combination with other reconstruction options, for the treatment of breast defects after tumor resection is gaining great popularity. In contrast to what was believed in the past, lipofilling of the breast is proven to be a safe, reliable method for the transposition of autologous fatty tissue in contour deformed areas of the breast.[40]

Fat injections into the breast can significantly improve small breast defects after limited lumpectomy. In larger excisions, partial breast reconstruction is preferred using the tissue replacement techniques described; however, autologous fat grafting is a useful adjunct to improve the final outcome. Fat injections can be considered primarily at the time of the breast conserving therapy to limit volume discrepancies between the two breasts, to add

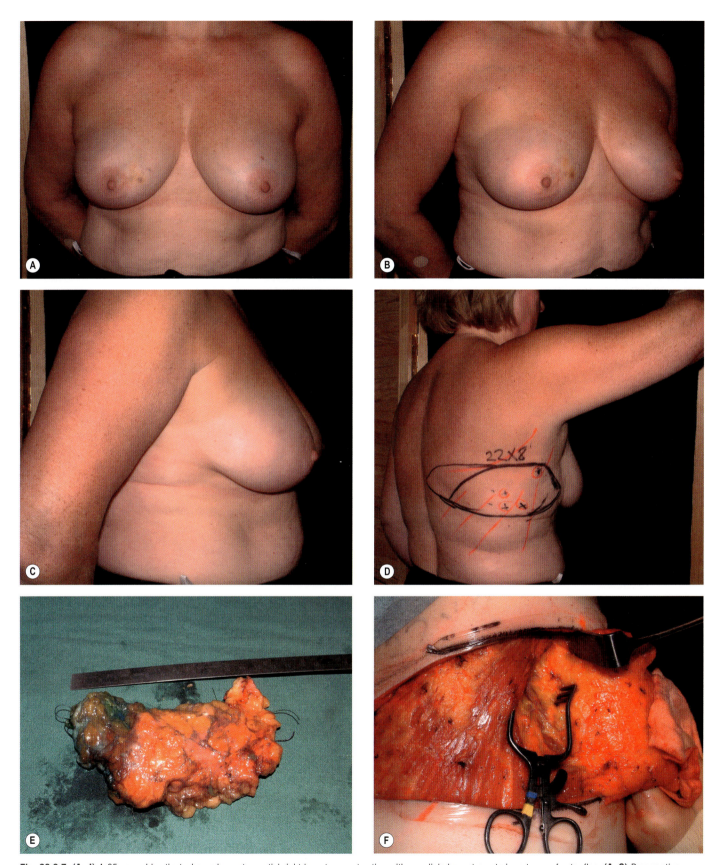

Fig. 23.3.7 (A–J) A 65-year-old patient who underwent a partial right breast reconstruction with a pedicled serratus anterior artery perforator flap. **(A–C)** Preoperative views. **(D)** A 22×8 cm flap was designed with marked perforators. **(E)** The quadrantectomy specimen (120 g). **(F)** The flap was based on the communication between serratus anterior and the intercostal perforator (arrow).

Continued

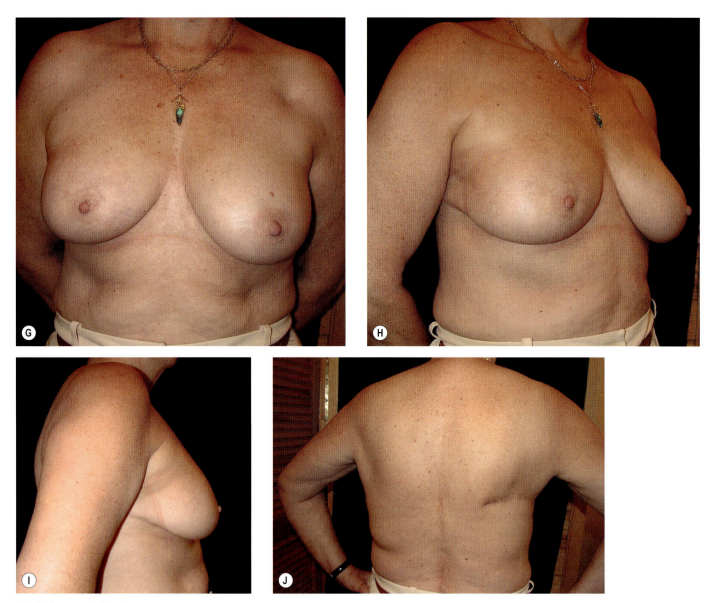

Fig. 23.3.7, cont'd (G–J) Postoperative views with the donor site at 3 years postoperatively.

superomedial fullness for an aesthetically pleasing breast cleavage or to correct the breast mound and shape; however, it is most often used secondarily. In second-stage procedures, fat grafting can be performed to refine volume, projection, or contour irregularities due to fat necrosis or flap contractures. Fat grafting has also demonstrated success in the treatment of skin atrophy of the breast after irradiation. The mechanism of action is postulated to be mediated by stem cells included with fat grafting in the intradermal plane. The major

limitation of this technique is that it is time consuming and prolongs operation time, especially in inexperienced hands and the requirement of staged applications. Some concerns about oncologic safety and monitoring of the breast have been raised. However, a recent meta-analysis demonstrated no difference in oncologic event rates after autologous fat grafting compared with non-autologous fat grafting patients.[41] However, fat necrosis after fat grafting on radiologic imaging might warrant a biopsy to rule out recurrences.

🌐 **Access the complete reference list online at**   **http://www.expertconsult.com**

1. Veronesi U, Cascinelli N, Mariani L, et al. Twenty-year follow-up of a randomized study comparing breast-conserving surgery with radical mastectomy for early breast cancer. *N Engl J Med*. 2002;347:1227–1232.

3. Clough KB, Kroll SS, Audretsch W. An approach to the repair of partial mastectomy defects. *Plast Reconstr Surg*. 1999;104:409–420.

7. McCready D, Holloway C, Shelley W, et al. Surgical management of early stage invasive breast cancer: a practice guideline. Breast

Cancer Disease Site Group of Cancer Care; Ontario's Program in Evidence-Based Care. *Can J Surg*. 2005;48:185–194.

9. Losken A, Dugal C, Styblo T, et al. A meta-analysis comparing breast conservation therapy alone to the oncoplastic technique. *Ann Plast Surg*. 2014;72:145–149.

16. Anderson BO, Masetti R, Silverstein MJ. Oncoplastic approaches to partial mastectomy: an overview of volume-displacement techniques. *Lancet Oncol*. 2005;6:145–157.

17. Kronowitz SJ, Kuerer HM, Buchholz TA, et al. A management algorithm and practical oncoplastic surgical techniques for repairing partial mastectomy defects. *Plast Reconstr Surg*. 2008;122:1631–1647.

19. Peters KK, Losken A. Applied anatomy and breast aesthetics: definition and assessment. In: Losken A, Hamdi M, eds. *Partial Breast Reconstruction: Techniques in Oncoplastic Surgery*. St. Louis: QMP Inc.; 2009:86.

28. Hamdi M, Van Landuyt K. Pedicled perforator flaps in breast reconstruction. In: Spear SI, Willey SC, Robb GL, et al., eds. *Surgery of the Breast: Principles and Art*. Philadelphia: Lippincott-Raven; 2006:833–844.

34. Hamdi M. Pedicled perforator flap reconstruction. In: Losken A, Hamdi M, eds. *Partial Breast Reconstruction: Techniques in Oncoplastic Surgery*. St. Louis: QMP Inc.; 2009:387.

36. Hamdi M. Oncoplastic and reconstructive surgery of the breast. *Breast*. 2013;22:S100–S105.

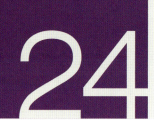

Fat grafting to the breast

Henry Wilson, Scott L. Spear†, and Maurice Y. Nahabedian

SYNOPSIS

- Autologous fat has demonstrated success when it comes to correcting mild to moderate contour deformities in reconstructed breasts.
- Fat grafting may be used safely and effectively for a variety of reconstructive indications.
- There is a variety of specific harvesting and processing techniques available.
- Fat grafting for breast augmentation is effective, but its precise role in the cosmetic plastic surgeon's armamentarium is yet to be defined.
- Fat grafting to the breast has become common practice for reconstructive and aesthetic breast surgery; however, it remains controversial for some indications.
- Complications are minor and infrequent if a proper technique is followed.
- External pre-expansion and adipose-derived stem cells hold promise for future enhancement of the results and treatment of difficult problems.

 Access the Historical Perspective section online at
http://www.expertconsult.com

Introduction

Autologous fat grafting to the female breast has a long history surrounded by a great deal of controversy. Over the past decade, there have been numerous clinical and scientific publications attesting to the risks and benefits.[4–24] Despite the paucity of high-quality published evidence and continued disagreement about the best technique, autologous lipofilling to the female breast continues to evolve. As with many fundamentally good ideas in plastic surgery, the concept is elegant in its simplicity: fat is removed from a location where it is

†Deceased

not needed and used to augment body contour in an area of need or desire. To be compelling, the procedure must have a reliable technique and not subject either the donor or recipient site to unacceptable risk.

This chapter examines the current use of autologous fat grafting of the breast for a variety of indications, including filling contour irregularities and supplementing other forms of breast reconstruction after mastectomy in both the radiated and non-radiated breast. Another indication is the correction of contour abnormalities following breast conserving therapy. Autologous fat has been used for reconstruction of the entire breast after mastectomy without requiring either an implant or a flap.[25] Fat grafting has also been described for correcting congenital anomalies of the breast such as Poland syndrome, pectus excavatum, and thoracic hypoplasia. Similarly, autologous fat can be used to correct acquired deformities of the breast other than after cancer treatment, such as might occur after previous implants or other breast surgery. The chapter concludes with an analysis of the controversy surrounding the use of autologous fat grafts for primary breast augmentation.[5,10,26–30]

Of the indications listed above, some are more widely accepted than others. The issues involving all of these applications are cost, efficacy, acute surgical risk, interference with the diagnosis, and treatment of breast cancer, and the remote possibility of increasing the risk of neoplasia. Fat grafting as a supplement to other forms of breast reconstruction after mastectomy is the most well-accepted application because of its excellent risk profile, its wide adoption by many surgeons, and the absence of negative reports.

In 2005, the authors reported on the use of autologous fat grafting to correct contour deformities in the reconstructed breasts of 37 patients.[4] Most of the 47 treated breasts (85%) experienced worthwhile improvement from the procedure, and only 8.5% of the treated breasts experienced a significant complication (one cellulitis and three cases of fat necrosis). Based on these results, fat injection was recommended as a "safe and effective tool for improving the cosmetic result of either autologous or implant breast reconstruction".

More recently, other retrospective reviews have found similarly good results and low complication rates. In a 2007 retrospective review by Missana et al.,[6] of 74 reconstructed breasts treated with fat grafting, the authors found good–excellent results in 86.5% and moderately–good results in an additional 13.5%. Their only complications were five cases of fat necrosis. In 2009, Kanchwala et al.[9] reported on fat grafting to 110 breast reconstruction patients, finding good–excellent results in 85% and reporting no complications other than "minor contour irregularities". Reporting in 2009 on 880 patients treated over 10 years for a variety of reconstructive and cosmetic breast concerns, Delay et al.[10] noted good–excellent results in the vast majority of patients with complications, including a 3% rate of fat necrosis and less than 1% infection. None of these review articles found any correlation of fat grafting with the development of a new or recurrent breast cancer, and mammographic abnormalities were confined to calcifications that were easy for experienced radiologists to distinguish from neoplastic patterns of calcification.

An understanding of the effective use of fat grafting in principle is fundamental to the use of fat grafting for any indication. For this reason, this chapter includes a detailed discussion of the treatment of generic contour deformities of the breast for which fat grafting is indicated. Contour deformities after reconstructive breast surgery for mastectomy are relatively common, and autologous fat has become a workhorse to correct them because of its relative simplicity, low cost, and lasting results.[4,5,10] The authors advise the surgeon to achieve success at fat grafting for these indications, prior to considering its use in the more controversial areas of lumpectomy deformities or cosmetic augmentation.

Basic science/disease process

Adipocytes are fragile. Unlike skin, muscle, or bone, fat lacks unit cohesion, which is perhaps why many early practitioners used dermal fat grafts. When fat is left attached to its overlying dermis, it is easier to work with, since it can be sutured into the desired location. Oxygen diffusion prior to revascularization remains a problem, however, so such grafts must be small and are best suited to craniofacial applications where the defects are small and the vascularity is high.

Autologous fat grafting with aspirated fat uses fat in a liquid form, which permits it to be harvested and deployed with minimal incisions. It also permits its injection in precise quantities into precisely the area it is needed, at least in theory. From the procurement at the donor site to deposition in the grafted area, there are several steps in processing that must be executed successfully. Each step introduces the potential for adipocyte trauma and technical error, so attention to technique is of paramount importance.

Stem cells and radiation deformities

Adipose-derived stem cells (ADSCs) were first described in the 1920s, with early research focusing on which cells survived transplantation and became new host fat cells, which helped to characterize the process and improve the survival of fat grafts. More recently, the regenerative qualities of ADSCs on damaged tissue were found, and they have potentially dramatic treatment implications for patients with radiation-induced injury.[31] As radiation is increasingly being used in the breast for aggressive indications, the average practitioner can be expected to encounter more and more of these deformities.

Radiation deformities are some of the most challenging problems the reconstructive breast surgeon encounters. Radiation-damaged breast tissue has a reduction of its capillary bed and is relatively hypoxic. The clinical picture is one of acute injury (radiodermatitis), followed by subcutaneous fibrosis and skin hyperpigmentation. There is substantial variability as to the extent to which an individual patient will exhibit these effects and their resolution over time. Common presenting problems after radiation include generalized fibrosis; scar retraction at lumpectomy defects; capsular contracture around prosthetic devices, and persistent skin hyperpigmentation. Uncommonly, radionecrosis occurs, resulting in a chronic wound.

Traditionally, little in the reconstructive armamentarium has been able to address the primary problem of tissue damage. Solutions have been centered around replacement techniques: flaps to replace a retracted lumpectomy defect or eliminate an implant with surrounding capsular contracture. The promise of ADSCs lies in their ability to reverse the fibrotic changes of radiation damage.[31] The future may bring more comprehensive solutions to breast reconstruction, such as ADSC-seeded biomaterial constructs[13] and fat grafting, combined with negative pressure external soft-tissue expansion.[25] Presently, the use of fat grafting augmented with expanded populations of ADSCs is limited to research institutions, but fat grafts harvested and processed with the traditional techniques may contain some stem cells.

Diagnosis/patient presentation

Patients present with contour deformities occurring after previous reconstructive or cosmetic breast surgery. Alternatively, a patient may request primary augmentation for hypomastia or congenital asymmetries such as tuberous breast or Poland syndrome. A potentially large patient population who may be served in the future is the post-mastectomy patient seeking total primary reconstruction with fat grafting.

Patient selection

Autologous fat grafting is indicated to restore normal contour in an area of deformity. These deformities occur commonly in breasts reconstructed with flaps or implants and also occur as undesirable sequelae of implants placed for cosmetic breast augmentation (Table 24.1). There now follows a discussion on specific indications, with examples of each.

Contour deformity after implant reconstruction

With implant reconstructions, thin overlying tissue can lead to sharp implant borders (Fig. 24.1) and visible rippling (Fig. 24.2), both of which can be effectively softened by fat grafting. These patients are often slender with relatively little subcutaneous fat, or are patients whose mastectomy flaps were left very thin by the breast surgeon. If the implant is very mobile in a large

pocket, an unnatural "trench" can form at the interface between the implant and the chest wall. This may be further accentuated medially by lateral shift of the implant when the patient is supine. Such deformities may require a combination of implant exchange to different size, capsulorrhaphy, capsular reinforcement with acellular dermal matrix, and fat grafting (see Fig. 24.4). These deformities are also encountered in the slender cosmetic patient, especially when implants are placed in the subglandular plane.

Contour deformity after flap reconstruction

In the case of flap reconstruction, the border of the flap is a common location for a depression, often occurring as a "step-off" where the flap ends and the normal residual tissue begins.[9] Characteristically, this deformity consists of skin flap directly over the chest wall muscle or bone, and reflects the step-off that can occur at the edge of a flap where it is inset to fill a mastectomy defect or from fat necrosis at the vulnerable edges of the reconstructive tissue (Figs. 24.3 & 24.4). Deformities intrinsic to the flap, such as areas of fat necrosis within the substance of the flap or the periumbilical tissue in a transverse rectus abdominus myocutaneous (TRAM), are also common indications and may occur within the flap substance or at the borders.

Contour deformities after implant or flap reconstructions in a radiated field

Suitable patients with radiation damage have a breast contour deformity secondary to implant or flap reconstruction after mastectomy, exacerbated by radiation changes such as those described in the radiation section above. These deformities may have components of these step-off or intrinsic flap deformities, in addition to the tissue fibrosis, skin changes, or capsular contracture brought about by radiation (Figs. 24.5 & 24.6). The complications of flap reconstructions that are the most difficult to correct tend to occur when the reconstruction was performed prior to the radiation.[34] These include volume loss, fat necrosis, delayed wound healing, and fibrosis. While the experience with fat grafting as an adjunct to other breast reconstructions has been largely favorable, the evidence is unclear and unconvincing, when looking specifically at the radiated breast. Radiation introduces added risks, complexities, and problems. The risks include an increased risk of infection and of non-healing of the surgical site. The complexities include the difficulty of creating space for the fat in a badly radiation-fibrosed recipient site, and the problems are the lack of both skin elasticity and a fertile recipient site conducive for the fat grafts to take.

Table 24.1 Specific indications for fat grafting		
Established indications: safe and effective	**Effective and probably safe[a]**	**Safe but not yet proven**
Flap border step-off	Deformity after lumpectomy and radiation	Primary reconstruction as the sole method[c]
Depression from fat necrosis		
Irregularities in mastectomy flap thickness	Cosmetic augmentation[b]	
Augmentation for inadequate flap volume	Augmentation deformities (rippling, visible deformities)	
Radiation deformity in flap reconstruction		
Sharp implant border (reconstruction)		
Implant rippling (reconstruction)		
[a]Detailed informed consent and IRB approval required. [b]Being evaluated in clinical trials.[25,32,33] [c]Being evaluated in clinical trials.[25]		

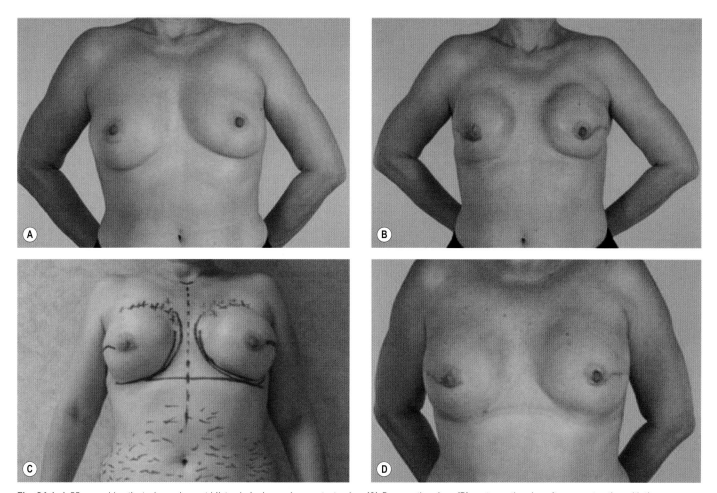

Fig. 24.1 A 55-year-old patient who underwent bilateral nipple-sparing mastectomies. **(A)** Preoperative view; **(B)** postoperative view after reconstruction with tissue expanders and acellular dermal matrix illustrates typical marginal contour deformities surrounding a prosthetic device. **(C)** Preoperative markings and **(D)** the 3-month postoperative result for fat grafting to margins with exchange of tissue expanders for permanent implants.

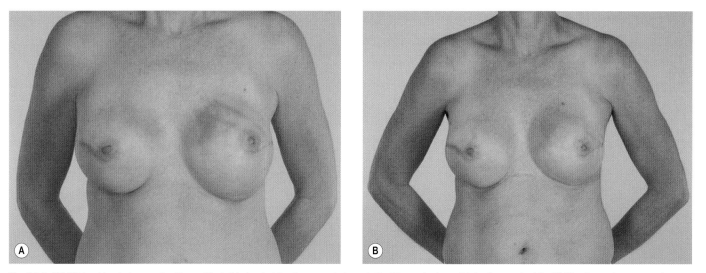

Fig. 24.2 **(A)** Bilateral implant reconstructions with visible implant borders superiorly on both sides and substantial rippling on the left. **(B)** The 6-month postoperative results after fat grafting superior poles bilaterally (80 cc right, 50 cc left) and left inferior capsulorrhaphy. Note softening of implant contour bilaterally and resolution of visible rippling on the left.

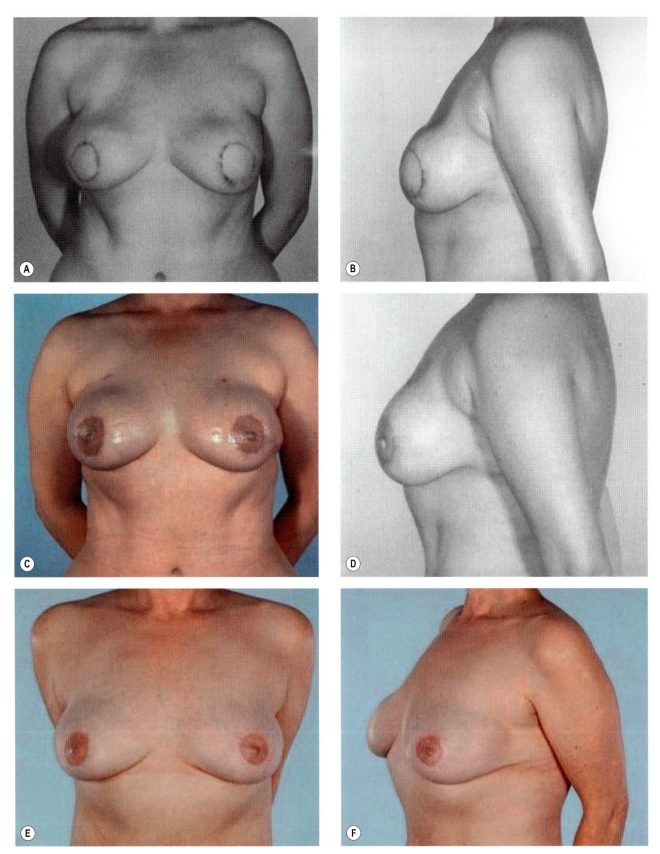

Fig. 24.3 (A,B) A 45-year-old patient with flap step-off deformities after bilateral immediate breast reconstruction with pedicled transverse rectus abdominus myocutaneous flaps. **(C,D)** At 11 months after bilateral nipple reconstruction with 120 cc of fat grafting to each superior pole. **(E,F)** The same patient 7 years after fat grafting to flap step-off deformities of the superior poles bilaterally.

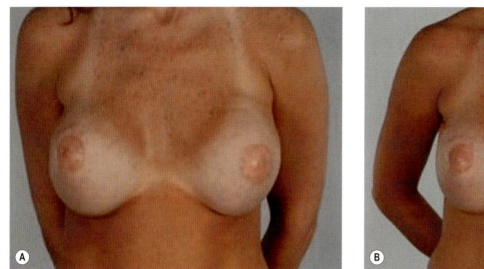
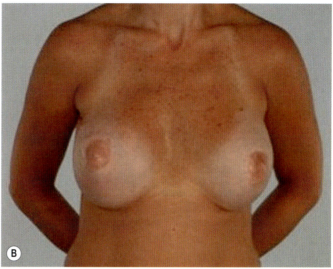

Fig. 24.4 A 33-year-old patient with bilateral step-off deformities (most pronounced on the left) treated by fat injection. **(A)** Preoperative view 2 years after bilateral breast reconstruction with latissimus flaps and implants. **(B)** The same patient 3 years after autologous fat grafting of 170 cc to the left upper pole and 50 cc to the right upper pole.

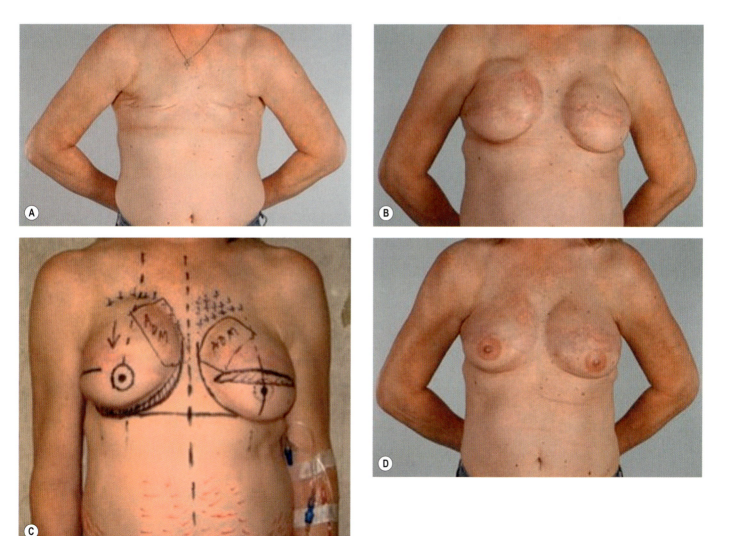

Fig. 24.5 A 51-year-old patient with history of bilateral modified radical mastectomies with postoperative radiation after each mastectomy. **(A)** The patient preoperatively, and **(B)** 3 months after bilateral reconstruction with latissimus flaps and tissue expanders. **(C)** Preoperative view prior to bilateral exchange of expanders for implants, nipple reconstructions, and treatment of bilateral upper pole contour deformities with fat grafting and acellular dermal matrix. **(D)** At 5 months after the operation.

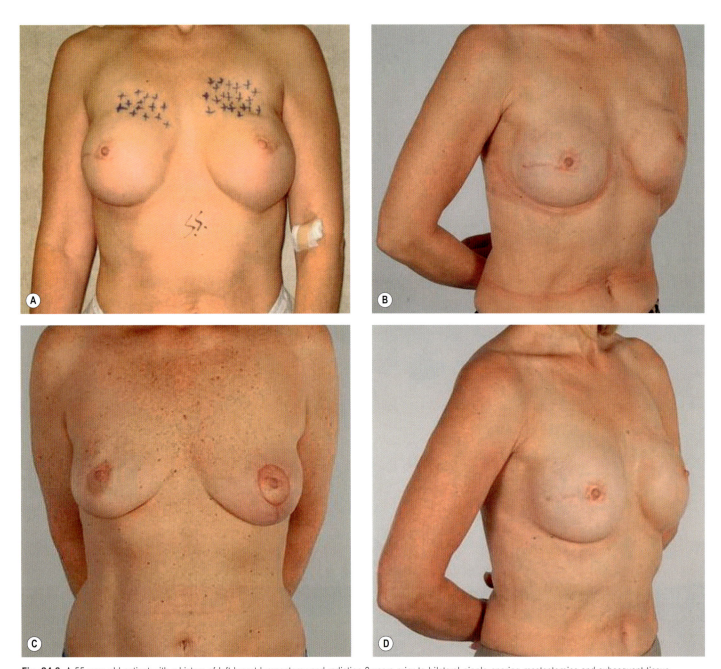

Fig. 24.6 A 55-year-old patient with a history of left breast lumpectomy and radiation 2 years prior to bilateral nipple-sparing mastectomies and subsequent tissue expander and implant reconstruction. Bilateral upper pole contour deformities **(A,B)** were treated with 35 cc right and 85 cc autologous fat injection. **(C,D)** At 1 year postoperatively.

A review of the literature indicates that experience with fat grafting in the radiated environment has only recently been addressed. The 2007 publication by Rigotti *et al.* details some cases showing dramatic improvements to both capsular contracture and impending implant exposure as a result of stem-cell enhanced autologous fat grafting.[31] In 2009, Delay *et al.* reported that fat grafting can improve the quality of radiation-damaged post-mastectomy skin contributing to an autologous reconstruction or permitting an implant reconstruction to be used where it may have previously been contraindicated.[10] Serra-Renom *et al.*

reported an innovative approach to the reconstruction of radiated mastectomy defects in 2009.[35] The authors reported on 65 patients, whom they reconstructed in three stages: tissue expander placement, expander exchange for permanent implant, and nipple reconstruction. At each stage, an average of 150 cc of autologous fat was grafted to enhance the volume of the reconstruction. The authors report excellent results, with no capsular contracture or other complications. They conclude that fat grafting enhanced the reconstruction by improving the skin quality and adding subcutaneous volume to the breasts.

Lumpectomy deformities

Lumpectomy deformities of up to 10–15% of the breast volume often result in satisfactory aesthetic results.[36] The actual resected percentage, however, may often be higher with re-excisions or a desire to avoid mastectomy on the part of the patient or breast surgeon. Although oncoplastic techniques may result in very good symmetry if performed at the time of lumpectomy, they are not universally utilized or available. Accordingly, lumpectomy with radiation results in suboptimal aesthetic outcomes of up to 30% (Fig. 24.7).[37] The idea of fat grafting these lumpectomy defects is very appealing because no other techniques are appropriate for most of these patients and what is missing is usually all, or in part, fat. Implants perform badly in a radiated environment, and flaps are often best reserved for total or subtotal mastectomy defects. The problems and challenges, however, are similar to those for radiation after mastectomy. Fibrosis, risk of infection, and a hostile environment for grafts make the radiated lumpectomy defect an uncertain, unproven application. This is magnified by the heightened concern for monitoring and detecting local breast cancer recurrence in these patients.

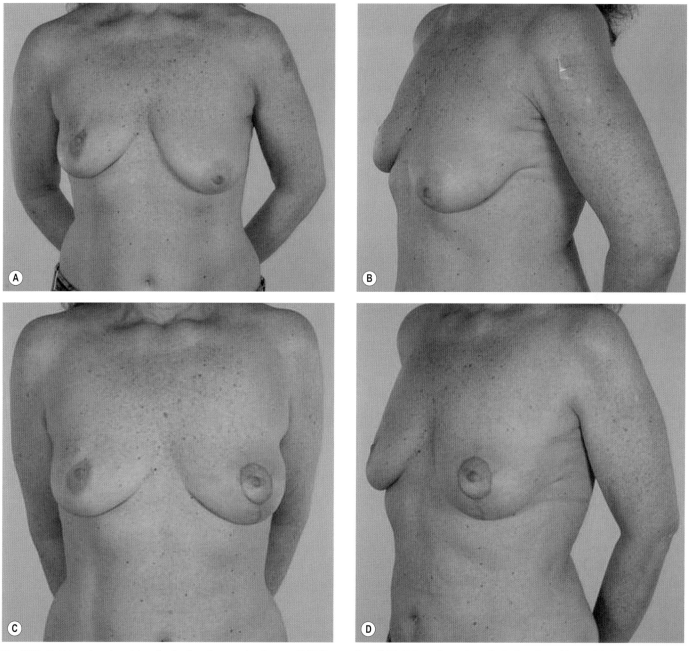

Fig. 24.7 Right breast contour deformity after breast-conserving therapy. **(A,B)** Preoperative. **(C,D)** At 2 months postoperatively, from fat grafting to right lumpectomy defect and left mastopexy. There has been a modest improvement in the right breast contour seen best on the oblique view.

There is little in the literature on lumpectomy deformities being reconstructed with autologous fat grafting. In his 2007 publication detailing the use of adipose-derived stem cells, Rigotti published impressive photographs of a patient whose radiated lumpectomy defect was dramatically improved by stem cell-enriched fat injection.[31] A 2009 report of experience by Delay *et al.* on 42 patients indicates that the fat grafting is valuable in the management of moderate deformities resulting from breast conservation.[10,38] The authors caution that the medico-legal environment surrounding fat grafting for this indication is treacherous, however, and they use a very strict protocol involving detailed pre- and post-procedure imaging, specially trained radiologists, and management of the patient within a multidisciplinary team. Delay recommends completing the "learning curve" for fat grafting prior to using it to reconstruct radiated lumpectomy defects.[10]

The concept of immediate fat grafting performed at the time of the partial mastectomy or lumpectomy has been described. Biazus *et al.* treated 20 patients with autologous fat injected in the subcutaneous and parenchymal layers immediately after excision and prior to radiation.[14] The average infiltrate was 121 cc that was usually twice the volume of the excised specimen. In total, 19 patients were classified as a BIRADs 2, and one as a BIRADs 3. Aesthetic outcome was graded as good to very good in the majority of cases at a minimum follow-up of 1 year.

Acquired breast deformities from trauma or surgery often occur in a setting without radiation damage. These patients may have problems beyond the scope of an implant correction but be unsuitable for a flap. Some may have had an implant and be unwilling to have another. For these patients, fat grafting offers the possibility of an autologous correction with minimal morbidity.

Congenital deformities

Just as the FDA recognized that certain non-mastectomy problems were surgically comparable with those caused by cancer treatment, it is recognized that some congenital and other acquired breast deformities can be and should be treated like those after mastectomy or breast-conserving therapy. These include Poland syndrome, pectus excavatum, thoracic hypoplasia, tuberous breasts, and major asymmetries. Some of these patients can be treated in whole or in part by other techniques, but fat grafting brings an additional powerful tool to help solve the problem, often where nothing else is practical. This has been shown for the deformity associated with the tuberous breast.[5] It has also been demonstrated for chest wall deformities where the upper pole is beyond the reach of the implant.[4]

Poland syndrome results in absence of the pectoralis muscles and underdevelopment of the breast gland. Provided the latissimus is present, an excellent reconstructive solution involves a latissimus flap with placement of an implant.[39] Postoperative deformities in the infraclavicular hollow may occur and respond well to fat grafting. Other candidates for fat injection present with unsatisfactory reconstruction after breast implant alone, usually with contour deformities laterally accentuated by the absence of the pectoralis. The deformity resulting from Poland syndrome can also be entirely reconstructed with fat grafting,[10] but it typically requires multiple sessions of grafting.

Anterior thoracic hypoplasia is characterized by a normal pectoralis muscle and sternal position, but a unilaterally depressed chest wall with hypoplastic breast and superiorly-displaced nipple areolar complex (NAC).[40] Treatment is typically with implant alone, though residual deformities may occur and respond well to fat grafting (Fig. 24.8).

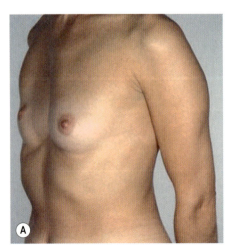 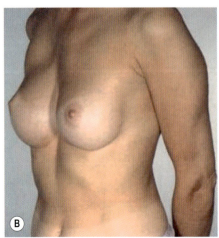 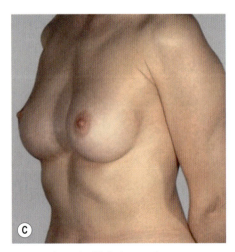

Fig. 24.8 **(A)** A patient with thoracic hypoplasia preoperatively. **(B)** A patient with thoracic hypoplasia after bilateral augmentation only. **(C)** At 2 years after two separate procedures of fat injection to right upper pole (140 cc and 150 cc, 14 months apart).

Tuberous breast deformity features a constricting ring though which developing tissue herniates, resulting in an enlarged NAC, narrow mammary base, elevation of the inframammary fold, and hypoplasia of one or more breast quadrants. Treatment depends on the presentation and may result in contour deformities that respond well to fat grafting. The tuberous breast has also been treated with fat grafting alone with impressive results.[5,10]

Primary breast augmentation

Perhaps most controversial is the use of autologous fat grafting for primary breast augmentation. While efficacy and safety are issues for all applications, here the issues are magnified. On the efficacy side, these patients are generally easily corrected with implants. With a high degree of reliability and certainty, a woman can enlarge her breast size by 200–500 cc (1 or 2 cup sizes) with a 1–2 h operation, with well known, well described, and definable risks. Regarding breast augmentation with lipofilling, however, the enlargement is less ambitious, less reliable, and less certain. The authors generally describe to the patient that it is the hope and intent to increase the breast by one half to one whole cup size. This result is clearly dependent on a number of things. The percentage of fat survival is key, but how to obtain that survival is still a work in progress. Defining the best candidate for lipo-breast augmentation is as important as the technique. Determining what type of fat to harvest, how to prepare it, where to inject it, and in what type of breast are all important questions. Regarding safety, the questions are equally important. These women have not had breast cancer, but they are at significant risk of developing breast cancer, resulting in concerns about radiographically obscuring or mimicking breast cancer. Of theoretical concern is the possibility of accelerating or inducing breast cancer in the younger at-risk women. Nevertheless, the concept of moving fat from less desirable areas such as the abdomen or thighs to more desirable areas such as a small breast is so seductive and compelling that it should be no surprise that academic-minded surgeons are studying it, entrepreneurial surgeons are marketing it, and many patients are very, very interested in it.

Safety issues apply for all of the non-cancer uses of autologous fat, but they are most acute in the purely cosmetic patient. For her, the indications for correction are so elective, the other options so good, and the risk of disturbance of her normal, healthy baseline are much greater than, e.g., the previously treated cancer patient. The authors have had a modest experience in primary breast augmentation with fat, most of it in a funded, IRB-approved, controlled clinical trial.[32] Our experience

prior to the trial in a handful of patients was mixed, with some having visually significant breast enhancement of up to one cup size (Figs. 24.9 & 24.10). Others had no discernible long-term benefit, despite several hours of hard work of obtaining, processing, and infiltrating the fat in front of and behind the breast parenchyma in several different planes (Fig. 24.11).

In a retrospective review published in 2007, Zheng et al. followed 66 Chinese patients treated with fat grafting for breast augmentation for an average of 37 months.[27] Fat grafts were harvested using 3 mm cannulas attached to a vacuum pump set to low negative pressure (−0.5 atm), washed with normal saline, and spun in a centrifuge at 600 rpm (26 g) for 2 min to isolate the middle layer, which was used as graft. Graft injection was performed with a one-holed 3 mm cannula through two injection sites (periareolar and inframammary), with an average of 174 mL of fat injected into each breast (101 mL subcutaneous; 73 mL subglandular). A total of 28 patients had one treatment; 21 patients were treated twice; and 17 patients three times. Results were judged by three independent plastic surgeons, who noted significant improvement in 28 patients (42.4%); improvement in 24 patients (36.4%); and no improvement in 14 patients (21.2%). A total of 27 patients (40.9%) were very satisfied; 26 patients (39.4%) were satisfied; and 13 (19.7%) were unsatisfied with the results. The only complications noted were fat necrosis or cyst formation in 11 patients (16.7%), none of which interfered with the final contour of the breast.

In another study published in 2008 of purely cosmetic breast augmentation with fat injection, Yoshimura et al. treated 40 Japanese patients using a protocol designed to increase the percentage of ADSCs in the grafted fat.[28] Adipose tissue was harvested using a 2.5 mm (inner) diameter cannula and conventional liposuction machine, after which half of the harvested fat was either washed and placed upright (25% of patients) or centrifuged unwashed at 700 g for 3 min (75% of patients). The other half of the liposuction aspirate was used to isolate the stromal vascular fraction in order to combine it with the fat to be grafted, a 90 min procedure designed to enhance the population of ADSCs in the fat graft. Injection was performed with 150 mm long 18-gauge needles into one of four injection sites (two periareolar, two inframammary) to distribute fat "on, around and under the mammary glands and also into the pectoralis muscles". An average of 273 mL of fat was grafted into each breast during a procedure that required, on average, over 4 h. Results were measured by the increase in chest circumference, which was between 4 and 8 cm at 6 months, corresponding to a 100–200 mL increase in the volume of each breast mound or "two to

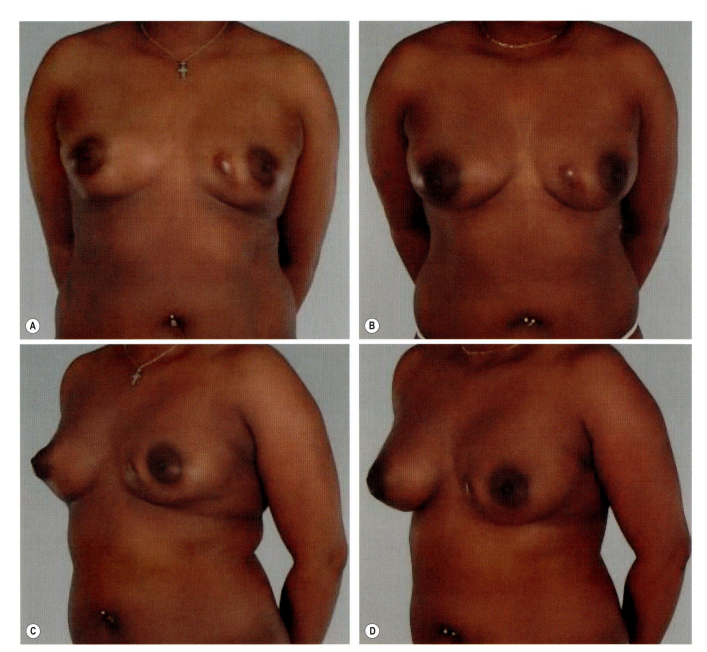

Fig. 24.9 A patient with approximately a one cup size increase after autologous fat grafting for breast augmentation. **(A,B)** Preoperative. **(C,D)** A 1-year postoperative view after one session of 300 cc of fat grafting to each breast.

three brassiere cup sizes". The authors state that "almost all" of the patients were satisfied with their enlarged breasts but did not quantify this and also did not have a separate panel to judge the results subjectively. MRI detected cysts in two patients, and mammography found two patients with microcalcifications at 24 months.

In 2008, Zocchi and Zuliani reported on 181 patients for breast augmentation with fat grafting.[41] They injected processed fat into the retroglandular and periglandular subcutaneous plane, using a disposable 2 mm cannula with a single hole for harvesting with negative pressure generated by a 60 mL syringe. Fat is "processed" only

by vibration of the upright syringes on a special vibrating table to stratify the fat into layers. Fat is then reimplanted into the above planes using special 2 mm cannulas: a flexible 27 cm-long one for the retroglandular plane and a stiffer 25 cm-long one for the subcutaneous plane. They injected an average of 325 mL or 375 mL of fat into each breast (two different numbers are reported in their article) and also utilized an external breast expansion device (BRAVA, Miami, FL) in some patients. The authors state that some patients did not comply with external expansion but do not reveal how many. Rating the aesthetic results, 38 patients (23%) judged them as excellent; 128 (72%) as good; 10 (6%) as

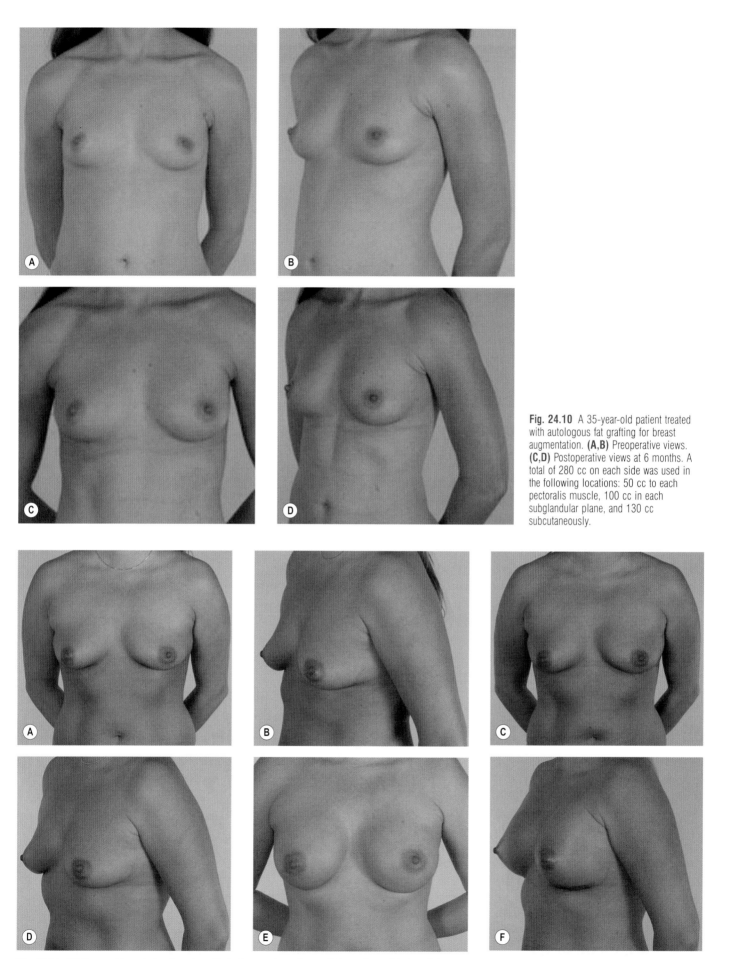

Fig. 24.10 A 35-year-old patient treated with autologous fat grafting for breast augmentation. **(A,B)** Preoperative views. **(C,D)** Postoperative views at 6 months. A total of 280 cc on each side was used in the following locations: 50 cc to each pectoralis muscle, 100 cc in each subglandular plane, and 130 cc subcutaneously.

Fig. 24.11 **(A)** Preoperative anterior view of a patient who experienced essentially no discernible benefit from fat grafting for breast augmentation. **(B)** Preoperative oblique view. **(C)** Postoperative anterior view of the patient 1 year after 165 cc autologous fat grafting to each breast. **(D)** A 1-year postoperative oblique view after grafting. **(E)** Anterior view of the patient 1 year postoperatively from bilateral prosthetic augmentation with 339 cc silicone implants. **(F)** A 1-year postoperative oblique view after implants.

fair; and five (3%) as insufficient. The surgeon judged them as excellent in 23 cases (13%); good in 123 (69%); fair in 25 (12%); and insufficient in 10 (6%). The authors state that an average of 55% of grafted volume persisted at 1 year but do not state how this was measured. Complications were not quantified, except to say they were "minimal and temporary" and that microcalcifications were found in some patients. While this study reports on a relatively large number of patients, it is mostly an informal report of cases.

With little quality data having been published on breast augmentation with fat grafting,[8] several clinical trials have been started in the US to better study the issue. Autologous fat grafting for cosmetic augmentation has been performed under research protocols in Miami,[25] Washington, DC,[32] and New Orleans.[33] Spear and Pittman have published a prospective evaluation of 10 women following lipoaugmentation as a sole modality.[42] The average amount of fat injected was 236 cc in the right breast and 250 cc in the left breast. The mean change in volume was 85 cc on the right and 98 cc on the left correlating to a retention volume of 36% and 39%, respectively. This was assessed using 3D imaging and MRI volume measurements. Mammographic imaging demonstrated a BIRADs score of 2 or higher in 50% of women.

Candidates for lipoaugmentation of the breast should have low risk factors for breast cancer. In addition, it is preferred that they have no personal history of benign breast disease. They must also have sufficient donor sites to support at least two stages of fat harvest for each session. Preoperative MRI is recommended as a baseline as well as a preoperative mammogram if the patient is aged 40 or over. Finally, a frank discussion with the patient about potential implications of fat grafting for cancer screening must occur, and a detailed informed consent should be included. The authors recommend that the surgeons performing breast augmentation with autologous fat grafting do so under Institutional Review Board oversight.

Total breast reconstruction

For the most ardent advocates of fat grafting of the breast, the next great opportunity is reconstructing the entire breast with autologous fat injections. The authors have never personally performed this, but total breast reconstruction for the patient with postmastectomy or congenital absence of the breast is possible. Anecdotal cases have been reported at various symposia and on websites by researchers involved in clinical trials.[25] Khouri *et al.* have recently reported their experience using external expansion and autologous fat grafting in 488 women and 616 breasts.[24] Of

these, 430 breasts were reconstructed using fat graft only. The average fat infiltration was 225 cc per session. The number of sessions was 2.7 for the non-radiated cohort of patients and 4.8 for the radiated cohort of patients. Complications included five pneumothoraces and 20 infections. Benign nodules were noted in 12% of non-radiated breasts and in 37% of radiated breasts. Patients reported normal and soft breasts with reasonable sensation.

Treatment/surgical technique

The defect is analyzed, using as much information as is available, including preoperative photographs, the contralateral normal breast, the original operative note, and pathology reports. The latter is especially valuable when reconstructing lumpectomy defects, since it typically contains a specimen weight, which can be used to plan the graft volume. Informed consent is obtained. Estimates of volume to be grafted are made to assist with determining what volume to harvest from the donor site.

The patient is marked in the standing position (Fig. 24.12), when areas of contour irregularity can be most clearly seen because of shadows created by overhead lighting. This most important step ensures that areas noticeable while standing are not overlooked when the patient is supine, with powerful surgical lights overhead that obscure shadows. The surgeon estimates the amount of fat needed for grafting and marks appropriate donor sites. After fat harvest and processing per the surgeon's preference, grafting is performed in a manner appropriate to the deformity being treated. Depressions are treated with multiple tunnels in a

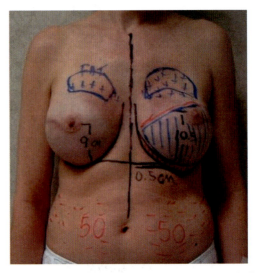

Fig. 24.12 Preoperative marking of the same patient as in Fig. 24.2. Areas for autologous fat grafting are denoted by the blue outline with "+" signs superiorly on each breast. The patient has also been marked for the left capsulorrhaphy.

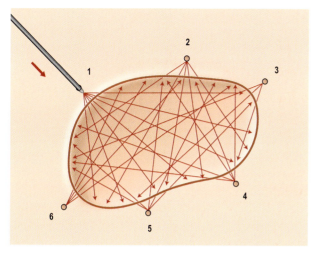

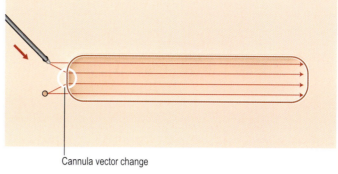

Fig. 24.15 Multiple longitudinal vectors used to treat longitudinal depressions (such as the edge of a flap or implant). Note vector change to permit multiple parallel treatment tunnels from a minimum of injection sites.

Fig. 24.13 Top view with defect borders marked with the bold line. Multiple criss-crossing tunnels across a typical small contour deformity, with six separate injection sites located at the periphery (1–6). Each tunnel may receive different amounts of graft along its length depending on the needs of the area and amounts already grafted by previous tunnels originating from other injection sites.

cross-hatch fashion (Figs. 24.13 & 24.14), while ridges and rippling respond best to a few long tunnels below the longitudinal depression (Fig. 24.15). Depressed areas with substantial scarring from fat necrosis or radiation damage may benefit from scar release with specialized cannulas that have cutting edges (Fig. 24.16). Care must be exercised when using these instruments – their effect can be quite destructive to an implant and catastrophic near a flap pedicle.

Multiple locations are selected as graft insertion sites. This may be as few as 4–8 around a lumpectomy defect or as many as 20 for breast augmentation. A blunt-tipped cannula attached to a 3 mL syringe is used to inject small volumes of fat during the withdrawal phase of the cannula movement. The cannula is passed repeatedly in a radial pattern from each injection site, with the goal being an interwoven mesh pattern of graft deposition at multiple levels. For breast augmentation, it is important

to attempt to stay within the subcutaneous plane and not within breast parenchyma during graft injection. Additional volume for augmentation may be grafted into the subglandular, intramuscular, and submuscular planes. Minimal "molding" is performed externally; the emphasis should be on correct and even graft deposition during cannula withdrawal. When the goal volume is reached, the injection sites are closed with adhesive strips and conforming dressing applied to the breast.

Notes on harvesting and processing fat

Appropriate donor site selection includes any area that has sufficient fat to donate, typically the abdomen, hips, and thighs. The site selected can be based on ease of harvest and patient preference, since no studies have demonstrated superiority of different sites in graft survival.[43]

Standard liposuction infiltration is performed with a dilute epinephrine-containing solution to minimize blood loss. To harvest the fat, all that is needed is an appropriate cannula attached to a means of suction and a collection container. Most practitioners use a 3 mm multi-hole cannula to harvest fat intended for use in the

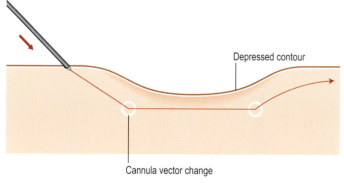

Fig. 24.14 A typical contour depression viewed from the side, with the cannula positioned at the top left near the injection site. Note the changes in directional vector the cannula must undergo as it traverses the bottom of the defect concavity. These depend on a rigid cannula and sometimes releasing underlying tethering scar tissue.

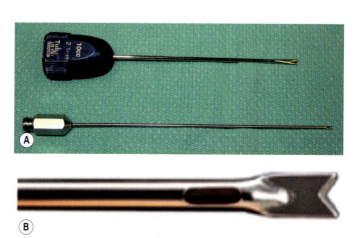

Fig. 24.16 (A,B) V-shaped dissectors. (©*Tulip, Byron Medical, with permission.*)

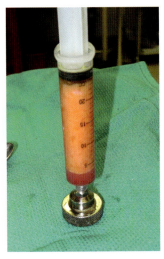

Fig. 24.17 Aspiration syringe standing upright. Note aqueous layer below aspirated fat and oil layer above aspirated fat.

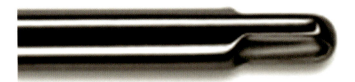

Fig. 24.19 Coleman aspiration cannula. (*©Byron Medical, with permission.*)

controversy surrounding the use of SVF is that *in vitro* studies have demonstrated that progenitor cells present in the breast have demonstrated enhanced growth in the presence of SVF.[46,47] Clinical studies that have assessed tumorigenesis in the setting of breast reconstruction and autologous fat grafting have been favorable, demonstrating a biopsy rate of 7.4% and no cases of locoregional cancer recurrence.[48]

Coleman's method

Coleman advocates using a cannula of his design, which has a blunt tip and two adjacent holes (Fig. 24.19). This is connected to a 10 mL syringe to which modest suction is applied when the surgeon's ring and small fingers pull back on the plunger. As the cannula is pushed through the harvest site, a combination of the curetting action of the cannula and the negative pressure pulls fat into the syringe. When the syringe is full, it is disconnected from the cannula, capped at the Luer connector end with a sterile cap, and the plunger is removed. The open end of the syringe may be covered with a Tegaderm (3M) to maintain sterility of syringe contents after plunger removal.[49] The syringe is placed into a sterile sleeve in a small centrifuge (Fig. 24.20). Other syringes are added, and the centrifuge spins the contents at 3000 rpm for 3 min.

breast. Next, the aspirated fat is refined by removing oil, blood, and infiltrate fluid. The simplest method of this is to allow the aspiration syringe to stand for 10–15 min (Fig. 24.17).[44] Finally, the processed fat is reinjected (Fig. 24.18) to the intended recipient site using a specialized injection cannula. Sydney Coleman, MD, was the earliest recent practitioner to codify and publish reliable steps, and his method is detailed below, followed by alternative methods that have been used successfully by other practitioners.

Some practitioners are considering the use of stromal vascular fraction (SVF) for fat infiltration. Essentially, this involves the enzymatic processing of fat to increase the concentration of ADSCs. The benefit of SVF is that the overall fat retention is enhanced and may approach 80% rather than the conventional 40–60%.[20,45] The

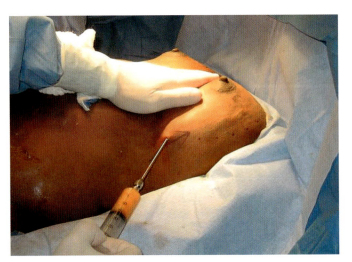

Fig. 24.18 Processed fat is grafted into the patient, in this case for breast augmentation.

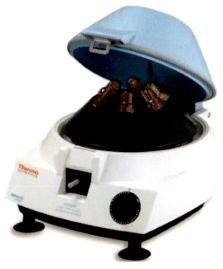

Fig. 24.20 Small centrifuge. (*Photo courtesy of Thermo Fisher Scientific, Inc. Reprinted with permission.*)

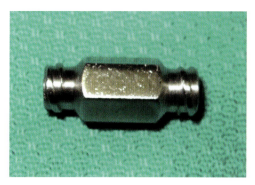

Fig. 24.21 Luer-to-Luer connector. (©Tulip, Byron Medical, with permission.)

After centrifugation, the syringe contents have been separated by density. The upper level of oil (ruptured adipocytes from aspiration) is removed by pouring it off and then removing any remainder with absorbent wicks of Telfa (Kendall). The bottom, densest level contains blood as well as infiltrate and is removed by briefly removing the cap and allowing it to drain. Using a Luer-to-Luer connector (Fig. 24.21), the prepared fat is transferred into 3 mL syringes ready for injection into the recipient site.

Alternative methods

Critics of Coleman's method point to the multiple small harvest syringes and two-hole cannula as unnecessarily time-consuming. Other practitioners therefore use larger syringes and multi-hole cannulas (available from Tulip Medical Products, San Diego, CA) or a modified liposuction set-up with a fat trap,[50,51] along with a cannula with multiple (10–12) holes to speed the process. A simple method of straining the fat is by using a sterilizable kitchen strainer (Fig. 24.22) to remove the aqueous and oil layers or standing the syringe up to allow the layers to separate as described above. The fat is then quickly (to prevent desiccation) transferred to a large syringe (using a sterile spoon or scalpel handle), from which point it is distributed to the smaller 3 cc or 1 cc syringes (using a Luer-to-Luer or 3-way connector) for grafting back into the patient.

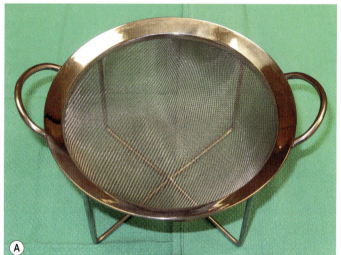

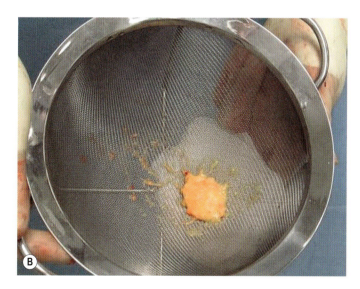

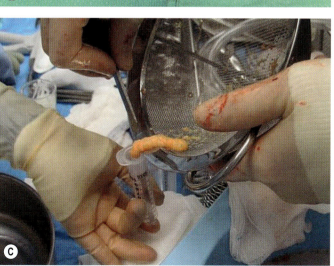

Fig. 24.22 (A) Sterilizable kitchen strainer. **(B)** A small amount of prepared fat after straining and washing. Note folded gauze against the fat beneath the strainer; this quickly wicks moisture from the strained graft. **(C)** Prepared fat is transferred to a 10 cc syringe for injection.

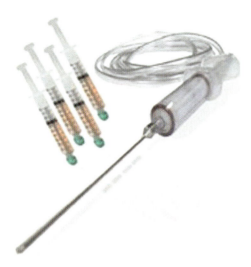

Fig. 24.23 LipiVage fat harvest system. (©*Genesis Biosystems, with permission.*)

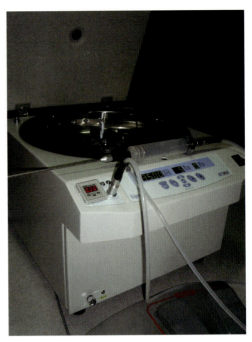

Fig. 24.25 Lipokit centrifuge. (©*Medi-Khan, with permission.*)

The harvesting and processing of fat is now being commercialized, with specialized systems available, which simplify many of the steps and provide "one-stop shopping" for the equipment necessary. These systems, such as those available from LipiVage (Fig. 24.23), Lipokit (Figs. 24.24 & 24.25), and Cytori (Fig. 24.26), promise substantial time savings for grafting. These systems provide standardization and simplicity and eliminate the need to collect the proper instruments, sometimes from several sources, to have an effective set-up. The drawbacks are that they are largely unproven and their cost is high.

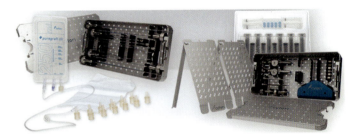

Fig. 24.26 Cytori Puregraft 250. (©*Cytori Therapeutics Inc, with permission.*)

Injection technique

Different cannulas are used for injection to those for harvesting. Typically, the injection cannula is a blunt cannula with a single hole for precise fat deposition (Fig. 24.27) and is available in different lengths and flexibilities. The cannula has a Luer connector for fitting to a syringe containing processed fat. If scarring is present

and needs to be released, a sharp cannula is used selectively (see Fig. 24.16). An 11-blade may be used to create the 2 mm hole for introduction of the injection cannula, which is advanced through an area of the intended fat grafting. As the cannula is withdrawn, slow and even pressure on the syringe plunger deposits a fine cylinder of fat into the tunnel created by introduction of the cannula.

The proper technique of depositing an even layer of fat one-handed during cannula withdrawal is a skilled practice. Some practitioners use an IV extension tubing to technically separate the process, permitting an assistant to focus only on plunger pressure while they focus

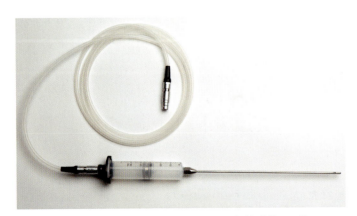

Fig. 24.24 Lipokit 60 cc syringe with suction tubing. (©*Medi-Khan, with permission.*)

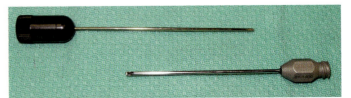

Fig. 24.27 Injection cannulae by Tulip (1.4 mm) and Byron (2 mm). (©*Byron Medical, with permission.*)

on a slow and even cannula withdrawal.[28] It is here also that the fat preparation technique may have implications for the consistent deposition of the grafted fat. The compression that results from a high-speed centrifuge or the existence of connective tissue clumps may create an obstacle to the even flow of grafted fat through the injection cannula. This leads some practitioners to prefer one preparation technique over another. Open straining permits removal of aspirated connective tissue clumps, and a low-speed centrifuge technique (Spingraft) packs the fat less tightly. Because increased pressure can sometimes clear a clump from the cannula, resulting in sudden focal overgrafting, it is best to avoid this situation entirely by stopping the procedure to clear a stoppage.[52]

The protocol of the senior author of this chapter (S.L. Spear) in a current clinical trial of breast augmentation with autologous fat at Georgetown is as follows: low-pressure vacuum aspiration is used with a 3-hole cannula to harvest fat from selected sites. Fat is transferred to 10 cc syringes for centrifuging, after which oil is decanted from the top and the aqueous component is poured out of the bottom of the syringe. Using periareolar and inframammary access incisions and a single-hole 2 mm cannula, fat is infiltrated into three planes: the subcutaneous, subglandular, and intramuscular. The exact amounts of grafting to each of these planes vary with the patient.

Brava

The Brava device (Brava LLC, Miami, FL) was initially developed as an external breast tissue expander, the goal of which was non-surgical breast augmentation.[53] The device consists of two semirigid polyurethane domes that are placed over each breast and seal at its periphery with silicone gel-filled donut bladders (Fig. 24.28). A small pump maintains 20 mmHg of negative pressure inside the domes, which are worn continuously for 10 h a day for a minimum of 10 weeks, if the device is used alone. One cup size increase can reasonably be expected, with the increase in size being maintained over time. The limited permanent size increase and compliance difficulties temper its more widespread use.

On the other hand, the device causes a temporary increase in the size of the breasts, past what can be expected to be maintained, due to swelling. This is effectively an expansion of the scaffold of soft tissues that comprise the breast, and is thought to have a salutary effect on fat graft survival. When used before autologous fat grafting for breast augmentation or reconstruction (for this indication, only 3–4 weeks is needed), it is thought to increase both the volume possible to graft and graft survival percentage. Studies are

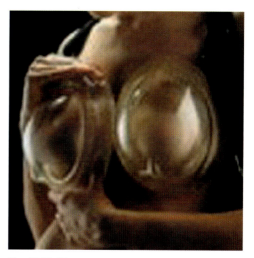

Fig. 24.28 BRAVA device. (©*BRAVA LLC, with permission.*)

presently underway to quantify these effects,[32,33] and initial results are encouraging.[30] If proven effective and reproducible, this technique may transform autologous breast reconstruction into a previously impossible minimally-invasive procedure for patients.

Postoperative care

Skin closure of the 2 mm access slits may be made with fine suture or adhesive strips, and a loosely supportive breast garment is fitted with cotton fluffs over grafted areas. Cool compresses reduce swelling, and the patient is encouraged to minimize arm movements for a week. The donor site is treated with a compressive garment similarly to any area of liposuction.

Acute swelling can be expected for 1–2 weeks but may persist for months. If a contour deformity remains after swelling has resolved, we recommend waiting at least 6 months prior to attempting another round of grafting. Physical examination and radiographic follow-up follow the same schedule as for any other breast surgery.

Hints and tips

- Use fat grafting on reconstructive contour deformities early in your experience, preferably while already performing a different procedure requiring general anesthesia.
- Basic instrumentation and techniques work well, are inexpensive, and provide an easy way to get started.
- Overgraft less if fat is centrifuged during processing.
- Appropriate patient expectations are important. Impressive results are possible but may require more than one session of grafting.

Outcomes, prognosis, and complications

Patient outcomes

Outcomes are illustrated in Figs. 24.1–24.11 for each of the indications listed above.

Graft survival

Early practitioners, using free *en bloc* fat grafts, noted substantial resorption of their free fat grafts and tried various measures to prevent this, such as transplanting fascia with the fat[54] or cutting the graft into several pieces.[55] Early reports of graft survival ranged from 25% to 50%, so early practitioners began to advocate the practice of overgrafting.[56,57] The modern method of transplanting fat by injecting it has not altered this recommendation, though there seems to be no consensus as to how much overgrafting should be done.

Graft survival percentage varies with the methods used to aspirate, prepare, and transplant the fat. It also varies with respect to the destination of the graft, with fat grafted into well-vascularized muscle surviving at a higher rate than fat grafted into a relatively oxygen-poor environment such as a depressed breast contour from fat necrosis of a TRAM flap. Some recent authors define the amount of overgrafting that should be performed in the breast; for example, Emmanuel Delay, grafting into reconstructed breasts, writes that he plans on 30% resorption rate and advocates overgrafting by 40%.[10] Kanchwala *et al.*[9] recommend overgrafting by no more than 10% to avoid fat necrosis and subsequent calcifications. These authors' experience supports overgrafting amounts in these approximate ranges for contour deformities. Preparation method matters; fat processed with washing and straining needs more overgrafting than centrifuged fat. Until more specific research is performed on the subject, there is no substitute from the personal experience of beginning conservatively. It is recommended that judicious overgrafting should be performed early in a surgeon's experience until one acquires a "feel" for how much overgrafting should be performed based on the technique being used and the quality of the recipient bed. Reconstructive contour deformities in non-radiated fields lend themselves well to this early experience.

Complications

There are risks in any surgical procedure, and autologous fat grafting to the female breast is no exception. Major complications are rare, and the ones reported in the literature are often the result of procedures being performed by poorly-trained practitioners.[58,59] Even when properly performed, however, there are certain events which occur with enough regularity to be highlighted in the informed consent.

Mammographic abnormalities[60–65] are relevant in patients who have not had a mastectomy. After breast augmentation with fat grafting, the most commonly seen abnormalities are calcifications. These come in the form of either coarse or fine microcalcifications and are thought to be the result of areas of fat necrosis. They can usually be readily distinguished from suspicious patterns by an experienced radiographer; those that cannot should be biopsied. Mammography can also detect oil cysts, which may also be palpable on exam. Preoperative mammography is recommended prior to autologous fat grafting to the breast for augmentation for comparison purposes in the event of any abnormality developing later. With respect to interference with breast cancer detection, the ASPS Fat Graft Task Force concluded, in its 2009 report: "Based on a limited number of studies with few cases, there appears to be no interference with breast cancer detection; however, more studies are needed to confirm these preliminary findings".[8]

Liponecrotic cysts or oil cysts, occur in areas of walled-off liquefaction necrosis. These can be multiple and small or, on occasion, quite large. A cyst is effectively treated by surgical excision. Their development probably correlates with improper technique of inadequately distributing the grafted fat – or attempting to graft too much fat into a particular area.[66,67] In his experience of 880 patients, Delay reports that approximately 15% of his patients developed oil cysts on mammogram.[10]

Infection may occur after fat injection and typically presents as painful swelling with erythema, warmth, and sometimes fever. The outcome of infection is variable, with reports of both loss of the grafted fat[4] and no effect on the results,[10] but abscess formation with sepsis has been reported in the literature.[68]

Persistent swelling. If swelling persists for over 2 months, it may signal the development of fat necrosis or a liponecrotic cyst. The index of suspicion for either of these complications is higher with higher volumes of grafted fat. Watchful waiting is the best course of action, since early imaging studies can be expected to show nonspecific inflammation. If a cyst is suspected, it may be detected with ultrasound.

Neoplasia risk is perhaps theoretical. The same qualities of ADSCs that make them regenerative (such as angiogenesis) might be shown in the future to increase the risk of breast cancer for the patient. In a literature review encompassing 283 patients undergoing fat grafting to the breast for cosmetic and reconstructive purposes, the ASPS Fat Graft Task Force report identified two cases of breast cancer.[8] One was in an area of the breast that was not grafted, and one was in an area potentially grafted, but there was no delay in diagnosis or treatment.[5] Only further study will prove or disprove any correlation between fat grafting and the development of subsequent breast cancer; until that time, the risk of neoplasia must be classified as unknown.

Secondary procedures

Fat grafting may need to be repeated, and it is often necessary to do so (Fig. 24.29). A recent retrospective review of 110 patients who underwent fat grafting for contour deformities in reconstructed breasts found that 55% of the patients required more than one session to satisfactorily correct the deformities.[9] More sessions can be expected in hostile environments such as irradiated fields.[31] Additional sessions may also be required for breast augmentation, depending on the goals of the patient, since there is a limit as to how much fat can be

realistically grafted into each breast at one time to expect reasonably good take of the graft. This limit varies patient-to-patient and is probably higher in patients who have undergone external pre-expansion.

Conclusions

Autologous fat grafting to the female breast is here to stay and will continue to evolve as practitioners continue to refine the technique and discover new applications of the grafted adipocyte. Established indications include contour deformities in breasts reconstructed by a variety of methods. No longer are practitioners debating whether fat grafting works; what is being discussed is the appropriate role of the more controversial indications, such as breast augmentation or total breast reconstruction. The next decade is likely to see more established protocols for these indications, as well as further progress defining the potential therapeutic power of ADSCs.

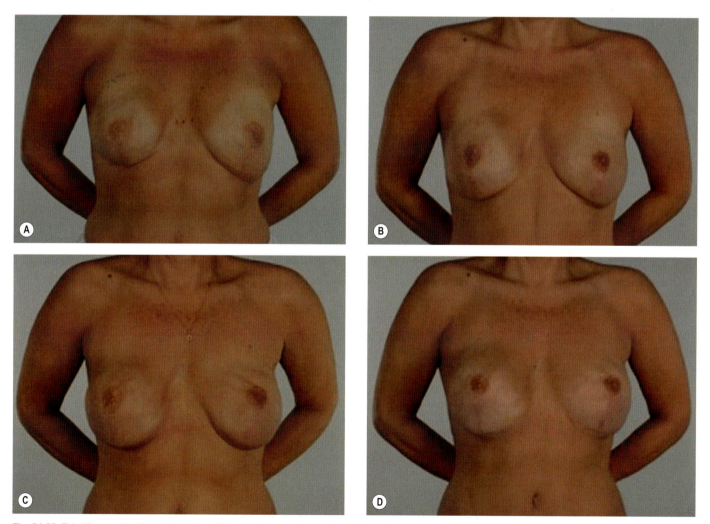

Fig. 24.29 This 49-year-old patient underwent multiple sessions of autologous fat grafting after bilateral nipple-sparing mastectomies with tissue expander reconstructions. **(A)** At 9 months after bilateral immediate breast reconstruction with tissue expanders. **(B)** The same patient 3 months after bilateral exchange of tissue expanders for 560 cc gel implants and fat grafting to superior poles; 80 cc right and 40 cc left. **(C)** A 4 months postoperative view after bilateral exchange to 650 cc gel implants and 75 cc fat grafting to the superomedial and inferomedial quadrants bilaterally. **(D)** At 9 months after bilateral breast scar revisions and fat grafting of 35 cc to each upper pole.

4. Spear S, Wilson H, Lockwood M. Fat injection to correct contour deformities in the reconstructed breast. *Plast Reconstr Surg.* 2005;116:1300–1305. *This article helped initiate the recent resurgence in interest in fat grafting to the breast and remains a good overview of real-world results and typical complications.*

5. Coleman SR, Saboeiro AP. Fat grafting to the breast revisited: safety and efficacy. *Plast Reconstr Surg.* 2007;119:775–785. *This comprehensive review with impressive results furthered the call to legitimize fat grafting to the breast and reverse the ASPS's 1987 condemnation of the practice.*

6. Missana MD, Laurent I, Barreau L, et al. Autologous fat transfer in reconstructive breast surgery: indications, technique and results. *Eur J Surg Oncol.* 2007;33:685–690.

8. Gutowski K. Current applications and safety of autologous fat grafts: a report of the ASPS Fat Graft Task Force. *Plast Reconstr Surg.* 2009;124:272–280. *The ASPS Fat Graft Task Force reports the results of a critical appraisal of the current literature on indications for autologous fat grafting and the risks associated with it.*

9. Kanchwala SK, Glatt BS, Conant EF, et al. Autologous fat grafting to the reconstructed breast: the management of acquired contour deformities. *Plast Reconstr Surg.* 2009;124:410–418.

10. Delay E, Garson S, Tousson G, et al. Fat injection to the breast: technique, results, and indications based on 880 procedures over 10 years. *Aesthetic Surg J.* 2009;29:360–376.

12. Mizuno M, Hyakusoku H. Fat grafting to the breast and adipose-derived stem cells: recent scientific consensus and controversy. *Aesthetic Surg J.* 2010;30:381–387. *An accessible current review article covering complications and ADSCs.*

31. Rigotti G, Marchi A, Galie M, et al. Clinical treatment of radiotherapy tissue damage by lipoaspirate transplant: a healing process mediated by adipose-derived adult stem cells. *Plast Reconstr Surg.* 2007;119:1409–1424. *A landmark article reporting on the efficacy of ADSCs at reversing radiation damage to the breast.*

35. Serra-Renom JM, Del Olmo JM, Serra-Mestre JM. Fat grafting in post mastectomy breast reconstruction with expanders and prosthesis in patients who have received radiotherapy: formation of new subcutaneous tissue. *Plast Reconstr Surg.* 2010;125:12–18.

58. Hyakusoku H, Ogawa R, Ono S, et al. Complications after autologous fat injection to the breast. *Plast Reconstr Surg.* 2009;123:360–370.

25

Radiation therapy considerations in the setting of breast reconstruction

Elizabeth Stirling Craig and Steven Kronowitz

Access video lecture content for this chapter online at expertconsult.com

SYNOPSIS

- Radiation therapy is a vital component of breast cancer multimodality treatment with proven benefits in decreasing local recurrence and improving long-term survival in select breast cancer patient populations.
- The negative effects of radiation therapy on short- and long-term complication rates, aesthetic outcomes, and patient satisfaction pose challenges for successful breast reconstruction in these patients.
- Irradiated skin and soft tissue are susceptible to delayed wound healing and often confer poor cosmetic outcomes and reconstructive failures.
- Radiation therapy protocols and specific strategies for breast cancer must be understood and considered in the treatment planning of patients who will undergo breast reconstruction.
- Breast reconstructive procedures, strategies, and techniques in the setting of radiation therapy must be fully considered in breast cancer patients to optimize outcomes.

Introduction

Despite the increasing incidence of breast cancer in the US over the past decade, early detection and more effective treatments have led to a steady decline in breast cancer mortality. Radiation therapy is a vital component of breast cancer multimodality treatment and has shown benefits in decreasing local recurrence and improving long-term survival in select breast cancer patient populations. However, the negative effects of radiation therapy on short- and long-term complication rates, aesthetic outcomes, and patient satisfaction all pose significant challenges for reconstructive surgeons in planning and performing breast reconstruction in patients who have had or may need radiation therapy. In this setting, understanding the specific radiation treatment protocols and strategies for breast cancer is paramount to managing the disease, minimizing complications, and maximizing aesthetic outcomes. Similarly, understanding the effects of radiation on specific breast reconstruction techniques, situations, and timing is crucial to planning, educating patients, and achieving the best result. This chapter discusses these important considerations for planning and delivering radiation therapy and for performing reconstructive procedures in patients with breast cancer.

Radiation therapy in breast cancer patients

The 2014 National Comprehensive Cancer Network (NCCN) Guidelines recommend post-mastectomy chest wall and nodal radiation for women at high risk for local recurrence of breast cancer, in particular those with close tumor margins (<1 mm), with T3 or T4 tumors, or with four or more positive axillary lymph nodes. Until recently, women with 1–3 positive nodes received variable recommendations for adjuvant radiation therapy. The NCIC-CTG MA.20 trial enrolled 1832 women (85% of which had 1–3 positive nodes) who underwent breast conservation, adjuvant chemotherapy, or endocrine therapy, and had received whole breast irradiation. The participants were then randomized to receive whole breast radiation therapy alone or in combination with regional nodal radiation therapy. There was significant improvement in disease-free interval and overall survival for patients who received the additional nodal radiation therapy. Although these data were derived from women who underwent breast-conserving surgery, its results are being extrapolated to include benefits for post-mastectomy patients. As a result, the new NCCN recommendations are for nodal irradiation for post-mastectomy women with 1–3 positive lymph nodes.

Breast conservation patients who undergo segmental mastectomy receive adjuvant whole breast irradiation as part of their standard treatment unless they are pregnant, received previous chest wall or breast radiation, or are older than 70 years of age and have hormone receptor-positive disease. Breast cancer patients who elect *not* to undergo adjuvant whole breast radiation have a three times higher risk of local recurrence and have a relative risk of death of 1.086, or an 8.6% increased chance of death when compared with those patients who *do* undergo adjuvant radiation therapy.

Locally advanced breast cancer is a collective term used to describe clinical stage III breast cancers, which represent either neglected primary tumors that slowly progress in unscreened patients or aggressive, high-grade tumors that rapidly proliferate between screening intervals. Understanding tumor biology and molecular subtype is paramount to providing targeted, effective therapy for all breast cancers, but in particular for locally advanced disease. Inflammatory breast cancer is the most aggressive subgroup of locally advanced breast cancers, with an elevated risk of local recurrence and distant metastasis. This patient population benefits most from multimodality treatment including neoadjuvant chemotherapy, surgery, radiation therapy, and endocrine therapy where indicated. Neoadjuvant chemotherapy is often necessary to convert these cancers into resectable tumors or to permit a breast-conserving approach, provided that the response to therapy is favorable.[1] In such cases, recommendations for adjuvant treatment, in particular radiation therapy, are made based on the tumor characteristics before chemotherapy, irrespective of tumor response. The majority, if not all, patients with locally advanced breast cancer are advised to receive adjuvant radiation to both the chest wall and nodal basins.

Radiation therapy during whole breast radiation is targeted towards the breast, subcutaneous tissue, chest wall, scar, and often drain sites. Computed tomography-based treatment planning assists in delivering the targeted dose of 45–50 Gy while minimizing radiation to the heart and lungs. Classic radiation techniques include using medial and lateral beams angled at tangents to reduce exposure to surrounding structures. Wedges, shielding blocks, and compensators were previously used to modify the intensity of the beams and reduce hot and cold spots; however, today these protective techniques have largely been replaced with the use of intensity-modulated radiation therapy (IMRT). IMRT modulates the intensity of multiple beams by using dynamic multileaf collimators that shield the various beams and allow for 3D conformal therapy. This technique delivers high precision radiation therapy and reduces treatment time.[2]

Nodal irradiation requires additional planning and is included based on previous stated NCCN recommendations. The lower axilla nodes (level I) are incidentally covered during standard breast and chest wall irradiation; however, levels II, III, and the internal mammary (IM) nodes are generally not included.[3] Patients with T3 or greater primary disease or those who had four or more positive lymph nodes and underwent axillary dissection of level I or II are at highest risk of disease recurrence in the level III (supraclavicular) area and should therefore receive targeted supraclavicular irradiation.[3] However, the apex of the lung receives a full dose of radiation when treating the supraclavicular area, and this should be taken into consideration with previous treatment plans to avoid a double dose of radiation.

Radiation therapy of the IM nodes is widely debated in the literature. Despite the Danish and British Columbia trials illustrating improved overall survival when treating the IM nodes of patients with 1–3 positive nodes, many radiation oncologists believe that IM node failures are rare and that the benefit of treatment is not warranted.[3] Treatment of IM nodes can be accomplished with either extra-wide tangent arrangements or use of an additional electron field, but both bear significant risks.[2] The concern with using extra-wide tangent techniques is the large radiation dose delivered to the underlying lung. Using a separate electron beam radiation for treating the IM nodes is an alternative technique to avoid extra-wide tangents, but does require a flat surface, has a limited depth of penetration, and can, therefore, be problematic in obtaining the necessary dose in cases of immediate breast reconstruction. Achieving an adequate radiation dose with the electron beam to the IM nodes while avoiding critical structures, such as those of the underlying breast reconstruction (tissue expander, implant, or flap), lung parenchyma, or the contralateral breast, can be particularly challenging.[2]

An additional radiation bolus dose of 10–16 Gy is often delivered to the tumor bed, scar, or the entire chest wall in select cases such as in patients with inflammatory breast cancer or those at highest risk of local recurrence (patients age <50 years, with positive nodes, with lymphovascular invasion, or with close tumor margins). Bolus doses can be delivered with photons, electrons, or less commonly, with brachytherapy. Controversy exists as to the optimal method to deliver a radiation boost.

Boost treatment is often associated with extensive fibrosis and, therefore, with compromised cosmesis.[2]

In an effort to minimize dose-related fibrosis and compromised cosmesis, hypofractionation and accelerated whole breast radiation have recently emerged as newer strategies for delivering radiation therapy.

Accelerated partial breast irradiation (APBI) involves treating the lumpectomy cavity and the surrounding 2 cm margin with larger daily fractions to achieve biologically equivalent total dosages. ABPI offers the advantages of sparing the remaining breast tissue and delivering an accelerated daily dose that truncates the necessary treatment time period. There is a theoretical concern that when using this technique, an occult foci of cancer in a remote location from the tumor cavity could be left untreated and thus increase the risk of local recurrence; however, fewer than 4% of recurrences are found distant to the tumor cavity.[4] Several techniques for delivering APBI are described: interstitial brachytherapy, balloon brachytherapy, 3D conformal radiation therapy, and intraoperative radiotherapy, all of which currently remain experimental with limited phase III data. The Radiation Therapy Oncology Group (RTOG)0413/National Surgical Adjuvant Breast and Bowel Project (NSABP) B-39 is a prospectively, randomized phase III trial comparing APBI with traditional whole breast radiation. Until these results are available, the American Society of Therapeutic Radiology and Oncology (ASTRO) has published guidelines for APBI patient selection (Table 25.1).[4]

Hypofractionated whole breast radiation entails the delivery of higher daily fraction doses over a shorter period of time to reach total doses bioequivalent to traditional whole breast radiotherapy. Until recently, conventional radiotherapy was delivered in small daily fractions to take advantage of the differential in sensitivity to fraction size between tumor cells and normal tissue. However, reports recently found conflicting evidence showing *similar* sensitivities to dose fraction size between normal tissue and tumor cells, thus negating the need for prolonged treatment that delivers small daily fractions. With the increasing demand for shorter therapy regimens, trials comparing hypofractionated regimens with traditional whole breast radiation have emerged, specifically in regard to local recurrence control and long-term toxicity. The FAST trial is a randomized trial aimed to compare conventional radiation with two hypofractionated regimens (30 Gy in five

Table 25.1 ASTRO guidelines for accelerated partial breast irradiation (APBI)

	Suitable	Cautionary	Unsuitable
Age (years)	≥60	50–59	<50
BRCA 1/2 mutation	Not present	–	Present
Tumor size (cm)	≤2	2.1–3	>3
T-stage	T1	T0 or T2	T3–4
Margins	Negative by at least 2 mm	Close (<2 mm)	Positive
Grade	Any	–	–
LVSI	No	Limited/focal	Extensive
ER status	Positive	Negative	–
Multicentricity	Unicentric only	–	Present
Multifocality	Unifocal	Clinically unifocal with total size 2.1–3 cm	Clinically multifocal or microscopically multifocal >3 cm
Histology	Invasive ductal, mucinous, tubular, or colloid	Invasive lobular	–
Pure DCIS	Not allowed	≤3 cm	If >3 cm in size
Extensive intraductal component	Not allowed	≤3 cm	If >3 cm in size
Associated LCIS	Allowed	–	–
N-stage	pN0 (i–, i+)	–	pN1, pN2, pN3
Nodal surgery	Sentinel lymph node biopsy or axillary lymph node dissection	–	None performed
Neoadjuvant therapy	Not allowed	–	If used

BRCA, breast cancer; DCIS, ductal carcinoma *in situ*; ER, estrogen receptor; LCIS, lobular carcinoma in situ; LVSI, lymphovascular space involvement.
(Reproduced with permission from Moran MS, Rowe BP. Accelerated Partial Breast Irradiation and Hypofractionated Whole Breast Radiation. *Oncology & Hematology Review (US)*. 2011;07(01):31.)

Table 25.2 Criteria for hypofractionation[a]	
1.	Age 50 years or older
2.	Pathologic stage T1–2N0 treated with breast-conserving surgery
3.	Not treated with systemic chemotherapy
4.	Within the breast along the central axis, minimum dose no less than 93% and maximum dose no greater than 107% of the prescription dose (±7%) (as calculated with 2D treatment planning without heterogeneity corrections)

[a]Patients should also be otherwise suitable for breast-conserving therapy (not pregnant, no history of certain collagen-vascular diseases, no prior radiotherapy to the breast, no multicentric disease).
(Reproduced with permission from Moran MS, Rowe BP. Accelerated partial breast irradiation and hypofractionated whole breast radiation. *Oncology & Hematology Review (US)*. 2011;07(01):31.)

fractions and 28.5 Gy in five fractions). Until sufficient phase III data are available, ASTRO has published guidelines for patient selection for hypofractionation radiation therapy (Table 25.2).

Despite the efforts to improve the precision of radiation treatment, irradiated skin and soft tissue remain highly susceptible to delayed wound healing, have decreased wound-break strength, and constitute the number one reason for poor aesthetic outcomes and reconstructive failures.[2] Radiation has acute and chronic side effects that are a result of the total dose and dose per fraction delivered. Acute toxicity is reversible damage that occurs during the daily radiation treatment as a result of DNA damage and manifests as skin erythema and desquamation. As a result of the DNA damage, free radicals are released that interfere with the normal tissues' ability to repair itself. Transforming growth factor-β (TGF-β) is then induced by the inflammatory cascade, resulting in long-term effects such as fibroblast differentiation, modulation of the extra-cellular matrix, and platelet aggregation. As platelets aggregate, they release more TGF-β, in turn setting off a self-perpetuating release of more TGF-β, thus contributing to the chronic fibroblastic state characteristic of the late effects of radiation injury.[2] Physiologically, the optimal time to operate on irradiated skin is the window between the time that acute reaction has resolved and before the development of extensive fibrosis.

Breast reconstruction and planning in the setting of radiation therapy

Repair of partial mastectomy defects

The evolution of oncoplastic techniques has dramatically changed the aesthetic results in patients undergoing partial mastectomy and whole breast radiation. As the population of the US becomes increasingly obese, extensive lumpectomy defects can be reasonably repaired with oncoplastic reductions, provided that there is remaining redundant breast tissue. This affords advantages to many patients who wish to preserve their breast and undergo a breast reduction in cases of macromastia. In addition to the cosmetic advantages, oncoplastic reduction in patients with macromastia facilitates the delivery of whole breast radiation without compromising the long-term oncologic risk.[5] In addition, recent studies have shown that obese patients who undergo breast conservation with oncoplastic reductions have fewer postoperative complications than do patients who undergo tissue expander reconstruction and autologous reconstructions.[5] As a result, breast conservation is increasing, and more extensive local resections are being classified in the category of partial mastectomy.[6]

Incorporating reparative techniques before adjuvant radiation therapy represents the ideal scenario in breast cancer patients; however, there are several important considerations in this patient population. A management algorithm published and described by Kronowitz *et al.* provides a useful guideline in the decision-making process for breast conservation patients (Fig. 25.1).[6]

For patients who present for breast reconstruction after partial mastectomy and adjuvant radiation therapy, the reconstructive method depends largely on the extent of the deformity, its location on the breast mound, and the remaining size of the breast. The advantage for these patients is that the reconstructive method is not reliant on margin status or on the risk of repeat excision, as these patients have already obtained negative margins. However, the tissues have been subjected to radiation (either partial or whole breast) and have pre-existing incisions from the excision, both of which interfere with the pliability of the tissues, wound healing, and potentially with the design of the dermoglandular pedicle and/or skin resection pattern. In addition, repair of partial mastectomy defects following radiation therapy with local tissue rearrangement or dermoglandular pedicles carries a 50% risk of complications. However, patients with smaller (size A or B cup) breasts are not candidates for oncoplastic reduction and benefit most from recruitment of regional non-irradiated soft tissue to fill in the defect with either a thoracodorsal artery perforator flap or latissimus dorsi flap.[6] While these flaps offer additional blood supply and improved wound healing, the cosmetic outcomes of these more extensive procedures tend to be inferior compared with immediate reconstruction that avoids retained skin paddles and a patchwork pattern with contrasting

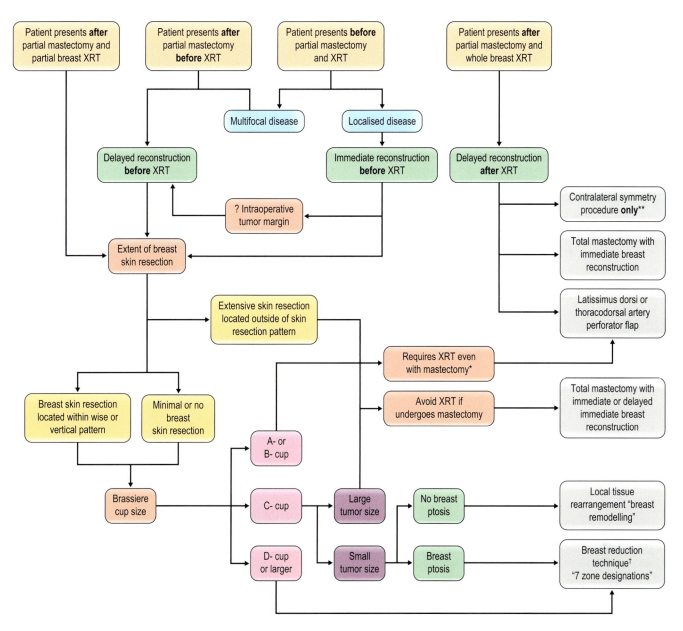

Fig. 25.1 Algorithm for oncoplastic reduction management based on XRT. *(Redrawn with permission from Kronowitz SJ, Kuerer HM, Buchholz TA, Valero V, Hunt KK. A management algorithm and practical oncoplastic surgical techniques for repairing partial mastectomy defects.* Plast Reconstr Surg. *Dec 2008;122(6):1631–1647.)*

color compared with the surrounding irradiated breast skin.[6] Patients who present with significant deformities that would necessitate a retained skin paddle may prefer instead to undergo completion mastectomy and total breast reconstruction as opposed to a partial repair.

Patients who present prior to partial mastectomy represent the ideal scenario for reconstruction; however,

there are several important considerations. The most important variable is tumor margin status. While it may seem intuitive to delay reconstruction until negative margins are confirmed, most patients are at low risk for positive margins (<5%), and delaying reconstruction would necessitate a potentially avoidable additional operation.[6] Patients who present with multifocal disease, however, do benefit from delayed reconstruction owing

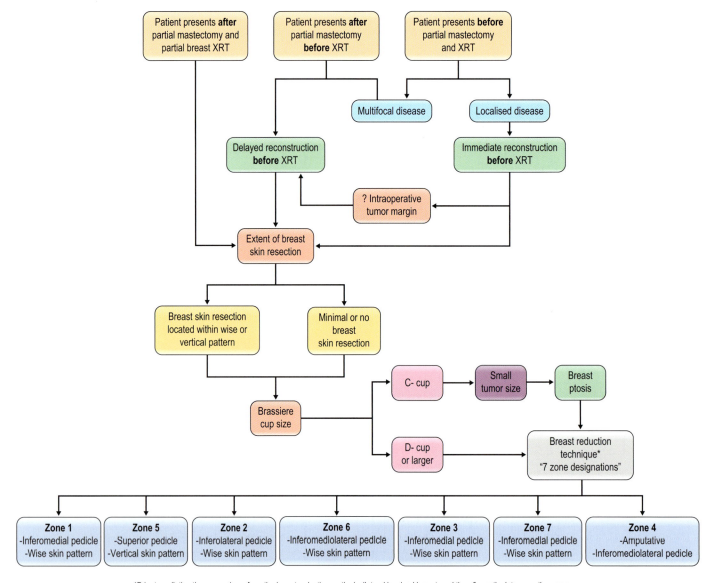

Fig. 25.2 Zones of defect and dermoglandular pedicles. *(Redrawn with permission from Kronowitz SJ, Kuerer HM, Buchholz TA, Valero V, Hunt KK. A management algorithm and practical oncoplastic surgical techniques for repairing partial mastectomy defects.* Plast Reconstr Surg. *Dec 2008;122(6):1631–1647.)*

to their elevated risk of positive margins and potential need for further excision.

Immediate reconstruction techniques for partial mastectomy defects are similar to techniques used in delayed partial breast reconstruction, but the former offer superior cosmetic results that maintain the color, texture, and wound healing capabilities of the non-radiated breast. The type of reconstruction will vary depending on the location of the defect, size of remaining breast, and anticipation of any resected breast skin. In general, large breasts with a moderate tumor size to breast:volume ratio are reconstructed with reduction pattern techniques that use dermoglandular pedicles to lift and reduce the nipple and breast,

respectively. Kronowitz *et al.* formulated zone designations and corresponding dermoglandular pedicles for reconstruction of partial mastectomy defects (Fig. 25.2).[6] Local tissue rearrangement is often used for reconstruction in moderate-sized breasts with minimal ptosis or small resultant defects and involves remodeling of the breast without transposing the nipple or reducing the breast size. Depending on the extent and location of the defect, the remaining breast parenchyma is mobilized from the surrounding area into the defect location to minimize the deformity. The mastectomy skin is often degloved from the underlying breast tissue, which remains attached to the underlying chest wall in order to maintain perfusion to the parenchyma. The skin envelope is then redraped over the recontoured breast mound.[6] Local tissue rearrangement can be limiting, in particular in cases of minimal remaining breast tissue. Patients should be advised regarding its limitations and consideration given to proceeding with a completion mastectomy and total breast reconstruction.

As part of the multidisciplinary approach, patients who elect to undergo breast conservation will be receiving adjuvant radiation treatment. There is no clinical evidence that suggests immediate repair of partial mastectomy defects interferes with adjuvant treatments; however, it is important that radiation oncology considerations are taken into account when deciding on the best approach for reconstruction. Whole breast radiation therapy is administered to the entire breast, with an additional boost given to the tumor bed cavity. Patients with large breasts can pose challenges when using whole breast radiation, which has a higher propensity for dose-inhomogeneity when compared with moderate breast patients.[7] These patients, therefore, benefit most from immediate reconstruction of partial mastectomy defects using reduction type techniques to reduce the overall size of the breast and improve dose homogeneity.[7] In these cases of immediate repair, the tumor bed needs to be appropriately marked with radio-opaque clips, as the tumor bed can be displaced during the reduction and thus can be hard to localize for adjuvant radiation treatment. On the other hand, patients for whom partial breast irradiation is planned should not be considered for immediate reconstruction, as this procedure interferes with adjuvant treatment. The advent of intraoperative partial breast radiation therapy, however, may make immediate repair a more feasible option in these patients.[6]

Reconstruction after total mastectomy

Following mastectomy, breast reconstruction involving the entire breast and/or nipple often requires multiple procedures. The optimal timing and technique of these procedures in patients requiring post-mastectomy radiation therapy are controversial and present many challenges. A thorough understanding of the adjuvant treatment plan is essential prior to deciding the best approach for reconstruction, particularly for patients needing adjuvant radiation.

Immediate breast reconstruction has a proven beneficial impact on psychosocial well-being, a reduced overall cost, and better aesthetic results compared with delayed reconstructions. The main factor in deciding whether a breast cancer patient is a candidate for immediate reconstruction is the patient's risk of needing adjuvant radiation therapy. Radiation therapy is the single most significant predictor of poor aesthetic outcomes and of increased risk of complications such as capsule contracture, fat necrosis, infection, seroma, and reconstructive failure. As discussed previously, tumor size and involvement of the axillary nodes together determine the risk of loco-regional recurrence and the need for adjuvant radiation therapy. Pre-mastectomy imaging can often be used to estimate tumor size; however, sentinel node biopsy is necessary to assess whether there is nodal involvement. Recently, consideration has been given to performing sentinel lymph node biopsies prior to mastectomy – so called "staged sentinel node biopsy" – in patients with tumors staged T2 or greater with unknown status of nodal involvement. Confirmation of nodal involvement or lack thereof may offer the opportunity for immediate reconstruction. However, the benefits of staged sentinel node biopsy need to be weighed against the risks of additional surgery and associated potential complications, increased cost, and patient inconvenience.[8]

An alternative to "staged sentinel lymph node biopsy" is "delayed-immediate" reconstruction, pioneered by Steven Kronowitz.[9] In this approach, patients who may need to receive adjuvant radiation therapy undergo immediate placement of a tissue expander at the time of mastectomy. Use of the tissue expander helps preserve the mastectomy skin and breast footprint for future definitive reconstruction and serves as a place-holder until the final pathology report is received. If the final pathology report indicates that adjuvant radiation therapy is needed, definitive reconstruction with either an implant or autologous reconstruction can be planned. If the IM nodes will be included in the radiation treatment protocol, the expander is often deflated prior to irradiation to allow for adequate dosimetry to the medial portion of the breast and chest wall. However, not all institutions treat the IM nodes and, therefore, deflation of the expander prior to irradiation may not be necessary. Tissue expanders with internal metal ports have not been shown to interfere with radiation treatment plans and are suitable for "delayed-immediate" reconstruction. Following completion of radiation therapy, expanders should be re-inflated rapidly to preserve the previously expanded breast envelope. Definitive reconstruction with an implant or autologous tissue is then planned once the irradiated skin has had sufficient time to heal and recover. The "delayed-immediate" approach offers the aesthetic advantage of immediate reconstruction without compromising the ability to perform adjuvant treatment.[9] However, irradiated tissue expanders do have a higher rate of complications than non-irradiated expanders, and patients should be counseled appropriately regarding this associated risk and the need to have easy access to medical care in case of an emergency.

Immediate definitive reconstruction with placement of an implant or autologous tissue in patients in whom adjuvant radiotherapy is indicated has been shown to result in poor aesthetic outcomes and, in some cases, to interfere with the delivery of radiation. Alterations in radiation treatment protocols have resulted in delivery of either higher doses to lung parenchyma and the heart or suboptimal doses to the targeted area.[3] The clinical significant of these findings, however, is unknown. Studies evaluating outcomes of two-stage breast reconstruction with tissue expanders consistently reveal high rates of wound healing complications, capsule contracture, and poor aesthetic outcomes in the setting or radiation. In one retrospective review of this population, authors noted a 45.4% complication rate with the use of irradiated tissue expanders and a 30% loss of permanent implants in the setting of PMRT.[10,11] Grades III and IV capsule contracture occurred twice as often in irradiated implants as in non-irradiated implants. Patients with a prior history of radiation therapy, such as previous breast-conserving therapy, were also associated with an elevated risk of complications and a need for explantation.[10] In a study of 482 patients who had implant reconstruction, both prior radiation therapy and post-mastectomy radiation therapy were found to have a negative effect on patient satisfaction ($p<0.001$ and $p=0.002$, respectively).[10,11]

Recently, acellular dermal matrix (ADM) was found to have potentially protective effects against explantation in patients with radiated tissue expanders. In a retrospective review by Seth and colleagues, irradiated expanders without ADM were found to have a three times higher complication rate than irradiated expanders with ADM.[8] In a larger study by Craig and colleagues that included 1376 tissue expander reconstructions, irradiated tissue expanders that used ADM had an associated higher rate of seromas (13.6% vs 10.9%, $p<0.001$), but a lower incidence of explantation (11.4% vs 20.4%, $p=0.0012$). During the body incorporation period, ADM is associated with higher rates of seroma and infection. However, if recognized early and treated appropriately, ADM that incorporates into the body may play a protective role in preventing explantation by serving as an additional vascularized barrier.[11] Further studies in this area are needed before definitive conclusions can be made, however.

Given the risks associated with reconstruction using irradiated expanders, attempts have been made to place implants *prior* to adjuvant radiation therapy;

however, this strategy is also associated with high rates of revision, capsule contracture, and implant loss.[11] In addition, patients who have received neoadjuvant chemotherapy and who will receive adjuvant radiation therapy 4–6 weeks following mastectomy pose a logistical challenge: performing a two-stage reconstruction in such a narrow time window. The small and select group of patients who are candidates for direct to implant (DTI) reconstruction at the time of mastectomy would be a more feasible population to undergoing adjuvant radiation therapy. However, we know from previous studies that DTI reconstruction patients are inherently at higher risk for wound healing problems and higher revision rates than are patients undergoing standard two-stage reconstructions. Thus, the use of adjuvant radiation therapy in DTI reconstruction patients would potentially magnify the revision rate in this high-risk radiation implant population. Autologous fat grafting has recently been implemented as a means to improve outcomes of irradiated prosthetic breast reconstructions. In a case–control series of patients with irradiated implants, Panettiere *et al.* compared outcomes of 61 patients who underwent fat grafting to outcomes of 41 patients who did not undergo fat grafting (control group).[12] Those patients who underwent fat grafting were found to have a significantly better aesthetic score than did control group patients.[12] Despite the aesthetic advantages of fat grafting in mastectomy patients, the theoretical risk of injecting stem cells into a breast with previous cancer remains. The safety of fat grafting in breast cancer patients is controversial, and patients should be educated about the potential risk of this strategy and the paucity of available oncologic data on this topic.

The gold standard for breast reconstruction in patients needing adjuvant radiation therapy is delayed autologous reconstruction. Optional donor sites include but are not limited to the latissimus flap, deep inferior epigastric artery perforator (DIEP) flap, profunda artery perforator (PAP) flap, transverse upper gracilis (TUG) flap, superior and inferior gluteal artery perforator (SGAP/IGAP) flaps, and lumbar artery perforator (LAP) flaps. Historically, autologous reconstruction has been performed after radiation therapy because of concerns for possible radiation-induced flap thrombosis and fat necrosis. In addition, immediate autologous reconstruction can theoretically interfere with radiation treatment planning in ways similar to the interference by inflated tissue expanders, but without the flexibility to "deflate" the autologous flap. However, recent data from Crisera and colleagues found immediate free flap breast reconstruction to be safe in oncologic settings.[13] Also, recent studies comparing irradiated with non-irradiated DIEP flaps revealed that use of the irradiated flaps yielded improved aesthetic outcomes with no statistical difference from the non-irradiated flaps in fat necrosis, volume loss, flap loss, or wound healing rates.[14–17]

The key factor in radiation therapy's effects on immediate autologous reconstruction outcomes is how the radiation treatment plan is carried out. Consideration and understanding of the radiation treatment plan is necessary to predict realistic outcomes for these breast cancer patients. For example, if the IM nodes or medial breast is targeted for therapy, and if that target is also the location of the flap anastomosis, then targeted therapy will likely result in flap thrombosis and in resultant volume deflation and fat necrosis. However, not all institutions target the IM node and not all surgeons use the IM artery as the recipient vessel for the flap. Choosing a recipient vessel that is outside the zone of targeted radiation therapy can help limit these radiation-induced flap changes and can optimize aesthetic outcomes in these select patients.

For patients who undergo standard delayed autologous free flap reconstruction, the optimal timing for definitive reconstruction remains controversial. Physiologically, the window between resolution of the acute phase of radiation injury and the initiation of extensive fibrosis would be ideal; however, it is often clinically difficult to ascertain where this window lies. Variability among institutions in techniques of radiation delivery, length of follow-up, and administration of systemic therapy limits the ability to adequately determine the optimal timing for reconstruction. A 2001 retrospective review by investigators at MD Anderson Cancer Center compared complication rates for irradiated immediate reconstruction transverse rectus abdominus myocutaneous (TRAM) flaps with rates for the non-irradiated TRAM flaps. While acute flap complications such as flap thrombosis or failure did not significantly differ between the two flap groups, late complications such as fat necrosis and volume loss were found to be significantly higher in the irradiated TRAM flap group than in the non-irradiated TRAM flap group.[18] As emphasized earlier, however, the radiation treatment plan at MD Anderson is noted to include the medial breast and often the IM nodes specifically; this therefore explains the higher rate of volume loss in the irradiated TRAM flap cohort. In general, delayed autologous free flap reconstruction is described as being performed safely as early as 6–9 months after a patient's completion of radiation therapy; however, the timing and use of this breast reconstruction technique should be determined on an individual basis.

Delayed pedicle autologous reconstruction such as latissimus flap reconstruction can theoretically be offered sooner than 6 months to patients because of the lack of concerns over radiation-induced recipient vessel injury. For patients who do not have available autologous tissue in free flap donor sites or patients who are deemed poor candidates for free flap reconstruction, pedicled latissimus flap reconstruction remains a valuable option to improve the breast contour and aesthetics, particularly in irradiated implant-based reconstruction.[3] In 2011, Selber was the first to describe the minimally invasive harvest of the latissimus muscle for breast reconstruction.[19] Since that time, subsequent studies of this technique have shown superior results with associated low rates of infection, delayed wound healing, and capsule contracture. However, there is a significant learning curve with the use of such techniques, and further studies are warranted before adopting these strategies into every plastic surgeon's armamentarium.

In a recent study evaluating rates of patient satisfaction with various breast reconstruction techniques, patients reported autologous reconstruction to be far superior to and more durable than implant-based reconstruction.[20,21] This finding is alarming, given that more than 80% of the breast reconstructions performed in the US are implant-based reconstructions. In addition, women who underwent implant reconstruction had satisfaction scores 8.6 points lower than did those patients who underwent breast-conserving therapy. It is not surprising that the softness of autologous tissue in reconstruction, even when irradiated as in breast-conserving therapy, is more desirable to patients than the palpability of implants are. Latissimus flap reconstruction received patient satisfaction scores similar to those for breast-conserving therapy and also remains a good option for thin patients who have a history of radiation therapy.[21] Given these findings, breast cancer patients should be educated about the long-term durability and aesthetic outcome of autologous and alloplastic breast reconstruction.

Conclusion

Radiation therapy is integral to multimodality treatment and decreasing local recurrence in select breast cancer patients. However, the effects radiation has on short- and long-term complication rates, aesthetic outcomes, and patient satisfaction pose significant challenges to reconstructive surgeons. Understanding radiation treatment protocols is paramount to minimizing complications and maximizing aesthetic outcomes.

Access the complete reference list online at   **http://www.expertconsult.com**

2. Kane GM. Therapeutic radiation: principles effects, and complications. In: Neligan PC, Gurtner GC, eds. *Plastic Surgery*. Vol. 1. 3rd ed. Principles. New York: Elsevier Saunders; 2013:654–675. *Comprehensive explanation of the physics and treatment plans for radiation therapy as it applies to breast cancer patients.*

3. Kronowitz SJ, Robb GL. Radiation therapy and breast reconstruction: a critical review of the literature. *Plast Reconstr Surg*. 2009;124:395–408. *A summary of the literature on radiation therapy and its impact on breast reconstruction outcomes.*

6. Kronowitz SJ, Kuerer HM, Buchholz TA, et al. A management algorithm and practical oncoplastic surgical techniques for repairing partial mastectomy defects. *Plast Reconstr Surg*. 2008;122:1631–1647.

Well-organized outline of how to approach oncoplastic reduction with regards to patient selection and surgical technique.

7. Lentz RB, Craig ES, Ross CC, et al. Does the left hand know what the right hand is doing? What plastic surgeons need to know about radiation therapy techniques. *Plast Reconstr Surg*. 2012;130:772e–773e. *Explanation of the common hurdles radiation oncologists face with treating breast cancer patients and its impact on outcomes.*

9. Kronowitz SJ. Delayed-immediate breast reconstruction: technical and timing considerations. *Plast Reconstr Surg*. 2010;125:463–474. *Well-organized summary of the commonly used delayed-immediate breast reconstruction approach to patients at risk for needing radiation therapy.*

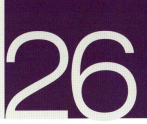

Surgical management of breast cancer-related lymphedema

Jaume Masià, Gemma Pons, and Elena Rodríguez-Bauzà

SYNOPSIS

- Breast cancer-related lymphedema (BCRL) is the result of impaired lymph drainage from the ipsilateral arm following surgical or radiotherapy treatment.
- BCRL develops in as many as 21% of women after breast cancer treatment. This disabling chronic condition has a high impact on quality of life and is a source of significant morbidity.
- Advances in imaging techniques have allowed us to better understand the anatomy and pathophysiology of the lymphatic system, and greater mastery of supermicrosurgical techniques has given us the opportunity to restore a dysfunctional lymphatic system in selected cases.
- As yet, no optimal treatment has been found, but the use of reconstructive approaches, and excisional or reductive techniques, mainly liposuction, allow us to improve the quality of life of patients in most cases.

Access the Historical Perspective section online at
http://www.expertconsult.com

Introduction

Breast cancer is the most frequent cause of lymphedema in western countries.[1] For many years, lymphedema treatment has been based on conservative physical and medical therapies. These treatments are often time-consuming, difficult to perform on a regular basis, and cumbersome, and such barriers lead to high rates of non-compliance and patient dissatisfaction.[2] Since the early 20th century, several surgical techniques have been described in an attempt to complement or provide a more effective alternative to these conservative treatments. Such surgical techniques are considered either reductive or reconstructive. Reductive techniques, such

as Brorson's liposuction,[3] aim to reduce the hypertrophic adipose and fibrotic tissue characterizing the intermediate and later lymphedema stages, while reconstructive techniques, such as autologous vascularized lymph node transfer (ALNT),[4] derivative lymphovenular techniques,[5] and lympholymphatic bypass,[6] aim to improve or restore the functionality of an impaired lymphatic system.

Nevertheless, no standardized protocol for lymphedema surgical treatment has yet been established. In this chapter, the authors describe their approach in surgical management of lymphedema, emphasizing the importance of the preoperative assessment.

Key points

- Preoperative assessment identifies potential candidates for reconstructive or reductive surgical techniques.
- ICG-lymphography is essential as the first step in the assessment to appraise the viability of the lymphatic system.
- Other imaging techniques help to determine the optimal surgical technique for every patient:
  - Lymphoscintigraphy is helpful to define the lymphedema pattern and to know how many lymph nodes remain active in the affected limb.
  - MR-lymphography provides a 3D reconstruction of the whole limb and shows both the superficial and the deep lymphatic system.
  - CT-angiography is crucial to minimize potential donor site morbidity when an autologous lymph node transfer is planned, especially when the flap is harvested from the inferior epigastric system.
  - Intraoperative ICG-lymphography improves precision when harvesting the lymph nodes at the donor site.

- Depending on the status of the axilla, in patients with active lymphatic channels, lymphatic-venous anastomosis (LVA) or LVA combined with autologous lymph node transfer (ALNT) is performed.
- If in the preoperative assessment, there are no active lymphatic channels and there is a non-pitting lymphedema with an excess of adipose and fibrotic tissue, the unique effective technique is the use of reductive surgery, especially the vibro-liposuction described by H. Brorson.[3]

Basic science/disease process

Lymphedema can be caused by an intrinsic fault in the lymph-conducting pathways (primary lymphedema) or by damage from events occurring outside the lymphatic system, such as surgical removal of lymph nodes. In BCRL, lymphedema occurs due to a mechanical disruption in outflow resistance and a rise in lymphatic pressure. The resulting lymphatic dilation is likely to cause valve incompetence, and hence explains the backflow of lymph, particularly towards the skin ("dermal backflow").[14]

The lymphatic walls undergo fibrosis, and fibrinoid thrombi accumulate within the lumen, obliterating many of the remaining lymph channels. Spontaneous lymphovenous shunts may form. Histologically, in the initial stage of lymphedema, both endothelial cells and smooth muscles cells in the proximal level of the lymphatic trunks become damaged. Occlusions of the lymphatic trunks and degeneration of the smooth muscle cells may start from the proximal regions of the limb.[15]

In recent years, work in BCRL has demonstrated that obstruction to lymph drainage following removal of axillary lymph nodes is too simple a mechanistic explanation.[16] It has become clear that other factors related to lymphedema are involved, such as obesity, destruction of pathways, and variability in the anatomy of the lymphatic system.

Diagnosis/patient presentation

Classically, the diagnosis of lymphedema was based on clinical evaluation supplemented by lymphoscintigraphy. Today, the current approach to diagnosis and preoperative planning should be made from another point of view, adding the results obtained by ICG-lymphography to the clinical evaluation.[17]

The key to success with surgical treatment is to identify patients who still have a functional lymphatic system and are potential candidates for reconstructive surgical techniques.

After an accurate clinical evaluation, an assessment using diagnostic imaging techniques is performed to study the functional and morphologic features of the lymphatic system so as to provide the best therapeutic option to each patient.

Clinical evaluation

A detailed anamnesis is essential to assess the cause of the lymphedema and its long-term course. This step differentiates between pitting and non-pitting edema, as non-pitting edema argues for an advanced stage of the disorder, characterized by severe fibrosis and hypertrophy of adipose tissue. It is also important to ask about antecedents of recurrent acute inflammatory episodes (cellulitis or erysipelas). Together with the anamnestic data, clinical evaluation determines the lymphedema stage according to the International Society of Lymphedema (Table 26.1).[18]

The clinical examination also involves measuring limb circumferences at predetermined anatomic levels and collecting photographic documentation. There are several methods of measurement. Volumetry is the most exact, but the circumference measurement is the easiest and most fundamental method. Since the 2nd European Conference on Supermicrosurgery in 2012, it was agreed that measures would be taken every 4 cm from the ulnar styloid process to the lateral malleolus in the elbow and up to the shoulder (Fig. 26.1).

Diagnostic imaging techniques

Diagnostic imagining techniques are essential tools to determine an appropriate therapeutic strategy for each patient and to assess the improvement after surgery. Our assessment protocol involves indocyanine green (ICG) lymphography, lymphoscintigraphy (LS), magnetic resonance (MR)-lymphography and, in some cases, computed tomography (CT)-angiography.

Table 26.1 International Society of Lymphology (ISL) staging

ISL stage	Features
0/IA	Subclinical condition where swelling is not evident despite impaired lymph transport
I	Accumulation of fluid, which subsides with limb elevation. Pitting may occur
II	Limb elevation alone rarely reduces tissue swelling. Pitting present, except in late stage II when more fibrosis occurs
III	Lymphostatic elephantiasis where pitting is absent and trophic skin changes (acanthosis, fat deposits, warty overgrowths) develop

(Reproduced with permission from Masia J, Pons G, Nardulli ML. Combined surgical treatment in breast cancer-related lymphedema. *J Reconstr Microsurg.* 2016;32:16–27.)

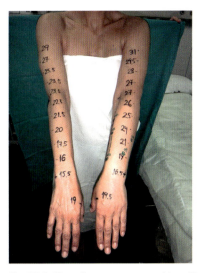

Fig. 26.1 Circumference measurement in a 45-year-old woman with stage II lymphedema. Measurements are taken every 4 cm from the ulnar styloid process to the lateral malleolus in the elbow to the shoulder.

Indocyanine green lymphography

ICG-lymphography is an essential test image performed as a diagnostic test in the authors' out-patient clinic during the first consultation. Depending on the results, further imaging studies are planned.

This study consists of injecting 0.1–0.2 mL of indocyanine green dye subcutaneously at the II and IV interdigital webspace in both hands. The dye is captured and transported by active lymphatic channels and can be visualized on real-time as fluorescent channels on a display. The entire exam is recorded (Fig. 26.2).

ICG-lymphography yields valuable information in assessment, providing a double evaluation. First, immediately after injection, it shows the velocity of the contrast ascending to the axilla, and after 5 min it shows where the contrast is stored, allowing evaluation of the dermal backflow. Second, it provides valuable pre-surgical data about the degree of impairment in the lymphatic system. It not only gives information about the number of enhanced lymphatic channels and their appearance but also shows the exact location of the active lymphatic channels and their transport capacity. This information is of crucial importance during the preoperative assessment because only a patient with active lymphatic channels can be considered a potential candidate for LVA surgery.

The procedure is limited by the possibility to only visualize lymphatics that are less than 2 cm deep with respect to the skin surface. As a result, the authors now combine ICG-lymphography with MR-lymphography, especially when a patient is a candidate for reconstructive surgery.

The preoperative planning assessment with ICG-lymphography is done the day before the LVA surgery or in the same day in the operating room. It provides a map of the lymphatic system, and the lymphatic channels are marked on the patient's skin surface. The preoperative mapping is completed with the information provided by MR-lymphography, as explained in more detail below (Fig. 26.3).

ICG-lymphography is also of paramount importance during ALNT surgery. It helps the understanding of the

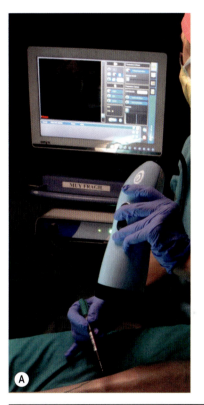

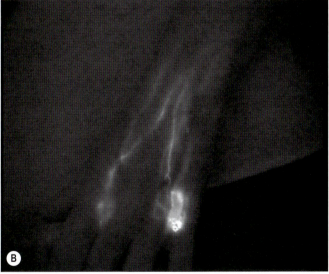

Fig. 26.2 IGC-lymphography. **(A)** ICG is captured by an infrared camera system, and **(B)** functioning lymphatic channels can be seen on a display device as fluorescent channels.

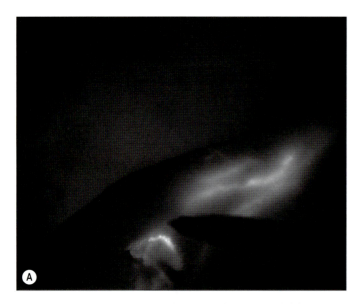

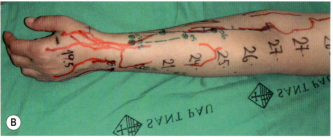

Fig. 26.3 (A) The lymphatic channels observed by IGC-lymphography and **(B)** drawn on the patient's skin thanks to the contrast medium (red color).

lymphatic pattern at the donor site limb. As the authors normally use the superficial inguinal nodes as donor-nodes for transplantation in the axilla, during ALNT surgery, ICG-lymphography allows us to locate the lymph nodes (LNs) draining the inferior limb and exclude these from the flap. This approach helps to reduce the risk of iatrogenic lower limb lymphedema.

Lymphoscintigraphy

Lymphoscintigraphy is a standardized imaging test that gives a global evaluation of the functionality of the lymphatic system. It also provides comparative information for the postoperative assessment. Images of the entire arm, the axilla, and the liver are taken over 40 min. Further images are captured 60, 120, and 180 min after the injection and interpreted. The main parameters evaluated are the tracer pathway, the time the tracer appears at the axilla, the presence or absence of major lymphatic collectors, visualization of nodes, and the presence or absence of dermal backflow. If tracer uptake in the axilla is absent, autologous lymph node transplantation to the axilla level can be planned. There is no reason for lymph node transfer in the axilla in a patient with lymph node functionality at the axillary region.

Despite its advantages, lymphoscintigraphy does not provide detailed morphologic and functional information about the lymphatic system, and information must be complemented with ICG-lymphography and MR-lymphography.

MR-lymphography

To overcome the limitations of ICG-lymphography, we use MR-lymphography to obtain a 3D reconstruction of the whole limb. It shows both the superficial and deep lymphatic system.

The authors perform MR-lymphography to obtain more information when planning the surgical technique. The data obtained not only assesses the lymphatic system of the limb but also helps to select the most suitable lymphatic channels for LVA. These can be distal to a dermal backflow area; a sign of lymphatic obstruction. Two coordinates are chosen for each lymphatic vessel and marked on the skin before LVA surgery. Combining the information provided by ICG-lymphography and MR-lymphography, the contractile vessels most likely to promote successful LVA can be located (Fig. 26.4).

Computed tomography-angiography

CT-angiography is performed when planning ALNT. It has become an essential tool to study the inferior epigastric donor area and to minimize potential donor site morbidity in the lower limb.

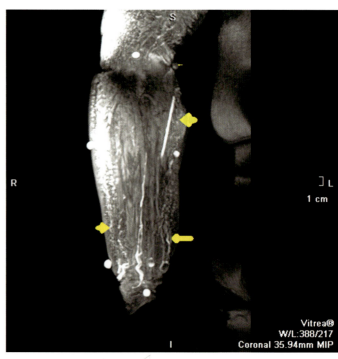

Fig. 26.4 Preoperative 3D coronal magnetic resonance lymphography showing several tortuous lymphatic channels in a right arm with lymphedema (yellow arrows).

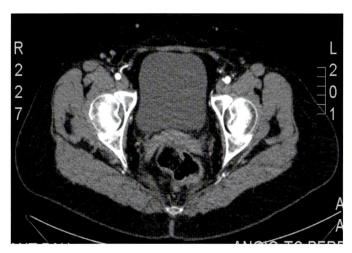

Fig. 26.5 Axial view of computed tomography angiography showing the right superficial inguinal lymph nodes (green arrows) and the nourishing superficial circumflex iliac vessels (blue arrows).

This technique is usually used to locate the abdominal perforators when performing an abdominal flap for breast reconstruction, and also to locate the lymph nodes in view of the high anatomic variability.

The most cranial and lateral inguinal nodes are selected. The first reason for this is that they are richly vascularized by the superficial epigastric system or the superficial circumflex iliac system, and the second reason is that this approach reduces the risk of secondary iatrogenic lymphedema.

CT-angiography is used to identify the number and location of the superficial inguinal nodes to be harvested in the LN flap, and to assess the LN vascular pedicle (superficial inferior epigastric system or superficial iliac circumflex iliac vessels) to determine its size, course, and exact location using exact coordinates, as described previously for abdominal perforator flaps (Fig. 26.5).[19]

Patient selection

The key point of BCRL treatment is patient selection. It is crucial to individualize the treatment for every patient independently of the clinical stage or the evolution time. A complete preoperative study will determine the possible success of the technique and establish the potentially effective technique.

Results from the preoperative clinical assessment and ICG-lymphography, lymphoscintigraphy, and MR-lymphography are of inestimable value in decision-making. Based on our experience to date, we have developed a treatment algorithm, the BLAST (Barcelona lymphedema algorithm for surgical treatment) (Fig. 26.6):

- If there is no evidence of active lymphatic channels (ICG assessment −/ lympho MRI −) and the lymphedema is advanced and non-pitting, we opt for a reductive technique such as liposuction according to the Brorson technique.

- If there is no evidence of active lymphatic channels (ICG assessment −/ lympho MRI −) and pitting lymphedema is present, intensive rehabilitation therapy is performed to re-assess the possibility of a reductive surgical technique.

- If there is evidence of a functioning lymphatic system (ICG assessment + and/or lympho MRI +), the authors choose a reconstructive technique according to the clinical characteristics of the axilla:

  • If the axillary area has good status, LVA is performed in the affected limb.

  • If the axillary area presents signs of impairment (i.e., radiodermitis, abundant fibrotic tissue), an ALNT approach is used in the armpit after fibrotic tissue release, complemented by LVA in the affected limb.

  • If the patient has amastia and requests breast reconstruction, ALNT with nodes included in the abdominal perforator flap (DIEP or SIEA) is opted for and LVA is performed distally on the affected limb. The authors call this procedure "T-BAR" (total breast anatomy restoration).

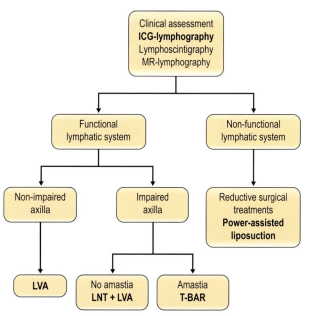

Fig. 26.6 Barcelona lymphedema algorithm for surgical treatment (BLAST). (Masià J, Pons G, Rodríguez-Bauzà E. Barcelona Lymphedema Algorithm for Surgical Treatment in Breast Cancer-Related Lymphedema. J Reconstr Microsurg. 2016;32:329–335.)

Treatment/surgical technique

Lymphatic-venular anastomosis (LVA)

The LVA procedure consists of performing skin incisions about 2 cm length in the affected limb in order to locate functional lymphatic vessels and to anastomose these to subdermal veins. The objective of this procedure is to redirect the lymph to the venous stream directly, without going through the thoracic duct. Both lymphatic and venule vessels have diameters of less than 0.8 mm, so the technique used is called "supermicrosurgery". The intervention is performed under general anesthesia to avoid patient discomfort in view of the lengthy procedure using high magnification microscope and specific supermicrosurgical instruments and sutures.

ICG-lymphography and MR-lymphography data help to locate the most functional lymphatic channels, which are likely to be anastomosed with superficial venules. These lymphatic channels are marked on the patient's skin just before surgery (Fig. 26.7).

The first lymphatic channels to be explored are those found at the coincident points obtained by these two techniques and preferably those located in the proximal region of the affected limb. In this way, if the anastomosis is feasible, it is possible to recruit a greater amount of lymph from the distal part of the limb. Most functioning lymphatic vessels, however, are found in the wrist and at the distal two-thirds of the arm, as the proximal vessels are normally damaged first.

At the selected cutaneous points and after injection of a small amount of local anesthetic with epinephrine to reduce bleeding, an approximately 2–3 cm skin incision is made. Lymphatic channels are carefully dissected and subsequently anastomosed end-to-end or end-to-side to subdermal venules of similar caliber, using 11-0 or 12-0 sutures. After performing the anastomosis, between 0.1 and 0.2 mL of Patent V Blue dye is injected about 2 cm distal to the incision. The dye is absorbed generally into the functional lymphatic channels, and the transport of the lymph can be seen and the permeability of the anastomosis can be verified (Figs. 26.8 & 26.9).

Autologous lymph node transfer

The procedure is based on the substitution of lymph nodes that have been previously surgically resected or damaged in the axilla, with a vascularized free tissue transfer flap containing a few LNs (between 3 and 6 nodes) from non-risk donor sites.

The donor area that used most often is the superficial inferior epigastric area with superficial circumflex iliac vessels. Morbidity at this site is low, and the final cosmetic result is satisfactory, as the scar is hidden. Other donor sites are the submental, supraclavicular region or the contralateral thoraco-dorsal axis. Before surgery, these areas are studied using angio-CT to assess where the superficial nodes and their vascular pedicle are. The authors also check the number and distribution of the deep lymph nodes, trying to make sure that the nodes to be removed are not disturbing normal lymphatic drainage of the lower limb.

ICG-lymphography allows us to locate the lymph nodes (LNs) draining the inferior limb. Before surgery, IGC is injected into the interdigital spaces of the lower limb to locate the lymphatic system draining the leg. This step reduces the risk of harvesting a flap containing these LNs, which would induce an iatrogenic lower limb lymphedema (Fig. 26.10).[20]

Before raising the flap (just before doing the skin incision), the authors inject 0.1–0.2 mL of ICG and 0.2–0.4 mL of 2.5% patent blue V dye (Guerbet, Roissy-Charles-de-Gaulle, France) intradermally in two or three spots above and below the inguinal fold in the potential drainage area to improve visibility of the superficial lymphatic vessels during dissection.

To reduce the risk of seroma, there is precise dissection, clipping, and cauterizing of the tiny lymphatic channels and side branches that are not included in the skin-adipose-LN flap.

Within the lymph node flap, the authors include a skin island of approximately 8×4 cm with some extra vascularized fat from the superficial circumflex iliac system. Its vascular pedicle is dissected with special care up to the femoral vessels. The adipose tissue surrounding the lymph nodes and the skin island included in the flap are useful to replace the fibrotic tissue in the axillary region and also to facilitate lymph absorption through the physiologic lymph-venous shunts.[14] The skin island makes postoperative monitoring easier (Fig. 26.11).

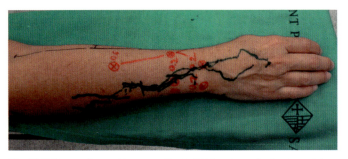

Fig. 26.7 Preoperative markings according to ICG-lymphography (green marks) and magnetic resonance lymphography (red marks) data in a 44-year-old woman with lymphedema in the right arm.

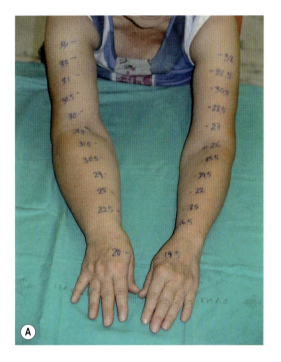

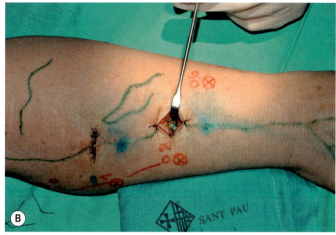

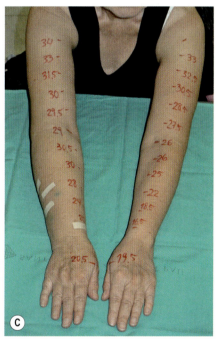

Fig. 26.8 A 55-year-old woman with right upper limb lymphedema who underwent lymphatico-venous anastomosis. **(A)** Preoperative markings; **(B)** intraoperative image; **(C)** postoperative markings.

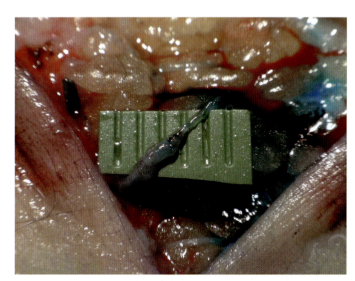

Fig. 26.9 Intraoperative view of the termino-terminal anastomosis between the proximal stump of the lymphatic vessel and the distal stump of the venule. The lymph fluid can be seen flowing through the anastomosis along the vein.

Once the flap is isolated, the donor site is closed using a quilting suture to avoid dead space, preferably a continuous spiral barbed suture. This is used to co-opt the walls of the donor site and prevent dead spaces, which could favor the accumulation of seroma. Before closing the area, a tissue sealant is applied to close the small lymphatic dissected collectors (Fig. 26.12). A suction drain is left in the donor area until the drainage is less than 15 cc/day, and external compression with a foam bandage is applied for 2 weeks.

As the site generally used for lymph node transfer is the axilla, anastomosis is normally performed between donor vessels of the circumflex scapular system, after debridement of fibrotic tissue.

It is essential to place the lymph nodes on the apex of the axilla in contact with the axillary tissue because this is where the afferent dominant lymphatic channels arrive from the arm.

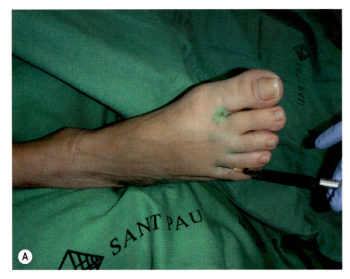

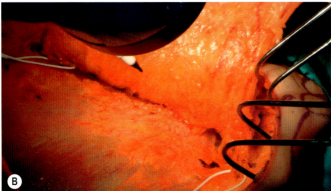

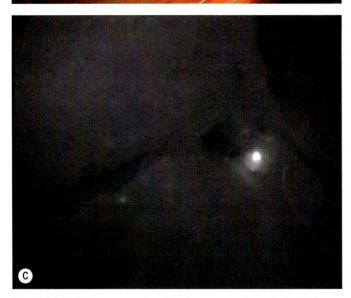

Fig. 26.10 (A–C) Reverse mapping of the leg to prevent donor site lymphedema.

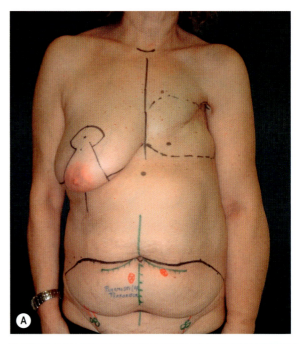

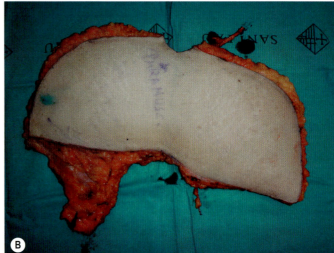

Fig. 26.11 (A) Preoperative markings of the flap and its nourishing vessels in a 57-year-old woman who underwent total breast anatomy restoration surgery for left breast amastia and upper limb lymphedema. **(B)** Shows the deep inferior epigastric artery perforator flap with the adipocutaneous flap containing the nodes.

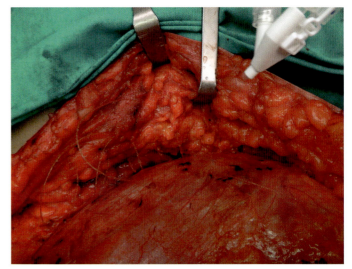

Fig. 26.12 Donor site closure using a quilting suture to avoid dead space.

If good lymphatic channels from the arm during dissection of the fibrotic tissue in the axilla are found, a lymph-lymphatic anastomosis can be performed to the afferent lymphatic channels from the transplanted skin-adipose-LN flap. It is also important to place the extra-vascularized adipose tissue making a bridge between the healthy fat from the proximal armpit; this is the way to use the physiologic L-V communications as an absorbing system for the lymph. At the same time, the contour of the anterior axilla line that normally is disrupted by the axillary clearance and the effect of the radiotherapy is improved.[21]

When the authors plan to approach lymphedema and autologous breast reconstruction simultaneously using an abdominal free flap, a compound abdominal (DIEAP/

SIEA) flap containing the LNs with double vascularization is raised, and in some cases, even with lymph-lymphatic anastomosis. This is the concept called T-BAR (total breast anatomy restoration), as noted above (Fig. 26.13).

Liposuction

Liposuction permits effective volume reduction in therapy-resistant lymphedema of the limbs.

Liposuction today is performed using power-assisted liposuction because the vibrating cannula facilitates the process. A tourniquet can be used to minimize blood loss. Liposuction is carried out following the technique described by Brorson.[3] This type of liposuction is performed circumferentially, step-by-step, from wrist to

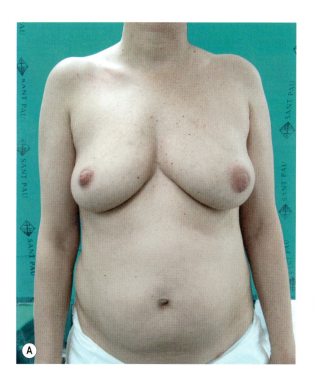

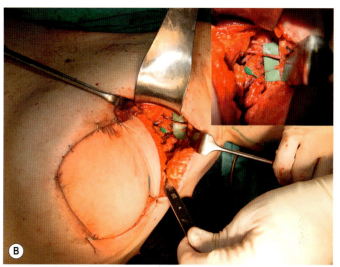

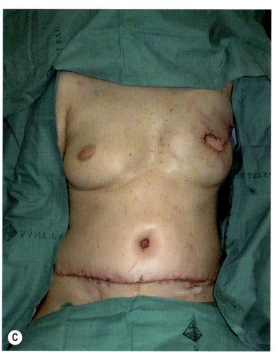

Fig. 26.13 T-bar (total breast anatomy restoration). **(A)** A 49-year-old woman who underwent immediate breast reconstruction with abdominal perforator flap and **(B)** lymph-lymphatic anastomosis between the upper limb lymphatic vessels and the afferent vessels from transplanted lymph nodes from the inguinal area. **(C)** The immediate postoperative result.

shoulder, and the hypertrophied fat is removed as completely as possible. The authors use 15 and 25 cm long cannulas with diameters of 3 and 4 mm.

When the arm distal to the tourniquet has been treated, a sterilized made-to-measure compression sleeve is applied to the arm to stem bleeding and reduce postoperative edema. The tourniquet is removed, and the proximal part of the compression sleeve is pulled up to compress the proximal part of the upper arm. The incisions are left open to drain through the sleeve (Fig. 26.14).

It is important to note that this therapy should be only be used in compliant patients who are committed to

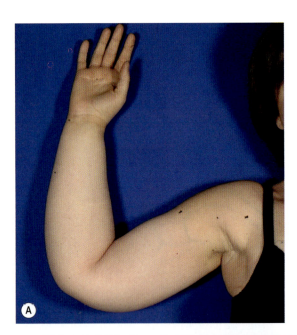

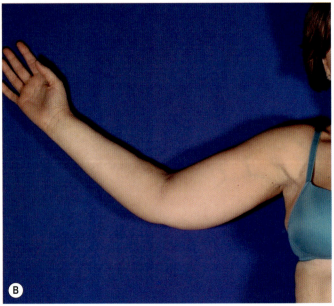

Fig. 26.14 A 55-year-old woman with advanced lymphedema and non-pitting who underwent liposuction according to the H. Brorson technique, with 670 cc of fat tissue extraction. **(A)** Preoperative images. **(B)** At 4 years postoperatively, with stable results.

wearing the lifelong compression garments. Such garments consist of two sets of a sleeve and glove, custommade from a template based on the healthy arm.

Postoperative care

Lymph-venous anastomosis

In the immediate postoperative period (first 48 h), the area where the LVA was performed is gently massaged every 2 h to promote drainage. It is also highly recommended to elevate the affected limb and decrease the amount of activity. On the 3rd postoperative day, patients start to activate muscles doing isometric exercises with a rubber handball. On the 15th day, patients can start a swimming or aquagym rehabilitation program three times a week for 1 year. Depending on the patient's personal circumstances, manual lymphatic drainage is recommended for at least 1 year, twice a week during the first 6 months and once a week during the last 6 months.

Autologous lymph node transfer

On the third postoperative day, muscle activation is initiated by doing isometric exercises with a rubber handball. On the 15th day, manual lymphatic drainage is recommend for 1 year, twice a week during the first 6 months and once a week during the second 6 months. Manual drainage should be directed towards the transplanted lymph nodes in order to stimulate neo-lymphogenesis. One month after surgery, the patient can start a swimming or aquagym rehabilitation program three times a week for 1 year. A light compression garment may be indicated for the first 6 months, depending on the patient's response.

Liposuction

In the immediate postoperative period, the arm is kept at heart level on a large pillow with the compression sleeve and glove in place. These garments are removed 3 days after surgery and replaced with a second set, while the first is washed and dried. This routine is repeated every 2 days for 2 weeks. After the 2-week control, the garments are changed every day. Washing is important because the shrinkage increases compression. The lifelong use of this compression is a prerequisite to maintaining the effect of liposuction.

Outcomes, prognosis, and complications

Outcomes and prognosis

Although various microsurgical procedures have been described to help reduce the severity of lymphedema, no consensus has yet been reached regarding the optimal treatment or benefits. Benefits described to date include a reduction in a limb volume reduction and/or improvements in subjective symptoms such as pain or heaviness.[8] Treatment, however, is not generally individualized, and most groups have applied the same technique in all stages of lymphedema.

In the authors' experience, after more than 10 years working with lymphedema, it is considered that with individualized treatment, following the BLAST algorithm, the degree of lymphedema and the subjective symptoms can be objectively improved. This of course depends on the degree of damage to the lymphatic system.

It has been found that microsurgical results are best when surgery is performed in the early stages of lymphedema following a rigorous preoperative study of the patient, as both LVA and ALNT need to be minimally functional to be successful. The preoperative study identifies patients who may benefit from a reconstructive microsurgical technique; patients with no severe fibrosis and a minimal residual functionality of their lymphatic system in the affected limb. On the contrary, those patients with dominant fibrosis of the limb and without a minimal residual functionality of their lymphatic system are more likely to benefit from reductive procedures such as liposuction.

Surgical complications

Although LVA is minimally invasive and an almost complication-free procedure, some side effects or minor complications have been described, such as the presence of retrograde blood flow, which reverses spontaneously within 48 h of surgery.

ALNT can be associated with certain complications and morbidity of the lymph node donor site.

Complications at the recipient site, such as those regarding arterial vascularization or venous drainage of the LN-flap, must be approached as for other microsurgical free flaps.

Specific complications of the ALNT procedure mainly affect the lymph node donor site. Seroma is a frequent complication at the LN-flap donor site and is mainly due to the dead space left in this area. Spraying a tissue sealant can be useful. To avoid dead spaces at the donor site after raising an LN-flap, a barbed monofilament strand can be used to perform a continuous spiral suture and close the donor site.

It is advisable to leave a suction drain in place until the drainage is less than 15 cc/day and to use compressive cycling garment for the first month. If seroma occurs despite these precautions, regular percutaneous aspiration must be performed and local compression should be increased until complete regression is achieved.

To minimize the risk of iatrogenic lymphedema, as mentioned earlier, care must be taken to harvest only the nodes located superficially and laterally to the common femoral vessels. These nodes can be preoperatively located by CT scan and more easily identified intraoperatively by performing ICG-lymphography of the donor site to assess nodes which must be spared. This assures us that we are not harvesting nodes draining the lower limb. Patent blue dye V is injected intradermally immediately above and below the anterior superior iliac spine, to assess those nodes which should be harvested.

Secondary procedures

Clinical postoperative assessment is performed by measuring limb circumferences the first month after surgery, every 3 months in the first year, and then twice per year, to verify the post-surgical improvement.

Limb lymphoscintigraphy (LS) is repeated 12 months after surgery. The technique and data interpretation are the same as those described for the preoperative exam. LS can verify whether an improvement in the lymphatic drainage has occurred respect to the preoperative exam. It can demonstrate the effectiveness of ALNT, as the viable transplanted nodes can be visualized in the recipient area and new lymph drainage pathways can appear. LS can also assess the patency of an LVA by means of indirect findings. For example, it can show the reduction of the dermal backflow or the disappearance of the tracer in a site of an LVA due to tracer passage into the blood circulation.

Postoperative ICG lymphography is repeated 1 year after surgery. The technique is the same as that described for the preoperative exam. Postoperatively, ICG-lymphography evaluates whether the lymphatic transport function has improved after lymphatic surgery compared with the preoperative exam. In addition, it helps to assess the patency of an LVA and to select new functional lymphatic channels when a secondary LVA surgery is planned. After ALNT, ICG-lymphography can sometimes integrate information provided by postoperative LS, as it can demonstrate the viability of autotransplanted lymph nodes, when sufficiently superficial (<2 cm of depth), because of the intrinsic limit of the exam.

If remnants of hypertrophic fatty tissue, without liquid, persist in the postoperative assessment, selective liposuction in the thickened area can be performed.

Access the complete reference list online at   **http://www.expertconsult.com**

1. DiSipio T, Rye S, Newman B, et al. Incidence of unilateral arm lymphoedema after breast cancer: a systematic review and meta-analysis. *Lancet Oncol.* 2013;14:500–515.

2. Mehrara BJ, Zampell JC, Suami H, et al. Surgical management of lymphedema: past, present, and future. *Lymphat Res Biol.* 2011;9:159–167.

3. Brorson H. Liposuction in lymphedema treatment. *J Reconstr Microsurg.* 2016;32:56–65.

4. Becker C, Assouad J, Riquet M, et al. Postmastectomy lymphedema: long-term results following microsurgical lymph node transplantation. *Ann Surg.* 2006;243:313–331.

5. Koshima I, Inagawa K, Urushibara K, et al. Supermicrosurgical lymphaticovenular -anastomosis for the treatment of lymphedema in the upper extremities. *J Reconstr Microsurg.* 2000;16: 437–442.

6. Baumeister R, Siuda S. Treatment of lymphedemas by microsurgical lymphatic grafting: what is proved? *Plast Reconstr Surg.* 1990;85: 64–74.

7. Suami H, Chang DW. Overview of surgical treatments for breast cancer-related lymphedema. *Plast Reconstr Surg.* 2010;126:1853–1863.

14. Mortimer PS. The pathophysiology of lymphedema. *Cancer.* 1998;83:2798–2802.

15. Koshima I, Kawada S, Moriguchi T, et al. Ultrastructural observations of lymphatic vessels in lymphedema in human extremities. *Plast Reconstr Surg.* 1996;97:397–407.

17. Masia J, Pons G, Nardulli ML. Combined surgical treatment in breast cancer-related lymphedema. *J Reconstr Microsurg.* 2016;32:16–27.

18. International Society of Lymphology. The diagnosis and treatment of peripheral lymphedema: 2013 consensus document of the International Society of Lymphology. *Lymphology.* 2013;46:1–11.

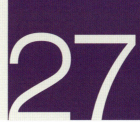

Reconstruction of the nipple areolar complex

Edward H. Davidson, Francesco M. Egro, and Kenneth C. Shestak

SYNOPSIS

- Nipple areolar complex (NAC) reconstruction completes breast reconstruction for many patients through a variety of approaches including, local "pull-out" flaps, skin/tissue composite grafts, tattooing in combination or isolation.
- The essential elements in successful post-mastectomy nipple reconstruction involve appropriate position, projection, and pigmentation of the reconstructed nipple and areola.
- Tattooing techniques have evolved to produce a remarkably natural appearance of the areola with an essentially non-invasive office-based procedure, albeit with the shortcoming of lack of nipple projection. With the introduction of "three-dimensional" (3D) tattooing, a remarkable facsimile of nipple projection can be created.
- To create a projected nipple, contralateral nipple sharing, tissue grafts from other sites, and local "pull-out" flaps can all be performed, with the latter constituting the current "state of the art".
- Local flaps usually require initial over-projection due to loss of projection over time, they do not recreate natural intermittent erectility and may be less desirable in reconstructed breasts with thin tissue overlying a prosthetic implant, or following radiation.
- Currently, no technique exists that restores erogenous or nursing function of the NAC.

Introduction

Reconstruction of the nipple areolar complex (NAC) for many women is perceived as the final battle in their war against breast cancer, completing the restoration of form that most closely resembles a native breast. Some breast reconstruction patients are content with a normal appearance in clothing following breast reconstruction alone and may choose not to pursue NAC reconstruction. In those who do pursue NAC reconstruction, there are the options of local flaps, skin grafts, tattooing, or some combination of the above. Though immediate NAC reconstruction, at the same time as the primary breast reconstruction procedure, has been described, it is more common to delay NAC reconstruction until the final shape of the reconstructed breast has stabilized to ensure correct and symmetrical positioning. Preservation of the NAC with NAC-sparing mastectomy, if oncologically sound, usually and more reliably achieves superior aesthetic results. Patients must be counseled that all current techniques of NAC preservation and reconstruction fail to confer native erogenous or nursing function. This chapter is focused on post-mastectomy NAC reconstruction in the female, but the considerations and approaches outlined herein may also be applied and indicated for NAC reconstruction in other scenarios, including following burns, trauma, congenital athelia (absence of nipple development), nipple loss after surgery, and in male as well as female patients.

Diagnosis/patient presentation

General considerations

The anatomy of the female nipple areolar complex can be as varied in shape, size, orientation, and color as the breasts on which they sit. Nonetheless, natural anatomic proportions between the breast and the nipple areolar complex have been suggested to be areola–breast and nipple–areola proportions of 1 : 3.4 and 1 : 3, respectively.[1] Classically, the aesthetic NAC position is described as at the point of maximal projection of the breast at some point above the inframammary fold.[2] Anatomic parameters for nipple position and areola diameter have also been described in males: nipple position 20 cm from the sternal notch and 18 cm from the midclavicular line; nipple to nipple distance of 21 cm and areolar diameter of 2.8 cm.[3] Alternatively, the male NAC position can be located using a technique based on the height of the patient and the chest circumference.[4] Adjusting the position of the NAC is difficult, and so aesthetic NAC reconstruction must therefore focus on position as well as projection and pigmentation.

When considering unilateral versus bilateral NAC reconstruction, the surgeon and patient can study the contralateral nipple position, base dimension, and projection to aid planning and selection of reconstructive technique. In planning for bilateral reconstruction, the surgeon, with patient assistance, must establish the position of the NAC without this luxury. Ignoring mastectomy scars and, for example, with the aid of an EKG lead pad, position is determined by the patient's "eye" with surgeon-led adjustment and explanation, as determined by the parameters outlined above. A unilateral reconstruction also affords the possibility of contralateral composite nipple–areola grafting, or "nipple sharing", especially if the native NAC is relatively large.[5]

NAC reconstruction is usually postponed until the final and stable setting of the reconstructed breast, optimally 3–4 months following breast reconstruction.[6] Some authors have proposed primary NAC reconstruction at the time of breast reconstruction in a single stage procedure.[7] Notably, this approach is limited to immediate autologous flap-based reconstruction, as opposed to implant-based reconstruction when the mastectomy flap blood supply is less robust. Furthermore, it is believed that NAC reconstruction at the time of expander/implant exchange should be avoided, as this may be associated with a higher rate of implant loss due to possible wound healing problems with the nipple reconstruction portion of the procedure, which may result in implant loss.

A plethora of methods of NAC reconstruction have been introduced, and while some have been consigned to history, others continue to evolve into the modern surgeon's armamentarium. Currently, reconstruction of the nipple is most often performed with local "pull-out" flaps, with tissue grafting (nipple sharing) having a lesser role. These flaps produce a projecting nipple, but a greater dimension of realism requires the introduction of pigment for both the nipple and more importantly for creation of the surrounding areola. For this reason, the areola is most commonly reconstructed with the use of an intradermal tattoo. This is especially true in nipple reconstruction techniques, where there is direct closure of the nipple flap donor area. A well-done tattoo provides shape, size, and color to the reconstructed areola.

At present, the ultimate in nipple "reconstruction" is preservation of the patient's native nipple in the form of a nipple-sparing mastectomy. Since its introduction, the inherent superior aesthetic result of NAC preservation compared with reconstructive techniques has contributed to the trend towards the increased popularity of this approach.

Etiology of athelia, absent nipple, may also influence the approach to reconstruction. Careful patient and tissue assessment is critical combined with good surgical judgment. For example, in reconstruction following burn injury or after post-mastectomy radiation, results with tissue grafts may be more predictable than local flaps.[8,9] Similarly, if thin mastectomy skin flaps are overlying a prosthetic breast implant then, again, surgical manipulation of compromised tissue to create a bed for a graft or to raise a flap may prove non-viable or even violate an implant capsule and result in reconstructive failure. In all these scenarios, tattooing and especially 3D tattooing may be a more prudent option.

Treatment/surgical technique

Tattooing

Intradermal tattooing of the nipple and/or areola has the advantage of being an essentially non-invasive office-based procedure. Results can vary, but in skilled hands this can produce a remarkably natural appearance of both nipple and areola.[10–12] The procedure has evolved from using emulsions that produced a painted experience to pigment gel suspensions which more closely resemble natural skin pigments and can provide the optical illusion of texture.[6,13] Optimal results are achieved by not using a darker pigment than the opposite areola where applicable, as well as use of alcohol skin prep, a short course of per oral antibiotics, and topical antibiotic ointment. Due to pigment fading, it has been our experience that tattooing will often need to be revised at 1 year.

This method of NAC reconstruction is an especially good idea if there is a paucity of tissue on pinch test and especially if there is an underlying implant, multiple scars, or previous radiation. The shortcoming of tattooing is the lack of nipple projection, and therefore, traditionally, this has served as a method for recreating the appearance of the areola and pigmentation of a reconstructed nipple. Tattooing can be performed before or after any nipple reconstruction, as determined by practitioner preference.

Newer, 3D tattooing techniques apply the artistic principles of light and shadow to create depth on a 2D surface. The 3D technique is essentially the inverse of the traditional NAC tattoo. Instead of using a darker inner circle to create the appearance of a nipple, a *lighter* inner circle is created with a dark border. This border is thickened inferiorly to create a shadow effect. The areola is created according to the patient's preferred diameter and color and is typically performed 3 months after breast reconstruction and takes approximately 45 min for a unilateral reconstruction. The introduction of professional tattoo artists to the reconstructive arena, adopting professional fundamentals of machine speed, needle type, and color mixing, as opposed to medical grade tattooing techniques, has also heralded improved pigment retention (Fig. 27.1).[14]

Tissue grafts for nipple and areola reconstruction

Although currently not the first-line treatment for most nipple reconstructions, composite grafts still have a role. The most popular method is that of contralateral nipple sharing, which affords the possibility of reconstruction by replacing "like with like". Many patients and surgeons are reluctant to risk the form and function of a healthy nipple, though others have shown erectile function and sensation of the donor nipple are unaffected by nipple sharing procedures.[15] However, as recently described by Zenn and Garofalo, this may be a particularly appealing option in the case of hypertrophied or large native nipples, and especially in irradiated or thin tissues in which local flaps may be precluded.[5]

Numerous donor sites for skin grafting to reconstruct the areola have been described including contralateral areola, thigh, groin, labia, eyelid, retroauricular skin, and oral mucous membrane, as well as testicular skin

in male NAC reconstruction. Thigh and groin skin have been suggested as a good color match for darker areolas with retroauricular skin, eyelid skin, and oral mucosa more suited to lighter areolas. Nonetheless, skin grafting from any of these sites may result in hyperpigmentation or more commonly fading of pigment in the skin that is hypopigmentation over time. Moreover and very importantly, skin grafting for areola reconstruction is of limited use at present and has fallen into disfavor by inherent donor site morbidity.[16-23] It has been supplanted by the use of the intradermal tattoo method of areola creation.

Local flaps

The concept of creation of a projected nipple through local dermal-fat flaps was introduced by Hartrampf in 1984, which in a real sense was the original skate flap (Fig. 27.2).[24] There are now many techniques, though most are variants or derivatives of the skate flap,[25] including the star flap (Fig. 27.3),[26] fishtail flap (Fig. 27.4),[27] H-flap,[28] bell flap,[29] C-V flap,[30] and arrow flap.[31] These flaps all obtain their vascular supply through the subdermal plexus, all share the challenge of maintaining long-term nipple projection and necessitate initial "over-correction", and for all donor site primary closure limits flap size or skin grafting is required.

Planning of the reconstruction

For unilateral nipple reconstruction, planning begins with a study of the opposite nipple including position and projection. Projection is best identified with the patient standing in front of a full-length mirror using an EKG lead pad with the central metal tab being nipple position. After placement, measurements from fixed landmarks such as the sternal midline and the suprasternal notch are made. It is important to realize that the ideal position of the nipple may be slightly different than it is on the patient's natural breast, depending on the size, projection, and position on the chest wall of the reconstructed breast. If the position selected by the patient is not aesthetically advisable, this is pointed out to the patient and corrections are made. The same exercise is undertaken for bilateral reconstruction.

Whenever possible, the design of the flap(s) in a unilateral nipple reconstruction should include dimensions (the width of the long limbs) which enable a reconstruction that is 40% larger than the patient's natural nipple to allow for loss of projection as a result of the contraction that occurs with healing. Projection of the reconstructed nipple is dependent on the design and the thickness and quality of the dermis of the skin

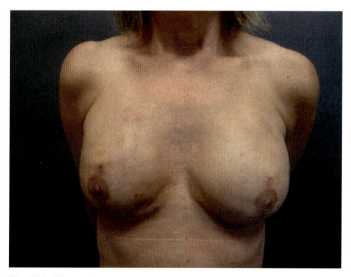

Fig. 27.1 3D tattooing can create a remarkably natural appearance of the areola and illusion of nipple projection.

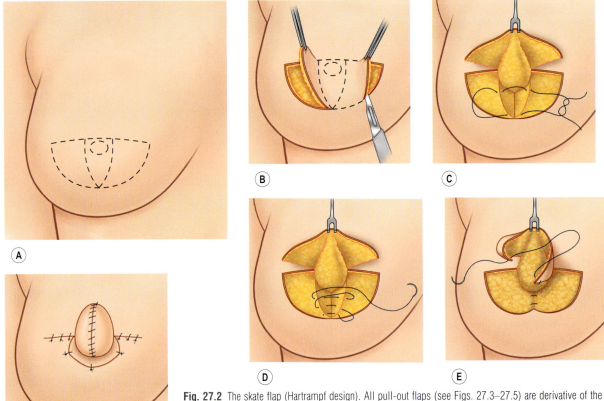

Fig. 27.2 The skate flap (Hartrampf design). All pull-out flaps (see Figs. 27.3–27.5) are derivative of the design. **(A)** The design of the flap. The base is superior to the inscribed circle; the wings are the lateral extensions. **(B)** The wings are elevated toward the central core at the deepest part of the dermis leaving a small thickness of the dermis. **(C)** The central core is elevated at a depth of 4–7 mm (depending on the size of the nipple required). **(D)** The lateral wings and central core resemble the fish called a "skate". The central fat donor area is closed. **(E)** The lateral wings are wrapped around the central core of elevated adipose tissue. **(F)** Flap closure routinely requires a skin graft over the dermis seen at the inferior aspect of the drawing.

utilized. For this reason, the latissimus dorsi flap is most ideal for creating nipples with excellent projection.

Planning and technique selection are also influenced by previous incisions on the reconstructed breast and their possible impact on the blood supply derived from the subdermal plexus.

Technique selection

Advantages and disadvantages

Selection of technique should consider blood supply and aesthetics in each clinical scenario. The skate flap (see Fig. 27.2) can create large nipples but often requires skin grafting for donor site closure. The star flap (see Fig. 27.3) more easily allows primary closure of the donor site. However, the disadvantage of this technique is that is results in lesser nipple projection and slight flattening of the breast contour that occurs when the local donor site is closed. Creation of significant nipple projection dictates lengthy lateral limbs that may extend beyond the ideal areola size. Nonetheless, the technique is extremely versatile for primary nipple reconstruction

and its reliability also renders it the senior author's (Ken Shestak) technique of choice for re-do nipple reconstruction.

The similar fishtail flap (see Fig. 27.4) also allows for primary closure of the donor site. The angle between the flaps can be varied, and so this has become the authors' technique of choice when the ideal nipple position is in or immediately adjacent to a mastectomy scar, as blood supply across the scar is not reliable. For this reason, the fishtail flap does not contain a "cap", and often the most anterior aspect of the reconstruct is left open to heal by secondary intention, since excessive folding of the flaps can impair their blood supply. Others have described successful incorporation of a pre-existing scar in the star flap technique; if the intended site of nipple reconstruction bisects through a vertical mastectomy scar, the star flap is designed as medially or laterally based, with its two lateral limbs lying adjacent to the scar and the transverse central component incorporating the vertical scar. On the other hand, if the selected site of nipple reconstruction passes into a horizontal scar, the flap is positioned inferiorly- or superiorly-based along the scar with its two lateral limbs adjacent to the scar

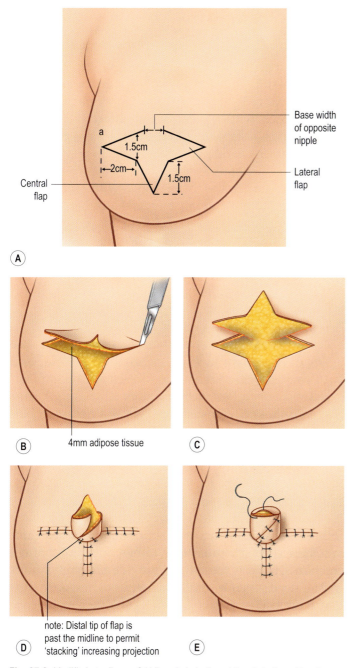

using a Bell flap, a modified star flap, or a skate flap with a full-thickness skin graft for areola reconstruction. Patients with ≤5 mm of nipple projection on the opposite breast were treated with either the Bell flap or the modified star flap. In patients where the areola complex exhibited significant projection, a bell flap was chosen

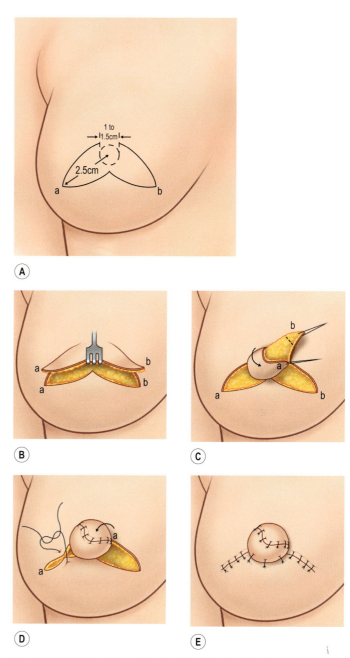

Fig. 27.3 Modified star flap or C-V flap. A derivative of the skate flap with primary closure of the donor area. **(A)** Flap planning. The base of the lateral flaps and central flap dimensions are illustrated. **(B)** The lateral and central flaps are elevated to a depth of 1 mm into the adipose tissue layer. **(C)** A central core of fat 5 mm thick is elevated at the base of the flap. **(D)** The lateral wings are wrapped around the central core and inset into the skin. **(E)** The cap of the flap is brought over the top of the overlapped lateral wings. The lateral and inferior skin flap donor areas are directly approximated.

Fig. 27.4 Fishtail flap. Also a derivative of the skate flap. There is a central pedicle, *but* unlike the modified star flap, there is no "cap" to cover the top of the nipple column. **(A)** A circle, which is the base of the flap. The length of the wings are variable, but most often, they are 2.5 cm in length. **(B)** The flaps are raised with 1–2 mm of adipose tissue on their deep surface. **(C)** The flaps are elevated towards their central core, with 3–5 mm of adipose tissue being raised around the central core. **(D)** The flaps are then wrapped around each other by stacking one upon the other. **(E)** The donor areas are closed by direct approximation. At times, the flaps may not allow closure of the most anterior part of the reconstructed nipple, and topical ointment applied daily will allow healing in 7–10 days. This is preferable to excessive folding or over-tightening of the delicate flaps.

and vertical central limb including the scar.[32] When designing the flap for reconstruction, whenever possible, superiorly-based flaps are preferred, as these appear more aesthetically pleasing to the patient; when she looks down, she does not see incisions on the nipple.

The authors have reported a comparative assessment of nipple and areola projection after reconstruction over the modified star flap. In those patients with >5 mm of nipple projection, reconstruction with a skate flap and full-thickness skin graft was performed. The best long-term nipple projection was obtained and maintained by the skate and star techniques. The major decrease in projection of the reconstructed nipple occurred during the first 3 months. After 6 months, the projection was stable. The loss of both nipple projections when using the Bell flap was so remarkable that the authors discourage the use of this procedure in virtually all patients.[33]

Several adjunctive strategies have been touted to improve maintenance of nipple projection with local flap reconstruction. Use of auricular cartilage, rib cartilage, acellular dermal matrix, calcium hydroxylapatite, and autologous fat grafting have all been described to augment flaps with varying success.[34–39] In the authors' opinion, all of these are salvage efforts that suffer from the effects of scarring of the bed and the inevitable consequence of attrition over time.

Though the impact on long-term projection, if any, is difficult to ascertain, most surgeons would advocate the use of a fenestrated/"donut" or stent-like dressing that protects/supports the newly reconstructed nipple as part of the postoperative regimen.[40–42]

The authors' preferred technique for local flap-based NAC reconstruction is the double opposing periareolar flap (Fig. 27.5).[43] A pull-out flap is also a derivative of the skate design. It is similar to the periareolar skate flap described by Hammond et al.[44] The nipple is derived as the lead edge of one of two opposing skin flaps contained in a circular design approximating the areola complex of the opposite breast. The larger flap gives rise to the nipple construct. Whenever possible, it is oriented with the larger flap having a superior location. The central nipple and the lateral and medial extensions are elevated just below the dermis with 1–2 mm of subdermal fat included with the skin flap elevation. As the dissection proceeds to the central area of the actual nipple, a core of additional subcutaneous fat (4–5 mm) is preserved deep to the dermis in the nipple (Fig. 27.5A,B) The central donor area is closed as the parent flap and opposing flap are incised at their peripheral margins (which correspond to the outline of the areola) with the incision made with a scalpel just through the dermis sparing the underlying subdermal plexus (Fig. 27.5C,D). The flaps are then easily advanced towards each other by sliding them on their subdermal plexus blood supply. The only undermined area is the nipple flap itself (Fig. 27.5E,F). There is no undermining of either the parent flap or the opposing flap or peripheral breast skin (and this is a key difference from the technique described by Hammond and

colleagues).[44] The dissection is straightforward, and the technique is rapid. After closure of the central flap donor area, a small de-epithelialization at the site of planned nipple position provides an excellent platform to inset the nipple upon, and this likely contributes to sustained projection. The resulting peripheral donor area is closed with a purse-string suture (Fig. 27.5G). Of particular advantage, all of the scars are contained within the peripheral periareolar incision and thus can be completely camouflaged by an intradermal tattoo. Nipple projection has been consistently maintained and appears similar to that of a skate flap (see Fig. 27.2). This is easiest to perform in the setting of an autologous tissue reconstruction but may be used following implant reconstruction after careful assessment of the skin flaps. In the case of a suboptimal mastectomy flap due to thin flap tissue, often encountered following tissue expansion, a simpler C-V or fishtail flap may be safer and preferable.

Caution must be adopted when considering the use of any of these flaps in thin irradiated tissues and/or if NAC reconstruction is being performed over an implant-based breast reconstruction rather than autologous tissue. In these circumstances, there is a risk of jeopardizing the implant, and therefore at the very least, the surgeon should be prepared to repair the capsule if violated and have a replacement implant available. Results of local flaps for nipple reconstruction can also be disappointing in radiated tissue.

A caveat to projected nipple creation with these techniques is that patients should be counseled regarding their constant projection rather than intermittent erectility. Nor can these flaps provide erogenous function. Indeed, even in more adventurous regional flaps that have been described such as the neurocutaneous island flap based on the medial antebrachial cutaneous nerve, though reportedly restoring sensibility, does not recapitulate erogenous sensation.[45]

Nipple areolar complex preservation

As prevention may be preferable to cure, so in the case of the NAC may preservation be preferable to reconstruction. Nipple preservation, either through tissue banking with delayed grafting or nipple–areola sparing mastectomy, if oncologically sound, may be an option to confer the best aesthetics to a reconstructed breast.

Millard first described NAC preservation by removal of the NAC at the time of mastectomy and saving or banking at the groin, buttocks, or abdomen with subsequent transfer to the breast after reconstruction.[46] However, even when oncologically safe, this technique has lost popularity owing to the aesthetic inadequacies

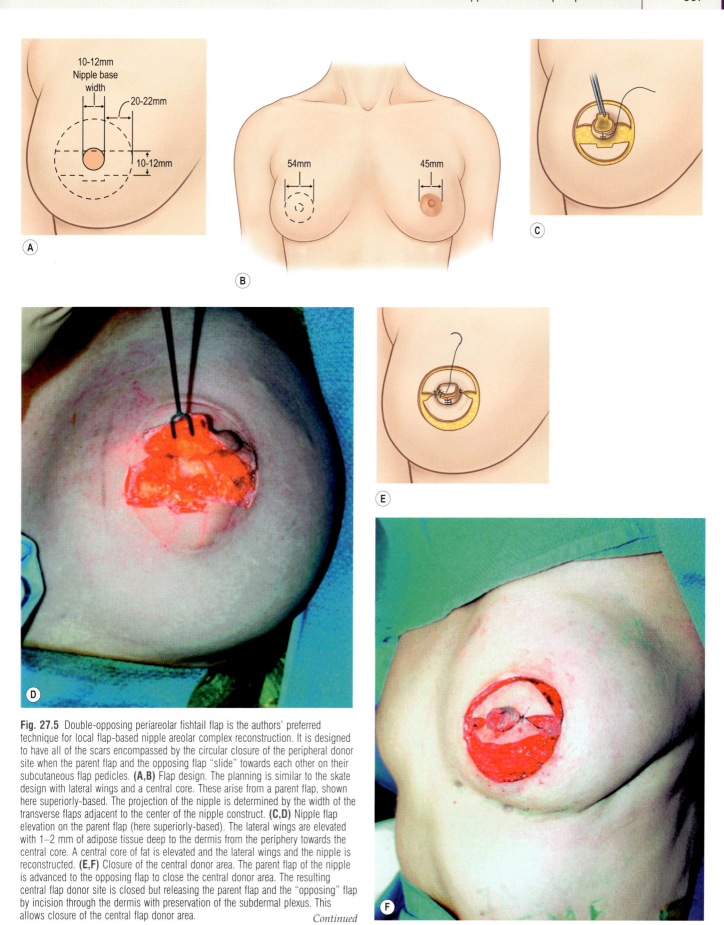

Fig. 27.5 Double-opposing periareolar fishtail flap is the authors' preferred technique for local flap-based nipple areolar complex reconstruction. It is designed to have all of the scars encompassed by the circular closure of the peripheral donor site when the parent flap and the opposing flap "slide" towards each other on their subcutaneous flap pedicles. **(A,B)** Flap design. The planning is similar to the skate design with lateral wings and a central core. These arise from a parent flap, shown here superiorly-based. The projection of the nipple is determined by the width of the transverse flaps adjacent to the center of the nipple construct. **(C,D)** Nipple flap elevation on the parent flap (here superiorly-based). The lateral wings are elevated with 1–2 mm of adipose tissue deep to the dermis from the periphery towards the central core. A central core of fat is elevated and the lateral wings and the nipple is reconstructed. **(E,F)** Closure of the central donor area. The parent flap of the nipple is advanced to the opposing flap to close the central donor area. The resulting central flap donor site is closed but releasing the parent flap and the "opposing" flap by incision through the dermis with preservation of the subdermal plexus. This allows closure of the central flap donor area. *Continued*

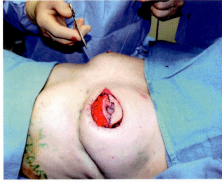

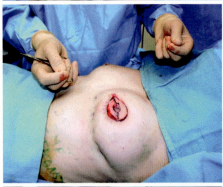

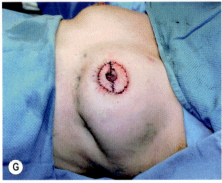

(G)

Fig. 27.5, cont'd **(G)** The resulting peripheral flap donor area is closed by a purse-string suture, and the skin is closed with a single layer of monofilament suture. A subsequent intradermal tattoo will disguise all of the incisions.

of pigment and projection loss associated with repeated harvest and grafting. More recent attempts at NAC banking with cryopreservation remain unproven.[47]

Nipple-sparing mastectomy, as the latest evolution of mastectomy technique, has proven to result in improved reconstructive and aesthetic outcomes in breast cancer care.[48] In an analysis of the way women expressed their reasons for choosing nipple-sparing mastectomy or NAC reconstruction, a clear psychological advantage of nipple-sparing mastectomy also emerged.[49]

The next paradigm shift in this arena is likely tissue engineering of the NAC, though at present, this approach is in its infancy.[50]

Conclusion

Nipple–areolar reconstruction requires an amalgamation of considerations of position, pigmentation, and projection. Many options for NAC reconstruction are available to the patient and surgeon, with the choice of technique dictated by aesthetic and tissue demands. Tattooing confers a higher dimension of realism to reconstruction and, with newer 3D techniques, these may ultimately replace tissue grafts and flaps in many situations, as well as being advantageous in thin and/or irradiated tissue as described herein. Tissue grafts and local flaps, however, in the absence of a clinical reality for tissue engineered or preserved NACs remain the mainstay for reconstructing a nipple with actual and sustained projection. More novel approaches are still required to restore erogenous and nursing functions of the reconstructed NAC.

Access the complete reference list online at **http://www.expertconsult.com**

1. Hauben DJ, Adler N, Silfen R, et al. Breast–areola–nipple proportion. *Ann Plast Surg*. 2003;50:510–513. *This anatomic study elegantly describes the anatomic geometry of the nipple areola complex. This may serve as a guide to reconstruction.*

2. Regnault P. Breast ptosis. Definition and treatment. *Clin Plast Surg*. 1976;3:193–203. *This is a landmark article classifying ptosis based on nipple position. Understanding of this is fundamental to NAC reconstruction in the context of its relation to the underlying breast.*

5. Zenn MR, Garofalo JA. Unilateral nipple reconstruction with nipple sharing: time for a second look. *Plast Reconstr Surg*. 2009;123:1648–1653. *This case series of over 50 patients is an excellent guide to the indications and techniques for nipple sharing.*

6. Farhadi J, Maksvytyte GK, Schaefer DJ, et al. Reconstruction of the nipple-areola complex: an update. *J Plast Reconstr Aesthet Surg*. 2006;59:40–53. *This is a comprehensive review that illustrates well the commonly adopted local tissue flaps in NAC reconstruction.*

14. Halvorson EG, Cormican M, West ME, et al. Three-dimensional nipple-areola tattooing: a new technique with superior results. *Plast Reconstr Surg*. 2014;133:1073–1075. *This is the definitive description of modern 3D tattooing of the NAC.*

24. Hartrampf CR Jr, Culbertson JH. A dermal-fat flap for nipple reconstruction. *Plast Reconstr Surg*. 1984;73:982–986. *A*

classic article from which all other pull-out flap designs have been derived.

33. Shestak KC, Gabriel A, Landecker A, et al. Assessment of long-term nipple projection: a comparison of three techniques. *Plast Reconstr Surg*. 2002;110:780–786. *A retrospective review of 68 patients and their nipple projection following reconstruction by either skate, modified star, or Bell flaps.*

43. Shestak KC, Nguyen TD. The double opposing periareola flap: a novel concept for nipple areola reconstruction. *Plast Reconstr Surg*. 2007;119:473–480. *This is the authors' preferred technique for local pull-out flap reconstruction of the NAC.*

48. Endara M, Chen D, Verma K, et al. Breast reconstruction following nipple-sparing mastectomy: a systematic review of the literature with pooled analysis. *Plast Reconstr Surg*. 2013;132:1043–1054. *A systemic review outlining the success and safety of nipple-sparing mastectomy. This surgical breakthrough can avoid the need for NSM altogether.*

49. Didier F, Arnaboldi P, Gandini S, et al. Why do women accept to undergo a nipple sparing mastectomy or to reconstruct the nipple areola complex when nipple sparing mastectomy is not possible? *Breast Cancer Res Treat*. 2012;132:1177–1184. *This article explores the relative benefits of NAC reconstruction and nipple-sparing mastectomy and identifies a clear benefit of the latter.*

28

Congenital breast deformities

Francesco M. Egro, Edward H. Davidson, James D. Namnoum, and Kenneth C. Shestak

SYNOPOSIS

- Congenital breast deformities are a relatively common problem and place an emotional burden on both the patient and their parents during puberty and adolescence.
- Breast deformities present unilaterally or bilaterally, as isolated anomalies, or more rarely, with other abnormalities affecting other organs. They can be broadly categorized as "hypoplastic" and "hyperplastic" disorders.
- Precise diagnosis and carefully timed surgical management is required to optimize outcomes and the social and psychosexual impact on patients and parents.

Introduction

Congenital breast deformities are a relatively common problem, which place a major emotional burden on both the patient and the parents, especially during puberty and adolescence. These deformities have the potential of causing anxiety, depression, peer rejection, and psychosexual dysfunction. This has a major impact on the patient's normal psychosocial development, participation in school activities, and social life. Breast deformities present unilaterally or bilaterally, as isolated anomalies, or more rarely with other abnormalities affecting other organs. They can be broadly categorized as "hypoplastic" and "hyperplastic disorders" (Table 28.1).[1] Each condition represents a unique challenge, which warrants consideration on an individual case basis. Surgical correction is dependent on the type of anomaly and involves decisions about timing and technique selection, with the goal to optimize the functional and aesthetic outcomes and best satisfy the psychological needs of the patient. This chapter discusses the most common congenital breast deformities and their surgical management.

Embryology

The breast is a modified apocrine sweat gland, which begins to develop at the 5th week of fetal development. Linear ectodermal ridges (also called "mammary ridges" or "milk lines") develop from 15–20 buds found bilaterally on the ventral surface of the embryo, extending from the axillary to the inguinal regions (Fig. 28.1). During the 7th week, some of these buds undergo apoptosis, leaving behind only a single pair of solid buds (primary mammary buds) at the level of the fourth or fifth intercostal space. Incomplete regression of the ectodermal ridge leads to the development of ectopic supernumerary nipples (polythelia) or breast tissue (polymastia) along the mammary ridge. The ectodermal primary mammary buds invade the underlying mesoderm, and by the 12th week, secondary mammary buds are formed, which will eventually form the mammary lobules. By the 5th month, the mammary ridge penetrates the underlying mesoderm, sending 15–20 epithelial branches into the developing breast. The areola also develops around the 5th month. During the 3rd trimester, these epithelial branches develop into primitive ducts under the influence of placental sex hormones, forming the lactiferous ducts and their branches. The lactiferous ducts converge to open into a mammary pit, which then becomes the nipple and starts protruding through the areola during infancy.[2] The breast parenchyma is contained within the superficial fascia, which is continuous with the superficial abdominal Camper's

Table 28.1 Summary of congenital hypoplastic and hyperplastic breast deformities

Hypoplastic	Hyperplastic
Breast hypoplasia and amazia	Gynecomastia
Athelia and amastia	Virginal mammary hypertrophy
Tuberous breast deformity	Giant fibroadenoma
Poland syndrome	Polythelia
Anterior thoracic hypoplasia	Polymastia

fascia. The superficial fascia consists of a superficial layer (outer layer covering the breast parenchyma) and a deep layer (posterior boundary of the breast parenchyma) that lies on the deep fascia of the pectoralis major and serratus anterior muscles. The deep layer is penetrated by the suspensory ligaments of Cooper, which extend from the breast dermis to the deep pectoral fascia, joining the two layers of the superficial fascia.[3] The formation of sweat glands, sebaceous glands, and apocrine glands occurs during the 2nd trimester. Breast tissue grows at the same rate as the rest of the body during childhood, as long as the estrogen levels are low. With the increase in estrogen levels during puberty, a series of morphologic stages occur, which are described by the Tanner classification.[4] Stage I (preadolescent) describes papilla elevation above the level of the chest wall. Stage II describes breast and papilla elevation, along with increased areola diameter. Stage III describes

ongoing enlargement of the breasts and areolae. Stage IV describes elevation of the areola and papilla above the breast mound. Lastly, stage V describes the appearance of a mature breast, with elevation of the papilla and regression of the areola. Most females achieve stage V by 16–18 years of age.[2]

Hypoplastic disorders

Breast hypoplasia and amazia

The mammary gland can either be underdeveloped (hypoplastic) or absent (amazia), and this may occur unilaterally or bilaterally, in isolation or in association with pectoral muscles defects. Breast asymmetry can be managed with various surgical options, including augmentation of the affected breast using implants (most commonly in the submuscular plane[5]) or myocutaneous flaps (e.g., latissimus dorsi myocutaneous flap); or most recently, by the use of autologous fat transfer (fat grafting), breast reduction mammaplasty, or mastopexy of the larger contralateral breast, or a combination of the above. Occasionally, the skin envelope needs to be expanded using a tissue expander prior to the insertion of a permanent implant. Minor corrections can safely be achieved by means of autologous adipose tissue transfer. The optimal timing for surgery depends on the degree of the deformity and its physical and psychological impact. It is probably optimal to temporize until the breast is fully developed whenever possible (usually by 18 years of age).[1,5,6] The simplest and most consistently successful method, when applicable, is mammaplasty – breast reduction and mastopexy as illustrated in Figs. 28.2 & 28.3.

Athelia and amastia

Athelia is defined as the absence of the nipple areolar complex (NAC) and usually occurs with amastia, which is defined as the absence of the whole breast unit including the NAC and the mammary gland. Athelia and amastia can be familial (autosomal dominant) and may occur unilaterally or bilaterally, in isolation or in association with amastia and other rare syndromes (e.g., scalp-ear-nipple syndrome, Al-Awadi/Raas-Rothschild syndrome, and Poland syndrome).[7] For this reason, patients need to be investigated to rule out other ectodermal abnormalities. The exact etiology is unknown, but a deficiency in parathyroid-related hormone might be the trigger to abnormal involution of the mammary ridge.[8] In 1965, Trier produced a classification of athelia, based on its association with amastia: Group 1 describes bilateral amastia with associated ectodermal congenital defects; Group 2 defines unilateral defects; Group 3

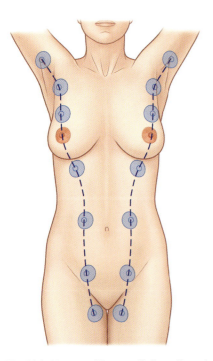

Fig. 28.1 Mammary ridges or milk lines. *(Reproduced with permission from Standring S. (ed.) Gray's Anatomy. 40th edn. London: Churchill Livingstone, Elsevier; 2008.)*

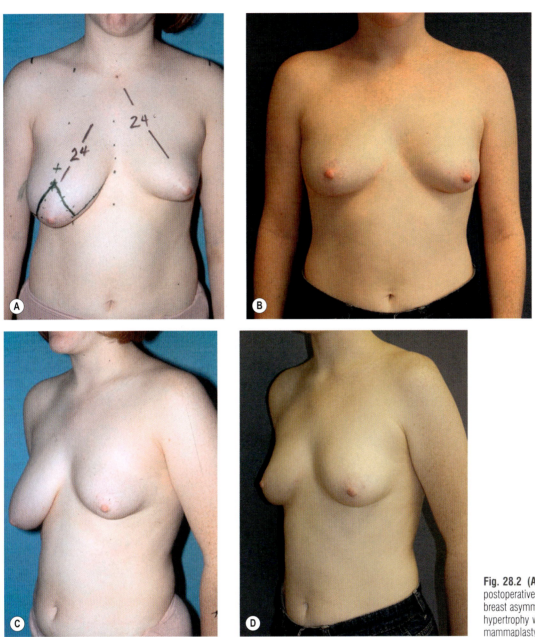

Fig. 28.2 **(A,C)** Preoperative and **(B,D)** 5-year postoperative images of a patient suffering from breast asymmetry caused by right unilateral breast hypertrophy who underwent right reduction mammaplasty.

defines bilateral amastia, with no other associated defects.[7] The surgical treatment depends on the presence of athelia, amastia, or both. The breast reconstruction can be performed using similar techniques to the ones described for hypoplastic or aplastic breasts. In cases where both NAC and mammary gland are absent, reconstruction of the nipple is delayed until breast reconstruction is completed. Nipple and areola reconstruction can be carried out using a combination of techniques including small local flaps, skin grafts, cartilage grafts, acellular dermal matrices, and/or NAC tattooing.[1,6]

Tuberous breast deformity

Tuberous breast deformity is a spectrum of aberrant breast shape, usually presenting in adolescence, and is characterized by a constricted base with a "high tight inframammary fold"; contracted skin envelope in both the vertical and horizontal dimensions; relative breast hypoplasia and asymmetry; enlarged diameter of the NAC and herniation of breast parenchyma through the NAC; and most often breast asymmetry. The exact incidence among the general population is uncertain, but most surgeons agree that it is not an uncommon condition.[9] DeLuca-Pytell *et al.* showed in their study that tuberous breast deformity was present in 88.8% of the women demonstrating asymmetry, and only 7% of those with symmetric breasts.[9] The exact etiology is controversial, but two hypotheses have been brought forward. In 2003, Mandrekas *et al.* described the constricted ring theory: a constricting ring is formed as a

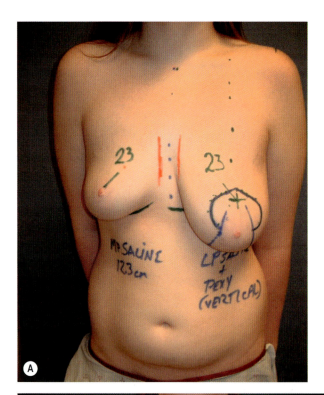

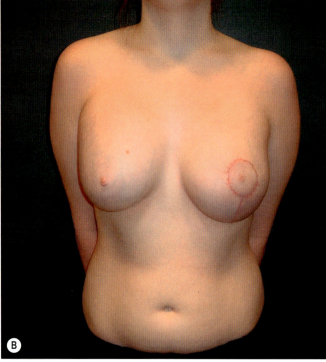

Fig. 28.3 (A) Preoperative and **(B)** at 4 months postoperative follow-up patient suffering from breast asymmetry caused by right breast hypoplasia and left breast hypertrophy, who underwent right partial subpectoral augmentation with a 360 cc smooth saline implant and left superior dermoglandular vertical mastopexy with 5 cm nipple transposition.

second hypothesis was brought forward by Costagliola *et al.* in 2013, who believe that the deformity is the result of a combination of factors: first, a congenital structural weakness and lack of elasticity of the NAC, and second, a hormonal imbalance between estrogen (horizontal thrust) and progesterone (vertical thrust) occurring during the breast growth period.[10] Multiple classifications have been brought forward to describe the extent of the deformity.[10–13] The most commonly used is a simplified version of the von Heimburg classification, introduced by Grolleau *et al.* in 1999 (Fig. 28.4): Type I describes hypoplasia of the lower medial quadrant;

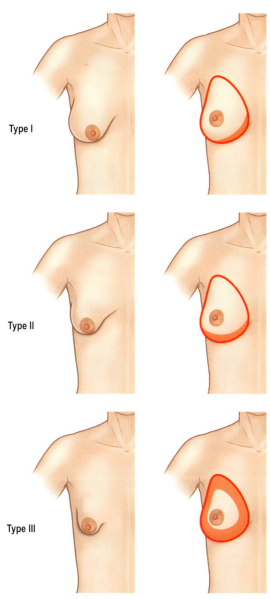

Fig. 28.4 Grolleau classification of tuberous breast deformity. Type I breasts have hypoplasia of the lower medial quadrant; Type II breasts have hypoplasia of both lower quadrants; Type III breasts have hypoplasia of all four quadrants. *(Redrawn after Grolleau JL et al. Breast base anomalies: treatment strategy for tuberous breasts, minor deformities, and asymmetry. Plast Reconstr Surg. 1999;104(7):2040–2048.)*

result of thickening of the superficial fascia at the level of the periphery of the NAC; this thickening prevents the expansion of the breast parenchyma inferiorly, which is instead rerouted towards the NAC, thus causing herniation through the missing fascia.[3] The

Type II describes hypoplasia of both lower quadrants; Type III describes hypoplasia of all four quadrants.[12]

One of the first procedures to correct tuberous breast deformity was described by Rees and Aston in 1976, who advocated widening of the constricted base by radial scoring.[14] Teimourian and Adham in 1983 described a combination of subpectoral augmentation, followed by donut-shaped periareolar de-epithelialization, excision of four wedges of breast tissue from below the new areola, and closure of the gaps to reduce both the herniated breast tissue and areola size.[15] Dinner and Dowden in 1987 advocated for a full-thickness incision through the skin with transposition of an inframammary skin flap to reconstruct the central breast, subcutaneous tissue, and breast parenchyma to release the cutaneous band causing the deformity.[16] Scheepers and Quaba in 1992 overinflated tissue expanders before exchange with a permanent implant.[17] Ribeiro et al. in 1998 transected the breast parenchyma horizontally and rearranged the inferior pole by unfolding the flap inwards or outwards.[18] Mandrekas et al. in 2003 described a similar approach to Ribeiro and colleagues, except that the constrictive band is divided vertically and the volume is obtained either by rearranging the two pillars or by placing an implant in the subglandular plane.[3] Pacifico and Kang in 2007 focused on areola reduction, subdermal undermining, and implant placement in the subglandular plane, without transecting the constrictive band.[19] Most recently, Kolker and Collins described their approach involving periareolar access; dissection to the new inframammary fold; glandular scoring; subpectoral implant placement; and mastopexy techniques.[20] Lastly, Coleman and Saboeiro reported the potential of lipoaugmentation by injecting autologous adipose tissue (370–380 cc per breast) into the subcutaneous tissue and pectoral muscle to enhance the contour aesthetics of the breast.[21]

Despite the variation in techniques, the general consensus advocates the use of a periareolar donut-type mastopexy pattern to adjust the size of the areola, followed by undermining, and division of the constriction bands by scoring or transection. The remaining flaps are rearranged to reconstruct the lower pole, and an implant can be inserted to add volume to the breast. A two-stage procedure, which entails initial tissue expander placement followed by implant insertion, is usually reserved for the most severe cases. The patient illustrated in Fig. 28.5 underwent a type III dual-plane release breast surgery with placement of synthetic implants beneath the pectoralis major muscle.

Complications reported in the literature derive mainly from small case series and include recurrence, asymmetry, delayed healing, scarring, loss of sensation, and implant-related complications, with capsular contracture and implant malposition being the most frequent of these.[22] Mandrekas et al. (n=11)[3] and Pacifico and Kang (n=11)[19] reported no complications. A more recent study by Kolker and Collins (n=26)[20] reported complication rates of 7.8%, with capsular contracture in 3.9% of the breasts and malposition in 3.9% of the breasts. Patient satisfaction and aesthetic outcomes were found to range from "good" to "excellent". Mandrekas et al. reported 100% patient satisfaction and 100% surgeon satisfaction.[3] Other studies confirmed patient satisfaction and identified aesthetic outcomes as "excellent" in 75% and "good" in 25% of the cases/patients.[19]

Poland syndrome

Poland syndrome is a rare congenital malformation with an incidence of 1 in 7000 to 1 in 100 000.[8] It was named after the anatomist Alfred Poland, a pathologist from Guy's Hospital in London, who described it in 1841. However, the condition was originally described by Lallemand in 1826.

Poland syndrome is characterized by various degrees of thoracic and ipsilateral upper extremity anomalies including some or all of the following: absence or hypoplasia of the breast; absence of the nipple; absence of the pectoralis major or minor; absence of adjacent muscles and sometimes costal cartilage; rib abnormalities; and upper extremity deformities (e.g., syndactyly, brachydactyly, or micromelia). The most obvious deformities are usually limb deformities in both females and males, and hypomastia in females. Breast deformities in women are variable, ranging from mild hypoplasia to aplasia. The typical breast deformity is characterized by loss of breast parenchyma, high inframammary fold, and a superiorly malpositioned and underdeveloped NAC.[6,8]

The etiology of Poland syndrome is unknown but is thought to be caused by hypoplasia of the subclavian artery and its branches, around the 4th and 6th week of gestation. This leads to vascular compromise of the internal thoracic artery affecting the development of the pectoralis major, and/or compromise of the branches of the brachial artery, potentially causing upper extremity deformities.[8] Poland syndrome has been associated with various pathologies and syndromes including breast cancer and other malignancies;[23,24] renal anomalies; and Mobius and Klippel–Feil syndromes.[25] Of note, familial cases have also been reported.[6]

Foucras et al.[26] introduced a classification to define the extent of Poland syndrome:

- *Grade 1*: Minor deformity consisting of pectoralis major hypoplasia. Women present with moderate breast hypoplasia and asymmetry. Men present with minor chest wall deformities. NAC is often small and elevated. No skeletal abnormalities are found.

■ *Grade 2*: Moderate deformity consisting of pectoralis major aplasia. Women present with significant breast asymmetry, hypoplasia, or aplasia. Patients present with moderate chest wall deformity. The NAC is hypoplastic or absent.

■ *Grade 3*: Severe deformities consisting of complete muscular and breast aplasia, as well as aplasia of other chest wall muscles, and major chest wall

deformity. This results in severe chest wall asymmetry. The NAC is also hypoplastic or absent.

The main goal of surgical intervention is to obtain breast symmetry, which can be achieved by rectifying the bone deformity, addressing soft-tissue deficiency, and reconstructing the breast. Usually reconstruction is considered a single-stage procedure in adults and a two-stage procedure in children, especially if chest wall reconstruction is needed. The best time for surgery is in the late teens, but operations can be performed from 11–12 years of age and onwards to help with self-esteem and

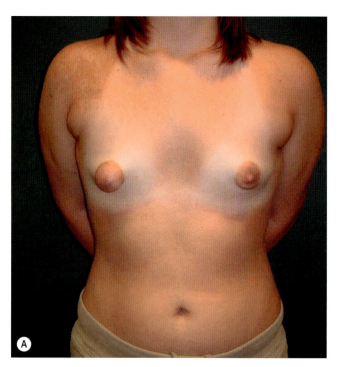

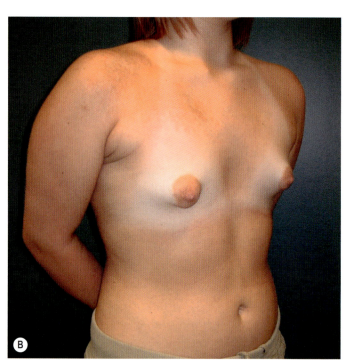

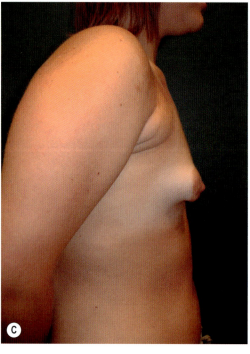

Fig. 28.5 (A–C) Preoperative and **(D–F)** 2-year postoperative follow-up images of an 18-year-old woman suffering from a bilateral breast tuberosity defect, who underwent type III dual-plane augmentation mammaplasty with subpectoral implant.

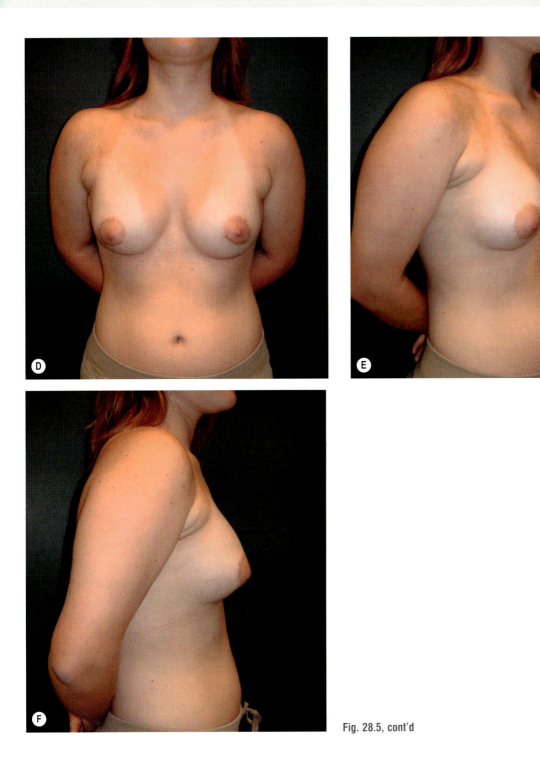

Fig. 28.5, cont'd

social and psychosexual growth. Reconstructive options usually include a combination of thoracic cage remodeling (e.g., bone grafts or prosthetic mesh), tissue expansion (subsequently replaced by permanent implants) or insertion of implant (shaped, round, or customized) in a dual-plane (if the pectoral muscle is normal), autologous fat transfer, contralateral mastopexy or reduction mammaplasty, and autologous free or pedicled muscle flaps. Commonly used flaps include latissimus dorsi, transverse rectus abdominis myocutaneous, deep inferior epigastric perforators, and superior or inferior gluteal artery perforator.[6,8,22] Pedicled latissimus dorsi myocutaneous flap reconstruction, with or without implant, has been considered a mainstay of the surgical management of moderate to severe chest wall deficiency and breast hypoplasia or aplasia. The benefits include ease of harvesting the flap, replacement of pectoralis major with similar tissue, and relative ease compared with microsurgical procedures. In the past in men, a customized silicone implant is preferred rather than an autologous flap. However, this technique has been associated with a high rate of complications, most notably seroma and implant malposition or migration, and most recently, it has been supplanted by autologous fat transfer (usually requiring two stages). In women, a two-stage reconstruction is preferred, starting with a tissue expander and followed by either an autologous flap (e.g., latissimus dorsi) with or without an implant, or a prosthetic device without flap coverage.[6,8,22]

Complications reported in the literature are primarily related to the reconstructive procedure itself. Implant insertion may be compromised because of capsular contracture, implant distortion, implant rupture, implant migration, and seroma formation.[22] Rocha *et al.* described the rare phenomena of costal reabsorption, parietal pericardium exposure, and mediastinal shift following prosthetic reconstruction.[27] Flap reconstruction may result in partial or total flap failure. Breast asymmetry is very common following unilateral reconstruction, which can be improved at a later stage by a secondary corrective procedure, either on the ipsilateral or contralateral side.[22]

Anterior thoracic hypoplasia

Anterior thoracic hypoplasia is a rare disorder, and separate from Poland syndrome. It presents with posterior displacement of ribs, anteriorly unilateral sunken chest wall, hypoplasia of the ipsilateral breast, and a superiorly displaced NAC. However, the sternum and pectoralis major are normal. Surgical management consists of augmentation mammaplasty using anatomic implants. A latissimus dorsi myocutaneous flap reconstruction is not usually considered because the pectoralis major is present, which provides coverage for the implant.[28,29]

Hyperplastic disorders

Gynecomastia

Gynecomastia is the most common form of pediatric hyperplastic disorder affecting up to 65% of pubescent boys.[30] Gynecomastia is defined as a benign proliferation of glandular tissue in the male breast. It is initially characterized by increased budding ducts and cellular stroma and usually resolves spontaneously without the need for surgery. Gynecomastia present for more than 1 year demonstrates extensive fibrosis and hyalinization with regression of the epithelial proliferation, thus increasing the need for surgical intervention. In normal male development, androgens produced by male gonadal tissue antagonize the effects of estrogen, which is responsible for the proliferation of breast tissue. Gynecomastia is typically a reflection of hormonal fluctuations with a relative predominance of estrogen.

In many instances, this is physiologic and commonly occurs during three periods of normal development: neonatal, caused by circulating maternal estrogens via the placenta; pubertal, caused by a relative excess of plasma estradiol versus testosterone; and elderly, caused by a decrease in circulating testosterone and peripheral aromatization of testosterone to estrogen. However, while gynecomastia is not itself a pathologic process, it can reflect an hormonal imbalance induced by underlying disease such as tumors (testicular, pituitary, adrenal); paraneoplastic tumors (colon, lung, and prostate); hypogonadism; Klinefelter's syndrome; idiopathic, iatrogenic secondary to medications (e.g., spironolactone, digoxin, ketoconazole); thyroid disease; granulomatous disease; renal failure; adrenal disease (Cushings, congenital adrenal hyperplasia); myotonic dystrophy; medications; HIV; marijuana use; liver disease; and alcoholism. The most common etiology in adolescents is idiopathic, while in patients over 40 years of age, it is due to medications. Given the varied etiology, surgery can be considered only if there is certainty that gynecomastia is not the presentation of an underlying pathology. For this reason, selected patients may require endocrinology and radiologic work-up (Fig. 28.6).

The severity of gynecomastia has been described using various classifications. Webster[31] based his classification on tissue type: type I describes the presence of glandular tissue; type II describes the presence of fatty and glandular mix; type III describes the presence of simple fatty tissue. Simon *et al.*[32] based their classification on the degree of tissue and skin excess: type I describes minor breast enlargement without skin excess; type II describes moderate breast enlargement without skin excess (IIa) or with minor skin redundancy (IIb); type III describes gross breast enlargement with skin excess creating a pendulous breast. Perhaps the most useful classification is that proposed by Rohrich *et al.*[30] who based their classification on glandular versus fibrous hypertrophy and degree of breast ptosis (skin excess): grade I describes minimal hypertrophy (<250 g) with no ptosis, primarily glandular (Ia) or fibrous (Ib); grade II describes moderate hypertrophy (250–500 g) with no ptosis, primarily glandular (IIa) or fibrous (IIb); grade III describes severe hypertrophy (>500 g) with grade I ptosis; grade IV describes severe hypertrophy (>250 g) with grade II or III ptosis.

Surgical management for gynecomastia is considered in those patients with absence of an underlying pathology, and persistence of breast enlargement for longer than 1 year (preferably more than 2 years). Surgical management targets removal of excess breast tissue and minimization of scars. Various methods have been used ranging from direct excision to suction-assisted

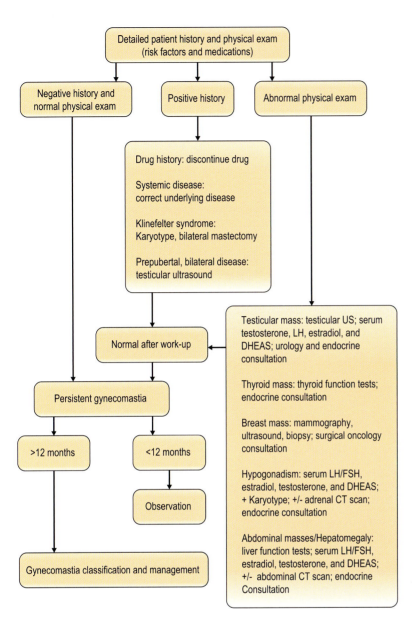

Fig. 28.6 A preoperative algorithm for gynecomastia is illustrated based on the possible etiologies. *(Redrawn from Rohrich RJ, Ha RY, Kenkel JM, Adams W. Classification and management of gynecomastia: defining the role of ultrasound-assisted liposuction.* Plast Reconstr Surg. *2003;111:909–923.)*

lipectomy, depending on the severity of gynecomastia. A major breakthrough was introduced by Courtiss, with the introduction of liposuction as the primary modality of treatment with surgical excision playing a secondary role. This dramatically decreased the incidence of post-surgical contour abnormalities and asymmetries.[33] Rohrich *et al.* advocate the use of ultrasound-assisted liposuction as a first-line technique in all grades of gynecomastia. If excess of skin or breast tissue persists, the authors advocate for a staged excision after 6–9 months, particularly in patients with Rohrich grade III and IV gynecomastia.[30] Lista and Ahmad reported the use of power-assisted liposuction in conjunction with a pull-through technique to sever the subdermal attachments of the fibroglandular breast tissue.[34] Prado and Castillo described the use of a power-assisted arthroscopic-endoscopic cartilage shaver as an alternative to the pull-through technique.[35] Other authors advocate the use of subcutaneous mastectomy or breast disk excision, with or without skin reduction, by means of a semicircular periareolar (Simmons grade I), submammary (Simmons grade I), circumareolar (Simmons grade II), or inverted T (Simmons grade III) incision pattern.[36] Lastly, severe cases of gynecomastia have been managed with transposition of the NAC on a dermoglandular pedicle, or rarely with reposition of the NAC as a full-thickness skin graft.[37] When there is uncertainty about the need to excise skin (grade III and IV), it is best to perform aggressive liposuction as the primary procedure while employing envelope modification if needed at a second stage.

Complications commonly reported in the literature include under-resection, over-resection, complex scars, and hematoma. Other complications that are not as frequent include wound dehiscence, excess skin, seroma, infection, partial nipple necrosis, pain, and loss of nipple sensation.[36] Rohrich *et al.* demonstrated that 86.9% of men that had undergone ultrasound-assisted liposuction for gynecomastia did not require additional procedures. The remaining 13.1% of patients (all grade III and IV) underwent a staged excision of skin and breast.[30] The main benefit of liposuction is the ability of increased breast volume reduction without the added scar burden. Although studies have shown high aesthetic outcomes, a recent study by Ridha *et al.* demonstrated that only 62.5% of patients within a cohort of 74 patients were "satisfied" or "very satisfied" with their result, and the postoperative satisfaction scores increased only moderately in all groups (liposuction alone, surgical excision alone, or a combination).[38] Surgical management for gynecomastia is therefore a decision to be taken after careful patient assessment and discussion of realistic expectations. Various approaches have been described, but no technique has yet gained universal acceptance by the surgical community.

Virginal mammary hypertrophy

Virginal mammary hypertrophy (also known as juvenile hypertrophy, juvenile macromastia, or gigantomastia) is a rare condition that results in a rapid, excessive, unilateral, or bilateral enlargement of breasts that usually presents in adolescents. Patients usually present with the typical symptoms of macromastia (bra-strap grooving, rashes, shoulder and neck pain) along with breast tenderness, thinned skin, dilated veins, and striae. Virginal mammary hypertrophy has been reported in both sporadic and familial forms; however, the etiology is unclear. The most popular theory is end-organ hypersensitivity to normal circulating levels of estrogen. Estrogen levels have been measured in patients with virginal mammary hypertrophy and have not been significantly elevated compared with controls.[39] Thus, receptor hypersensitivity might occur due to increased receptor density, receptor signaling, or another unidentified compound that binds to estrogen receptors.[40] Virginal mammary hypertrophy is a diagnosis of exclusion, and other conditions such as phyllodes tumor, virginal fibroadenoma, fibrocystic disease, and endocrine conditions must be ruled out.

Dancey *et al.* proposed a classification of virginal mammary hypertrophy based on body mass index (BMI), pubescent status, and the presence of an inciting pharmacologic agent: type 1a describes idiopathic, spontaneous, excessive breast growth in a patient with a BMI >30; type 1b describes idiopathic, spontaneous, excessive breast growth in a patient with a BMI <30; type 2a describes excessive breast growth related to an imbalance of endogenous hormone production occurring during puberty; type 2b describes excessive breast growth related to an imbalance of endogenous hormone production occurring during pregnancy; and type 3 describes excessive breast growth induced by a pharmacologic agent.[41]

The standard treatment of virginal mammary hypertrophy is surgical resection. Early recognition of this condition is key to minimize the extent of the surgery and its associated morbidity. Reduction mammaplasty is most commonly performed either as a pedicle-based procedure or with a free nipple-graft. This technique is usually preferred because of the ability to preserve lactation, and has better aesthetic and psychological outcomes. Pharmacologic management has also been employed, but potential side effects have limited their use. The medications reported in the literature include tamoxifen, dydrogesterone, medroxyprogesterone acetate, danazol, and bromocriptine.[40]

Giant fibroadenomas

Giant fibroadenomas are benign, unilateral, fast growing breast masses that usually present during puberty. As with virginal mammary hypertrophy, giant fibroadenomas result from breast tissue hypersensitivity to normal estrogen levels. The diagnosis is confirmed by breast tissue biopsy. The standard treatment of giant fibroadenomas is reduction mammaplasty, and the timing is dictated by the onset of the rapid growth phase. The pattern is designed in such a way as to incorporate the fibroadenoma in the excision segment, and the pedicle in the location of the greatest amount of normal breast tissue to preserve breast fullness. A secondary surgery can be performed to achieve symmetry including a matching contralateral reduction mammaplasty or a delayed mastopexy and/or augmentation mammaplasty.

Polythelia

Polythelia (also known as accessory, supernumerary, or third nipples) is a benign condition that presents with additional nipples or NACs and is a result of failure of the mammary ridge to regress *in utero*. Thus they are located along the milk line (see Fig. 28.1), extending from the axilla to the pubic region. Polythelia has an incidence up to 5.6%, and although normally presents sporadically, familial cases have also been reported. In rare cases, polythelia can be associated to renal anomalies, which require further investigation (urinalysis and ultrasound). Surgical excision is a treatment of choice. Before puberty, pigmented lesions along the milk lines should be excised; after puberty, a wider tissue excision may be required, especially in women, because of the growth of associated glandular breast tissue. The NAC can easily be removed using an elliptical excision.[8,28]

Polymastia

Polymastia (also known as accessory or supernumerary breasts, multiple breast syndrome, or mammae erraticae) is a benign condition identified in 1–2% of live births and presenting with additional breasts and NACs located along the milk line (most commonly in the axilla). Polymastia is usually sporadic, but familial cases have also been reported. In rare cases, it can be associated with renal anomalies, which require further investigation. Unlike polythelia, which is usually identified at birth, polymastia is often not noted until puberty or pregnancy, when hormonal influences enlarge the supernumerary breast tissue. The treatment of choice is surgical excision of the accessory gland and primary closure.[8,28]

Conclusion

This chapter has outlined the most common congenital breast deformities and their surgical management. Precise diagnosis and carefully timed surgical management is required to optimize outcomes and the social and psychosexual impact on patients. It is a field where the plastic surgeon must treat the patient by selecting both the most appropriate procedure and timing for the surgical intervention, and manage the family. The variety and heterogeneity of these conditions tests the surgeon's knowledge, experience, and skill in the arena of breast surgery challenges. The surgery offers the surgeon the rewarding opportunity to work with a highly motivated group of young people and follow them for many years during an important time in their lives.

Access the complete reference list online at **http://www.expertconsult.com**

1. Sadove AM, van Aalst JA. Congenital and acquired pediatric breast anomalies: a review of 20 years' experience. *Plast Reconstr Surg.* 2005;115:1039–1050.

3. Mandrekas AD, Zambacos GJ, Anastasopoulos A, et al. Aesthetic reconstruction of the tuberous breast deformity. *Plast Reconstr Surg.* 2003;112:1099–1109.

8. Latham K, Fernandez S, Iteld L, et al. Pediatric breast deformity. *J Craniofac Surg.* 2006;17:454–467. *This article provides a solid review of the most common congenital breast disorders describing the diagnosis, work-up, and management. It also provides key references related to congenital breast disorders.*

10. Costagliola M, Atiyeh B, Rampillon F. Tuberous breast: revised classification and a new hypothesis for its development. *Aesthetic Plast Surg.* 2013;37:896–903.

12. Grolleau JL, Lanfrey E, Lavigne B, et al. Breast base anomalies: treatment strategy for tuberous breasts, minor deformities, and asymmetry. *Plast Reconstr Surg.* 1999;104:2040–2048. *This article presents the most commonly used classification of tuberous breast deformity.*

21. Coleman SR, Saboeiro AP. Fat grafting to the breast revisited: safety and efficacy. *Plast Reconstr Surg.* 2007;119:775–787.

22. Nahabedian MY. Breast deformities and mastopexy. *Plast Reconstr Surg.* 2011;127:91e–102e.

30. Rohrich RJ, Ha RY, Kenkel JM, et al. Classification and management of gynecomastia: defining the role of ultrasound-assisted liposuction. *Plast Reconstr Surg.* 2003;111:909–925. *This article provides a strong review of the etiology, pathophysiology, diagnosis, and treatment of gynecomastia. Furthermore, it offers a clear algorithm of the evaluation and treatment of gynecomastia based on a classification developed by the authors.*

40. Hoppe IC, Patel PP, Singer-Granick CJ, et al. Virginal mammary hypertrophy: a meta-analysis and treatment algorithm. *Plast Reconstr Surg.* 2011;127:2224–2231. *This article offers a thorough meta-analysis examining published case reports and presents a cumulative algorithm for the diagnosis and treatment of virginal mammary hypertrophy.*

41. Dancey A, Khan M, Dawson J, et al. Gigantomastia – a classification and review of the literature. *J Plast Reconstr Aesthet Surg.* 2008;61:493–502. *This article presents a classification of virginal mammary hypertrophy based on the cause, management, and prognosis of the disease.*

Index

Page numbers followed by "*f*" indicate figures, "*t*" indicate tables, "*b*" indicate boxes, and "*e*" indicate online content.